# Hematologic Malignancies: Hodgkin Lymphoma

Andreas Engert
Sandra J. Horning
Editors

# Hematologic Malignancies: Hodgkin Lymphoma

## A Comprehensive Update on Diagnostics and Clinics

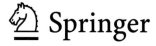 Springer

Andreas Engert
Universität Köln
Klinik I für Innere Medizin
Joseph-Stelzmann-Str. 9
50924 Köln
Germany
a.engert@uni-koeln.de

Sandra J. Horning
Stanford University
Department of Medicine
Medical School Office Bldg.
Stanford, CA 94305-5479
USA
sandra.horning@stanford.edu

ISBN: 978-3-642-12779-3    e-ISBN: 978-3-642-12780-9

DOI: 10.1007/978-3-642-12780-9

Springer Heidelberg Dordrecht London New York

Library of Congress Control Number: 2010932936

*Cover design*: eStudio Calamar, Figueres/Berlin

Printed on acid-free paper

Springer is part of Springer Science+Business Media (www.springer.com)

Hodgkin lymphoma is one of the best curable malignancies both in adult and pediatric oncology. Today, more than 80% of all patients can be cured with risk-adapted treatment including chemotherapy and radiotherapy. This progress is largely due to the development of multiagent chemotherapy more than 40 years ago and the improvements in radiotherapy. Since then, this fascinating disease has been in the focus of scientific and clinical research. Major more recent achievements were the definite proof that Hodgkin lymphoma is a true malignancy despite its peculiar histology with the Hodgkin and Reed–Sternberg cells derived from "crippled" B-lymphocytes. Establishing immortal cell lines from patients with end-stage disease initiated a variety of different research activities into the pathophysiology, immunology, and treatment. The discovery of the Ki-1 antigen that was expressed in high density on H-RS cells substantially improved the prognostic precision since nearly all malignant cells in Hodgkin lymphoma tissue are strongly expressing this antigen, which was later designated to the CD30 cluster. Monoclonal antibodies against this antigen were not only being successfully used for immunophenotyping but also exploited therapeutically. After a number of nonsuccessful clinical trials with antibody constructs or fully human monoclonal antibodies targeting CD30, this story now seems to come full circle with the advent of an anti-CD30 antibody–drug conjugate that has given remarkable responses in end-stage Hodgkin lymphoma patients.

Due to the substantially improved prognosis and the generally young age of patients affected, Hodgkin lymphoma has also become a model to study long-term effects of successful radiotherapy and chemotherapy. Today, more patients die from treatment-related long-term toxicity than from uncontrolled Hodgkin lymphoma. We must thus very carefully balance our attempts to further improve disease control with the need to keep the risk of long-term consequences as low as possible. In addition, there are also a number of relevant physical and psychosocial issues that need to be further exploited including the risk of infertility, and fatigue. Fortunately, after more than 20 years of standstill, we now experience the development of new-targeted treatment also for patients with Hodgkin lymphoma. This hopefully might result in more individualized and less toxic treatments for our patients.

This book should give you an overview on past and current achievements in the area of Hodgkin lymphoma with a special emphasis on late effects and new treatment options. We would like to express our sincere gratitude to all those who have contributed to this project.

Cologne and Stanford, October 2010

Andreas Engert
Sandra Horning

# Contents

**Part**

**I**

**From Hodgkin's Disease
to Hodgkin Lymphoma**

# Epidemiology

**1**

Sally L. Glaser, Ellen T. Chang, Christina A. Clarke, and Theresa H. Keegan

## Contents

## Abbreviations

| | |
|---|---|
| CI | Confidence interval |
| COX | Cyclooxygenase |
| EA | Early antigen |
| EBNA | Epstein–Barr nuclear antigen |
| EBV | Epstein–Barr virus |
| HL | Hodgkin lymphoma |
| HLA | Human leukocyte antigen |
| HRS | Hodgkin Reed–Sternberg |
| IL | Interleukin |
| IM | Infectious mononucleosis |
| OR | Odds ratio |
| RR | Relative risk |
| SEER | Surveillance, Epidemiology, and End Results |
| SES | Socioeconomic status |
| US | United States |
| UVR | Ultraviolet radiation |
| VCA | Viral capsid antigen |

Hodgkin lymphoma (HL) is a relatively rare malignancy, occurring in the United States (US) at approximately 1/20th the rate of lung cancer, and 1/7th the rate of non-Hodgkin lymphoma in 2006 [1]. Yet, it has inspired a high degree of scientific interest because of the heterogeneity of its clinical presentation and behavior, with some aspects characteristic of malignancy but others recalling an infectious process; the complexity of its histology, including the infrequent malignant Hodgkin Reed–Sternberg (HRS) cell in an otherwise normal reactive infiltrate, and the variability of cell surface markers [2]; and its unusual occurrence in children and young adults, in whom it is one of the most common cancers [1], as well as in older persons. Motivated by these characteristics and MacMahon's seminal papers on the epidemiology of HL in 1957 and

S.L. Glaser (✉), E.T. Chang, C.A. Clarke, and T.H. Keegan
Cancer Prevention Institute of California (formerly the Northern California Cancer Center), 2201 Walnut Avenue, Suite 300, Fremont, CA 94538, USA
e-mail: sally.glaser@cpic.org

A. Engert and S.J. Horning (eds.), *Hodgkin Lymphoma*,
DOI: 10.1007/978-3-642-12780-9_1, © Springer-Verlag Berlin Heidelberg 2011

1966 [3, 4], epidemiologists have worked to disentangle the complexity of this disease so as to arrive at a clear understanding of its pathogenesis and etiology. However, even as findings from this research have helped elucidate some aspects of HL etiology, they have continued to reveal significant epidemiologic heterogeneity across patient groups that recalls the disease's clinical and pathologic complexity. This heterogeneity complicates the interpretation of epidemiologic research conducted for HL as a single entity and perhaps challenges the classification of what is currently categorized as HL. Indeed, in 1999, HL was split into two main groups – classical HL, which comprises the majority of the subtypes, and lymphocyte-predominant HL, an uncommon disease considered a B-cell lymphoma despite HRS cell presence [5]. Regardless, the central feature of classical HL epidemiology is the very consistent observation of heterogeneity in its occurrence and risk factors.

Therefore, this chapter will provide an overview of the epidemiology of HL with particular attention to its etiologic heterogeneity. It will do so for several areas of established relevance: incidence patterns, timing of exposure to common infections, the role of Epstein–Barr virus (EBV), familial aggregation and heritability, altered immune function, and selected lifestyle practices. Where possible, it focuses on classical HL.

## 1.1 Incidence Patterns

HL has a low and relatively stable incidence with a slight male excess. Worldwide, estimated age-adjusted incidence rates for 2002 were 1.2 and 0.8 per 100,000 males and females, respectively [6]. Over time, HL incidence has changed minimally in the US: cancer registry data showed a nonsignificant 0.01% annual percent decrease in incidence rates between 1975 and 2006, in stark contrast to the significant and rapid 3.6% annual percent increases in non-Hodgkin lymphoma rates between 1975 and 1991 [1], years encompassing the AIDS epidemic.

### 1.1.1 Heterogeneity of Incidence Patterns

When examined across relatively homogeneous population groups, HL incidence follows complex patterns.

Rates vary internationally: estimated 2002 incidence rates ranged from 2.3 and 1.9 per 100,000 males and females in more developed regions, to 1.0 and 0.5 per 100,000 males and females in less developed regions [6]. Moreover, rates in the US were 3.2 and 2.4 per 100,000 males and females (based on 5,037 and 3,820 cases), whereas rates in China were 0.2 and 0.1 per 100,000, respectively (based on 1,690 and 720 cases) [6]. The latter international difference alludes to additional incidence variation by race/ethnicity. Indeed, within the US, average annual age-adjusted incidence rates per 100,000 for 2002–2006 were 3.1 in non-Hispanic Whites (hereafter referred to as Whites), 2.5 in Blacks, 2.3 in Hispanics, and 1.3 in Asians [7]. Despite the temporal stability of HL incidence in the US overall and for Whites, rates in Asians increased significantly at 3.3% annually since 1992 [1], suggesting additional group-specific influences on disease occurrence.

Arguably, the hallmark of HL epidemiology is its variation in occurrence by age at diagnosis. The appearance of the disease in young as well as older persons was first noted in 1902 by Dorothy Reed, for whom the HRS cell was named in part, when she wrote, "The disease occurs in more than half the instances in early life; probably the majority of cases are in children" [8]. In 1966, MacMahon described the young-adult incidence peak as "…a distinct bump, almost as though a separate group of cases with a symmetrical age distribution around age 25–29 had been superimposed on the basic lymphoma pattern" [4]. Figure 1.1 shows that this

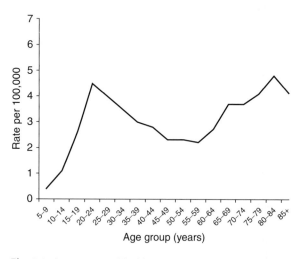

**Fig. 1.1** Average annual incidence rates of Hodgkin lymphoma (HL) per 100,000 persons by age group, 2002–2006, United States [7]

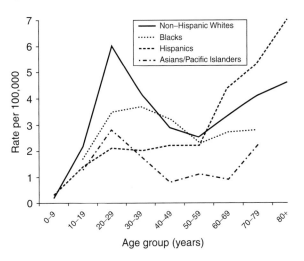

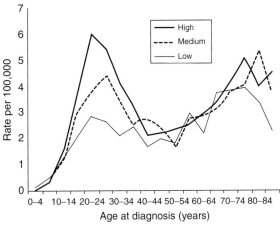

**Fig. 1.2** Average annual incidence rates of Hodgkin lymphoma (HL) per 100,000 persons by age group and race/ethnicity, 2002–2006, United States [7]

**Fig. 1.3** Average annual incidence rates of Hodgkin lymphoma (HL) per 100,000 persons by age group and tertile of neighborhood socioeconomic status, 1988–1992, CA [15]

bimodal curve was still apparent in US data for 2002–2006 [7]. However, while the bimodal curve remains a defining epidemiologic feature of HL, its shape varies substantially by race, geography, time, sex, and tumor characteristics. Figure 1.2 shows that the young-adult peak in the same US data was most pronounced in Whites, intermediate in Blacks, and lowest in Hispanics and Asians [7]. In 1971, Correa and O'Conor showed by compiling international data that the magnitude of the young-adult peak was directly correlated with regional economic status [9]. Updating this analysis in 1995, Macfarlane et al. determined that this correlation had weakened as international economic differentials narrowed over time [10]; indeed, rates in young adults have risen in populations experiencing improved standards of living, as noted in Singapore over time [11] and in comparisons of Asians in Asia to those who migrated from Asia to the US [12] and Canada [13]. Nevertheless, the age-specific social-class gradient persists both internationally [14] and within the US. Figure 1.3 illustrates how rates based on population-based cancer registry data for the 3,794 HL patients diagnosed in California from 1988 to 1992 varied with neighborhood socioeconomic status (SES) for young but not older adults [15]; these gradients further differed by racial/ethnic group, being strongest for Hispanic and Asian females (Table 1.1).

The age-specific variation in HL incidence rates also differs by sex. Despite an overall male excess, HL is more common in young women than men

diagnosed at ages 20 through 34 years – an uncommon pattern in cancers – but consistently more common in older men than women, typical of malignant disease (Fig. 1.4) [7]. Furthermore, increases in rates of young-adult HL over time were more pronounced in women than men in Connecticut [16], and in Singapore after 1995 [11]. HL rates also differ markedly by recognized histologic subtypes overall and across ages (Fig. 1.5) [7]. Nodular sclerosis HL, the most common subtype (average annual age-adjusted incidence rate of 1.6 per 100,000 in the US in 2002–2006 [7]), primarily affects young adults. In contrast, mixed cellularity, the next most common subtype (average annual age-adjusted incidence rate of 0.3 per 100,000 in the US in 2002–2006 [7]), has a slight young-adult peak and rates that rise with older age. The positive associations of neighborhood SES with HL incidence in Californian young adults noted in Fig. 1.3 occurred primarily for the nodular sclerosis histologic subtype [15].

Thus, the descriptive epidemiology of HL clearly illustrates variation in its incidence across a range of demographic factors and tumor characteristics. While some clustering of characteristics (e.g., young-adult HL primarily comprising the nodular sclerosis subtype) suggests etiologically distinct subgroups of HL, the inconsistency of many such associations (e.g., the occurrence of mixed cellularity HL in some young adults) prevents the clean assignment of subcategories of HL based on these characteristics.

**Table 1.1** Average annual age-adjusted[a] incidence rates of Hodgkin lymphoma (HL) per 100,000 person-years, by race/ethnicity, age group, tertiles of neighborhood socioeconomic status (SES), and sex, 1988–1992, CA [15]

| Race/ ethnicity | Ages 15–44 years at diagnosis | | | | | | | | | | | | Ages ≥45 at diagnosis | | | | | | | | | | | |
|---|---|---|---|---|---|---|---|---|---|---|---|---|---|---|---|---|---|---|---|---|---|---|---|---|
| | High SES | | | | Medium SES | | | | Low SES | | | | High SES | | | | Medium SES | | | | Low SES | | | |
| | Male | | Female | | Male | | Female | | Male | | Female | | Male | | Female | | Male | | Female | | Male | | Female | |
| | N | Rate | N | Rate | N | Rate | N | Rate | N | Rate | N | Rate | N | Rate | N | Rate | N | Rate | N | Rate | N | Rate | N | Rate |
| Whites | 437 | 4.88 | 400 | 4.61 | 352 | 4.44 | 319 | 4.28 | 160 | 4.00 | 136 | 3.50 | 256 | 4.24 | 169 | 2.37 | 169 | 3.61 | 142 | 2.32 | 106 | 4.07 | 80 | 2.25 |
| Blacks | 18 | 3.92 | 14 | 3.30 | 29 | 2.93 | 24 | 2.62 | 42 | 3.44 | 35 | 2.45 | <5 | – | 10 | 4.53 | 13 | 4.23 | 9 | 2.61 | 17 | 3.06 | 13 | 1.54 |
| Hispanics | 31 | 2.16 | 39 | 2.95 | 75 | 2.32 | 46 | 1.67 | 116 | 1.69 | 62 | 1.03 | 24 | 5.71 | 9 | 1.58 | 31 | 4.37 | 25 | 3.19 | 42 | 3.16 | 34 | 2.25 |
| Asians | 17 | 1.19 | 20 | 1.34 | 14 | 0.95 | 8 | 0.57 | 12 | 1.28 | 5 | 0.44 | 11 | 2.38 | 5 | 0.84 | 13 | 3.12 | <5 | – | 11 | 2.60 | <5 | – |

[a]Standardized to the 2000 US age standard

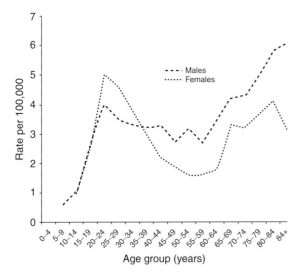

**Fig. 1.4** Average annual incidence rates of Hodgkin lymphoma (HL) per 100,000 persons by age group and sex, 2002–2006, United States [7]

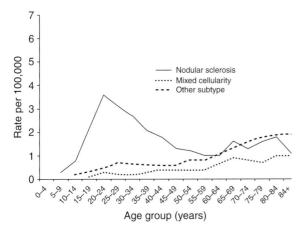

**Fig. 1.5** Average annual incidence rates of Hodgkin lymphoma (HL) per 100,000 persons by age group and histologic subtype, 2002–2006, United States [7]

## 1.2 Timing of Exposure to Common Infections

From his early observations of epidemiologic heterogeneity in HL by age, MacMahon proposed an infectious etiology for young-adult HL [4]. Noting similarities between HL and paralytic polio, prior to the availability of the polio vaccine, in the way that their incidence increased with age in young adults,

Gutensohn and Cole proposed that HL at these ages resulted from late infection with a common agent [17]. This "delayed-infection" hypothesis was supported by three lines of evidence: (1) the association between social class and HL rates described above and elsewhere [15, 17–20], and a twofold or greater increased risk of HL in young adults with a higher personal SES and educational level [17, 21–26], which suggested that environmental conditions regulating exposure to infections impacted disease risk; (2) the increased HL risk in young adults associated with having an early birth order, coming from a small family, having a more highly educated mother, and, more recently, not attending nursery school [22, 25, 27–31], which suggested a role of protected childhood environments and thus reduced or delayed exposure to infectious agents; and (3) the consistent finding of an approximately threefold elevated risk of HL in young adults reporting a history of infectious mononucleosis (IM) [32–39], a manifestation of primary EBV infection occurring in adolescence or young adulthood rather than childhood (the more usual age at infection).

### 1.2.1 Heterogeneity of Effect

The hypothesis that timing of infection relates to HL development itself arose from the observation of age variation in HL incidence, and subsequent research has borne it out. In the 1970s, Gutensohn et al. found differences across broad age groups in the direction of some childhood environment associations [25, 40, 41]. In young adults (ages 15–39 years), HL risk was associated with having fewer siblings, living in a single- vs. multiple-family house, and having better educated parents, whereas in children (ages 0–14 years) and older adults (ages 55 years and older), risk increased with measures of more rather than fewer social exposures in childhood. These age differences in risk patterns, supported by numerous later studies [22, 27–29, 31], were interpreted to suggest three etiologic forms of HL – childhood, young-adult, and older-adult – an important initial paradigm of HL epidemiology. In recent case–control studies, many of the previously reported childhood social-class risk factors have not been associated with HL risk [24, 30, 36, 42], suggesting that temporal demographic changes, such as decreasing family size, may have altered some of the childhood exposures most relevant to the development of HL [24, 30].

## 1.3 Role of Epstein–Barr Virus

The inference from the IM-HL association that EBV, a ubiquitous B-lymphotropic oncogenic virus that establishes latent infection [43], might have a direct role in HL etiology has been supported by serologic and tumor findings. After HL patients were noted to have elevated anti-EBV titers compared to controls (e.g., [44]), Mueller et al. were the first to demonstrate that EBV titers were altered before HL diagnosis, with patterns that suggest viral reactivation and enhanced replication (relative risks (RR) of HL with elevated levels of IgG and IgA antibodies against viral capsid antigen (VCA) of 2.6 (90% confidence interval (CI) 1.1–6.1) and 3.7 (95% CI 1.4–9.3), respectively, and with elevated levels of IgG antibodies against Epstein–Barr nuclear antigen (EBNA) and early antigen (EA) diffuse component of 4.0 (95% CI 1.4–11.4) and 2.6 (95% CI 1.1–6.1), respectively) [45]. These findings are consistent with defective immunological surveillance and control of infection with EBV leading to viral reactivation and, potentially, a higher risk of B-cell transformation and the development of HL. In the late 1980s, this possibility was further supported by the detection in some HL tumors of EBV gene products that were monoclonal and expressed by all HRS cells, indicating infection prior to malignant expansion [46]. However, contrary to expectation from the epidemiologic evidence that EBV might be an etiologic agent for all HL, the virus was found only in a proportion of tumors.

### 1.3.1 Heterogeneity of Effect

The proportion of tumors with evidence of EBV (hereafter called EBV-positive) has been shown to vary substantially by patient demographic and tumor characteristics, providing strong evidence of the virus' varying role across subsets of HL [47, 48]. Among 1,546 patients assembled from 14 international studies, the percentages of tumors that were EBV-positive were 34 and 64% in developed and less developed countries, 23 and 70% for nodular sclerosis and mixed cellularity histologies, 48 and 22% in males and females, 36 and 60–65% in Whites and most non-Whites, respectively, and higher in children (57%) and older adults (52%) than in young adults (32%) [47]. Similar differences in associations of EBV and HL by age, sex, and race/ethnicity emerged in more uniformly collected population-based data from 1,032 US cases (Table 1.2) [49] and from 537 UK cases [50]. When compared to the graphs in Fig. 1.5, the estimated incidence rate curves for EBV-positive and EBV-negative HL in the UK (Fig. 1.6) also show the close resemblance between age-incidence curves for EBV-positive HL and mixed cellularity HL, and for EBV-negative HL and nodular sclerosis HL. Altogether, these descriptive differences in EBV-positive and EBV-negative HL are consistent with their being separate pathogenic entities.

Subsequent analytic research has supported the hypothesis that EBV-positive and EBV-negative HL have different pathologies. Studies to relate risk of

**Table 1.2** Numbers of Hodgkin lymphoma (HL) cases and percentages with Epstein–Barr virus (EBV)-positive tumors by patient age group, race/ethnicity, and sex, California regions, 1988–1997 [49]

| Age group (years) | White | | | | Hispanic | | | |
|---|---|---|---|---|---|---|---|---|
| | Males | | Females | | Males | | Females | |
| | N | % EBV-positive | N | % EBV-positive | N | % EBV-positive | N | % EBV-positive |
| 0–14 | 10 | 50.0 | 11 | 9.1 | 20 | 70.0 | 9 | 88.9 |
| 15–34 | 137 | 25.6 | 189 | 13.2 | 55 | 38.2 | 47 | 12.8 |
| 35–54 | 88 | 19.3 | 84 | 9.5 | 23 | 47.8 | 28 | 39.3 |
| 55+ | 34 | 49.3 | 26 | 38.2 | 20 | 85.0 | 17 | 76.5 |
| Total | 304 | 29.9 | 352 | 17.1 | 118 | 53.4 | 101 | 37.6 |

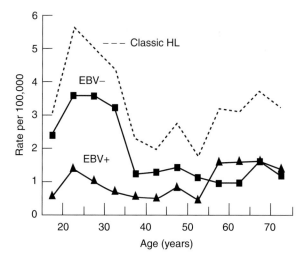

**Fig. 1.6** Age-specific incidence rates of Hodgkin lymphoma per 100,000 person-years and Epstein–Barr virus (EBV) tumor status, 1993 to mid-1997, ages 16–74 years, Scotland and Northern England [50]

## 1.4 Familial Aggregation and Heritability

Genetic predisposition to HL is supported by substantial evidence of family aggregation and, increasingly, associations with specific genes. Case studies have shown that families of HL probands can have affected first-, second-, and third-degree members with HL [59, 60]; other hematologic malignancies [61–66] and solid tumors [67–70]; can share human leukocyte antigen (HLA) haplotypes [71]; and can be consanguineous [67, 72] – all consistent with an inherited predisposition to HL. HL risk was found to be nearly 100-times higher in identical than fraternal twins [73], indicating a substantially stronger effect of shared genes than shared environment. Case–control and cohort studies consistently have reported a threefold to sevenfold increased risk of HL in first-degree relatives of patients [66, 68, 72, 74–83] and familial associations with other hematopoietic malignancies [75, 84–86]. Data from linkages of population-based cancer and family record registries, which are the least vulnerable to bias in studies of family aggregation, have produced similar results [63, 87]. They also have shown a higher risk for siblings than for parents of cases [63], a younger age at diagnosis for familial than nonfamilial cases [87–89] (although possibly due to various biases [90]), and an elevated occurrence of other lymphomas (particularly diffuse large B-cell lymphoma [91]) and other malignancies [92], as well as some autoimmune diseases (e.g., multiple sclerosis [93, 94]). Genetic predisposition to HL also is suggested by the consistent observations of higher rates in Jews and lower rates in Asians unexplained by differences in SES [12, 18, 24, 25, 30].

In affected families, analyses of candidate susceptibility genes have implicated the HLA region of chromosome 6 and polymorphisms of various cytokine genes, as reviewed below. The single published genome-wide association scan to date found strong linkage consistent with recessive inheritance on chromosome 4p, as well as on chromosomes 2, 4q, 7, 11, and 17 in 44 high-risk families [95].

### 1.4.1 Heterogeneity of Effect

Risk of familial HL and lymphoma related to HL has been reported to vary by age, sex, and degree of

EBV-positive HL to a history of IM, a strong EBV-related risk factor for HL in early studies, produced mixed findings due, in part, to reliance on a self-reported (and thus possibly inaccurate) history of IM [30, 51–56]. However, in prospective data linking serologically confirmed IM with HL diagnoses from a population-based cancer registry, Hjalgrim et al. observed that IM was associated only with risk of EBV-positive HL (estimated RR=4.0, 95% CI 3.4–4.5), with an estimated median time from IM to HL of 4.1 years (95% CI 1.8–8.3) [34]. Chang et al. showed that the antibody response to EBV differed significantly between EBV-positive and EBV-negative HL patients, with EBV-positive patients more likely to be EBV carriers in general and to have more prevalent and elevated EBV antibody titers against both lytic and latent virus antigens [57]. Together, these findings support an aberrant immune response to EBV and thus abnormal immunity in patients with EBV-positive HL, relative to those with EBV-negative HL. Further, differences have been identified in other risk factors for EBV-positive and EBV-negative HL, as shown for selected studies in Table 1.3. From the accumulated evidence, Jarrett suggested that HL represents four disease entities: one in children, which is EBV-associated; one in young adults with a history of late EBV infection and EBV-positive tumors; one in young adults, which is EBV-negative; and one in older persons, which is EBV-associated [58].

**Table 1.3** Risk factor patterns for Hodgkin lymphoma (HL) subclassified by tumor Epstein–Barr virus (EBV) status, selected studies

| Risk factor | Study | Patient group | Adjusted odds ratios (95% confidence intervals) | | |
|---|---|---|---|---|---|
| | | | EBV-positive HL vs. controls | EBV-negative HL vs. controls | EBV-positive vs. EBV-negative HL |
| *Social class measures* | | | | | |
| Lower vs. higher education | [57][a] | All adults | | | 0.8 (0.6–1.0) |
| Single vs. shared bedroom, age 11 | [53][b] | Young adult women | 4.0 (1.1–14.4) | 1.0 (0.7–1.6) | |
| *N* of older siblings (trend per sibling) | [36][c] | Young adults | 0.77 (0.56–1.05) | 1.01 (0.83–1.22) | 0.65 (0.45–0.95) |
| *N* of older siblings (trend per sibling) | | Older adults | 1.35 (1.06–1.70) | 0.84 (0.68–1.03) | 1.60 (1.12–2.29) |
| *EBV infection* | | | | | |
| Elevated antibody to VCA | [57][a] | All adults | | | 3.6 (1.4–8.7) |
| Anti-EBNA-1: Anti EBNA-2 ≤1.0 | | | | | 3.2 (1.1–9.0) |
| IM | [36][d] | Young adults | 3.96 (2.19–7.18) | 1.36 (0.81–2.26) | 2.68 (1.40–5.12) |
| Years since IM: 1–4 | | | 11.86 (3.10–45.3) | 0.41 (0.04–3.75) | |
| *Smoking* | | | | | |
| ≥10 packs of cigarettes during life | [57][a] | All adults | | | 1.8 (1.1–3.0) |
| Ever vs. never | [157][e] | All adults | 1.62 (1.08–2.43) | 1.13 (0.86–1.49) | |
| Current vs. never | | | 2.36 (1.51–3.71) | 1.43 (1.05–1.97) | |

[a]$N$=95 EBV-positive HL cases, 303 EBV-negative HL cases (OR adjusted for age, sex, education level)

[b]Ages 19–44: $N$=24 EBV-positive HL cases, 187 EBV-negative HL cases; ages 45–79: $N$=13 EBV-positive HL cases, 44 EBV-negative HL cases (OR for EBV-positive HL vs. controls adjusted for age, race/ethnicity, Catholic religion, ever smoking, childhood household size, birth order, bedroom sharing at age 11, number of playmates at age 8; OR for EBV-negative HL vs. controls adjusted for age, race/ethnicity, Catholic religion, lactation, birthplace, living in a rented family home at age 8, childhood household size, birth order, bedroom sharing at age 11, number of playmates at age 8)

[c]Ages 18–44: $N$=85 EBV-positive HL cases, 253 EBV-negative HL cases; ages 45–74: $N$=57 EBV-positive HL cases, 104 EBV-negative HL cases (OR adjusted for age, gender, country, history of IM, maternal education)

[d]$N$=95 EBV-positive HL cases, 303 EBV-negative HL cases (OR adjusted for age, sex, education level, smoking status, elevated VCA IgG and IgA, and EA IgA, and EBNA-1:EBNA-2≤1.0)

[e]Ages 18–74: $N$=142 EBV-positive HL cases, 357 EBV-negative HL cases (OR adjusted for age, gender, country, number of younger and older siblings, history of IM, mother's age at subject's birth, maternal education, subject's education, family history of hematopoietic cancer)

familial relationship. In linked Swedish registry data, Goldin et al. found the risk of HL higher for families of probands vs. controls under 40 years (RR=4.25, 95% CI 1.85–9.77) than those older than 40 years (RR=2.56, 95% CI 0.90–7.25) [63]. Other studies found higher risks of familial lymphoma for HL patients younger than 60 years at diagnosis [84] and for offspring diagnosed under age 50 years [96]. Studies also noted higher HL risk for male relatives of patients, particularly brothers; for same-sex siblings; and for siblings compared with parents of cases [63, 78, 87, 97, 98]. Horwitz et al. proposed that the same-sex concordance of HL in families suggested a susceptibility gene in the pseudoautosomal regions of the sex chromosomes [99, 100], but these patterns also are consistent with a role for shared environmental exposures in familial aggregation of HL and other lymphomas. Anecdotal reports have identified multiplex families with EBV-positive HL [101]; however, tumors in familial cases do not appear consistently to be concordant for EBV [60].

## 1.5 Immune Function

A role for immune function in HL pathogenesis is anticipated, as HL is a B-cell malignancy characterized by immune dysregulation and, within the tumor, by a reactive inflammatory infiltrate and abnormal cytokine expression [2]. Indeed, the etiologic importance of immune function has been demonstrated directly by associations of HL risk with diseases involving immune dysregulation or inflammation, with serum cytokine profiles, and with polymorphisms of immune-function genes. In fact, the strongest risk factors reported for HL include HIV infection (which depletes T-helper cell populations), iatrogenic immunosuppression posttransplantation, and autoimmune conditions, as described below.

### 1.5.1 Immunodeficiency Disorders and HIV

Risk of HL is strongly increased in persons with primary immune deficiencies [102] and with acquired immune deficiency following HIV infection or bone marrow transplantation [103]. From large linkages of US population-based AIDS and cancer registries, risk of HL in HIV-infected populations was estimated at 11.5-fold (95% CI 10.6–12.5) higher than in the general population, with greater risks for the mixed cellularity (RR = 18.3, 95% CI 15.9–20.9) and lymphocytic depletion (RR = 35.3, 95% CI 24.7–48.8) histologic subtypes [104]. Compared to HIV-unrelated HL, HIV-HL is clinically more aggressive, portends poorer survival, and is almost uniformly EBV-positive [105]. Among HIV-infected persons, risk of HL varies by the degree of immunodeficiency, with rates higher for those with CD4 cell counts of 150–199 cells/μL than for those with fewer than 50 cells/μL [106]. This implies that risk of HL is greater with moderate than with severe immunodeficiency. Accordingly, HIV-HL rates have increased since the introduction of highly active antiretroviral therapies in 1996 [107], presumably because of related improvements in average CD4 counts. In one study of patients who had bone marrow transplantation, the incidence of HL was estimated at nearly 15-fold higher than expected (standardized incidence ratio = 14.8, 95% CI 3.9–32.9) [108].

### 1.5.2 Autoimmune Conditions

HL risk is increased in persons with autoimmune diseases. Although such evidence is impacted by the often-small sample sizes given the rarity of these conditions, and by the possibility of reverse causality [109], a large Scandinavian database linking disease registries showed that risk of HL ($n$ = 9,314 cases compared with 37,069 controls) was increased twofold for systematic autoimmune disease overall, with significantly elevated ORs ranging from 2 to 5 for rheumatoid arthritis, systemic lupus erythematosus, Sjögren's syndrome, and sarcoidosis [110]. In 1,155 HL cases over age 67 years at diagnosis from the Surveillance, Epidemiology and End Results (SEER)-Medicare data and controls from the Medicare files, HL risk was similarly elevated among those with a history of lupus, scleroderma, or rheumatoid arthritis [111]. The positive association between autoimmune disease and HL risk irrespective of age may be explained by a number of mechanisms. These include autoantigen-mediated chronic B-cell stimulation, leading to the emergence of a malignant clone (perhaps further enabled by acquired resistance to apoptosis in autoimmune disorders) [112], immunosuppressive treatment for autoimmune disorders, and shared environmental and/or genetic risk factors for both autoimmunity and HL [109]. Evidence of immunologic differences between EBV-positive and EBV-negative HL suggests that risk associations with autoimmune disorders also may differ by tumor EBV status, but studies to date have not examined this possibility.

### 1.5.3 Inflammation

Cytokines, which are produced by HRS cells and believed to act as autocrine growth factors and maintainers of the tumor inflammatory infiltrate [2], have been linked to HL risk through observations of elevated serum/plasma levels of interleukin (IL)-2 [113]; IL-6 [114–116], including before treatment [114, 117]; IL-10 [118, 119]; IL-12 [113]; CC chemokine ligand (CCL)117 and CCL22 [120]; and inflammatory marker YKL-40 [114].

A role for chronic and perhaps, subclinical, inflammation in HL etiology was suggested by reduced risks of HL with routine aspirin use (OR = 0.60, 95% CI

0.42–0.85) in a large US case–control study [121] and with >2 vs. ≤2 prescriptions of low-dose aspirin (OR=0.7, 95% CI 0.5–1.2) in a prospective nested case–control study in linked Danish cancer registry and prescription databases [122]. Aspirin may exert a protective effect by triggering HL cell death through inhibition of the transcription factor NF-κB [123, 124], which helps regulate the expression of immune, inflammatory, and apoptotic genes, and is constitutively activated in and required for survival by HRS cells [125–128]. Aspirin also may protect against HL through its irreversible binding to the active site of cyclooxygenase (COX)-1 and -2 [129], potent mediators of inflammation and tumor growth that are overexpressed in HL [130, 131].

### 1.5.4 Immune Gene Polymorphisms

The highly polymorphic HLA system, which plays a role in infection control by encoding cell-surface molecules that present antigenic peptides to T-cells [132], has been associated with HL risk for decades [59, 133–135]. Early research linked HLA serologic types A1, B5, B8, and B18 to HL risk [136]. In family studies, various HLA class II polymorphisms, including the *DRB5-0101* allele, the haplotype *DRB\*1501-DQA1\*0102-DQB1\*0602*, and a *TAP1* allele, were associated with HL risk [134]. In population studies, HL risk has been related to various HLA genotypes, with considerable patient subgroup specificity as described in Sect. 1.5.5 below. While the findings regarding HLA generally suggest recessive inheritance and additional genetic and environmental factors [71, 133, 137, 138], it is unclear whether the identified associations involve true susceptibility alleles or reflect the strong linkage disequilibrium in the HLA region [139].

Among cytokine genes, several single nucleotide polymorphisms in *IL6* have been associated with HL risk [140], including a promoter region polymorphism (rs1800795, 174G>C) in young adults [115]; other associations were detected with polymorphisms in *IL1R1* (involved in activation of NF-κB) and *IL4R* (expressed on HRS cells) [140]. Cozen et al. found *IL12* +1,188A>C associated with elevated risk for HL in 90 case twins vs. 90 convenience controls (OR=2.9, 95% CI 1.1–7.30) [113]. Several common polymorphisms in *IL10* have been linked to risk of HL [119],

with the association of the −1,082 GG genotype possibly restricted to EBV-positive cases [141]; further, IL-10 plasma levels were elevated for individuals homozygous for *IL10* promotor alleles −592 and −1,082 [119]. A single nucleotide polymorphism in *NFKB1* was recently associated with increased risk of HL (rs1585215 GG vs. AA: OR=3.5, 95% CI 2.2–5.7, $P_{trend}=1.7\times10^{-8}$), as were *NFKB1* haplotypes ($P_{global}=6.0\times10^{-21}$) [142].

### 1.5.5 Heterogeneity of Effects

The impact of some aspects of immune function on risk of HL appears to be relatively unvaried across patient subgroups. The lack of variation in the associations of aspirin use and the related *NFKB1* polymorphism with HL risk by age group, sex, and tumor EBV status suggests that inflammation represents an essential underlying component of HL pathogenesis [122, 142]. For autoimmune disease, the associated risk of HL appeared stronger for the mixed cellularity subtype in a subset of Swedish HL patients (*N*=9,314) for whom histologic subtype information was available [110]. Baecklund et al. found that the risk of HL with rheumatoid arthritis did not vary by tumor histologic subtype or EBV presence [143]. However, all of these analyses were limited by relatively low statistical power for stratified analyses, which may also explain the apparent lack of heterogeneity.

For associations of HL risk with HLA genotype, findings consistently have revealed heterogeneity. In race-specific analysis, risk was found to be increased for HLA class II *DPB1\*0301* in Whites [144–147] but decreased for *DPB1\*0201* [144] and for *DPB1\*0401* in Asians using population-stratified controls [145]. *DPB1\*0301* associations were further restricted to nodular sclerosis HL in one study [148] and to EBV-positive tumors in young adults in another [149]; the risk association with a *TAP1* allele was limited to the nodular sclerosis subtype [134]. Evaluating the entire HLA region, Diepstra, Niens, and colleagues identified associations that were dependent on EBV tumor status: for EBV-positive HL, risk was significantly elevated with specific class I A microsatellite markers (D6S265, D6S510) [150] (ORs of 6.0, 95% CI 1.7–22.1, to 9.8, 95% CI 2.7–34.9, for seven SNPs), whereas for EBV-negative HL, it was associated with one class III marker

(D6S273) [151]. Subsequent work detected associations of *HLA-A*01* with increased risk and *HLA-A*02* with decreased risk of EBV-positive HL, and significantly lower prevalence of *HLA-A*02* patients among 152 EBV-positive patients (35.5%) than 322 EBV-negative patients (50.9%) [152]. As HLA-A molecules present EBV peptides to T-cells, it is feasible that SNPs with low affinity for EBV and thus an inefficient immune response could be linked to risk of EBV-positive HL [132, 151]. Observations linking risk of IM in young adults with various class I polymorphisms (including markers D6S510 and D6S265) strengthen support for a role for management of EBV infection in the etiology of EBV-positive HL [153].

## 1.6 Selected Life-Style and Environmental Risk Factors

### 1.6.1 Smoking

In a 2002 study of men, Briggs et al. reported a near-doubling of HL risk with current cigarette smoking, with significant dose–response effects for intensity and duration of exposure, and risk highest for the mixed cellularity subtype (OR = 3.4, 95% CI 1.8–6.4) [154]. Subsequent case–control and cohort studies consistently have found risks elevated for current smoking [52, 57, 155–162] and, in some studies, limited to the mixed cellularity subtype [154, 156]. Three studies also found the elevated risk restricted to EBV-positive tumors (which are often of mixed cellularity histology) [156, 157, 162]; Hjalgrim et al. reported a significant doubling of risk of EBV-positive HL irrespective of patient age or tumor histologic subtype but with the effect apparently stronger in males than females [157]. Tobacco smoke may impact HL pathogenesis through its associated immunosuppression [163], especially that permitting reactivation of latent EBV infection.

### 1.6.2 Alcohol Consumption

Moderate alcohol consumption has been associated repeatedly with reduced risk of HL. Five case–control studies from various countries reported a significant halving of risk of HL for drinkers at most levels of total alcohol intake [22, 155, 160, 164, 165], while four others reported nonsignificantly protective or null associations [158, 162, 166, 167]. Few of these studies had sufficient numbers of cases to assess level of drinking by relevant HL subtypes, although one study reported null associations for both EBV-positive and -negative disease [162]. However, because most of these studies used nondrinkers as reference groups, their findings may be biased by the well-reported phenomenon of prediagnostic "alcohol-related pain" [168] that could have led to voluntary cessation of alcohol consumption. A prospective cohort study that was able to measure alcohol consumption prior to HL diagnosis reported protective (albeit statistically insignificant) effects of alcohol similar to those reported by case–control studies [159]; however, this study used nondrinkers as opposed to lifetime abstainers as a reference group. Alcohol could influence lymphomagenesis through its established immunologic effects [169].

### 1.6.3 Ultraviolet Radiation Exposure

Increased exposure to ultraviolet radiation (UVR) may decrease risk of HL. A large, population-based case–control study in Sweden and Denmark detected a consistent inverse association, with significant inverse dose–response trends, between risk of HL and UVR exposure, as measured by sunbathing habits, sunburn history, sun vacations abroad, and solarium visits [170]. Grandin et al. found that having phenotypic features that may be associated with reduced sun exposure (i.e., fair complexion or a high propensity to sunburn) increased HL risk [171]. Likewise, a European case–control study reported that increasing skin sensitivity to sun exposure was associated with elevated risk of HL [172]. However, the latter two studies did not find a significant association of HL risk with artificial sun lamp use [171, 172], frequency of outdoor activities [171], or non-working days during childhood or adulthood [172]. Nevertheless, the OR estimates of association with outdoor activities and non-working days were below 1.0, whereas the associations with school/work days were above 1.0, consistent with a protective effect of UVR exposure. The putative inverse association between UVR exposure and HL risk may be a consequence of activation of vitamin D production by UVR [173]. Evidence supports a protective effect of vitamin D against HL development, including the fact that it promotes differentiation and inhibits proliferation of lymphoma cells in vitro [174] and maintains homeostasis of normal B cells [175].

### 1.6.4 Body Size and Physical Activity

HL patients have been found to be significantly heavier at birth and heavier and taller as children than controls matched on age, sex, and social class [176]; some studies also noted HL patients were taller in adulthood [25, 177, 178], but others did not [159, 179–181]. Adult height could be associated with HL risk because of better nutrition [182, 183], which, like HL risk, is likely related to higher childhood socioeconomic status [184, 185], common genetic determinants [95, 148, 150, 182], or promotion of nascent HL tumors in taller persons by higher circulating levels of insulin-like growth factors and other growth hormones [182, 186]. Obesity has been associated with a nearly two [180, 182] to threefold [181, 187] increased risk in men but not in women [181, 187–189], although one study found a nonsignificant association in both sexes [159]. The stronger relationship between obesity and HL risk in men may be a result of their greater tendency to visceral adiposity [181]. Larger birth weight and higher levels of body mass index were associated with increased HL risk in young-adult women but reduced risks in older women [178]. Larger body size could influence risk of HL by triggering higher levels of the cytokine IL-6 [115], insulin resistance, compensatory hyperinsulinemia, or increased production of growth factors, including estrogens [190].

### 1.6.5 Parity

The change in gender patterns of HL incidence from female-dominated in young adulthood to male-dominated in later adulthood suggests that reproductive events or their correlates might contribute to the declining risk of HL in women vis-à-vis men after their early 20s [20, 191]. One registry-based study in Norway identified a significant inverse relationship between HL risk and parity in young-adult women, with an RR of 0.46 among women with 3+ births compared with nulliparous women [192]. Subsequent studies described a slight to moderate decrease in HL risk with higher parity, with some finding a more protective apparent effect in women of reproductive age [21, 193–196]. These data, and findings of lower HL risk with nursing, exogenous hormone use, and a history of endometriosis [197], suggest an effect of steroid or other hormones on HL pathogenesis, possibly through influences on regulation of immune system development or function.

### 1.7 Summary

The epidemiology of HL provides consistent evidence of a disease with complex pathogenesis, as illustrated by the distinctive patterns of its incidence rates and risk profiles by age, race/ethnicity, sex, economic level, and tumor characteristics. From MacMahon's early observations, efforts to interpret and summarize these heterogeneous findings have resulted in models of multiple-disease etiologies, with the most recent hypothesis proposing four diseases based on integration of two primary determinants of heterogeneity – age and tumor EBV status [58]. However, efforts to further understand possible etiologic pathways have been hampered by two challenges. One is the relatively recent observation that some markers of childhood social class initially predictive of risk no longer are associated with HL [24, 30]. This change leaves few established risk factors for HL, especially for the largest subgroup of patients, i.e., young adults with EBV-negative HL [198]. Moreover, those factors shown to strongly impact risk (e.g., HIV infection) have low population prevalence, and few novel ones have been identified. Thus, epidemiologic research into the etiology of HL currently is without strong leads, especially for EBV-negative young-adult disease.

The other challenge to advancing the epidemiology of HL, rooted in its heterogeneity, is the problem of conducting adequately powered studies in meaningful patient subgroups of this relatively uncommon disease. To date, research points to the importance for HL etiology not only of age and tumor EBV status, but also of histologic subtype, genetic predisposition, and environmental exposures. To be informative, therefore, epidemiologic studies must be large enough to examine and disentangle the joint contributions of these factors to HL development.

The accumulated epidemiologic evidence points to HL as an uncommon outcome in susceptible individuals of immune dysfunction provoked by early and concurrent environmental exposures. Beyond this, however, our understanding of HL etiology remains poor. To meet the ultimate public health goal of disease prevention, epidemiologic research into HL must be focused in novel directions and involve study populations of substantial size in order to address its etiologic heterogeneity.

**Acknowledgments**  The authors thank Kari Fish, Sarah Shema, and June Kristine Winters for help with this chapter. The collection of cancer incidence data used in this chapter was supported by the California Department of Health Services as part of the statewide cancer reporting program mandated by California Health and Safety Code Section 103885; the National Cancer Institute's Surveillance, Epidemiology and End Results Program under contract N01-PC-35136 awarded to the Northern California Cancer Center (now the Cancer Prevention Institute of California), contract N01-PC-35139 awarded to the University of Southern California, and contract N02-PC-15105 awarded to the Public Health Institute; and the Centers for Disease Control and Prevention's National Program of Cancer Registries, under agreement #U55/CCR921930-02 awarded to the Public Health Institute. The ideas and opinions expressed herein are those of the authors and endorsement by the State of California, Department of Health Services, the National Cancer Institute, and the Centers for Disease Control and Prevention or their contractors and subcontractors is not intended nor should be inferred.

# References

1. Homer MJ, Ries LAG, Krapcho M, et al., editors. SEER Cancer Statistics Review, 1975-2006. Bethesda, MD: National Cancer Institute; 2009.
2. Mani H, Jaffe ES. Hodgkin lymphoma: An update on its biology with new insights into classification. Clin Lymph Res. 2009;9:206–16.
3. MacMahon B. Epidemiological evidence on the nature of Hodgkin's disease. Cancer. 1957;10:1045–54.
4. MacMahon B. Epidemiology of Hodgkin's disease. Cancer Res. 1966;26(6):1189–201.
5. Harris NL, Jaffe ES, Diebold J, et al. World Health Organization classification of neoplastic diseases of the hematopoietic and lymphoid tissues: report of the Clinical Advisory Committee meeting-Airlie House, Virginia, November 1997 [see comments]. J Clin Oncol. 1999;17(12): 3835–49.
6. Ferlay J, Bray F, Pisani P, et al. GLOBOCAN 2002: Cancer incidence, mortality and prevalence worldwide. In: IARC CancerBase No 5 version 20. Lyon: IARC Press; 2004.
7. Surveillance, Epidemiology, and End Results (SEER) Program (www.seer.cancer.gov) SEER*Stat Database: Incidence – SEER 17 Regs Limited-Use + Hurricane Katrina Impacted Louisiana Cases, Nov 2008 Sub (2000-2006) <Katrina/Rita Population Adjustment> – Linked To County Attributes - Total U.S., 1969–2006 Counties, National Cancer Institute, DCCPS, Surveillance Research Program, Cancer Statistics Branch, released April 2009, based on the November 2008 submission.
8. Reed DM. On the pathological changes in Hodgkin's disease, with especial reference to its relation to tuberculosis. Johns Hopkins Hosp Rep. 1902;10:133–396.
9. Correa P, O'Conor GT. Epidemiologic patterns of Hodgkin's disease. Int J Cancer. 1971;8(2):192–201.
10. Macfarlane G, Evstifeeva T, Boyle P, et al. International patterns in the occurrence of Hodgkin's disease in children and young adult males. Int J Cancer. 1995;61(2):165–9.
11. Hjalgrim H, Seow A, Rostgaard K, et al. Changing patterns of Hodgkin lymphoma incidence in Singapore. Int J Cancer. 2008;123(3):716–9.
12. Glaser SL, Hsu JL. Hodgkin's disease in Asians: incidence patterns and risk factors in population-based data. Leuk Res. 2002;26:261–9.
13. Au WY, Gascoyne RD, Gallagher RE, et al. Hodgkin's lymphoma in Chinese migrants to British Columbia: a 25-year survey. Ann Oncol. 2004;15(4):626–30.
14. Caporaso NE, Goldin LR, Anderson WF, et al. Current insight on trends, causes, and mechanisms of Hodgkin's lymphoma. Cancer J. 2009;15:117–23.
15. Clarke CA, Glaser SL, Keegan THM, et al. Neighborhood socioeconomic status and Hodgkin lymphoma incidence in California. Cancer Epidemiol Biomark Prev. 2005;14:1441–7.
16. Chen YT, Zheng T, Mei-Chu C, et al. The increase in Hodgkin's disease incidence among young adults. Experience in Connecticut, 1935–1992. Cancer. 1997;79:2209–18.
17. Gutensohn N, Cole P. Epidemiology of Hodgkin's disease in the young. Int J Cancer. 1977;19(5):595–604.
18. Cozen W, Katz J, Mack TM. Risk patterns of Hodgkin's disease in Los Angeles vary by cell type. Cancer Epidemiol Biomark Prev. 1992;1(4):261–8.
19. Glaser SL. Regional variation in Hodgkin's disease incidence by histologic subtype in the US. Cancer. 1987;60:2841–7.
20. Grufferman S, Delzell E. Epidemiology of Hodgkin's disease. Epidemiol Rev. 1984;6:76–106.
21. Abramson JH, Pridan H, Sacks MI, et al. A case-control study of Hodgkin's disease in Israel. J Natl Cancer Inst. 1978;61: 307–14.
22. Bernard SM, Cartwright RA, Darwin CM, et al. Hodgkin's disease: case control epidemiological study in Yorkshire. Br J Cancer. 1987;55(1):85–90.
23. Cohen BM, Smetana HF, Miller RW. Hodgkin's disease: Long survival in a study of 388 World War II army cases. Cancer. 1964;17:856–66.
24. Glaser SL, Clarke CA, Nugent RA, et al. Social class and risk of Hodgkin's disease in young-adult women in 1988-94. Int J Cancer. 2002;98:110–7.
25. Gutensohn N, Cole P. Childhood social environment and Hodgkin's disease. New Engl J Med. 1981;304:135–40.
26. Serraino D, Franceschi S, Talamini R, et al. Socio-economic indicators, infectious diseases and Hodgkin's disease. Int J Cancer. 1991;47:352–7.

27. Alexander FE, Ricketts TJ, McKinney PA, et al. Community lifestyle characteristics and incidence of Hodgkin's disease in young people. Int J Cancer. 1991;48(1):10–4.

28. Bonelli L, Vitale V, Bistolfi F, et al. Hodgkin's disease in adults: association with social factors and age at tonsillectomy. A case-control study. Int J Cancer. 1990;45(3):423–7.

29. Chang ET, Montgomery SM, Richiardi L, et al. Number of siblings and risk of Hodgkin's lymphoma. Cancer Epidemiol Biomark Prev. 2004;13(7):1236–43.

30. Chang ET, Zheng T, Weir EG, et al. Childhood social environment and Hodgkin's lymphoma: new findings from a population-based case-control study. Cancer Epidemiol Biomark Prev. 2004;13(8):1361–70.

31. Westergaard T, Melbye M, Pedersen JB, et al. Birth order, sibship size and risk of Hodgkin's disease in children and young adults: a population-based study of 31 million person-years. Int J Cancer. 1997;72:977–81.

32. Carter CD, Brown Jr TM, Herbert JT, et al. Cancer incidence following infectious mononucleosis. Am J Epidemiol. 1977; 105(1):30–6.

33. Connelly RR, Christine BW. A cohort study of cancer following infectious mononucleosis. Cancer Res. 1974;34 (5):1172–8.

34. Hjalgrim H, Askling J, Sorensen P, et al. Risk of Hodgkin's disease and other cancers after infectious mononucleosis. J Natl Cancer Inst. 2000;92(18):1522–8.

35. Hjalgrim H, Askling J, Rostgaard K, et al. Characteristics of Hodgkin's lymphoma after infectious mononucleosis. N Engl J Med. 2003;349:1324–32.

36. Hjalgrim H, Smedby KE, Rostgaard K, et al. Infectious mononucleosis, childhood social environment, and risk of Hodgkin lymphoma. Cancer Res. 2007;67:2382–8.

37. Kvåle G, Høiby EA, Pedersen E. Hodgkin's disease in patients with previous infectious mononucleosis. Int J Cancer. 1979;23:593–7.

38. Miller RW, Beebe GW. Infectious mononucleosis and the empirical risk of cancer. J Natl Cancer Inst. 1973;50: 315–21.

39. Rosdahl N, Larsen SO, Thamdrup AB. Infectious mononucleosis in Denmark. Epidemiological observations based on positive Paul-Bunnell reactions from 1940-1969. Scand J Infect Dis. 1973;5(3):163–70.

40. Gutensohn NM. Social class and age at diagnosis of Hodgkin's disease: new epidemiologic evidence for the "two-disease hypothesis". Cancer Treat Rep. 1982;66(4): 689–95.

41. Gutensohn NM, Shapiro DS. Social class risk factors among children with Hodgkin's disease. Int J Cancer. 1982;30(4): 433–5.

42. Glaser SL, Clarke CA, Stearns CB, et al. Age variation in Hodgkin's disease risk factors in older women: evidence from a population-based case-control study. Leuk Lymphoma. 2001;42:997–1004.

43. IARC Working Group on the Evaluation of Carcinogenic Risks to Humans. Epstein-Barr virus and Kaposi's sarcoma herpesvirus/human herpesvirus8, vol. 7. Lyon: International Agency for Research on Cancer; 1997.

44. Evans AS, Gutensohn NM. A population-based case-control study of EBV and other viral antibodies among persons with Hodgkin's disease and their siblings. Int J Cancer. 1984;34: 149–57.

45. Mueller N, Evans A, Harris NL, et al. Hodgkin's disease and Epstein-Barr virus. Altered antibody pattern before diagnosis. N Engl J Med. 1989;320(11):689–95.

46. Weiss LM, Movahed LA, Warnke RA, et al. Detection of Epstein-Barr viral genomes in Reed-Sternberg cells of Hodgkin's disease. N Engl J Med. 1989;320:502–6.

47. Glaser SL, Lin RJ, Stewart SL, et al. Epstein-Barr virus-associated Hodgkin's disease: epidemiologic characteristics in international data. Int J Cancer. 1997;70:375–82.

48. Jarrett RF. Risk factors for Hodgkin's lymphoma by EBV status and significance of detection of EBV genomes in serum of patients with EBV-associated Hodgkin's lymphoma. Leuk Lymphoma. 2003;44 Suppl 3:S27–32.

49. Glaser SL, Gulley ML, Clarke CA, et al. Racial/ethnic variation in EBV-positive classical Hodgkin lymphoma in California populations. Int J Cancer. 2008;123:1499–507.

50. Jarrett RF, Krajewski AS, Angus B, et al. The Scotland and Newcastle epidemiological study of Hodgkin's disease: impact of histopathological review and EBV status on incidence estimates. J Clin Pathol. 2003;56:811–6.

51. Alexander FE, Lawrence DJ, Freeland J, et al. An epidemiologic study of index and family infectious mononucleosis and adult Hodgkin's disease (HD): evidence for a specific association with EBV+ve HD in young adults. Int J Cancer. 2003;107(2):298–302.

52. Cozen W, Hamilton AS, Zhao P, et al. A protective role for early oral exposures in the etiology of young adult Hodgkin lymphoma. Blood. 2009;114(19):4014–20.

53. Glaser SL, Keegan THM, Clarke CA, et al. Exposure to childhood infections and risk of EBV-defined Hodgkin's lymphoma in women. Int J Cancer. 2005;115:599–605.

54. Montella M, Maso LD, Crispo A, et al. Do childhood diseases affect NHL and HL risk? A case-control study from northern and southern Italy. Leuk Res. 2006;30(8):917–22.

55. Newton R, Crouch S, Ansell P, et al. Hodgkin's lymphoma and infection: findings from a UK case-control study. Br J Cancer. 2007;97(9):1310–4.

56. Sleckman BG, Mauch PM, Ambinder RF, et al. Epstein-Barr virus in Hodgkin's disease: correlation of risk factors and disease characteristics with molecular evidence of viral infection. Cancer Epidemiol Biomark Prev. 1998;7: 1117–21.

57. Chang ET, Zheng T, Lennette ET, et al. Heterogeneity of risk factors and antibody profiles in Epstein-barr virus genome-positive and -negative Hodgkin lymphoma. J Infect Dis. 2004;189:2271–81.

58. Jarrett RF. Viruses and Hodgkin's lymphoma. Ann Oncol. 2002;13 Suppl 1:23–9.

59. Hors J, Steinberg G, Andrieu JM, et al. HLA genotypes in familial Hodgkin's disease. Excess of HLA identical affected sibs. Eur J Cancer. 1980;16(6):809–15.

60. Lin AY, Kingma DW, Lennette ET, et al. Epstein-Barr virus and familial Hodgkin's disease. Blood. 1996;88(8):3160–5.

61. Bjerrum OW, Hasselbalch HC, Drivsholm A, et al. Non-Hodgkin malignant lymphomas and Hodgkin's disease in first-degree relatives. Evidence for a mutual genetic predisposition? Scand J Haematol. 1986;36(4):398–401.

62. Donhuijsen-Ant R, Abken H, Bornkamm G, et al. Fatal Hodgkin and non-Hodgkin lymphoma associated with persistent Epstein-Barr virus in four brothers. Ann Intern Med. 1988;109(12):946–52.

63. Goldin LR, Pfeiffer RM, Gridley G, et al. Familial aggregation of Hodgkin lymphoma and related tumors. Cancer. 2004;100:1902–8.

64. Lynch HT, Marcus JN, Weisenburger DD, et al. Genetic and immunopathological findings in a lymphoma family. Br J Cancer. 1989;59(4):622–6.

65. Padua L, Palmisani MT, Di Trapani G, et al. Myasthenia gravis and thymic Hodgkin's disease associated in one patient with familial lymphoproliferative disorders. Clin Neuropathol. 1994;13(5):292–4.

66. Razis DV, Diamond HD, Craver LF. Familial Hodgkin's disease: its significance and implications. Ann Intern Med. 1959;51(5):933–71.

67. Buehler SK, Firme F, Fodor G, et al. Common variable immunodeficiency, Hodgkin's disease, and other malignancies in a Newfoundland family. Lancet. 1975;1(7900):195–7.

68. Grufferman S, Ambinder RF, Shugart YY, et al. Increased cancer risk in families of children with Hodgkin's disease. Am J Epidemiol. 1998;147(11):S8.

69. Lynch HT, Marcus JN, Lynch JF. Genetics of Hodgkin's and non-Hodgkin's lymphoma: a review. Cancer Invest. 1992;10(3):247–56.

70. McKeen EA, Mulvihill JJ, Levine PH, et al. The concurrence of Saethre-Chotzen syndrome and malignancy in a family with in vitro immune dysfunction. Cancer. 1984;54 (12):2946–51.

71. Chakravarti A, Halloran SL, Bale SJ, et al. Etiological heterogeneity in Hodgkin's disease: HLA linked and unlinked determinants of susceptibility independent of histological concordance. Genet Epidemiol. 1986;3(6):407–15.

72. Haim N, Cohen Y, Robinson E. Malignant lymphoma in first-degree blood relatives. Cancer. 1982;49(10):2197–200.

73. Mack TM, Cozen W, Shibata DK, et al. Concordance for Hodgkin's disease in identical twins suggesting genetic susceptibility to the young-adult form of the disease. N Engl J Med. 1995;332:413–8.

74. Brown JR, Neuberg D, Phillips K, et al. Prevalence of familial malignancy in a prospectively screened cohort of patients with lymphoproliferative disorders. Br J Haematol. 2008;143(3):361–8.

75. Chang ET, Smedby KE, Hjalgrim H, et al. Family history of hematopoietic malignancy and risk of lymphoma. J Natl Cancer Inst. 2005;97(19):1466–74.

76. Friedman DL, Kadan-Lottick NS, Whitton J, et al. Increased risk of cancer among siblings of long-term childhood cancer survivors: a report from the Childhood Cancer Survivor Study. Cancer Epidemiol Biomark Prev. 2005;14(8):1922–7.

77. Goldgar DE, Easton DF, Cannon-Albright LA, et al. Systematic population-based assessment of cancer risk in first-degree relatives of cancer probands. J Natl Cancer Inst. 1994;86:1600–8.

78. Grufferman S, Cole P, Smith PG, et al. Hodgkin's disease in siblings. N Engl J Med. 1977;296(5):248–50.

79. Hemminki K, Czene K. Attributable risks of familial cancer from the Family-Cancer Database. Cancer Epidemiol Biomark Prev. 2002;11:1638–44.

80. Kerzin-Storrar L, Faed MJ, MacGillivray JB, et al. Incidence of familial Hodgkin's disease. Br J Cancer. 1983;47(5):707–12.

81. McDuffie H, Pahwa P, Karunanayake C, et al. Clustering of cancer among families of cases with Hodgkin Lymphoma (HL), Multiple Myeloma (MM), Non-Hodgkin's Lymphoma (NHL), Soft Tissue Sarcoma (STS) and control subjects. BMC Cancer. 2009;9(1):70.

82. Pang D, Alston RD, Eden TOB, et al. Cancer risks among relatives of children with Hodgkin and non-Hodgkin lymphoma. Int J Cancer. 2008;123(6):1407–10.

83. Rudant J, Menegaux F, Leverger G, et al. Family history of cancer in children with acute leukemia, Hodgkin's lymphoma or non-Hodgkin's lymphoma: the ESCALE study (SFCE). Int J Cancer. 2007;121(1):119–26.

84. Casey R, Brennan P, Becker N, et al. Influence of familial cancer history on lymphoid neoplasms risk validated in the large European case-control study epilymph. Eur J Cancer. 2006;42(15):2570–6.

85. Chatterjee N, Hartge P, Cerhan JR, et al. Risk of non-Hodgkin's lymphoma and family history of lymphatic, hematologic, and other cancers. Cancer Epidemiol Biomark Prev. 2004;13(9):1415–21.

86. Wang SS, Slager SL, Brennan P, et al. Family history of hematopoietic malignancies and risk of non-Hodgkin lymphoma (NHL): a pooled analysis of 10 211 cases and 11 905 controls from the International Lymphoma Epidemiology Consortium (InterLymph). Blood. 2007;109(8):3479–88.

87. Altieri A, Hemminki K. The familial risk of Hodgkin's lymphoma ranks among the highest in the Swedish Family-Cancer Database. Leukemia. 2006;20(11):2062–3.

88. Paltiel O, Schmit T, Adler B, et al. The incidence of lymphoma in first-degree relatives of patients with Hodgkin disease and non-Hodgkin lymphoma: results and limitations of a registry-linked study. Cancer. 2000;88(10):2357–66.

89. Shugart YY, Hemminki K, Vaittinen P, et al. Apparent anticipation and heterogeneous transmission patterns in familial Hodgkin's and non-Hodgkin's lymphoma: report from a study based on Swedish cancer database. Leuk Lymphoma. 2001;42:407–15.

90. Daugherty SE, Pfeiffer RM, Mellemkjaer L, et al. No evidence for anticipation in lymphoproliferative tumors in population-based samples. Cancer Epidemiol Biomark Prev. 2005;14(5):1245–50.

91. Goldin LR, Björkholm M, Kristinsson SY, et al. Highly increased familial risks for specific lymphoma subtypes. Br J Haematol. 2009;146(1):91–4.

92. Hemminki K, Li X. Familial risk in testicular cancer as a clue to a heritable and environmental aetiology. Br J Cancer. 2004;90(9):1765–70.

93. Hjalgrim H, Rasmussen S, Rostgaard K, et al. Familial clustering of Hodgkin lymphoma and multiple sclerosis. J Natl Cancer Inst. 2004;96(10):780–4.

94. Landgren O, Kerstann KF, Gridley G, et al. Re: Familial clustering of Hodgkin lymphoma and multiple sclerosis. J Natl Cancer Inst. 2005;97(7):543–4.

95. Goldin LR, McMaster ML, Ter-Minassian M, et al. A genome screen of families at high risk for Hodgkin lymphoma: evidence for a susceptibility gene on chromosome 4. J Med Genet. 2005;42:595–601.

96. Hemminki K, Li X, Czene K. Familial risk of cancer: data for clinical counseling and cancer genetics. Int J Cancer. 2004;108:109–14.

97. Hemminki K, Li X. Cancer risks in twins: results from the Swedish family-cancer database. Int J Cancer. 2002; 99(6):873–8.

98. Swerdlow AJ, De Stavola B, Maconochie N, et al. A population-based study of cancer risk in twins: relationships to birth order and sexes of the twin pair. Int J Cancer. 1996; 67(4):472–8.

99. Horwitz M, Wiernik PH. Pseudoautosomal linkage of Hodgkin disease. Am J Hum Genet. 1999;65(5):1413–22.

100. Horwitz MS, Mealiffe ME. Further evidence for a pseudoautosomal gene for Hodgkin's lymphoma: Reply to "The familial risk of Hodgkin's lymphoma ranks among the highest in the Swedish Family-Cancer Database" by Altieri A and Hemminki K. Leukemia. 2006;21(2):351.

101. Kamper PM, Kjeldsen E, Clausen N, et al. Epstein-Barr virus-associated familial Hodgkin lymphoma: paediatric onset in three of five siblings. Br J Haematol. 2005;129(5): 615–7.

102. Mueller NE, Grufferman S. Hodgkin lymphoma. In: Schottenfeld D, Fraumeni JF, editors. Cancer epidemiology and prevention. 3rd ed. New York: Oxford University Press; 2006. p. 872–97.

103. Rowlings PA, Curtis RE, Passweg JR, et al. Increased incidence of Hodgkin's disease after allogeneic bone marrow transplantation. J Clin Oncol. 1999;17(10):3122–7.

104. Frisch M, Biggar RJ, Engels EA, et al. Association of cancer with AIDS-related immunosuppression in adults. JAMA. 2001;285(13):1736–45.

105. Berenguer J, Miralles P, Ribera JM, et al. Characteristics and outcome of AIDS-related Hodgkin lymphoma before and after the introduction of highly active antiretroviral therapy. JAIDS. 2008;47(4):422–8.

106. Biggar RJ, Jaffe ES, Goedert JJ, et al. Hodgkin lymphoma and immunodeficiency in persons with HIV/AIDS. Blood. 2006;108(12):3786–91.

107. Engels EA, Pfeiffer RM, Goedert JJ, et al. Trends in cancer risk among people with AIDS in the United States 1980–2002. AIDS. 2006;20(12):1645–54.

108. Baker KS, DeFor TE, Burns LJ, et al. New malignancies after blood or marrow stem-cell transplantation in children and adults: incidence and risk factors. J Clin Oncol. 2003;21(7):1352–8.

109. Smedby KE, Baecklund E, Askling J. Malignant lymphomas in autoimmunity and inflammation: a review of risks, risk factors, and lymphoma characteristics. Cancer Epidemiol Biomark Prev. 2006;15:2069–77.

110. Kristinsson SY, Landgren O, Sjoberg J, et al. Autoimmunity and risk for Hodgkin's lymphoma by subtype. Haematologica. 2009;94(10):1468–9.

111. Anderson LA, Gadalla S, Morton LM, et al. Population-based study of autoimmune conditions and the risk of specific lymphoid malignancies. Int J Cancer. 2009;125: 398–405.

112. Eguchi K. Apoptosis in autoimmune diseases. Intern Med. 2001;40:275–84.

113. Cozen W, Gill PS, Salam MT, et al. Interleukin-2, interleukin-12, and interferon-{gamma} levels and risk of young adult Hodgkin lymphoma. Blood. 2008;111(7):3377–82.

114. Biggar RJ, Johansen JS, Ekström Smedby K, et al. Serum YKL-40 and interleukin 6 levels in Hodgkin lymphoma. Clin Cancer Res. 2008;14(21):6974–8.

115. Cozen W, Gill PS, Ingles SA, et al. IL-6 levels and genotype are associated with risk of young adult Hodgkin lymphoma. Blood. 2004;103(8):3216–21.

116. Gause A, Scholz R, Klein S, et al. Increased levels of circulating interleukin-6 in patients with Hodgkin's disease. Hematol Oncol. 1991;9(6):307–13.

117. Gause A, Keymis S, Scholz R, et al. Increased levels of circulating cytokines in patients with untreated Hodgkin's disease. Lymphokine Cytokine Res. 1992;11(2):109–13.

118. Herling M, Rassidakis GZ, Medeiros LJ, et al. Expression of Epstein-Barr virus latent membrane protein-1 in Hodgkin and Reed-Sternberg cells of classical Hodgkin's lymphoma: associations with presenting features, serum interleukin 10 levels, and clinical outcome. Clin Cancer Res. 2003;9(6): 2114–20.

119. Hohaus S, Giachelia M, Massini G, et al. Clinical significance of interleukin-10 gene polymorphisms and plasma levels in Hodgkin lymphoma. Leuk Res. 2009;33(10): 1352–6.

120. Niens M, Visser L, Nolte IM, et al. Serum chemokine levels in Hodgkin lymphoma patients: highly increased levels of CCL17 and CCL22. Br J Haematol. 2008;140(5):527–36.

121. Chang ET, Zheng T, Weir EG, et al. Aspirin and the risk of Hodgkin's lymphoma in a population-based case-control study. J Natl Cancer Inst. 2004;96:305–15.

122. Chang ET, Cronin-Fenton DP, Friis S, et al. Aspirin and other nonsteroidal anti-inflammatory drugs in relation to Hodgkin lymphoma risk in northern Denmark. Cancer Epidemiol Biomark Prev. 2010;19:59–64.

123. Baeuerle PA, Baltimore D. NF-kappa B: ten years after. Cell. 1996;87(1):13–20.

124. Yamamoto Y, Yin MJ, Lin KM, et al. Sulindac inhibits activation of the NF-kappaB pathway. J Biol Chem. 1999; 274(38):27307–14.

125. Bargou RC, Leng C, Krappmann D, et al. High-level nuclear NF-kappa B and Oct-2 is a common feature of cultured Hodgkin/Reed-Sternberg cells. Blood. 1996;87(10): 4340–7.

126. Bargou RC, Emmerich F, Krappmann D, et al. Constitutive nuclear factor-kappaB-RelA activation is required for proliferation and survival of Hodgkin's disease tumor cells. J Clin Invest. 1997;100(12):2961–9.

127. Hinz M, Loser P, Mathas S, et al. Constitutive NF-kappaB maintains high expression of a characteristic gene network, including CD40, CD86, and a set of antiapoptotic genes in Hodgkin/Reed-Sternberg cells. Blood. 2001;97(9): 2798–807.

128. Izban KF, Ergin M, Huang Q, et al. Characterization of NF-kappaB expression in Hodgkin's disease: inhibition of constitutively expressed NF-kappaB results in spontaneous caspase-independent apoptosis in Hodgkin and Reed-Sternberg cells. Mod Pathol. 2001;14(4):297–310.

129. Van Der Ouderaa FJ, Buytenhek M, Nugteren DH, et al. Acetylation of prostaglandin endoperoxide synthetase with acetylsalicylic acid. Eur J Biochem. 1980;109(1):1–8.

130. Goodwin JS, Messner RP, Bankhurst AD, et al. Prostaglandin-producing suppressor cells in Hodgkin's disease. N Engl J Med. 1977;297(18):963–8.

131. Hsu SM, Hsu PL, Lo SS, et al. Expression of prostaglandin H synthase (cyclooxygenase) in Hodgkin's mononuclear and Reed-Sternberg cells. Functional resemblance between

H-RS cells and histiocytes or interdigitating reticulum cells. Am J Pathol. 1988;133(1):5–12.

132. Diepstra A, Niens M, te Meerman GJ, et al. Genetic susceptibility to Hodgkin's lymphoma associated with the human leukocyte antigen region. Eur J Haematol Suppl. 2005;75(66):34–41.

133. Berberich FR, Berberich MS, King MC, et al. Hodgkin's disease susceptibility: linkage to the HLA locus demonstrated by a new concordance method. Hum Immunol. 1983;6:207–17.

134. Harty LC, Lin AY, Goldstein AM, et al. HLA-DR, HLA-DQ, and TAP genes in familial Hodgkin disease. Blood. 2002;99:690–3.

135. Lynch HT, Saldivar VA, Guirgis HA, et al. Familial Hodgkin's disease and associated cancer. Cancer. 1976; 38:2033–41.

136. Hors J, Dausset J. HLA and susceptibility to Hodgkin's disease. Immunol Rev. 1983;70:167–92.

137. Paltiel O. Family matters in Hodgkin lymphoma. Leuk Lymph. 2008;49(7):1234–5.

138. Shugart YY, Hemminki K, Vaittinen P, et al. A genetic study of Hodgkin's lymphoma: an estimate of heritability and anticipation based on the familial cancer database in Sweden. Hum Genet. 2000;106:553–6.

139. Ahmad T, Neville M, Marshall SE, et al. Haplotype-specific linkage disequilibrium patterns define the genetic topography of the human MHC. Hum Mol Genet. 2003;12(6): 647–56.

140. Liang X, Caporaso N, McMaster ML, et al. Common genetic variants in candidate genes and risk of familial lymphoid malignancies. Br J Haematol. 2009;146(4):418–23.

141. da Silva GN, Bacchi MM, Rainho CA, et al. Epstein-Barr virus infection and single nucleotide polymorphisms in the promoter region of interleukin 10 gene in patients with Hodgkin lymphoma. Arch Pathol Lab Med. 2007;131: 1691–6.

142. Chang ET, Birmann BM, Kasperzyk JL, et al. Polymorphic variation in NFKB1 and other aspirin-related genes and risk of Hodgkin lymphoma. Cancer Epidemiol Biomark Prev. 2009;18(3):976–86.

143. Baecklund E, Iliadou A, Askling J, et al. Association of chronic inflammation, not its treatment, with increased lymphoma risk in rheumatoid arthritis. Arthritis Rheum. 2006;54:692–701.

144. Bodmer JG, Tonks S, Oza AM, et al. HLA-DP based resistance to Hodgkin's disease. Lancet. 1989;333(8652): 1455–6.

145. Oza AM, Tonks S, Lim J, et al. A clinical and epidemiological study of human leukocyte antigen-DPB alleles in Hodgkin's disease. Cancer Res. 1994;54(19):5101–5.

146. Taylor GM, Gokhale DA, Crowther D, et al. Increased frequency of HLA-DPB1*0301 in Hodgkin's disease suggests that susceptibility is HVR-sequence and subtype-associated. Leukemia. 1996;10:854–9.

147. Taylor GM, Gokhale DA, Crowther D, et al. Further investigation of the role of HLA-DPB1 in adult Hodgkin's disease (HD) suggests an influence on susceptibility to different HD subtypes. Br J Cancer. 1999;80:1405–11.

148. Klitz W, Aldrich CL, Fildes N, et al. Localization of predisposition to Hodgkin disease in the HLA class II region. Am J Hum Genet. 1994;54(3):497–505.

149. Alexander FE, Jarrett RF, Cartwright RA, et al. Epstein-Barr Virus and HLA-DPB1-*0301 in young adult Hodgkin's disease: evidence for inherited susceptibility to Epstein-Barr Virus in cases that are EBV(+ve). Cancer Epidemiol Biomark Prev. 2001;10:705–9.

150. Diepstra A, Niens M, Vellenga E, et al. Association with HLA class I in Epstein-Barr-virus-positive and with HLA class III in Epstein-Barr-virus-negative Hodgkin's lymphoma. Lancet. 2005;365:2216–24.

151. Niens M, van den Berg A, Diepstra A, et al. The human leukocyte antigen class I region is associated with EBV-positive Hodgkin's lymphoma: HLA-A and HLA complex group 9 are putative candidate genes. Cancer Epidemiol Biomark Prev. 2006;15:2280–4.

152. Niens M, Jarrett RF, Hepkema B, et al. HLA-A*02 is associated with a reduced risk and HLA-A*01 with an increased risk of developing EBV-positive Hodgkin lymphoma. Blood. 2007;110:3310–5.

153. McAulay KA, Higgins CD, Macsween KF, et al. HLA class I polymorphisms are associated with development of infectious mononucleosis upon primary EBV infection. J Clin Invest. 2007;117:3042–8.

154. Briggs NC, Hall HI, Brann EA, et al. Cigarette smoking and risk of Hodgkin's disease: a population-based case-control study. Am J Epidemiol. 2002;156:1011–20.

155. Besson H, Brennan P, Becker N, et al. Tobacco smoking, alcohol drinking and Hodgkin's lymphoma: a European multi-centre case-control study (EPILYMPH). Br J Cancer. 2006;95(3):378–84.

156. Glaser SL, Keegan TH, Clarke CA, et al. Smoking and Hodgkin lymphoma risk in women United States. Cancer Causes Control. 2004;15(4):387–97.

157. Hjalgrim H, Ekström-Smedby K, Rostgaard K, et al. Cigarette smoking and risk of Hodgkin lymphoma: a population-based case-control study. Cancer Epidemiol Biomark Prev. 2007;16:1561–6.

158. Klatsky AL, Li Y, Baer D, et al. Alcohol consumption and risk of hematologic malignancies. Ann Epidemiol. 2009;19(10):746–53.

159. Lim U, Morton LM, Subar AF, et al. Alcohol, smoking, and body size in relation to incident Hodgkin's and non-Hodgkin's lymphoma risk. Am J Epidemiol. 2007;166(6): 697–708.

160. Nieters A, Deeg B, Becker N. Tobacco and alcohol consumption and risk of lymphoma: results of a population-based case-control study in Germany. Int J Cancer. 2006; 118(2):422–30.

161. Nieters A, Rohrmann S, Becker N, et al. Smoking and lymphoma risk in the European Prospective Investigation into Cancer and Nutrition. Am J Epidemiol. 2008;167(9): 1081–9.

162. Willett EV, O'Connor S, Smith AG, et al. Does smoking or alcohol modify the risk of Epstein-Barr Virus-positive or -negative Hodgkin lymphoma? Epidemiology. 2007;18(1): 130–6.

163. Sopori ML, Kozak W. Immunomodulatory effects of cigarette smoke. J Neuroimmunol. 1998;83(1–2):148–56.

164. Gorini G, Stagnaro E, Fontana V, et al. Alcohol consumption and risk of Hodgkin's lymphoma and multiple myeloma: a multicentre case-control study. Ann Oncol. 2007;18(1):143–8.

165. Kanda J, Matsuo K, Kawase T, et al. Association of alcohol intake and smoking with malignant lymphoma risk in Japanese: a hospital-based case-control study at Aichi Cancer Center. Cancer Epidemiol Biomark Prev. 2009; 18(9):2436–41.

166. Monnereau A, Orsi L, Troussard X, et al. Cigarette smoking, alcohol drinking, and risk of lymphoid neoplasms: results of a French case–control study. Cancer Causes Control. 2008;19(10):1147–60.

167. Tavani A, Pregnolato A, Negri E, et al. Diet and risk of lymphoid neoplasms and soft tissue sarcomas. Nutr Cancer. 1997;27(3):256–60.

168. Bobrove AM. Alcohol-related pain and Hodgkin's disease. West J Med. 1983;138(6):874–5.

169. Diaz LE, Montero A, Gonzalez-Gross M, et al. Influence of alcohol consumption on immunological status: a review. Eur J Clin Nutr. 2002;56 Suppl 3:S50–3.

170. Ekström Smedby K, Hjalgrim H, Melbye M, et al. Ultraviolet radiation exposure and risk of malignant lymphomas. J Natl Cancer Inst. 2005;97(3):199–209.

171. Grandin L, Orsi L, Troussard X, et al. UV radiation exposure, skin type and lymphoid malignancies: results of a French case-control study. Cancer Causes Control. 2008; 19(3):305–15.

172. Boffetta P, van der Hel O, Kricker A, et al. Exposure to ultraviolet radiation and risk of malignant lymphoma and multiple myeloma – a multicentre European case-control study. Int J Epidemiol. 2008;37(5):1080–94.

173. Guyton KZ, Kensler TW, Posner GH. Vitamin D and vitamin D analogs as cancer chemopreventive agents. Nutr Rev. 2003;61(7):227–38.

174. Hickish T, Cunningham D, Colston K, et al. The effect of 1, 25-dihydroxyvitamin D3 on lymphoma cell lines and expression of vitamin D receptor in lymphoma. Br J Cancer. 1993;68(4):668–72.

175. Chen S, Sims GP, Chen XX, et al. Modulatory effects of 1, 25-dihydroxyvitamin D3 on human B cell differentiation. J Immunol. 2007;179(3):1634–47.

176. Isager H, Andersen E. Pre-morbid factors in Hodgkin's disease. I. Birth weight and growth pattern from 8 to 14 years of age. Scand J Haematol. 1978;21:250–5.

177. Hancock BW, Mosely R, Coup AJ. Height and Hodgkin's disease (letter). Lancet. 1976;2:1364.

178. Keegan THM, Glaser SL, Clarke CA, et al. Body size, physical activity and risk of Hodgkin lymphoma in women. Cancer Epidemiol Biomark Prev. 2006;15:1095–101.

179. La Vecchia C, Negri E, Parazzini F, et al. Height and cancer risk in a network of case-control studies from northern Italy. Int J Cancer. 1990;45(2):275–9.

180. Paffenbarger Jr RS, Wing AL, Hyde RT. Characteristics in youth indicative of adult-onset Hodgkin's disease. J Natl Cancer Inst. 1977;58(5):1489–91.

181. Willett EV, Roman E. Obesity and the risk of Hodgkin lymphoma (United Kingdom). Cancer Causes Control. 2006;17:1103–6.

182. Gunnell D, Okasha M, Smith GD, et al. Height, leg length, and cancer risk: a systematic review. Epidemiol Rev. 2001;23(2):313–42.

183. Silventoinen K. Determinants of variation in adult body height. J Biosoc Sci. 2003;35(2):263–85.

184. Mueller N. Hodgkin's disease. In: Schottenfeld D, Fraumeni Jr JF, editors. Cancer epidemiology and prevention. 2nd ed. New York, NY: Oxford University Press; 1996. p. 893–919.

185. Mueller N, Grufferman S. The epidemiology of Hodgkin's disease. In: Mauch PM, Armitage JO, Diehl V, et al., editors. Hodgkin's disease. Philadelphia: Lippincott Williams & Wilkins; 1999. p. 61–77.

186. Okasha M, Gunnell D, Holly J, et al. Childhood growth and adult cancer. Best Pract Res Clin Endocrinol Metab. 2002;16(2):225–41.

187. Wolk A, Gridley G, Svensson M, et al. A prospective study of obesity and cancer risk (Sweden). Cancer Causes Control. 2001;12(1):13–21.

188. Bosetti C, Dal Maso L, Negri E, et al. Re: Body mass index and risk of malignant lymphoma in Scandinavian men and women. J Natl Cancer Inst. 2005;97(11):860–1.

189. Chang ET, Hjalgrim H, Smedby KE, et al. Body mass index and risk of malignant lymphoma in Scandinavian men and women. J Natl Cancer Inst. 2005;97(3):210–8.

190. Bianchini F, Kaaks R, Vainio H. Overweight, obesity, and cancer risk. Lancet Oncol. 2002;3(9):565–74.

191. Glaser SL. Reproductive factors in Hodgkin's disease in women: a review. Am J Epidemiol. 1994;139:237–46.

192. Kravdal O, Hansen S. Hodgkin's disease: The protective effect of childbearing. Int J Cancer. 1993;55:909–14.

193. Kravdal O, Hansen S. The importance of childbearing for Hodgkin's disease: new evidence from incidence and mortality models. Int J Epidemiol. 1996;25(4):737–43.

194. Lambe M, Hsieh CC, Tsaih S-W, et al. Childbearing and the risk of Hodgkin's disease. Cancer Epidemiol Biomark Prev. 1998;7:831–4.

195. Tavani A, Pregnolato A, La Vecchia C, et al. A case-control study of reproductive factors and risk of lymphomas and myelomas. Leuk Res. 1997;21:885–8.

196. Zwitter M, Zakelj MP, Kosmelj K. A case-control study of Hodgkin's disease and pregnancy. Br J Cancer. 1996; 73:246–51.

197. Glaser SL, Clarke CA, Nugent RA, et al. Reproductive risk factors in Hodgkin's disease in women. Am J Epidemiol. 2003;158:553–63.

198. Hjalgrim H, Engels EA. Infectious aetiology of Hodgkin and non-Hodgkin lymphomas: a review of the epidemiological evidence. J Int Medicine. 2008;264(6):537–48.

# The Role of Viruses in the Genesis of Hodgkin Lymphoma

**2**

Ruth F. Jarrett

## Contents

## Abbreviations

| | |
|---|---|
| BART | BamHI A rightward transcripts |
| cHL | Classical Hodgkin lymphoma |
| EBER | EBV-encoded small RNAs |
| EBNA | EBV nuclear antigen |
| EBV | Epstein–Barr virus |
| HHV | Human herpesvirus |
| HL | Hodgkin lymphoma |
| HLA | Human leukocyte antigen |
| HRS | Hodgkin and Reed–Sternberg |
| LMP | Latent membrane protein |
| MCV | Merkel cell polyomavirus |
| MV | Measles virus |
| SNP | Single nucleotide polymorphism |
| TTV | Torque teno virus |

## 2.1 Introduction

Hodgkin lymphoma (HL) is a heterogeneous condition. Seminal papers published in 1957 and 1966 suggested that HL in younger and older adults had different etiologies and further suggested an infectious etiology for young adult HL [1, 2]. Subsequent epidemiological studies provide broad support for these hypotheses [3, 4]. Data linking young adult HL with a high standard of living in early childhood and lack of child–child contact suggest that delayed exposure to common childhood infections may be involved in the etiology of this group of cases [5, 6]. There is now compelling evidence that a proportion of cases of HL are associated with the Epstein–Barr virus (EBV). Paradoxically, older adult and childhood cases of HL are more likely to be EBV-associated than young adult cases [7–9].

R.F. Jarrett
LRF Virus Centre, Institute of Comparative Medicine,
University of Glasgow, Glasgow G61 1QH, UK
e-mail: r.f.jarrett@vet.gla.ac.uk

A. Engert and S.J. Horning (eds.), *Hodgkin Lymphoma*,
DOI: 10.1007/978-3-642-12780-9_2, © Springer-Verlag Berlin Heidelberg 2011

In this chapter, I will review studies on viral involvement in HL with a focus on classical HL (cHL), since nodular lymphocyte predominance HL is considered a separate disease entity. The association with EBV will be discussed with an emphasis on recent data and findings that support a causal role for EBV in this malignancy. Studies investigating involvement of other candidate viruses in this disease will be summarized.

## 2.2 Hodgkin Lymphoma and Epstein–Barr Virus

EBV is a gamma-herpesvirus with a worldwide distribution [10, 11]. Over 90% of healthy adults are infected by EBV and, following primary infection, the virus establishes a persistent infection with a reservoir in memory B-cells [12]. Although EBV is an extremely efficient transforming agent, the virus is kept under tight control by cell-mediated immune responses, and both primary and persistent infection are usually asymptomatic [11].

EBV infection can be lytic or latent. Lytic infection is associated with expression of a large number of viral genes, production of progeny virus and death of the infected cell; in contrast, latent infection is associated with expression of a small number of EBV genes, persistent infection and growth transformation [11]. In B-cells transformed by EBV in vitro, six EBV nuclear antigens (EBNA-1, -2, -3a, -3b, -3c, and LP; also called EBNA-1–6) are expressed alongside three latent membrane proteins (LMP1, LMP2A, and LMP2B) [10]. In addition, noncoding viral RNAs are expressed in all latently infected cells [10]. These include two small nonpolyadenylated transcripts, the EBERs, and a large number of viral microRNAs derived from the BARTs (*BamH*I A rightward transcripts) and the primary EBNA transcript [10, 13–16]. Expression of the full set of latent genes is known as latency type III and is associated with transformation of B-cells [10]. EBV gene expression in EBV-positive lymphomas occurring in the context of immunosuppression frequently follows this pattern; however, more restricted patterns of EBV gene expression are also observed [11]. The EBNA-3 family proteins are immunodominant and the other latent antigens elicit only subdominant or weak cell-mediated immune responses [17, 18]. The pattern of gene expression in

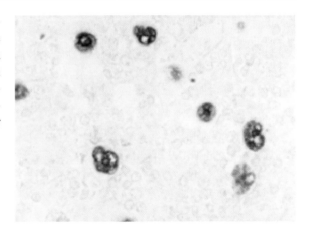

**Fig. 2.1** Epstein–Barr virus (EBV)-encoded small RNA (EBER) in situ hybridization staining of EBV-positive Hodgkin and Reed–Sternberg (HRS) cells. The characteristic staining pattern is observed in the nuclei of HRS cells

EBV-associated malignancies most probably depends on both the lineage and stage of differentiation of the infected tumor cells and the host EBV-specific immune response.

In EBV-associated HL, the Hodgkin and Reed–Sternberg (HRS) cells are infected by EBV and the infection is clonal, i.e., all the tumor cells are derived from a single infected cell [19–22]. The virus is present in all the HRS cells and EBNA-1, LMP1, LMP2A, and 2B as well as the EBER RNAs and BARTs are expressed; the remaining EBNAs are downregulated [20, 22–25]. This pattern of gene expression is referred to as latency type II [11]. EBV infection of HRS cells can be readily demonstrated in sections of routinely fixed, paraffin-embedded material using either EBER in situ hybridization or LMP1 immunohistochemistry (Fig. 2.1). Reagents for both assays are commercially available.

### 2.2.1 EBV and the Pathogenesis of Hodgkin Lymphoma

The molecular pathogenesis of HL and the origin of HRS cells are described in detail in the following chapter 3. Briefly, HRS cells have clonally rearranged immunoglobulin genes with evidence of somatic hypermutation, indicating a derivation from B-cells that have participated in a germinal center reaction [26, 27]. A pathognomonic feature of these cells is the global suppression of

B-cell signature genes and inappropriate expression of genes usually associated with other hemopoietic lineages [28, 29]. Importantly, HRS cells do not express B-cell receptors. Survival of germinal center B-cells normally requires signaling through both B-cell receptors and CD40; HRS cells must therefore have acquired a non-physiological survival mechanism. Functional studies of EBV, and LMP1 and LMP2A, in particular, support a role for the virus in HRS cell survival.

In 2005, three independent groups published data showing that germinal center B-cells lacking B-cell receptors could survive and be immortalized by EBV [30–32]. In elegant experiments, Mancao and Hammerschmidt [33] later showed that this survival function was dependent on LMP2A expression. A series of in vivo and in vitro studies from the Longnecker laboratory have further defined LMP2A function [34–36], and shown that this viral protein can mimic an activated B-cell receptor and provide a survival signal to B-cell-receptor-negative B-cells [35]. LMP2A expression in B-cells also results in downregulation of B-cell specific genes and induction of genes associated with proliferation and inhibition of apoptosis, a gene expression profile similar to that seen in HL-derived cell lines [37]. Constitutive activation of Notch1 by LMP2A, and subsequent inhibition of E2A and downregulation of EBF, two transcription factors that regulate B-cell development, appear to be involved in both survival signaling and transcriptional regulation [34]. Thus, LMP2A is likely to play a key role in both the survival and reprogramming of EBV-positive HRS cells.

Survival of germinal center B-cells requires signaling through surface CD40 as well as B-cell receptors. LMP1 is an integral membrane protein that interacts with several signal transduction pathways to activate NF-κB, Jun N-terminal kinase (JNK), and p38 mitogen-activated protein [38–42]. In this way, LMP1 mimics a constitutively active CD40 molecule, although providing a more potent and sustained signal [10, 11]. Activation of the NF-κB pathway, which is a feature of HRS cells, leads to upregulation of antiapoptotic genes, including c-FLIP and XIAP, which are likely to contribute to HRS cell survival [43–45].

The EBV genome is normally maintained as an episome in infected cells, i.e., it does not integrate. The EBNA-1 protein is responsible for maintenance of the genome in an episomal form, and also for genome replication and partitioning during mitosis [10, 46]. EBNA-1 can also influence both viral and cellular gene expression and appears to confer a B-cell survival advantage, although the impact of EBNA-1 on oncogenesis in vivo is controversial [10, 47–50]. Interestingly, in the context of HL, overexpression of EBNA-1 in vitro leads to the appearance of multinucleated cells [49]. The precise function of the EBER transcripts is also unclear but expression of these small RNAs appears important for efficient EBV-induced B-cell growth and transformation [10, 51].

The function of the BARTs, which are expressed by HRS cells, remained elusive for many years but recent data show that these complex transcripts contain two clusters of microRNAs [13–16, 23]. Expression of the BART microRNAs has been most studied in relation to nasopharyngeal carcinoma, an EBV-associated malignancy that shares a similar pattern of EBV gene expression to cHL [13–16], and profiling of these transcripts in cHL has not been reported to date. Little information about the targets of these potent gene regulators is currently available but they are likely to have an important role in oncogenesis. In addition to encoding microRNAs, EBV regulates the expression of cellular microRNAs; EBV infection of primary B-cells leads to a conspicuous downregulation of many microRNAs with the notable exception of mIR-155, which is highly expressed by both EBV-positive and -negative HRS cells [52, 53].

## 2.2.2  Risk Factors for EBV-Associated Hodgkin Lymphoma

It is clear that EBV is associated with only a proportion of cHL cases, around one third in industrialized countries [7, 8, 54]. EBV-associated cHL cases are not randomly distributed among all cHL cases, and the demographic features and risk factors for development of EBV-positive and -negative HL show distinctive features [7, 8]. Children (<10 years) and older adults (50+ years) are more likely to be EBV-associated than young adult cases (15–34 years) [8, 9, 54]. Among EBV-associated cases, males predominate with a ratio of approximately 2:1 whereas males and females are more evenly represented among EBV-negative cases [7, 54]. In developing countries, where childhood HL is more common, a higher proportion of cases are EBV-associated [7, 8]. Material deprivation is associated with an increased proportion of EBV-positive childhood cHL cases in industrialized countries, and there is some evidence that this also holds true for older adult cases [54, 55].

EBV infection usually occurs in childhood, and in many parts of the world there is almost universal infection by the age of 5 years. If infection is delayed until adolescence, as is increasingly occurring in industrialized countries, primary EBV infection manifests as infectious mononucleosis in around 25% of individuals [56]. Infectious mononucleosis is associated with an increased risk of cHL, and this increase is focused in EBV-associated cases [57–60]. The increased risk appears short-lived with a median time interval between infectious mononucleosis and HL of approximately 3–4 years [59, 60]. Thus, in both developing and developed countries there appears to be a period following primary EBV infection, probably lasting several years, in which risk of EBV-associated cHL is increased. On the basis of the above data, we have proposed an extension of MacMahon's model of HL that divides cHL into four subgroups on the basis of EBV-association, age at diagnosis, and age at infection by EBV (Fig. 2.2) [2, 61].

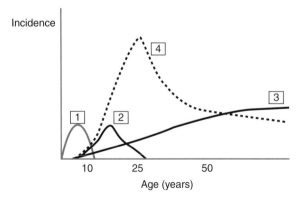

**Fig. 2.2** The four disease model of classical Hodgkin lymphoma (cHL). This model divides cHL into four subgroups on the basis of EBV-association, age at diagnosis, and age at EBV infection. Three groups of EBV-associated disease are recognized: (1) a childhood disease, usually occurring below the age of 10 years, which is more common in developing countries; (2) a disease, most commonly seen in young adults, which occurs following infectious mononucleosis; (3) a disease associated with poor control of EBV infection, which is typified by the older adult cases but can occur at other ages, particularly in the context of immunosuppression. (4) Superimposed on these is a single group of EBV-negative cHL cases, which accounts for the young adult age-specific incidence peak seen in industrialized countries. The incidence of each of these four disease subgroups will determine the overall shape of the age-specific incidence curve in any particular geographical locale

Racial and ethnic differences in proportions of EBV-associated cHL suggest that genetic factors also contribute to risk of developing EBV-associated cHL [7, 62]. It is now apparent that there are strong associations between human leukocyte antigen (HLA) class I genes and EBV-associated cHL. HL was, in fact, the first malignant disease to be associated with HLA class I, and early studies showed that HLA-A1 was associated with increased susceptibility [63]. At this time the association between EBV and HL was not known and the increased risk associated with HLA-A1 was modest [63]. Recent genotyping studies investigating markers across the entire HLA region initially revealed that microsatellite markers and single nucleotide polymorphisms (SNPs) in the HLA class I region were strongly associated with EBV-positive cHL [64, 65]. The informative markers are in linkage disequilibrium with HLA-A*01 and HLA-A*02, and it was subsequently demonstrated that HLA-A*01 is associated with an increased and HLA-A*02 with a decreased risk of EBV-associated HL [66]. Risk is independently associated with HLA-A*01 and HLA-A*02, i.e., the increased risk associated with HLA-A*01 is not simply due to lack of HLA-A*02, and is dependent on the copy number of each of these alleles [67]. As a result, there is an almost tenfold variation in odds of EBV-associated cHL between HLA-A*01 homozygotes and HLA-A*02 homozygotes [67]. Cytotoxic T-cell responses, restricted through HLA class I, are critical for the control of EBV infection, and HLA-A*02 is known to present a wide range of peptides derived from EBV lytic and latent antigens, including those expressed by HRS cells [17, 18]. In contrast, there are no well-characterized HLA-A*01-restricted EBV epitopes [68]. The described associations with HLA-A, therefore, seem biologically plausible. However, HLA-A*01 is in strong linkage disequilibrium with HLA-B*08, which is associated with immunodominant EBV-specific cytotoxic T-cell responses; therefore, the biological basis of the increased risk associated with HLA-A*01 is not straightforward and requires further investigation. Further work is also necessary to determine whether the critical HLA-A-restricted cell-mediated immune responses are directed towards EBV-infected HRS cells, or whether it is the control of persistent EBV infection, and the host−virus equilibrium, which is all important. Given the failure to expand and accumulate EBV-specific cytotoxic T-cells in cHL tumors, and the counterintuitive association between increased cytotoxic T-cells and inferior outcome, the latter possibility appears more likely [69–72].

As mentioned above, prior infectious mononucleosis is associated with an increased risk of EBV-positive HL [57–60]. Propensity to develop infectious mononucleosis has been associated with the same genotypic markers (microsatellites and SNPs) that were originally associated with EBV-positive HL, albeit with lesser statistical significance [73]. It therefore appeared possible that the association between infectious mononucleosis and EBV-associated HL could result from shared genetic susceptibility rather than a temporal association. HLA class I typing of over 700 cHL cases, with available self-reported history of infectious mononucleosis, revealed that prior infectious mononucleosis was independently associated with EBV-associated HL after adjusting for the effects of HLA-A alleles [67]. In addition, a statistically significant interaction between prior infectious mononucleosis and HLA-A*02 was detected; the effect of this was to abrogate the increased risk of EBV-associated HL following infectious mononucleosis in HLA-A*02-positive individuals [67]. These results suggest that infectious mononucleosis is associated with an increased risk of EBV-associated cHL and that this risk is modified by the EBV-specific cytotoxic T-cell response restricted through HLA-A*02.

These data are consistent with the idea that there is a window of time following primary EBV infection when there is an increased risk of EBV-associated HL. Genetic factors, specifically HLA-A genotype, can modify risk and this most probably reflects the strength and breadth of EBV-specific cytotoxic T-cell responses. EBV-associated cHL patients have higher numbers of EBV-infected cells than patients with EBV-negative disease [74], and infectious mononucleosis patients have very high numbers of circulating EBV-infected B-cells, which decrease over time [75]. These findings suggest that the total number of EBV-infected cells may be a critical determinant of risk of EBV-associated cHL. If this is indeed the case, then it would theoretically be possible to decrease the risk of EBV-positive cHL by EBV vaccination or by treatment of infectious mononucleosis. EBV-associated cHL occurring in older adults most probably results from reactivation of viral infection; in this situation it is plausible that an age-related decline in immune function is associated with an increased number of EBV-infected B-cells.

### 2.2.3 EBV and Hodgkin Lymphoma: A Causative Association?

In the absence of prevention of EBV infection, it is difficult to prove that the association between EBV and cHL is causal; however, consideration of the viral, molecular, and epidemiological data provides support for this idea. (1) In healthy individuals, EBV infects 1–50 per million B-cells [76]. EBV is consistently associated with a significant proportion of cHL cases; therefore, it is unlikely that EBV is simply a passenger virus in an HRS cell that has arisen from an EBV-infected B-cell transformed by other mechanisms. (2) In EBV-associated cases, the viral infection is clonal and all HRS cells are infected. Although EBNA-1 facilitates both synchronous replication of the viral episome with cellular DNA and genome partitioning, this process is not 100% efficient [46]. If the virus is not required for maintenance of the transformed phenotype, one would expect to see a gradual loss of viral genomes from the tumor cells. (3) LMP1 and LMP2A have plausible biological function in the pathogenesis of cHL, as described above. (4) Crippling mutations of immunoglobulin genes have been described in a quarter of cHL cases but almost all of these cases have been EBV-positive [77]. This suggests that EBV is required to rescue HRS cells (or precursors) that have destructive mutations of their immunoglobulin genes. (5) Deleterious mutations of the TNFAIP3 gene, a negative regulator of NF-κB, are much more frequent in HRS cells from EBV-negative compared to EBV-positive cases (see Chap. 3) [78]. Likewise, mutations of the gene encoding the NF-κB inhibitor, Iκ-Bα, have been described only in EBV-negative cases [79–82]. This suggests that HRS cells in EBV-negative cHL have developed alternative strategies to constitutively activate NF-κB. (6) EBV-associated cHL cases share risk factors for disease development, which are distinct from those associated with EBV-negative cHL. (7) Development of EBV-associated cHL is temporally related to primary EBV infection in some cases [59, 60].

## 2.2.4 EBV and the Clinicopathological Features of Hodgkin Lymphoma

Although differences in the molecular pathogenesis of EBV-associated and nonassociated cHL are emerging, the phenotypic expression of both processes appears remarkably similar. Mixed cellularity HL cases are significantly more likely to be EBV-associated than nodular sclerosis HL cases [7, 8]. In most series, around 60–70% of mixed cellularity HL cases are associated with EBV, compared to ~25% of nodular sclerosis HL cases [7, 8]. Despite these differences, it is clear that "barn door" nodular sclerosis HL cases can be EBV-positive, and so the lack of a complete correlation between histological subtype and EBV status is not simply due to the criteria used in histological subtyping of cHL. In industrialized countries, nodular sclerosis is more common than mixed cellularity HL, and in our experience the majority (just) of EBV-positive cases are in fact nodular sclerosis HL and not mixed cellularity HL. Gene expression profiling has been successfully applied to the study of HRS cells [28, 29]. Although no systematic comparison of EBV-positive and -negative cases has been reported thus far, there is no evidence that expression profiles of the two groups of cases cluster differently (Ralf Kuppers, personal communication).

Early studies investigating clinical outcome in relation to EBV status in cHL appeared conflicting but a more consistent picture is now emerging [83–86]. Among young adult cases, aged 15–34 years, there appears to be no significant difference in overall survival by EBV status. In contrast, EBV-positivity is associated with inferior outcome among older adult cases, aged 50 years or over. It is not clear whether this difference is related to the disease process itself or whether it is a reflection of the underlying co-morbidity or immune dysregulation that potentially predisposes to EBV-associated cHL. Further studies investigating this issue and alternative treatment options in EBV-positive older patients are required.

## 2.3 Non-EBV-Associated Hodgkin Lymphoma Cases

As mentioned above, young adult cHL cases are the group of cases least likely to be associated with EBV and yet it is for these cases that there is most epidemiological evidence pointing to viral involvement. Early studies reported consistent associations between young adult HL and correlates of a high standard of living in early childhood [87]. Recent studies have generally not detected associations with the same social class variables and this probably relates to secular changes in living standards; however, one study observed an increased risk of young adult HL in individuals with ≤1 year of preschool attendance [5, 60]. Together, the data suggest that diminished social contact in early childhood is associated with an increased risk of this disease. From this it is inferred that young adult HL may be associated with delayed exposure to a common childhood infection. Interview and questionnaire data generally support the idea that young adult HL patients have experienced fewer common infections in childhood [57, 88].

It has frequently been suggested that EBV is involved in all cases of HL but uses a hit-and-run mechanism in "EBV-negative" cases. This possibility is very difficult to exclude but the available data indicate that this mechanism cannot account for all cases in which EBV is not detected. Importantly, not all cases are EBV infected; in fact, we found that EBV-negative cHL cases in the 15–24 year age group were more likely to be EBV-seronegative than age-matched controls [89]. In addition, there is no evidence for retention of fragments of integrated EBV genomes in "EBV-negative" HL biopsies [89, 90].

We therefore believe that another viral agent is involved in EBV-negative HL. This agent is likely to be a virus that infects many people early in life; therefore, candidate agents include herpesviruses and polyomaviruses. These are discussed in further detail below. The Anellovirus genus, which includes Torque teno virus (TTV) and related viruses, also fit these criteria. zur Hausen and de Villiers [91] have suggested that TTVs and TTV-like viruses could play a role in the development of leukemias and lymphomas that are associated with a "protected childhood environment." In their model, it is postulated that TTVs and related anelloviruses increase the risk of chromosomal abnormalities and that anellovirus load is increased in individuals who have experienced fewer infections. TTVs have been detected in HL [92–94]; however, further knowledge of these extremely common and genomically diverse viruses is required before their potential involvement in HL can be evaluated.

### 2.3.1  Hodgkin Lymphoma and Herpesviruses Other than EBV

At present, there are eight known human herpesviruses (HHVs), including EBV (officially HHV-4). With the exception of herpes simplex virus 2 and HHV-8, all are widespread in distribution and most adults are infected. Like EBV, HHV-8 is a gamma-herpesvirus that is associated with human lymphomas, but there is no evidence that this virus is associated with cHL [95–97]. The α-herpesviruses, herpes simplex virus 1 and varicella zoster virus, have also not been detected in HL biopsies [96]. In contrast, genomes of the β-herpesviruses, human cytomegalovirus, HHV-6, and HHV-7 have been detected in HL tumors using sensitive molecular assays. Schmidt et al. [97] detected human cytomegalovirus genomes by PCR in 8/86 HL biopsies, although smaller case series failed to identify this virus in tumor samples [96, 98–100]. HHV-7 has been detected in 20–53% of HL biopsies by PCR [96–98]; however, using Southern blot analysis, which is much less sensitive than PCR but would still be expected to detect a virus present in all HRS cells, negative results have been obtained [101]. There is, therefore, no evidence that HHV-7 is directly involved in HL pathogenesis.

HHV-6 deserves special mention because serological studies have shown that HHV-6 antibody titers and, in some studies, seroprevalence are higher in HL cases than controls [102–104]. Furthermore, we found that young adults with non-EBV-associated HL had higher titers of HHV-6 antibodies than age-matched cases with EBV-associated disease (unpublished results). HHV-7 antibody titers were similar in the two groups of cases suggesting a specific association between HHV-6 and cHL. HHV-6 has been consistently detected in HL biopsies using PCR, with detection rates varying from 12.5 to 79% [96–98, 105–107]; however, studies of reactive lymph nodes have reported similar detection frequencies [98, 107]. There is no evidence from in situ hybridization and immunohistochemical studies that the virus is localized to HRS cells [107–109], and Southern blot studies have largely been negative following exclusion of cases with integrated HHV-6 [95, 104, 107, 110]. Current data do not, therefore, favor a direct role for HHV-6 in disease pathogenesis. It remains possible that HHV-6 is a marker for another virus that is associated with HL. The ability of HHV-6 to integrate into chromosomal DNA also suggests novel mechanisms in which this virus could interact with the host genome and contribute to oncogenesis [110, 111].

In order to search for novel members of the herpesvirus family, we and others have designed degenerate PCR assays that amplify herpesvirus polymerase and glycoprotein B gene sequences [96, 112]. The primer sequences in degenerate assays are derived from well-conserved peptide motifs in amino acid sequences of proteins; therefore, these assays should have the ability to detect genomes from known and currently unknown viruses [113]. Using herpesvirus polymerase assays we did not detect novel herpesviruses in HL tumors although the assays had sufficient sensitivity to detect EBV in EBV-associated cases, and to pick up HHV-6 and HHV-7 sequences in a significant minority of cases [96].

### 2.3.2  Polyomaviruses and Hodgkin Lymphoma

There are currently five known human polyomaviruses, namely JCV, BKV, KIV, WUV, and Merkel cell polyomavirus (MCV or MCPyV) [114–116]. JCV and BKV were discovered almost 40 years ago but the latter viruses have all been discovered since 2007 with the advent of modern molecular techniques for virus discovery. Recent seroprevalence studies suggest that the majority of adults are infected by BKV, KIV, WUV, and MCV and a significant minority (35–39%) are infected by JCV [117–119]. Infection generally occurs in early childhood, with infection by JCV occurring slightly later than infection with the other viruses [117]. MCV is detectable in around 80% of Merkel cell carcinomas and is the only human polyomavirus to be unambiguously associated with a specific malignancy [115, 120]; however, other polyomaviruses clearly have oncogenic potential.

Using sensitive quantitative PCR assays, we found no evidence of JCV or BKV genomes in 35 cHL biopsies [121]. Hernandez-Losa et al. [98] detected JCV in 1/20 and BKV in 2/20 cHL samples using a multiplex, nested PCR. Similarly, Shuda et al. [122] detected MCV in only 1/30 HL samples examined by quantitative PCR. To date, there have been no reports on KIV or WUV prevalence in adult cHL samples. Degenerate PCR assays based on conserved sequences in the T antigen and structural proteins of polyomaviruses have been applied to the study of HL [121, 123]. Volter et al. [123] examined five cases of HL using a degenerate PCR assay based on the viral VP1 protein but did not detect any evidence of polyomavirus infection. We examined 35 cases of cHL, including 23 EBV-negative cases, using three degenerate polyomavirus assays based on the large T antigen and, similarly, obtained negative results [121]. The latter assays were designed before the discovery of KIV, WUV, and MCV; sequence alignment suggests that the assays would be able to detect KIV and WUV but not MCV. Overall, these results provide no evidence for polyomavirus involvement in the pathogenesis of cHL but it remains possible that an unknown polyomavirus has escaped detection using the available assays.

### 2.3.3 Measles Virus and Hodgkin Lymphoma

In 2003, Benharroch et al. reported an association between measles virus (MV) and cHL [124]. They subsequently reported that MV proteins were detectable by immunohistochemistry, using at least two antibodies, in HRS cells from the majority of HL cases [125]. MV RNA was also detected by RT-PCR and in situ hybridization in a significant minority of the cases examined [125]. Subsequent studies have failed to confirm these associations [126, 127]. Our group found no evidence of MV in 97 cHL cases examined by immunohistochemistry and 20 cHL cases investigated using RT-PCR [127]. Similarly, Maggio et al. found no evidence of MV genomes or transcripts in HRS cells microdissected from biopsies from 18 German and 17 Israeli HL cases [126]; the latter cases had previously scored positive for MV antigens [125]. Epidemiological studies have also failed to show that MV infection is a risk factor for development of cHL; on the contrary, the data suggest a mild protective effect of prior MV infection [57, 88].

### 2.4 Conclusions

While the evidence suggesting a causal relationship between EBV and a proportion of cHL cases appears strong, current data do not show a consistent and specific association between any virus and EBV-negative HL. This does not exclude viral involvement. HL is a notoriously difficult disease to investigate, and virus discovery studies present particular challenges. The difficulty of obtaining large numbers of highly enriched HRS cells has precluded the use of certain techniques, such as representational difference analysis, in the analysis of HL [113]. Next generation sequencing methods have opened new avenues for virus discovery and have led to the identification of several novel viruses in the last few years [115, 116, 128]. Digital transcriptome subtraction [115], the technique used in the discovery of MCV, is now being applied to the study of HL. It is likely that, in the not too far distant future, complete sequencing of HRS cell DNA will also be performed. These techniques provide our best hope of discovering a new virus in EBV-negative HRS cells. It is possible that cellular mutations substitute for the functions of EBV genes in EBV-negative HRS cells. Deleterious mutations of inhibitors of the NF-κB pathway, including genes encoding A20 and IκBα, appear to be present in the HRS cells of many cases of EBV-negative HL (see Chap. 5) [78–82], and it is possible that these mutations substitute for LMP1. However, there is no obvious link between these mutations and the epidemiological features of cHL and involvement of another virus still appears attractive. Identification of a virus in EBV-negative cHL would open up possibilities for disease prevention as well as novel therapeutic targets, and so it is important to resolve whether, or not, such an agent exists. Exciting times are ahead.

**Acknowledgments** To Scamp, my faithful old feline friend who died during the preparation of this manuscript. Thanks to Tina Rich for reading the manuscript. Work in our laboratory is supported by the Leukaemia Lymphoma Research and the Kay Kendall Leukaemia Fund.

### References

1. MacMahon B. Epidemiological evidence of the nature of Hodgkin's disease. Cancer. 1957;10:1045–54.
2. MacMahon B. Epidemiology of Hodgkin's disease. Cancer Res. 1966;26:1189–201.
3. Alexander FE, McKinney PA, Williams J, et al. Epidemiological evidence for the "two-disease hypothesis" in Hodgkin's disease. Int J Epidemiol. 1991;20:354–61.

4. Gutensohn NM. Social class and age at diagnosis of Hodgkin's disease: new epidemiologic evidence for the "two-disease hypothesis". Cancer Treat Rep. 1982;66: 689–95.

5. Chang ET, Zheng T, Weir EG, et al. Childhood social environment and Hodgkin's lymphoma: new findings from a population-based case-control study. Cancer Epidemiol Biomark Prev. 2004;13:1361–70.

6. Gutensohn NM, Shapiro DS. Social class risk factors among children with Hodgkin's disease. Int J Cancer. 1982;30: 433–5.

7. Glaser SL, Lin RJ, Stewart SL, et al. Epstein-Barr virus-associated Hodgkin's disease: epidemiologic characteristics in international data. Int J Cancer. 1997;70:375–82.

8. Jarrett RF, Armstrong AA, Alexander E. Epidemiology of EBV and Hodgkin's lymphoma. Ann Oncol. 1996;7: S5–S10.

9. Jarrett RF, Gallagher A, Jones DB, et al. Detection of Epstein-Barr virus genomes in Hodgkin's disease: relation to age. J Clin Pathol. 1991;44:844–8.

10. Kieff E, Rickinson AB. Epstein-Barr virus and its replication. In: Knipe DM, Howley PM, editors. Fields virology. Philadelphia: Lippincott Williams & Wilkins; 2007. p. 2603–54.

11. Rickinson AB, Kieff E. Epstein-Barr virus. In: Knipe DM, Howley PM, editors. Fields virology. 5th ed. Philadelphia: Lippincott Williams & Wilkins; 2007. p. 2655–700.

12. Babcock GJ, Decker LL, Volk M, et al. EBV persistence in memory B cells in vivo. Immunity. 1998;9:395–404.

13. Cai X, Schafer A, Lu S, Bilello JP, Desrosiers RC, Edwards R, et al. Epstein-Barr virus microRNAs are evolutionarily conserved and differentially expressed. PLoS Pathog. 2006;2:e23.

14. Cosmopoulos K, Pegtel M, Hawkins J, et al. Comprehensive profiling of Epstein-Barr virus microRNAs in nasopharyngeal carcinoma. J Virol. 2009;83:2357–67.

15. Edwards RH, Marquitz AR, Raab-Traub N. Epstein-Barr virus BART microRNAs are produced from a large intron prior to splicing. J Virol. 2008;82:9094–106.

16. Zhu JY, Pfuhl T, Motsch N, et al. Identification of novel Epstein-Barr virus microRNA genes from nasopharyngeal carcinomas. J Virol. 2009;83:3333–41.

17. Hislop AD, Taylor GS, Sauce D, et al. Cellular responses to viral infection in humans: lessons from Epstein-Barr virus. Annu Rev Immunol. 2007;25:587–617.

18. Khanna R, Burrows SR. Role of cytotoxic T lymphocytes in Epstein-Barr virus-associated diseases. Annu Rev Microbiol. 2000;54:19–48.

19. Gledhill S, Gallagher A, Jones DB, et al. Viral involvement in Hodgkin's disease: detection of clonal type A Epstein-Barr virus genomes in tumour samples. Br J Cancer. 1991;64:227–32.

20. Pallesen G, Hamilton-Dutoit SJ, Rowe M, et al. Expression of Epstein-Barr virus latent gene products in tumour cells of Hodgkin's disease. Lancet. 1991;337:320–2.

21. Weiss LM, Strickler JG, Warnke RA, et al. Epstein-Barr viral DNA in tissues of Hodgkin's disease. Am J Pathol. 1987;129:86–91.

22. Wu TC, Mann RB, Charache P, et al. Detection of EBV gene expression in Reed-Sternberg cells of Hodgkin's disease. Int J Cancer. 1990;46:801–4.

23. Deacon EM, Pallesen G, Niedobitek G, et al. Epstein-Barr virus and Hodgkin's disease: transcriptional analysis of virus latency in the malignant cells. J Exp Med. 1993;177: 339–49.

24. Grasser FA, Murray PG, Kremmer E, et al. Monoclonal antibodies directed against the Epstein-Barr virus-encoded nuclear antigen 1 (EBNA1): immunohistologic detection of EBNA1 in the malignant cells of Hodgkin's disease. Blood. 1994;84:3792–8.

25. Niedobitek G, Kremmer E, Herbst H, et al. Immunohistochemical detection of the Epstein-Barr virus-encoded latent membrane protein 2A in Hodgkin's disease and infectious mononucleosis. Blood. 1997;90:1664–72.

26. Kuppers R. Molecular biology of Hodgkin lymphoma. Hematology Am Soc Hematol Educ Program. 2009:491–6.

27. Kuppers R. The biology of Hodgkin's lymphoma. Nat Rev Cancer. 2009;9:15–27.

28. Kuppers R, Klein U, Schwering I, et al. Identification of Hodgkin and Reed-Sternberg cell-specific genes by gene expression profiling. J Clin Invest. 2003;111:529–37.

29. Schwering I, Brauninger A, Klein U, et al. Loss of the B-lineage-specific gene expression program in Hodgkin and Reed-Sternberg cells of Hodgkin lymphoma. Blood. 2003;101:1505–12.

30. Bechtel D, Kurth J, Unkel C, et al. Transformation of BCR-deficient germinal-center B cells by EBV supports a major role of the virus in the pathogenesis of Hodgkin and post-transplantation lymphomas. Blood. 2005;106:4345–50.

31. Chaganti S, Bell AI, Pastor NB, et al. Epstein-Barr virus infection in vitro can rescue germinal center B cells with inactivated immunoglobulin genes. Blood. 2005;106: 4249–52.

32. Mancao C, Altmann M, Jungnickel B, et al. Rescue of "crippled" germinal center B cells from apoptosis by Epstein-Barr virus. Blood. 2005;106:4339–44.

33. Mancao C, Hammerschmidt W. Epstein-Barr virus latent membrane protein 2A is a B-cell receptor mimic and essential for B-cell survival. Blood. 2007;110:3715–21.

34. Anderson LJ, Longnecker R. Epstein-Barr virus latent membrane protein 2A exploits Notch1 to alter B-cell identity in vivo. Blood. 2009;113:108–16.

35. Caldwell RG, Brown RC, Longnecker R. Epstein-Barr virus LMP2A-induced B-cell survival in two unique classes of EmuLMP2A transgenic mice. J Virol. 2000;74:1101–13.

36. Portis T, Longnecker R. Epstein-Barr virus LMP2A interferes with global transcription factor regulation when expressed during B-lymphocyte development. J Virol. 2003;77:105–14.

37. Portis T, Dyck P, Longnecker R. Epstein-Barr Virus (EBV) LMP2A induces alterations in gene transcription similar to those observed in Reed-Sternberg cells of Hodgkin lymphoma. Blood. 2003;102:4166–78.

38. Devergne O, Cahir McFarland ED, Mosialos G, et al. Role of the TRAF binding site and NF-κB activation in Epstein-Barr virus latent membrane protein 1-induced cell gene expression. J Virol. 1998;72:7900–8.

39. Eliopoulos AG, Gallagher NJ, Blake SM, et al. Activation of the p38 mitogen-activated protein kinase pathway by Epstein-Barr virus-encoded latent membrane protein 1 coregulates interleukin-6 and interleukin-8 production. J Biol Chem. 1999;274:16085–96.

40. Eliopoulos AG, Young LS. Activation of the cJun N-terminal kinase (JNK) pathway by the Epstein-Barr virus-encoded latent membrane protein 1 (LMP1). Oncogene. 1998;16: 1731–42.

41. Izumi KM, Kieff ED. The Epstein-Barr virus oncogene product latent membrane protein 1 engages the tumor necrosis factor receptor-associated death domain protein to mediate B lymphocyte growth transformation and activate NF-κB. Proc Natl Acad Sci U S A. 1997;94: 12592–7.

42. Kieser A, Kilger E, Gires O, et al. Epstein-Barr virus latent membrane protein-1 triggers AP-1 activity via the c-Jun N-terminal kinase cascade. EMBO J. 1997;16:6478–85.

43. Bargou RC, Emmerich F, Krappmann D, et al. Constitutive nuclear factor-κB-RelA activation is required for proliferation and survival of Hodgkin's disease tumor cells. J Clin Invest. 1997;100:2961–9.

44. Dutton A, O'Neil JD, Milner AE, et al. Expression of the cellular FLICE-inhibitory protein (c-FLIP) protects Hodgkin's lymphoma cells from autonomous Fas-mediated death. Proc Natl Acad Sci U S A. 2004;101:6611–6.

45. Kashkar H, Haefs C, Shin H, et al. XIAP-mediated caspase inhibition in Hodgkin's lymphoma-derived B cells. J Exp Med. 2003;198:341–7.

46. Nanbo A, Sugden A, Sugden B. The coupling of synthesis and partitioning of EBV's plasmid replicon is revealed in live cells. EMBO J. 2007;26:4252–62.

47. Kang MS, Lu H, Yasui T, et al. Epstein-Barr virus nuclear antigen 1 does not induce lymphoma in transgenic FVB mice. Proc Natl Acad Sci U S A. 2005;102:820–5.

48. Kang MS, Soni V, Bronson R, et al. Epstein-Barr virus nuclear antigen 1 does not cause lymphoma in C57BL/6J mice. J Virol. 2008;82:4180–3.

49. Kennedy G, Komano J, Sugden B. Epstein-Barr virus provides a survival factor to Burkitt's lymphomas. Proc Natl Acad Sci U S A. 2003;100:14269–74.

50. Wilson JB, Bell JL, Levine AJ. Expression of Epstein-Barr virus nuclear antigen-1 induces B cell neoplasia in transgenic mice. EMBO J. 1996;15:3117–26.

51. Yajima M, Kanda T, Takada K. Critical role of Epstein-Barr Virus (EBV)-encoded RNA in efficient EBV-induced B-lymphocyte growth transformation. J Virol. 2005;79: 4298–307.

52. Godshalk SE, Bhaduri-McIntosh S, Slack FJ. Epstein-Barr virus-mediated dysregulation of human microRNA expression. Cell Cycle. 2008;7:3595–600.

53. van den Berg A, Kroesen BJ, Kooistra K, et al. High expression of B-cell receptor inducible gene BIC in all subtypes of Hodgkin lymphoma. Genes Chromosom Cancer. 2003;37: 20–8.

54. Jarrett RF, Krajewski AS, Angus B, et al. The Scotland and Newcastle epidemiological study of Hodgkin's disease: impact of histopathological review and EBV status on incidence estimates. J Clin Pathol. 2003;56:811–6.

55. Flavell K, Constandinou C, Lowe D, et al. Effect of material deprivation on Epstein-Barr virus infection in Hodgkin's disease in the West Midlands. Br J Cancer. 1999;80:604–8.

56. Crawford DH, Macsween KF, Higgins CD, et al. A cohort study among university students: identification of risk factors for Epstein-Barr virus seroconversion and infectious mononucleosis. Clin Infect Dis. 2006;43:276–82.

57. Alexander FE, Jarrett RF, Lawrence D, et al. Risk factors for Hodgkin's disease by Epstein-Barr virus (EBV) status: prior infection by EBV and other agents. Br J Cancer. 2000; 82:1117–21.

58. Alexander FE, Lawrence DJ, Freeland J, et al. An epidemiologic study of index and family infectious mononucleosis and adult Hodgkin's disease (HD): evidence for a specific association with EBV+ve HD in young adults. Int J Cancer. 2003;107:298–302.

59. Hjalgrim H, Askling J, Rostgaard K, et al. Characteristics of Hodgkin's lymphoma after infectious mononucleosis. N Engl J Med. 2003;349:1324–32.

60. Hjalgrim H, Smedby KE, Rostgaard K, et al. Infectious mononucleosis, childhood social environment, and risk of Hodgkin lymphoma. Cancer Res. 2007;67:2382–8.

61. Jarrett RF. Viruses and Hodgkin's lymphoma. Ann Oncol. 2002;13(S1):23–9.

62. Glaser SL, Gulley ML, Clarke CA, et al. Racial/ethnic variation in EBV-positive classical Hodgkin lymphoma in California populations. Int J Cancer. 2008;123:1499–507.

63. Hors J, Dausset J. HLA and susceptibility to Hodgkin's disease. Immunol Rev. 1983;70:167–92.

64. Diepstra A, Niens M, Vellenga E, et al. Association with HLA class I in Epstein-Barr-virus-positive and with HLA class III in Epstein-Barr-virus-negative Hodgkin's lymphoma. Lancet. 2005;365:2216–24.

65. Niens M, van den Berg A, Diepstra A, et al. The human leukocyte antigen class I region is associated with EBV-positive Hodgkin's lymphoma: HLA-A and HLA complex group 9 are putative candidate genes. Cancer Epidemiol Biomark Prev. 2006;15:2280–4.

66. Niens M, Jarrett RF, Hepkema B, et al. HLA-A*02 is associated with a reduced risk and HLA-A*01 with an increased risk of developing EBV-positive Hodgkin lymphoma. Blood. 2007;110:3310–5.

67. Hjalgrim H, Rostgaard K, Johnson PC, et al. HLA-A alleles and infectious mononucleosis suggest critical role for cytotoxic T-cell response in EBV-related Hodgkin lymphoma. Proc Natl Acad Sci U S A. 2010;107(14):6400–5.

68. Brennan RM, Burrows SR. A mechanism for the HLA-A*01-associated risk for EBV+ Hodgkin lymphoma and infectious mononucleosis. Blood. 2008;112:2589–90.

69. Alvaro T, Lejeune M, Salvado MT, et al. Outcome in Hodgkin's lymphoma can be predicted from the presence of accompanying cytotoxic and regulatory T cells. Clin Cancer Res. 2005;11:1467–73.

70. Chapman AL, Rickinson AB, Thomas WA, et al. Epstein-Barr virus-specific cytotoxic T lymphocyte responses in the blood and tumor site of Hodgkin's disease patients: implications for a T-cell-based therapy. Cancer Res. 2001;61: 6219–26.

71. Kelley TW, Pohlman B, Elson P, et al. The ratio of FOXP3+ regulatory T cells to granzyme B+ cytotoxic T/NK cells predicts prognosis in classical Hodgkin lymphoma and is independent of bcl-2 and MAL expression. Am J Clin Pathol. 2007;128:958–65.

72. Oudejans JJ, Jiwa NM, Kummer JA, et al. Activated cytotoxic T cells as prognostic marker in Hodgkin's disease. Blood. 1997;89:1376–82.

73. McAulay KA, Higgins CD, Macsween KF, et al. HLA class I polymorphisms are associated with development of infectious

mononucleosis upon primary EBV infection. J Clin Invest. 2007;117:3042–8.

74. Khan G, Lake A, Shield L, et al. Phenotype and frequency of Epstein-Barr virus-infected cells in pretreatment blood samples from patients with Hodgkin lymphoma. Br J Haematol. 2005;129:511–9.

75. Hochberg D, Souza T, Catalina M, et al. Acute infection with Epstein-Barr virus targets and overwhelms the peripheral memory B-cell compartment with resting, latently infected cells. J Virol. 2004;78:5194–204.

76. Khan G, Miyashita EM, Yang B, et al. Is EBV persistence in vivo a model for B cell homeostasis? Immunity. 1996;5:173–9.

77. Brauninger A, Schmitz R, Bechtel D, et al. Molecular biology of Hodgkin's and Reed/Sternberg cells in Hodgkin's lymphoma. Int J Cancer. 2006;118:1853–61.

78. Schmitz R, Hansmann ML, Bohle V, et al. TNFAIP3 (A20) is a tumor suppressor gene in Hodgkin lymphoma and primary mediastinal B cell lymphoma. J Exp Med. 2009;206 (5):981–9.

79. Cabannes E, Khan G, Aillet F, et al. Mutations in the IkBa gene in Hodgkin's disease suggest a tumour suppressor role for IκB α. Oncogene. 1999;18:3063–70.

80. Emmerich F, Meiser M, Hummel M, et al. Overexpression of IκBα without inhibition of NF-κB activity and mutations in the IκBα gene in Reed-Sternberg cells. Blood. 1999;94:3129–34.

81. Jungnickel B, Staratschek-Jox A, Brauninger A, et al. Clonal deleterious mutations in the IκBα gene in the malignant cells in Hodgkin's lymphoma. J Exp Med. 2000;191: 395–402.

82. Lake A, Shield LA, Cordano P, et al. Mutations of NFKBIA, encoding IκBα, are a recurrent finding in classical Hodgkin lymphoma but are not a unifying feature of non-EBV-associated cases. Int J Cancer. 2009;125:1334–42.

83. Clarke CA, Glaser SL, Dorfman RF, et al. Epstein-Barr virus and survival after Hodgkin disease in a population-based series of women. Cancer. 2001;91:1579–87.

84. Diepstra A, van Imhoff GW, Schaapveld M, et al. Latent Epstein-Barr virus infection of tumor cells in classical Hodgkin's lymphoma predicts adverse outcome in older adult patients. J Clin Oncol. 2009;27(23):3815–21.

85. Jarrett RF, Stark GL, White J, et al. Impact of tumor Epstein-Barr virus status on presenting features and outcome in age-defined subgroups of patients with classic Hodgkin lymphoma: a population-based study. Blood. 2005;106: 2444–51.

86. Keegan TH, Glaser SL, Clarke CA, et al. Epstein-Barr virus as a marker of survival after Hodgkin's lymphoma: a population-based study. J Clin Oncol. 2005;23:7604–13.

87. Gutensohn N, Cole P. Epidemiology of Hodgkin's disease in the young. Int J Cancer. 1977;19:595–604.

88. Glaser SL, Keegan TH, Clarke CA, et al. Exposure to childhood infections and risk of Epstein-Barr virus-defined Hodgkin's lymphoma in women. Int J Cancer. 2005;115(4): 599–605.

89. Gallagher A, Perry J, Freeland J, et al. Hodgkin lymphoma and Epstein-Barr virus (EBV): no evidence to support hit-and-run mechanism in cases classified as non-EBV-associated. Int J Cancer. 2003;104:624–30.

90. Staratschek-Jox A, Kotkowski S, Belge G, et al. Detection of Epstein-Barr virus in Hodgkin-Reed-Sternberg cells: no evidence for the persistence of integrated viral fragments in Latent membrane protein-1 (LMP-1)-negative classical Hodgkin's disease. Am J Pathol. 2000;156:209–16.

91. zur Hausen H, de Villiers EM. Virus target cell conditioning model to explain some epidemiologic characteristics of childhood leukemias and lymphomas. Int J Cancer. 2005; 115:1–5.

92. Figueiredo CP, Franz-Vasconcelos HC, Giunta G, et al. Detection of Torque teno virus in Epstein-Barr virus positive and negative lymph nodes of patients with Hodgkin lymphoma. Leuk Lymphoma. 2007;48:731–5.

93. Garbuglia AR, Iezzi T, Capobianchi MR, et al. Detection of TT virus in lymph node biopsies of B-cell lymphoma and Hodgkin's disease, and its association with EBV infection. Int J Immunopathol Pharmacol. 2003;16:109–18.

94. Jelcic I, Hotz-Wagenblatt A, Hunziker A, et al. Isolation of multiple TT virus genotypes from spleen biopsy tissue from a Hodgkin's disease patient: genome reorganization and diversity in the hypervariable region. J Virol. 2004;78:7498–507.

95. Armstrong AA, Shield L, Gallagher A, et al. Lack of involvement of known oncogenic DNA viruses in Epstein-Barr virus-negative Hodgkin's disease. Br J Cancer. 1998;77:1045–7.

96. Gallagher A, Perry J, Shield L, et al. Viruses and Hodgkin disease: no evidence of novel herpesviruses in non-EBV-associated lesions. Int J Cancer. 2002;101:259–64.

97. Schmidt CA, Oettle H, Peng R, et al. Presence of human β- and gamma-herpes virus DNA in Hodgkin's disease. Leuk Res. 2000;24:865–70.

98. Hernandez-Losa J, Fedele CG, Pozo F, et al. Lack of association of polyomavirus and herpesvirus types 6 and 7 in human lymphomas. Cancer. 2005;103:293–8.

99. Lin SH, Yeh HM, Tzeng CH, et al. Immunoglobulin and T cell receptor β chain gene rearrangements and Epstein-Barr viral DNA in tissues of Hodgkin's disease in Taiwan. Int J Hematol. 1993;57:251–7.

100. Samoszuk M, Ravel J. Frequent detection of Epstein-Barr viral deoxyribonucleic acid and absence of cytomegalovirus deoxyribonucleic acid in Hodgkin's disease and acquired immunodeficiency syndrome-related Hodgkin's disease. Lab Invest. 1991;65:631–6.

101. Berneman ZN, Torelli G, Luppi M, et al. Absence of a directly causative role for human herpesvirus 7 in human lymphoma and a review of human herpesvirus 6 in human malignancy. Ann Hematol. 1998;77:275–8.

102. Ablashi DV, Josephs SF, Buchbinder A, et al. Human B-lymphotropic virus (human herpesvirus-6). J Virol Meth. 1988;21:29–48.

103. Clark DA, Alexander FE, McKinney PA, et al. The seroepidemiology of human herpesvirus-6 (HHV-6) from a case-control study of leukaemia and lymphoma. Int J Cancer. 1990;45:829–33.

104. Torelli G, Marasca R, Luppi M, et al. Human herpesvirus-6 in human lymphomas: identification of specific sequences in Hodgkin's lymphomas by polymerase chain reaction. Blood. 1991;77:2251–8.

105. Collot S, Petit B, Bordessoule D, et al. Real-time PCR for quantification of human herpesvirus 6 DNA from lymph nodes and saliva. J Clin Microbiol. 2002;40:2445–51.

106. Lacroix A, Jaccard A, Rouzioux C, et al. HHV-6 and EBV DNA quantitation in lymph nodes of 86 patients with Hodgkin's lymphoma. J Med Virol. 2007;79:1349–56.

tumor cells in LPHL, which are termed lymphocyte predominant (LP) cells according to the new WHO classification (previously called L&H cells, for lymphocytic and/or histiocytic Reed–Sternberg (RS) cell variants), carry one large nucleus that is often multilobated ("popcorn cell") (Fig. 3.1a). In contrast to classic HRS cells, the number of nucleoli is increased, but they are usually less prominent and less eosinophilic. LP cells are found in a nodular or follicular background that is dominated by small B lymphocytes that usually express IgD, but a more diffuse growth pattern can also be encountered, especially during progression. The follicular infiltration pattern is highlighted by the presence of CD21-positive follicular dendritic cells that tend to form a well-developed meshwork in the nodules. Immunohistochemically, LP cells demonstrate a complete B cell phenotype with expression of CD20, CD75, and, frequently, CD79a (Fig. 3.1b; Table 3.1). Moreover, the essential B cell transcription factors BOB.1 and OCT-2 are usually positive, and the expression of BCL6 and activation-induced cytidine deaminase (AID) is well in line with a germinal center (GC) derivation of the tumor cells, although CD10 is generally negative [1–3]. The negativity of the tumor cells for CD30, CD15, and Epstein–Barr virus (EBV) helps to distinguish LP cells from HRS cells in cHL, although occasionally a weak positivity for CD30 can be present in LP cells (Table 3.1). Whereas in initial lesions small B cells dominate the background, histiocytes and T cells may become more prominent during the evolution of LPHL, to an extent

that LPHL may be hardly distinguishable from T cell/histiocyte-rich large B cell lymphoma (THRLBCL). A prominent feature of LPHL, however, is the often impressive rosetting of LP cells by T cells that belong to the subset of follicular T helper cells and therefore express CD57 and PD-1 [4–6].

### 3.1.2 Classical Hodgkin Lymphoma: The HRS Cells

The characteristic tumor cell of cHL, the RS cell, is large and contains at least two nuclear lobes or nuclei, usually with a prominent nuclear membrane (Fig. 3.2a). In contrast to LP cells in LPHL, the nucleoli of RS cells are often eosinophilic. The mononuclear variant of RS cells is termed the Hodgkin cell. However, the morphological spectrum of the tumor cell population in cHL can be broad and includes variants such as lacunar cells and mummified cells. In general, the tumor cells in cHL are called Hodgkin and Reed/Sternberg cells. Immunohistochemically, the HRS cells stain positive for CD30 (Fig. 3.2c), and CD15 is coexpressed in the majority of cases, occasionally with prominent staining of the Golgi area of the tumor cell. However, CD15 is negative in a significant proportion of cHL (20–25%) and therefore not required to establish the diagnosis of cHL [1]. CD45 is usually negative, as are the B cell transcription factors BOB.1 and OCT-2. In the vast

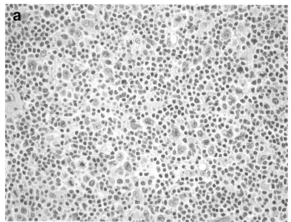
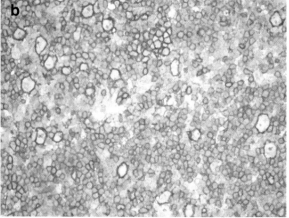

Fig. 3.1 Nodular lymphocyte-predominant Hodgkin lymphoma (LPHL). (a) HE-stained lymph node infiltrate showing multiple characteristic, multilobated tumor cells – termed lymphocyte predominant (LP) cells – in a background of small lymphocytes and histiocytes (×400). (b) Strong CD20 expression in LP cells,

but also in reactive, small B cells in the background (×400). Note that some of the tumor cells show rosetting by a CD20-negative lymphocyte population. These cells are T cells that often express the follicular T-helper cell marker PD-1

**Table 3.1** Genetic and phenotypic features of HRS and LP cells

| Feature | HRS cells | LP cells |
| --- | --- | --- |
| Phenotype | | |
| CD30 expression | Yes | Rare |
| CD15 expression | Yes (~70%)[a] | No |
| B cell receptor expression | No | Yes |
| Loss of most B cell markers | Yes | Modest |
| Expression of germinal center (GC) B cell markers (e.g., BCL6, activation-induced cytidine deaminase (AID)) | Rarely | Yes |
| Expression of markers for non-B cells (e.g., CD3, granzyme B, CCL17) | Frequently | No |
| Putative cell of origin | Defective, pre-apoptotic germinal center B cell | Germinal center B cell |
| EBV positivity | Yes (~40%) | No |
| Signaling pathways | | |
| NF-κB activation | Yes | Yes |
| JAK/STAT activation | Yes | Yes |
| Aberrant expression of multiple RTKs | Yes (60–100%) | Yes (~40%) |
| Genetic lesions | | |
| NFKBIA mutations | Yes (10–20%) | No |
| NFKBIE mutations | Yes (~10%) | n.a. |
| TNFAIP3 mutations | Yes (~40%) | No |
| REL gains/amplifications | Yes (~50%) | No |
| BCL6 translocations | Rare | Yes (~50%) |
| JAK2 gains/amplification | Yes (~30%) | No |
| SOCS1 mutations | Yes (~40%) | Yes (~50%) |

*n.a.* not analyzed; *RTK* receptor tyrosine kinase
[a]Numbers in brackets refer to the percentage of positive cases

majority of cases, the derivation of the tumor cells from the B cell lineage is indicated by a nuclear positivity for the B cell specific activator protein PAX5/BSAP, but the staining is usually weaker compared to the staining intensity in the small reactive B cell population in the background of the infiltrate [7]. CD20 expression can be observed in HRS cells in 30–40% of cases, but the expression is frequently restricted to a subset of the tumor cell population, and even within one HRS cell it is of varying intensity in different parts of the cell membrane. In comparison to CD20 expression, CD79a expression is observed less frequently [8, 9]. An EBV association, either demonstrated by immunohistochemical staining for LMP1 (latent membrane protein 1; Fig. 3.2d) or by EBER in situ hybridization, is found in a significant proportion of cHL, but the frequency varies considerably between different histological subtypes and across geographical areas [1]. Whether cHL cases exist with a *bona fide* derivation from the T cell lineage is currently a matter of debate. Single cases have been reported, in which a T cell receptor rearrangement could be proven in the HRS cells [10, 11], but others argue that such cases might represent only mimics of cHL which are not to be included in a disease entity that – based on fundamental principles of current lymphoma classification schemes – is of B cell derivation [12]. HRS cells reside in a cellular background that varies among the different histological subtypes of cH,L which will be discussed in the following sections.

### 3.1.2.1 Nodular Sclerosis Classical Hodgkin Lymphoma

In NSCHL, affected lymph nodes frequently show a markedly thickened capsule and a nodular infiltrate whereby individual nodules are surrounded by broad collagen bands (Fig. 3.2b). HRS cells are present in a background of small lymphocytes and other non-neoplastic cells such as histiocytes and eosinophils. The number of HRS cells can vary significantly between NSCHL cases and also within a single infiltrated lymph node. Occasionally, HRS cells can form sheets that can be associated with necrosis and an intense fibrohistiocytic reaction. Morphologically, HRS cells in NSCHL often show a retraction artifact of the cytoplasmic membrane that appears to be a consequence of formalin fixation, which has led to the term "lacunar cell variant" of HRS cells. The immunohistochemical phenotype of HRS cells in NSCHL as described above is the classic phenotype, however, association with EBV is less common as compared to other cHL subtypes, especially MCCHL.

### 3.1.2.2 Mixed Cellularity Classical Hodgkin Lymphoma

HRS cells in MCCHL usually have a classic morphological appearance and are scattered in a background that can contain small lymphocytes, eosinophils, neutrophils, plasma cells, and histiocytes. The infiltration pattern can

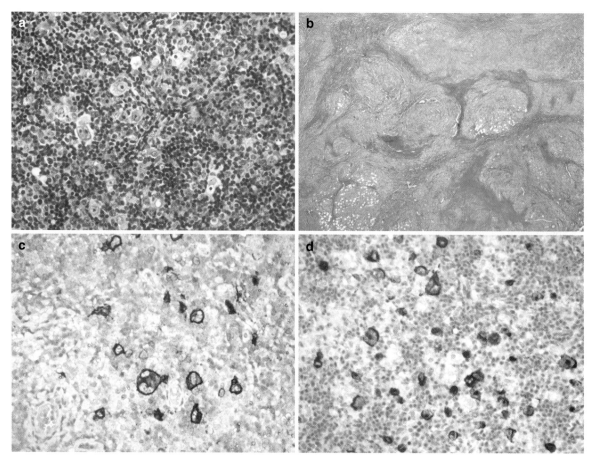

**Fig. 3.2** Classical Hodgkin lymphoma (cHL). (**a**) Characteristic Hodgkin and Reed–Sternberg (HRS) cells in a mixed background of small lymphocytes, histiocytes, and eosinophils in a mixed cellularity cHL (MCCHL) (HE, ×400). (**b**) Nodular sclerosis subtype of cHL that demonstrates thick collagen bands surrounding the nodular infiltrates (PAS, ×20). (**c**) CD30 expression in HRS cells (×400). (**d**) Immunohistochemical staining for latent membrane protein 1 (LMP1) shows Epstein–Barr virus (EBV) association of HRS cells (×400)

be diffuse or vaguely nodular; sometimes, the lymph node architecture and especially some B cell areas are partially preserved leading to an interfollicular infiltration pattern. The characteristic features of other histologic cHL subtypes (e.g., the formation of nodular collagen bands) are absent and, thus, MCCHL is sometimes considered as the "wastebasket" of cHL. The EBV association of HRS cells is the highest among all cHL subtypes and can reach 75% [1].

### 3.1.2.3 Lymphocyte-Depleted Classical Hodgkin Lymphoma

LDCHL is the rarest histological subtype of cHL (<1% of cases) and probably the most problematic one to define. It is characterized by an increased number of

HRS cells present in the infiltrate and/or depletion of small lymphocytes in the non-neoplastic background population. In some cases, HRS cells are of anaplastic appearance and in other cases, the background is composed of extensive diffuse fibrosis. However, if the pattern of fibrosis is nodular and therefore characteristic of NSCHL, a given case should be classified as NSCHL, regardless of whether there is a high number of HRS cells. Since the definition of LDCHL has changed over the past decades, some of the established clinical and biological features appear outdated in the context of the current definition. Moreover, with the increase in knowledge and the development of additional immunohistochemical markers, some of the cHL cases that were previously assigned to the LDCHL category would nowadays be included into borderline categories or even different entities [1].

### 3.1.2.4 Lymphocyte-Rich Classical Hodgkin Lymphoma

In LRCHL, the HRS cells are present in a lymphocyte-rich background that can be nodular or, rarely, diffuse. Often, B cell follicles are partially preserved with recognizable GC, and HRS cells can be found in expanded mantle and marginal zones thus providing a B cell rich background. HRS cells in LRCHL may resemble LP cells in LPHL morphologically to such an extent that they are indistinguishable from each other without additional immunohistochemical characterization. It is of significance that eosinophils and neutrophils should be absent from the nodular infiltrates and may only be found in low numbers in interfollicular zones and close to vascular structures. The immunophenotype of the HRS cells is classic, and an EBV association is occasionally observed, though at a lower frequency compared to MCCHL [1].

## 3.2 Differential Diagnosis

In most instances, the diagnosis of LPHL and cHL is unambiguous on the basis of morphological, clinical, and, especially, immunohistochemical features (Table 3.1). However, a gray area between cHL and diffuse large B cell lymphoma (DLBCL), specifically with primary mediastinal large B cell lymphoma (PMBL), has long been known, and the most recent WHO classification introduced the category of "B cell lymphoma, unclassifiable, with features intermediate between DLBCL and classical Hodgkin lymphoma" [1]. It is important to note that lymphomas falling into this category are not considered a separate disease entity; rather, it was felt that lymphomas in which there is a discordance between morphological aspects of the infiltrate and the expected immunophenotype should be labeled as "intermediate" to allow a more precise definition of biological and clinical features of these lymphomas in the future. Frequently, these borderline lymphomas present with large mediastinal masses. Morphologically, they consist of large, pleomorphic B cells that grow in a sheet-like pattern in a background of a fibrotic stroma. A subset of the tumor cells may resemble HRS cells, specifically the lacunar variant, and parts of the infiltrate may correspond to the growth pattern of cHL, particularly the nodular sclerosis subtype. Immunophenotypically, there is often a preserved expression program of cHL including expression of CD30 and CD15, while markers of the B cell lineage that are often downregulated in cHL, such as CD20 and CD79a, are equally expressed in the tumor cells [1]. It is important to note that these gray zone lymphomas appear to be more common in male patients, in contrast to NSCHL and PMBL that are more frequent in females [13]. Clinically, these tumors may behave more aggressively than NSCHL and PMBL; it has to be determined in the future whether treatment regimens for aggressive B cell lymphomas or for cHL are more beneficial.

The differential diagnosis between cHL and Alk-negative anaplastic large cell lymphoma (ALCL) of T cell lineage can usually be resolved using an appropriate panel of immunohistochemical markers including T cell, cytotoxic, and other markers. Problems arise when morphological features favor cHL, but tumor cells lack PAX5/BSAP expression while cytotoxic markers are expressed. As discussed above, it is a matter of current debate whether such cases should be grouped into the cHL category or diagnosed as ALCL. Remarkably, a recent global gene expression study revealed surprisingly few consistent differences in the gene expression of HRS cells and Alk-negative ALCL cells [14].

Finally, EBV-associated lymphoproliferations, e.g., in the context of a coexisting T cell non-HL as well as EBV-associated DLBCL of the elderly, a subgroup of DLBCL introduced in the new WHO classification [1], can harbor HRS or HRS-like cells and therefore mimic cHL [15]. Besides other morphological and immunohistochemical features and information on the clinical setting, the pattern of EBV infection, determined by LMP1 staining or EBER in situ hybridization, might help to distinguish between these tumors.

## 3.3 Histogenesis of HRS and LP Cells

### 3.3.1 Cellular Origin of HRS and LP Cells

The unusual immunophenotype of HRS cells, which does not resemble any normal hematopoietic cell, has hampered the identification of the cellular origin of these cells considerably. Moreover, only few cell lines were available for detailed genetic studies, and the rarity of the HRS cells in the tissue posed a problem for their molecular analysis. Finally, by microdissection of HRS cells from tissue sections and single-cell polymerase chain reaction analysis of these cells, it was clarified that HRS cells derive from B cells in nearly all cases [16, 17]. This is because rearranged immunoglobulin (Ig) heavy (IgH) and light (IgL) chain gene rearrangements were detected in these cells. The detection of identical IgV gene rearrangements in the HRS cells of a given HL case also established the monoclonal nature of these cells, a hallmark of malignant cancer cells. With a few exceptions, somatic mutations were detected in the rearranged V genes of HRS cells [16–19]. As the process of somatic hypermutation, which generates such mutations, is specifically active in antigen-activated mature B cells proliferating in the GC microenvironment in the course of T-dependent immune responses [20], the presence of mutated IgV genes in the HRS cells established their derivation from GC-experienced B cells. A surprising finding was that about 25% of cases of cHL showed destructive IgV gene mutations, such as nonsense mutations or deletions causing frameshifts that rendered originally functional V region genes non-functional [16]. When such mutations happen in normal GC B cells, these cells quickly undergo apoptosis. On this basis, it was proposed that HRS cells in these cases derive from preapoptotic GC B cells that were rescued from apoptosis because they harbored or acquired some transforming events [16, 21]. It is important to note that crippling mutations, such as those generating premature stop codons, represent only a small fraction of disadvantageous IgV gene mutations that cause apoptotic death of GC B cells, and it is therefore likely that also most or even all other cases of cHL are derived from preapoptotic GC B cells. Even a few HL with unmutated IgV genes may derive from these precursors, because GC founder cells proliferating in GC become prone to apoptosis before the onset of somatic hypermutation activity [22]. The GC B cell origin of HRS cells was further supported by the molecular analysis of composite lymphomas, composed of a cHL and a B cell non-HL. Such cases are often clonally related and show an intriguing pattern of shared as well as distinct somatic V gene mutations [23–25]. This pattern supports the assumption that both lymphomas were derived from distinct members of a proliferating GC B cell clone.

A few cases of cHL appear to originate from T cells, because T cell receptor gene rearrangements were detected in some cases diagnosed as HL and expressing some typical T cell molecules [10, 11]. However, it is debated whether these are true HL (see above). Remarkably, among HL cases with expression of one or more T cell markers, the majority nevertheless derives from B cells [10, 11].

The expression of multiple B cell markers by LP cells of LPHL already indicated a B cell derivation of these cells. Moreover, LP cells express several markers typically expressed by GC B cells, such as BCL6, AID, centerin, and hGAL, and the cells grow in a follicular pattern in close association with typical constituents of normal GC, i.e., follicular dendritic cells and GC-type T helper cells [2–5, 26, 27]. This pointed to a close relationship between LP cells and GC B cells. This is indeed supported by the detection of clonally related and somatically mutated IgV genes in these cells [17, 28–30]. As opposed to cHL, the V genes are selected for functionality and a fraction of cases shows ongoing somatic hypermutation during clonal expansion, a hallmark of GC B cells [17, 28, 29]. Thus, these findings altogether indicate a GC B cell origin of LP cells. A recent large-scale gene expression profiling of isolated LP cells in comparison to the main subsets of mature B cells has led to a further specification of the derivation of LP cells by showing that the gene expression pattern of LP cells resembles that of GC B cells that have already acquired some features of post-GC memory B cells [31].

### 3.3.2 Relationship of Hodgkin Cells and Reed–Sternberg Cells and Putative HRS Cell Precursors

The relationship of the mononucleated Hodgkin cells to the multinuclear RS cells and the potential existence of HRS precursor cells has been a matter of debate. Based on the "mixed" phenotype of HRS cells and many numerical chromosomal aberrations in these cells, it has been speculated that HRS cells as such or, specifically, the RS cells may derive from cell fusions. However, a detailed study of antigen receptor loci revealed that HRS cells do not carry more than two different alleles of these loci, which strongly supports the assumption that these cells do not derive from cell fusions [32]. Several studies of HL cell lines showed that the mononuclear Hodgkin cells give rise to the RS cells, and that the latter have little proliferative activity [33, 34]. This presumably happens through endomitosis, i.e., nuclear division without cell division.

Another debated issue relates to the question whether the CD30+ typical HRS cells represent the entire tumor clone in HL, or whether members of the HRS cell clones exist among small CD30− cells. An initial study for numerical chromosomal abnormalities indeed suggested that such CD30− clone members might exist [35]. However, trisomies of chromosomes as studied in that work are not a stringent clonal marker. Moreover, a molecular analysis of EBV-positive HL cases for members of the malignant clones among small, CD30− EBV+ B cells in the HL lymph nodes suggested that the small EBV+ B cells rarely, if at all, belong to the HRS cell clones [36]. Recently, two HL cell lines were reported to contain small subpopulations of CD20+CD30−Ig+ B cells coexpressing the stem cell marker aldehyde dehydrogenase (ALDH) [37]. These cells had clonogenic potential and gave rise to the typical HRS cells of these lines. It is important to note that ALDH$^{high}$ cells were also detectable in the peripheral blood of most HL patients, and it was reported that these cells were often clonally related to the HRS cells [37]. However, the clonal relationship between the HRS cells and ALDH$^{high}$ peripheral blood B cells was not clearly shown [38], so it remains to be clarified whether ALDH$^{high}$ B cells indeed represent precursors of the HRS cell clones. A previous study using a highly sensitive PCR for HRS cell-specific Ig gene rearrangements failed to detect members of the HRS cell clone in the peripheral blood or bone marrow of two HL patients [39].

## 3.4  Genetic Lesions

HRS cells have a much higher number of chromosomal aberrations, including multiple numerical as well as structural abnormalities, than most other lymphomas [40]. However, it is still unclear whether this is mostly a side-effect of some type of genetic instability, and whether the expression of specific oncogenes or tumor suppressor genes is recurrently affected by these lesions. When the B cell origin of HRS cells became clear, HRS cells were studied for the presence of chromosomal translocations involving the Ig loci, as such translocations are a hallmark of many B cell lymphomas. Fluorescence in situ hybridization (FISH) studies indeed provided evidence for such translocations in about 20% of cases, but most of the translocation partners involved remain to be identified [41, 42]. In a few cases, the translocation partners were BCL2, BCL3, REL, BCL6, or MYC [41–44]. In LPHL, translocations of the BCL6 gene have been found in about 30% of cases [45, 46]. These translocations can involve the Ig loci, but also multiple other partners [47].

Due to the difficulty to analyze the few HRS and LP cells for mutations in oncogenes and tumor suppressor genes, only relatively few of such genes have been analyzed so far in these cells. There was a major interest to understand the apoptosis resistance of HRS cells, but it turned out that mutations in the CD95 gene, an important death receptor, as well as in members of the CD95 signaling pathway (FADD, caspase 8, caspase 10) were rare or not found at all [48–50]. Likewise, no mutations were found in the BCL2 family member BAD, and also ATM lesions are very rare [51–53]. The TP53 tumor suppressor gene was mutated in less than 10% of cases where the exons of TP53 usually carrying mutations were studied in isolated HRS cells [54, 55]. However, recent studies of HL cell lines indicate that HRS cells may additionally carry untypical TP53 mutations and that the frequency of TP53 mutations may therefore be higher than previously thought [56]. MDM2, a negative regulator of TP53, frequently shows gains in HRS cells, which might contribute to impaired functions of TP53 in these cells [57].

HRS cells show constitutive activity of the NF-κB transcription factor (see below), which is essential for the survival of these cells. The mechanisms of this activation were originally not understood. Consequently, members and regulators of this signaling pathway were studied for genetic lesions (Table 3.1). Inactivating mutations in the main NF-κB inhibitor NFKBIA (IκBα) were found in about 10–20% of HL cases and also in several HL cell lines (Fig. 3.3) [58–61]. One study also detected mutations in another NF-κB inhibitor, NFKBIE (IκBε), in a few cases [62]. Moreover, HRS cells frequently harbor genomic gains or amplifications of the REL gene [63–65], encoding an NF-κB family member, and a correlation between such gains and strong REL protein expression was found [66]. Also the IκB family member BCL3, which acts as a positive regulator of NF-κB activity, is affected by chromosomal gains or translocations in a small fraction of cHL [67, 68]. Recently, somatic and clonal inactivating mutations were found in the TNFAIP3 gene in about 40% of cHL [69, 70]. TNFAIP3 encodes

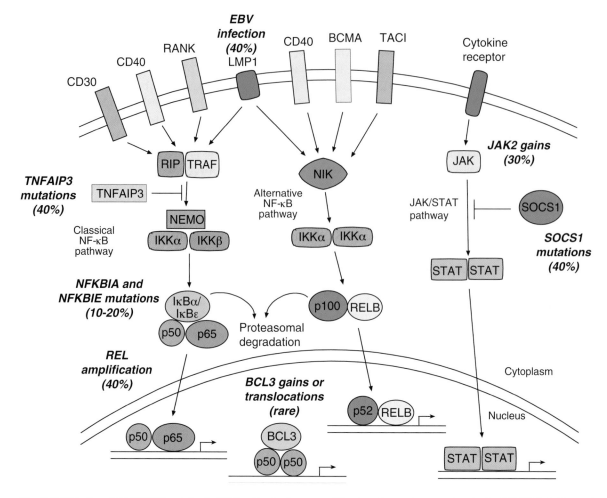

**Fig. 3.3** NF-κB and JAK/STAT activity in HRS cells. In the classical NF-κB signaling pathway, stimulation of numerous receptors leads via TNF receptor associated factors (TRAFs), which are often associated with the receptor interacting protein (RIP), to activation of the IKK complex, which is composed of IKKα, IKKβ, and NEMO. The IKK complex subsequently phosphorylates the NF-κB inhibitors IκBα and IκBε. This marks them for ubiquitination and subsequent proteasomal degradation. Thereby the NF-κB transcription factors (p50/p65 or p50/REL heterodimers) are no longer retained in the cytoplasm and translocate into the nucleus, where they activate multiple genes. The signal transduction from TRAFs/RIP to the IKK complex can be inhibited by TNFAIP3, which removes activating ubiquitins from RIP and TRAFs and additionally links ubiquitins to these molecules to mark them for proteasomal degradation. In the alternative NF-κB pathway, activation of receptors such as CD40, BCMA, and TACI causes stimulation of the kinase NIK, which then activates an IKKα complex. Activated IKKα processes p100 precursors to p52 molecules, which translocate as active p52/RELB NF-κB heterodimers into the nucleus. HRS cells show constitutive activity of the classical and alternative NF-κB signaling pathway. This activity is probably mediated by diverse mechanisms, including receptor signaling through CD40, RANK, BCMA, and TACI; genomic REL amplification; destructive mutations in the TNFAIP3, IκBα, and IκBε genes; and signaling through the EBV-encoded LMP1. The role of CD30 signaling in HRS cells is controversially discussed. HRS cells may also harbor nuclear BCL3/(p50)$_2$ complexes, and in a few cases the strong BCL3 expression appears to be mediated by genomic gains or chromosomal translocations. The JAK/STAT pathway is the main signaling pathway for cytokines. Upon binding of cytokines to their receptors, members of the JAK kinase family become activated by phosphoylation. The activated JAKs then phosphorylate and thereby activate STAT transcription factors. These phosphorylated factors homo- or heterodimerize and translocate into the nucleus where they activate target genes. Main inhibitors of the JAK/STAT pathway are SOCS (suppressor of cytokine signaling) factors, which function by binding to JAK molecules and inhibiting their enzymatic activity, and additionally by inducing proteasomal JAK degradation. In HRS cells, STAT3, -5, and -6 are constitutively active. Besides activation of cytokine receptors (e.g., IL13 receptor and IL21 receptor) through cytokines, activation of this pathway is mediated by genomic gains of the JAK2 gene and frequent inactivating mutations in the SOCS1 gene. The frequency of genetic lesions and viral infections affecting NF-κB or STAT activity in classical Hodgkin lymphoma (HL) cases is indicated

for the A20 protein, which is a dual ubiquitinase and deubiquitinase that functions as a negative regulator of NF-κB. It inhibits signaling from the receptor interacting protein (RIP) and TNF receptor associated factors (TRAF) to the IKK kinases, which are essential mediators of NF-κB signaling. TNFAIP3 mutations were mainly found in EBV-negative cases. Nearly 70% of EBV⁻ cases carried TNFAIP3 mutations, indicating that EBV infection and A20 inactivation are alternative pathogenetic mechanisms in HL [70]. As LMP1 of EBV, which is expressed in EBV-positive HRS cells, mimics an active CD40 receptor and signals through NF-κB [71, 72], LMP1 may replace the role of A20 inactivation in EBV⁺ HL.

As it was recently revealed that also the LP cells of LPHL show strong constitutive NF-κB activity [31], also these cells were studied for mutations in NFKBIA and TNFAIP3, but clonal destructive mutations were not found (Table 3.1) [73].

Genetic lesions were also found in members of the JAK/STAT pathway, which is constitutively activated in HRS and LP cells. In about 40% of cases analyzed, both HRS and LP cells showed somatic mutations in the SOCS1 gene, which encodes a main inhibitor of STAT signaling (Fig. 3.3) [74, 75]. Furthermore, a fraction of cHL cases show genomic gains or amplifications of the JAK2 locus, which encodes one of the kinases activating the STAT factors (Table 3.1) [64, 76].

## 3.5 Deregulated Transcription Factor Networks and Signaling Pathways

### 3.5.1 The Lost B Cell Phenotype

Early immunohistochemical studies already revealed that HRS cells usually do not express typical B cell markers, such as CD20, CD79b, or the BCR [9, 77–79]. This lack of expression of B cell markers was indeed one of the reasons why the B cell origin of HRS cells was not revealed until genetic studies for Ig gene rearrangements unequivocally demonstrated a B cell identity of these cells (see above). Gene expression profiling studies of HRS cells in comparison to normal B cells then showed that there is a global loss of the B cell typical gene expression in HRS cells [80]. This downregulation involved all types of genes with important

functions in these cells, for example, cell surface receptors (CD37, CD53), components of signaling pathways (SYK, BLK, SLP-65), and transcription factors (PU.B, A-MYB, SPI-B). Remarkably, however, HRS cells have retained expression of molecules that are involved in antigen-presenting functions and the interaction with CD4⁺ T helper cells. HRS cells usually express MHC class II, CD40, CD80, and CD86 [80, 81]. This indicates that an interaction with T helper cells is important for HRS cell survival. In line with this view, HRS cells are typically surrounded by CD40L expressing CD4⁺ T cells [82].

We are now beginning to understand which factors contribute to the lost B cell phenotype of HRS cells. First, several transcription factors that positively regulate the expression of multiple genes in B cells are downregulated, including OCT-2, PU.1, and BOB.1 [77, 78, 83]. Second, although E2A, a master regulator of the B cell transcription program, is still expressed, HRS cells also show deregulated expression of ID2 and ABF1 [84–86], which bind to E2A and inhibit its function [85]. The physiological role of ABF1 is poorly understood, but ID2 is normally expressed in dendritic cells and natural killer cells, and supports the generation of these cells concomitant with suppression of B cell development [87, 88]. Third, HRS cells express activated Notch-1, which normally induces T cell differentiation in lymphocyte precursors and suppresses a B lineage differentiation of such cells [89, 90]. Activation of Notch-1 is probably caused by interaction with its ligand Jagged-1, which is expressed by other cells in the HL microenvironment [90]. Moreover, HRS cells have downregulated the Notch-1 inhibitor Deltex1 [89]. Fourth, STAT5A and STAT5B are activated in HRS cells and have been reported to induce an HRS cell-like phenotype in normal B cells [91]. Constitutive active STAT5 induced expression of CD30 and of the T cell transcription factor GATA3 in the B cells and led to downregulation of BCR expression. Fifth, the downregulation of multiple B cell genes in HRS cells is further mediated by epigenetic mechanisms, as DNA methylation has been detected for numerous such genes [92, 93]. Sixth, HRS cells express several transcription factors that have important roles in hematopoietic stem cells and early lymphoid precursors, including GATA2, BMI1, RING1, and RYBP [94–97]. The expression of these factors may contribute to a "dedifferentiated" phenotype of HRS cells.

Surprisingly, PAX5, the main B lineage commitment and maintenance factor, is still expressed in HRS cells, albeit at reduced levels [7]. As many of its direct target genes are not expressed, it is likely that PAX5 activity is inhibited. Notch-1 is a candidate for this inhibition [89]. It may also be that PAX5 target genes are not expressed because other transcription factors needed for the efficient expression of these genes are missing.

The downregulation of many B cell transcription factors that also suppress the expression of non-B lineage genes, combined with the upregulated expression of genes promoting expression of genes of other hematopoietic cell types (e.g., Notch-1, ID2), not only explains the lost B cell phenotype of HRS cells, but also the heterogenous expression of genes specifically expressed by dendritic cells, T cells, or other cell types. It is an intriguing question whether the lost B cell phenotype of HRS cells is related to their origin from crippled GC B cells. Perhaps, due to the stringent selection of B cells for expression of a functional BCR (a high-affinity one in the GC), there is a selection in HRS cell pathogenesis downregulating the B cell gene expression program to escape the selectional forces that induce apoptosis in GC B cells with unfavorable IgV gene mutations. However, the lost B cell phenotype could also be a side-effect of so far unknown transforming events.

### 3.5.2 Constitutive Activation of Multiple Signaling Pathways

It is obvious that tumor cells need to activate and deregulate signaling pathways and transcription factors that promote their survival and proliferation. Nevertheless, it is striking how many of such pathways are constitutively activated in HRS cells, and cHL appears to be rather unique among lymphoid malignancies in the extent to which multiple signaling pathways contribute to the survival and expansion of HRS cells. It has already been mentioned above that HRS cells show constitutive NF-κB activity. This activity is essential for HRS cell survival [98], and is most likely not only mediated by genetic lesions (see above), but also by signaling through receptors. NF-κB factors of both the canoncial pathway (p50/p65) and the non-canonical NF-κB pathway (p52/RelB) are activated (Fig. 3.3). HRS cells express the TNF receptor family members CD30, CD40, RANK, TACI, and BCMA, which activate NF-κB, and cells expressing the respective ligands are found in the HL microenvironment

[82, 99–103]. There are, however, conflicting data about the role of CD30 in NF-κB activation [104, 105]. In EBV-positive cases of cHL, the virally encoded LMP1 mimics an active CD40 receptor and hence also contributes to NF-κB activation [106].

Another central signaling pathway, which is like NF-κB activated both by genetic lesions as well as by ligand-mediated receptor triggering, is the JAK/STAT pathway (Fig. 3.3). This is the main signaling pathway for cytokines. Activation of cytokine receptors causes activation of JAK kinases which in turn phosphorylate and thereby activate STAT transcription factors. The phosphorylated STAT factors dimerize and then translocate into the nucleus where they activate transcription of target genes. HRS cells show activation of STAT3, STAT5, and STAT6 [91, 107–109]. The activation of STAT6 is at least partly mediated by signaling through IL13. As HRS cells express IL13 and its receptor, STAT6 activation can be mediated through an autocrine stimulation loop [110, 111]. Signaling through the IL21 receptor contributes to STAT3 and STAT5 activation in HRS cells, which is also enhanced by the NF-κB activity in the cells [91, 112, 113]. As mentioned above, STAT5 activity may contribute to the lost B cell phenotype of HRS cells. Inhibition of STAT activity in HL cell lines resulted in reduced proliferation of the cells, further supporting an important pathogenetic role of this signaling pathway [107, 108, 110].

Receptor tyrosine kinases (RTK) are important regulators of cell growth, survival, and proliferation. In multiple cancers, specific RTK are activated, often by somatic mutations [114]. In contrast, HRS cells show multiple activated RTK, and their activation does not appear to be due to activating mutations but at least partly to ligand-mediated stimulation [115]. RTK that are often expressed in varying combinations in HRS cells include PDGFRA, DDR2, EPHB1, RON, TRKA, TRKB, and MET [115, 116]. The expression of most of these is aberrant, as they are not expressed by normal GC B cells [115]. They are also usually not expressed by other B cell non-HL, showing that this is a specific feature of HL among B cell lymphomas [115, 117]. Expression of multiple RTKs is most pronounced in EBV-negative cases of cHL, suggesting that EBV activates pathways in HRS cells replacing the function of RTKs [118]. For PDGFRA and TRKA, a growth-inhibitory effect has been shown upon their inhibition in HL cell lines, giving a first indication that the activity of RTKs is important for HRS cell proliferation [115, 119].

Signaling through various receptors is mediated by the mitogen-activated protein kinase (MAPK)/ERK pathway. In HRS cells, the serine/threonine kinases ERK1, ERK2, and ERK5 are activated [120, 121]. Inhibition of their activity has antiproliferative effects on HL cell lines [121]. Signaling through CD30, CD40, and RANK may contribute to the stimulation of this pathway [121].

The transcription factor AP-1 acts as homo- or heterodimers of Jun, Fos, and ATF components. In HRS cells, c-Jun and Jun-B are overexpressed and constitutively active [122]. The overexpression of Jun-B is mediated by NF-κB [122]. AP-1 induces many target genes and promotes proliferation of HRS cells. Target genes of AP-1 include CD30 and galectin-1, the latter of which has immunomodulatory functions [123, 124].

Finally, also the phosphatidylinositol-3-kinase (PI3K)/AKT pathway, which is a main promoter of cell survival, shows activity in HRS cells [125, 126]. AKT is a serine/threonine kinase that is activated in HRS cells, as evident from its phosphorylated state and phosphorylation of known target proteins [125, 126]. Inhibition of AKT in HL cell lines causes cell death, suggesting an important role of active AKT in HRS cell survival [125, 126]. PI3K may be activated in HRS cells by signaling through CD30, CD40, RANK, and RTK.

While we have a relatively detailed insight into signaling pathways active in HRS cells, less is known about signaling pathways constitutively active in LP cells of LPHL. However, LP cells also show a high constitutive activity of NF-κB [31]. RTKs are partly also aberrantly expressed by these cells [115], and activation of the JAK/STAT pathway has been observed [74].

In conclusion, HRS cells are characterized by the deregulated and constitutive activation of multiple signaling pathways and transcription factors that contribute to the survival and proliferation of these cells. The multitude of different stimulated pathways appears to be rather unique among human B cell lymphomas. Often, these pathways are activated by common mechanisms, and they may interact in numerous ways.

## 3.6 Antiapoptotic Mechanisms

With a presumed origin from pre-apoptotic GC B cells, it is critical to understand through which mechanisms HRS cell escape from apoptosis. A number of factors contributing to HRS cell survival have already been discussed in the previous section: constitutive activity of NF-κB, STAT, PI3K, Notch1, AP-1, RTK, and ERK. Several specific inhibitors of the two main apoptosis pathways deserve specific mentioning. Although HRS cells express the CD95 death receptor of the extrinsic apoptosis pathway as well as its activating ligand, HL cell lines are resistant to CD95-mediated death induction, suggesting a specific inhibition of this pathway [127–129]. As mentioned above, this resistance is neither due to mutations in the CD95 receptor itself, nor in its interaction partners FADD, caspase 8, or caspase 10. However, HRS cells show strong expression of the CD95 inhibitor cFLIP (cellular FADD-like interleukin 1β-converting enzyme-inhibitory protein), and this factor impairs CD95 signaling in HRS cells [127, 128]. Inhibition of the intrinsic (mitochondrial) apoptosis pathway is probably mediated through strong expression of the anti-apoptotic factors BCLXL and XIAP (X-linked inhibitor of apoptosis) [130, 131]. BCLXL inhibits apoptosis at the level of the mitochondrial apoptosis induction, whereas XIAP inhibits activity of caspases 3 and 9, which are downstream executioners of the mitochondrial apoptosis program. Although HRS cells also express proapoptotic Smac, which can inhibit XIAP, the cells show an impaired release of Smac from the mitochondria into the cytoplasm [132]. As mentioned above, HRS cells express high levels of the pro-apoptotic TP53 factor, but resistance to TP53-mediated apoptosis appears to be rarely due to inactivating mutations in the TP53 gene. An important factor for the inhibition of TP53 activity is MDM2, which is expressed at high levels in HRS cells [133]. The functional role of MDM2 as an TP53 inhibitor in HRS cells is supported by the fact that HL cell lines expressing wild-type TP53 are rendered apoptosis-sensitive toward pharmacological apoptosis inducers upon inhibition of MDM2 by its antagonist nutlin 3 [134, 135].

## References

1. Swerdlow SH, Campo E, Harris NL, Jaffe ES, Pileri SA, Stein H, et al. Classification of tumours of haematopoietic and lymphoid tissues, 4th ed. Lyon: IARC Press; 2008.
2. Carbone A, Gloghini A, Gaidano G, Franceschi S, Capello D, Drexler HG, et al. Expression status of BCL-6 and syndecan-1 identifies distinct histogenetic subtypes of Hodgkin's disease. Blood. 1998;92:2220-8.

3. Greiner A, Tobollik S, Buettner M, Jungnickel B, Herrmann K, Kremmer E, et al. Differential expression of activation-induced cytidine deaminase (AID) in nodular lymphocyte-predominant and classical Hodgkin lymphoma. J Pathol 2005;205:541-7.

4. Hansmann ML, Fellbaum C, Hui PK, Zwingers T. Correlation of content of B cells and Leu7-positive cells with subtype and stage in lymphocyte predominance type Hodgkin's disease. J Cancer Res Clin Oncol. 1988;114:405-10.

5. Kamel OW, Gelb AB, Shibuya RB, Warnke RA. Leu 7 (CD57) reactivity distinguishes nodular lymphocyte predominance Hodgkin's disease from nodular sclerosing Hodgkin's disease, T-cell-rich B-cell lymphoma and follicular lymphoma. Am J Pathol. 1993;142:541-6.

6. Nam-Cha SH, Roncador G, Sanchez-Verde L, Montes-Moreno S, Acevedo A, Dominguez-Franjo P, et al. PD-1, a follicular T-cell marker useful for recognizing nodular lymphocyte-predominant Hodgkin lymphoma. Am J Surg Pathol. 2008;32:1252-7.

7. Foss HD, Reusch R, Demel G, Lenz G, Anagnostopoulos I, Hummel M, et al. Frequent expression of the B-cell-specific activator protein in Reed-Sternberg cells of classical Hodgkin's disease provides further evidence for its B-cell origin. Blood. 1999;94:3108-13.

8. Korkolopoulou P, Cordell J, Jones M, Kaklamanis L, Tsenga A, Gatter KC, et al. The expression of the B-cell marker mb-1 (CD79a) in Hodgkin's disease. Histopathology. 1994;24:511-5.

9. Kuzu I, Delsol G, Jones M, Gatter KC, Mason DY. Expression of the Ig-associated heterodimer (mb-1 and B29) in Hodgkin's disease. Histopathology. 1993;22:141-4.

10. Müschen M, Rajewsky K, Bräuninger A, Baur AS, Oudejans JJ, Roers A, et al. Rare occurrence of classical Hodgkin's disease as a T cell lymphoma. J Exp Med. 2000; 191:387-94.

11. Seitz V, Hummel M, Marafioti T, Anagnostopoulos I, Assaf C, Stein H. Detection of clonal T-cell receptor gamma-chain gene rearrangements in Reed-Sternberg cells of classic Hodgkin disease. Blood. 2000;95:3020-4.

12. Mani H, Jaffe ES. Hodgkin lymphoma: an update on its biology with new insights into classification. Clin Lymphoma Myeloma 2009;9:206-6.

13. Traverse-Glehen A, Pittaluga S, Gaulard P, Sorbara L, Alonso MA, Raffeld M, et al. Mediastinal gray zone lymphoma: the missing link between classic Hodgkin's lymphoma and mediastinal large B-cell lymphoma. Am J Surg Pathol. 2005; 29:1411-21.

14. Eckerle S, Brune V, Döring C, Tiacci E, Bohle V, Sundstrom C, et al. Gene expression profiling of isolated tumour cells from anaplastic large cell lymphomas: insights into its cellular origin, pathogenesis and relation to Hodgkin lymphoma. Leukemia 2009;23(11):2129-38.

15. Asano N, Yamamoto K, Tamaru J, Oyama T, Ishida F, Ohshima K, et al. Age-related Epstein-Barr virus (EBV)-associated B-cell lymphoproliferative disorders: comparison with EBV-positive classic Hodgkin lymphoma in elderly patients. Blood. 2009;113:2629-36.

16. Kanzler H, Küppers R, Hansmann ML, Rajewsky K. Hodgkin and Reed-Sternberg cells in Hodgkin's disease represent the outgrowth of a dominant tumor clone derived from (crippled) germinal center B cells. J Exp Med. 1996;184:1495-505.

17. Küppers R, Rajewsky K, Zhao M, Simons G, Laumann R, Fischer R, et al. Hodgkin disease: Hodgkin and Reed-Sternberg cells picked from histological sections show clonal immunoglobulin gene rearrangements and appear to be derived from B cells at various stages of development. Proc Natl Acad Sci USA. 1994;91:10962-6.

18. Marafioti T, Hummel M, Foss H-D, Laumen H, Korbjuhn P, Anagnostopoulos I, et al. Hodgkin and Reed-Sternberg cells represent an expansion of a single clone originating from a germinal center B-cell with functional immunoglobulin gene rearrangements but defective immunoglobulin transcription. Blood. 2000;95:1443-50.

19. Müschen M, Küppers R, Spieker T, Bräuninger A, Rajewsky K, Hansmann ML. Molecular single-cell analysis of Hodgkin- and Reed-Sternberg cells harboring unmutated immunoglobulin variable region genes. Lab Invest. 2001;81:289-5.

20. Küppers R, Zhao M, Hansmann ML, Rajewsky K. Tracing B cell development in human germinal centres by molecular analysis of single cells picked from histological sections. EMBO J. 1993;12:4955-67.

21. Küppers R, Rajewsky K. The origin of Hodgkin and Reed/Sternberg cells in Hodgkin's disease. Annu Rev Immunol. 1998;16:471-93.

22. Lebecque S, de Bouteiller O, Arpin C, Banchereau J, Liu YJ. Germinal center founder cells display propensity for apoptosis before onset of somatic mutation. J Exp Med. 1997;185:563-71.

23. Bräuninger A, Hansmann ML, Strickler JG, Dummer R, Burg G, Rajewsky K, et al. Identification of common germinal-center B-cell precursors in two patients with both Hodgkin's disease and Non-Hodgkin's lymphoma. N Engl J Med. 1999;340:1239-47.

24. Küppers R, Sousa AB, Baur AS, Strickler JG, Rajewsky K, Hansmann ML. Common germinal-center B-cell origin of the malignant cells in two composite lymphomas, involving classical Hodgkin's disease and either follicular lymphoma or B-CLL. Mol Med. 2001;7:285-92.

25. Marafioti T, Hummel M, Anagnostopoulos I, Foss HD, Huhn D, Stein H. Classical Hodgkin's disease and follicular lymphoma originating from the same germinal center B cell. J Clin Oncol. 1999;17:3804-9.

26. Montes-Moreno S, Roncador G, Maestre L, Martinez N, Sanchez-Verde L, Camacho FI, et al. Gcet1 (centerin), a highly restricted marker for a subset of germinal center-derived lymphomas. Blood. 2008;111:351-8.

27 Natkunam Y, Lossos IS, Taidi B, Zhao S, Lu X, Ding F, et al. Expression of the human germinal center-associated lymphoma (HGAL) protein, a new marker of germinal center B-cell derivation. Blood. 2005;105:3979-86.

28. Braeuninger A, Küppers R, Strickler JG, Wacker HH, Rajewsky K, Hansmann ML. Hodgkin and Reed-Sternberg cells in lymphocyte predominant Hodgkin disease represent clonal populations of germinal center-derived tumor B cells. Proc Natl Acad Sci USA. 1997;94:9337-42.

29. Marafioti T, Hummel M, Anagnostopoulos I, Foss HD, Falini B, Delsol G, et al. Origin of nodular lymphocyte-predominant Hodgkin's disease from a clonal expansion of highly mutated germinal-center B cells. N Engl J Med. 1997;337:453-8.

30. Ohno T, Stribley JA, Wu G, Hinrichs SH, Weisenburger DD, Chan WC. Clonality in nodular lymphocyte-predominant Hodgkin's disease. N Engl J Med. 1997;337:459-65.

31. Brune V, Tiacci E, Pfeil I, Döring C, Eckerle S, van Noesel CJM, et al. Origin and pathogenesis of nodular lymphocyte-predominant Hodgkin lymphoma as revealed by global gene expression analysis. J Exp Med. 2008;205:2251-68.

32. Küppers R, Bräuninger A, Müschen M, Distler V, Hansmann ML, Rajewsky K. Evidence that Hodgkin and Reed-Sternberg cells in Hodgkin disease do not represent cell fusions. Blood. 2001;97:818-21.

33. Drexler HG, Gignac SM, Hoffbrand AV, Minowada J. Formation of multinucleated cells in a Hodgkin's-disease-derived cell line. Int J Cancer. 1989;43:1083-90.

34. Newcom SR, Kadin ME, Phillips C. L-428 Reed-Sternberg cells and mononuclear Hodgkin's cells arise from a single cloned mononuclear cell. Int J Cell Cloning. 1988;6:417-31.

35. Jansen MP, Hopman AH, Bot FJ, Haesevoets A, Stevens-Kroef MJ, Arends JW, et al. Morphologically normal, CD30-negative B-lymphocytes with chromosome aberrations in classical Hodgkin's disease: the progenitor cell of the malignant clone? J Pathol. 1999;189:527-32.

36. Spieker T, Kurth J, Küppers R, Rajewsky K, Bräuninger A, Hansmann ML. Molecular single-cell analysis of the clonal relationship of small Epstein-Barr virus-infected cells and Epstein-Barr virus-harboring Hodgkin and Reed/Sternberg cells in Hodgkin disease. Blood. 2000;96:3133-8.

37. Jones RJ, Gocke CD, Kasamon YL, Miller CB, Perkins B, Barber JP, et al. Circulating clonotypic B cells in classic Hodgkin lymphoma. Blood. 2009;113:5920-6.

38. Küppers R. Clonogenic B cells in classic Hodgkin lymphoma. Blood. 2009;114(18):3970-1.

39. Vockerodt M, Soares M, Kanzler H, Küppers R, Kube D, Hansmann ML, et al. Detection of clonal Hodgkin and Reed-Sternberg cells with identical somatically mutated and rearranged VH genes in different biopsies in relapsed Hodgkin's disease. Blood. 1998;92:2899-907.

40. Weber-Matthiesen K, Deerberg J, Poetsch M, Grote W, Schlegelberger B. Numerical chromosome aberrations are present within the CD30+ Hodgkin and Reed-Sternberg cells in 100% of analyzed cases of Hodgkin's disease. Blood. 1995;86:1464-8.

41. Martin-Subero JI, Klapper W, Sotnikova A, Callet-Bauchu E, Harder L, Bastard C, et al. Chromosomal breakpoints affecting immunoglobulin loci are recurrent in Hodgkin and Reed-Sternberg cells of classical Hodgkin lymphoma. Cancer Res. 2006;66:10332-8.

42. Szymanowska N, Klapper W, Gesk S, Küppers R, Martin-Subero JI, Siebert R. BCL2 and BCL3 are recurrent translocation partners of the IGH locus. Cancer Genet Cytogenet. 2008;186:110-4.

43. Gravel S, Delsol G, Al Saati T. Single-cell analysis of the t(14;18)(q32;p21) chromosomal translocation in Hodgkin's disease demonstrates the absence of this transformation in neoplastic Hodgkin and Reed-Sternberg cells. Blood. 1998;91:2866-74.

44. Poppema S, Kaleta J, Hepperle B. Chromosomal abnormalities in patients with Hodgkin's disease: evidence for frequent involvement of the 14q chromosomal region but infrequent bcl-2 gene rearrangement in Reed-Sternberg cells. J Natl Cancer Inst. 1992;84:1789-93.

45. Renné C, Martin-Subero JI, Hansmann ML, Siebert R. Molecular cytogenetic analyses of immunoglobulin loci in nodular lymphocyte predominant Hodgkin's lymphoma reveal a recurrent IGH-BCL6 juxtaposition. J Mol Diagn. 2005;7:352-6.

46. Wlodarska I, Nooyen P, Maes B, Martin-Subero JI, Siebert R, Pauwels P, et al. Frequent occurrence of BCL6 rearrangements in nodular lymphocyte predominance Hodgkin lymphoma but not in classical Hodgkin lymphoma. Blood. 2003;101:706-10.

47. Wlodarska I, Stul M, De Wolf-Peeters C, Hagemeijer A. Heterogeneity of BCL6 rearrangements in nodular lymphocyte predominant Hodgkin's lymphoma. Haematologica. 2004;89:965-72.

48. Maggio EM, van den Berg A, de Jong D, Diepstra A, Poppema S. Low frequency of FAS mutations in Reed-Sternberg cells of Hodgkin's lymphoma. Am J Pathol. 2003;162:29-35.

49. Müschen M, Re D, Bräuninger A, Wolf J, Hansmann ML, Diehl V, et al. Somatic mutations of the CD95 gene in Hodgkin and Reed-Sternberg cells. Cancer Res. 2000;60:5640-3.

50. Thomas RK, Schmitz R, Harttrampf AC, Abdil-Hadi A, Wickenhauser C, Distler V, et al. Apoptosis-resistant phenotype of classical Hodgkin's lymphoma is not mediated by somatic mutations within genes encoding members of the death-inducing signaling complex (DISC). Leukemia. 2005;19:1079-82.

51. Bose S, Starczynski J, Chukwuma M, Baumforth K, Wei W, Morgan S, et al. Down-regulation of ATM protein in HRS cells of nodular sclerosis Hodgkin's lymphoma in children occurs in the absence of ATM gene inactivation. J Pathol. 2007;213:329-36.

52. Lespinet V, Terraz F, Recher C, Campo E, Hall J, Delsol G, et al. Single-cell analysis of loss of heterozygosity at the ATM gene locus in Hodgkin and Reed-Sternberg cells of Hodgkin's lymphoma: ATM loss of heterozygosity is a rare event. Int J Cancer. 2005;114:909-16.

53. Schmitz R, Thomas RK, Harttrampf AC, Wickenhauser C, Schultze JL, Hansmann ML, et al. The major subtypes of human B-cell lymphomas lack mutations in BCL-2 family member BAD. Int J Cancer. 2006;119:1738-40.

54. Maggio EM, Stekelenburg E, Van den Berg A, Poppema S. TP53 gene mutations in Hodgkin lymphoma are infrequent and not associated with absence of Epstein-Barr virus. Int J Cancer. 2001;94:60-6.

55. Montesinos-Rongen M, Roers A, Küppers R, Rajewsky K, Hansmann M-L. Mutation of the p53 gene is not a typical feature of Hodgkin and Reed-Sternberg cells in Hodgkin's disease. Blood. 1999;94:1755-60.

56. Feuerborn A, Moritz C, Von Bonin F, Dobbelstein M, Trümper L, Sturzenhofecker B, et al. Dysfunctional p53 deletion mutants in cell lines derived from Hodgkin's lymphoma. Leuk Lymphoma. 2006;47:1932-40.

57. Küpper M, Joos S, Von Bonin F, Daus H, Pfreundschuh M, Lichter P, et al. MDM2 gene amplification and lack of p53 point mutations in Hodgkin and Reed-Sternberg cells: results from single-cell polymerase chain reaction and molecular cytogenetic studies. Br J Haematol. 2001;112:768-75.

58. Cabannes E, Khan G, Aillet F, Jarrett RF, Hay RT. Mutations in the IkBa gene in Hodgkin's disease suggest a tumour suppressor role for IkBa. Oncogene. 1999;18:3063-70.

59. Emmerich F, Meiser M, Hummel M, Demel G, Foss HD, Jundt F, et al. Overexpression of I kappa B alpha without inhibition of NF-kappaB activity and mutations in the I kappa B alpha gene in Reed-Sternberg cells. Blood. 1999;94:3129-34.

60. Jungnickel B, Staratschek-Jox A, Bräuninger A, Spieker T, Wolf J, Diehl V, et al. Clonal deleterious mutations in the ikBa gene in the malignant cells in Hodgkin's disease. J Exp Med. 2000;191:395-401.

61. Lake A, Shield LA, Cordano P, Chui DT, Osborne J, Crae S, et al. Mutations of NFKBIA, encoding IkappaBalpha, are a recurrent finding in classical Hodgkin lymphoma but are not a unifying feature of non-EBV-associated cases. Int J Cancer. 2009;125:1334-42.

62. Emmerich F, Theurich S, Hummel M, Haeffker A, Vry MS, Döhner K, et al. Inactivating I kappa B epsilon mutations in Hodgkin/Reed-Sternberg cells. J Pathol. 2003;201:413-20.

63. Joos S, Granzow M, Holtgreve-Grez H, Siebert R, Harder L, Martin-Subero JI, et al. Hodgkin's lymphoma cell lines are characterized by frequent aberrations on chromosomes 2p and 9p including REL and JAK2. Int J Cancer. 2003;103: 489-95.

64. Joos S, Menz CK, Wrobel G, Siebert R, Gesk S, Ohl S, et al. Classical Hodgkin lymphoma is characterized by recurrent copy number gains of the short arm of chromosome 2. Blood. 2002;99:1381-7.

65. Martin-Subero JI, Gesk S, Harder L, Sonoki T, Tucker PW, Schlegelberger B, et al. Recurrent involvement of the REL and BCL11A loci in classical Hodgkin lymphoma. Blood. 2002;99:1474-7.

66. Barth TF, Martin-Subero JI, Joos S, Menz CK, Hasel C, Mechtersheimer G, et al. Gains of 2p involving the REL locus correlate with nuclear c-Rel protein accumulation in neoplastic cells of classical Hodgkin lymphoma. Blood. 2003;101:3681-6.

67. Martin-Subero JI, Wlodarska I, Bastard C, Picquenot JM, Höppner J, Giefing M, et al. Chromosomal rearrangements involving the BCL3 locus are recurrent in classical Hodgkin and peripheral T-cell lymphoma. Blood. 2006;108:401-2.

68. Mathas S, Jöhrens K, Joos S, Lietz A, Hummel F, Janz M, et al. Elevated NF-kappaB p50 complex formation and Bcl-3 expression in classical Hodgkin, anaplastic large-cell, and other peripheral T-cell lymphomas. Blood. 2005;106:4287-93.

69. Kato M, Sanada M, Kato I, Sato Y, Takita J, Takeuchi K, et al. Frequent inactivation of A20 in B-cell lymphomas. Nature. 2009;459:712-6.

70. Schmitz R, Hansmann ML, Bohle V, Martin-Subero JI, Hartmann S, Mechtersheimer G, et al. TNFAIP3 (A20) is a tumor suppressor gene in Hodgkin lymphoma and primary mediastinal B cell lymphoma. J Exp Med. 2009;206:981-9.

71. Mosialos G, Birkenbach M, Yalamanchili R, VanArsdale T, Ware C, Kieff E. The Epstein-Barr virus transforming protein LMP1 engages signaling proteins for the tumor necrosis factor receptor family. Cell. 1995;80:389-99.

72. Uchida J, Yasui T, Takaoka-Shichijo Y, Muraoka M, Kulwichit W, Raab-Traub N, et al. Mimicry of CD40 signals

by Epstein-Barr virus LMP1 in B lymphocyte responses. Science. 1999;286:300-3.

73. Schumacher MA, Schmitz R, Brune V, Tiacci E, Döring C, Hansmann ML, et al. Mutations in the genes coding for the NF-{kappa}B regulating factors I{kappa}B{alpha} and A20 are uncommon in nodular lymphocyte-predominant Hodgkin lymphoma. Haematologica. 2009;95(1):153-7.

74. Mottok A, Renné C, Willenbrock K, Hansmann ML, Bräuninger A. Somatic hypermutation of SOCS1 in lymphocyte-predominant Hodgkin lymphoma is accompanied by high JAK2 expression and activation of STAT6. Blood. 2007;110:3387-90.

75. Weniger MA, Melzner I, Menz CK, Wegener S, Bucur AJ, Dorsch K, et al. Mutations of the tumor suppressor gene SOCS-1 in classical Hodgkin lymphoma are frequent and associated with nuclear phospho-STAT5 accumulation. Oncogene. 2006;25:2679-84.

76. Joos S, Küpper M, Ohl S, von Bonin F, Mechtersheimer G, Bentz M, et al. Genomic imbalances including amplification of the tyrosine kinase gene JAK2 in CD30+ Hodgkin cells. Cancer Res. 2000;60:549-52.

77. Re D, Müschen M, Ahmadi T, Wickenhauser C, Staratschek-Jox A, Holtick U, et al. Oct-2 and Bob-1 deficiency in Hodgkin and Reed Sternberg cells. Cancer Res. 2001;61:2080-4.

78. Stein H, Marafioti T, Foss HD, Laumen H, Hummel M, Anagnostopoulos I, et al. Down-regulation of BOB.1/ OBF.1 and Oct2 in classical Hodgkin disease but not in lymphocyte predominant Hodgkin disease correlates with immunoglobulin transcription. Blood. 2001;97:496-501.

79. Watanabe K, Yamashita Y, Nakayama A, Hasegawa Y, Kojima H, Nagasawa T, et al. Varied B-cell immunophenotypes of Hodgkin/Reed-Sternberg cells in classic Hodgkin's disease. Histopathol. 2000;36:353-61.

80. Schwering I, Bräuninger A, Klein U, Jungnickel B, Tinguely M, Diehl V, et al. Loss of the B-lineage-specific gene expression program in Hodgkin and Reed-Sternberg cells of Hodgkin lymphoma. Blood. 2003;101:1505-12.

81. Poppema S. Immunology of Hodgkin's disease. Baillieres Clin Haematol. 1996;9:447-57.

82. Carbone A, Gloghini A, Gruss HJ, Pinto A. CD40 ligand is constitutively expressed in a subset of T cell lymphomas and on the microenvironmental reactive T cells of follicular lymphomas and Hodgkin's disease. Am J Pathol. 1995;147: 912-22.

83. Torlakovic E, Tierens A, Dang HD, Delabie J. The transcription factor PU.1, necessary for B-cell development is expressed in lymphocyte predominance, but not classical Hodgkin's disease. Am J Pathol. 2001;159:1807-14.

84. Küppers R, Klein U, Schwering I, Distler V, Bräuninger A, Cattoretti G, et al. Identification of Hodgkin and Reed-Sternberg cell-specific genes by gene expression profiling. J Clin Invest. 2003;111:529-37.

85. Mathas S, Janz M, Hummel F, Hummel M, Wollert-Wulf B, Lusatis S, et al. Intrinsic inhibition of transcription factor E2A by HLH proteins ABF-1 and Id2 mediates reprogramming of neoplastic B cells in Hodgkin lymphoma. Nature Immunol. 2006;7:207-15.

86. Renné C, Martin-Subero JI, Eickernjager M, Hansmann ML, Küppers R, Siebert R, et al. Aberrant expression of

ID2, a suppressor of B-cell-specific gene expression, in Hodgkin's lymphoma. Am J Pathol. 2006;169:655-64.

87. Hacker C, Kirsch RD, Ju XS, Hieronymus T, Gust TC, Kuhl C, et al. Transcriptional profiling identifies Id2 function in dendritic cell development. Nat Immunol. 2003;4:380-6.

88. Yokota Y, Mansouri A, Mori S, Sugawara S, Adachi S, Nishikawa S, et al. Development of peripheral lymphoid organs and natural killer cells depends on the helix-loop-helix inhibitor Id2. Nature. 1999;397:702-6.

89. Jundt F, Acikgoz O, Kwon SH, Schwarzer R, Anagnostopoulos I, Wiesner B, et al. Aberrant expression of Notch1 interferes with the B-lymphoid phenotype of neoplastic B cells in classical Hodgkin lymphoma. Leukemia. 2008;22(8):1587-94.

90. Jundt F, Anagnostopoulos I, Förster R, Mathas S, Stein H, Dörken B. Activated Notch 1 signaling promotes tumor cell proliferation and survival in Hodgkin and anaplastic large cell lymphoma. Blood. 2001;99:3398-403.

91. Scheeren FA, Diehl SA, Smit LA, Beaumont T, Naspetti M, Bende RJ, et al. IL-21 is expressed in Hodgkin lymphoma and activates STAT5; evidence that activated STAT5 is required for Hodgkin lymphomagenesis. Blood. 2008;111:4706-15.

92. Doerr JR, Malone CS, Fike FM, Gordon MS, Soghomonian SV, Thomas RK, et al. Patterned CpG methylation of silenced B cell gene promoters in classical Hodgkin lymphoma-derived and primary effusion lymphoma cell lines. J Mol Biol. 2005;350:631-40.

93. Ushmorov A, Leithäuser F, Sakk O, Weinhausel A, Popov SW, Möller P, et al. Epigenetic processes play a major role in B-cell-specific gene silencing in classical Hodgkin lymphoma. Blood. 2005;107:2493-500.

94. Dukers DF, van Galen JC, Giroth C, Jansen P, Sewalt RG, Otte AP, et al. Unique polycomb gene expression pattern in Hodgkin's lymphoma and Hodgkin's lymphoma-derived cell lines. Am J Pathol. 2004;164:873-81.

95. Raaphorst FM, van Kemenade FJ, Blokzijl T, Fieret E, Hamer KM, Satijn DP, et al. Coexpression of BMI-1 and EZH2 polycomb group genes in Reed-Sternberg cells of Hodgkin's disease. Am J Pathol. 2000;157:709-15.

96. Sanchez-Beato M, Sanchez E, Garcia JF, Perez-Rosado A, Montoya MC, Fraga M, et al. Abnormal PcG protein expression in Hodgkin's lymphoma. Relation with E2F6 and NFkappaB transcription factors. J Pathol. 2004;204:528-37.

97. Schneider EM, Torlakovic E, Stuhler A, Diehl V, Tesch H, Giebel B. The early transcription factor GATA-2 is expressed in classical Hodgkin's lymphoma. J Pathol. 2004;204:538-45.

98. Bargou RC, Emmerich F, Krappmann D, Bommert K, Mapara MY, Arnold W, et al. Constitutive nuclear factor-kappaB-RelA activation is required for proliferation and survival of Hodgkin's disease tumor·cells. J Clin Invest. 1997;100:2961-9.

99. Carbone A, Gloghini A, Gattei V, Aldinucci D, Degan M, De Paoli P, et al. Expression of functional CD40 antigen on Reed-Sternberg cells and Hodgkin's disease cell lines. Blood. 1995;85:780-9.

100. Chiu A, Xu W, He B, Dillon SR, Gross JA, Sievers E, et al. Hodgkin lymphoma cells express TACI and BCMA receptors and generate survival and proliferation signals in response to BAFF and APRIL. Blood. 2007;109:729-39.

101. Fiumara P, Snell V, Li Y, Mukhopadhyay A, Younes M, Gillenwater AM, et al. Functional expression of receptor activator of nuclear factor kappaB in Hodgkin disease cell lines. Blood. 2001;98:2784-90.

102. Molin D, Fischer M, Xiang Z, Larsson U, Harvima I, Venge P, et al. Mast cells express functional CD30 ligand and are the predominant CD30L-positive cells in Hodgkin's disease. Br J Haematol. 2001;114:616-23.

103. Schwab U, Stein H, Gerdes J, Lemke H, Kirchner H, Schaadt M, et al. Production of a monoclonal antibody specific for Hodgkin and Sternberg-Reed cells of Hodgkin's disease and a subset of normal lymphoid cells. Nature. 1982;299:65-7.

104. Hirsch B, Hummel M, Bentink S, Fouladi F, Spang R, Zollinger R, et al. CD30-induced signaling is absent in Hodgkin's cells but present in anaplastic large cell lymphoma cells. Am J Pathol. 2008;172:510-20.

105. Horie R, Watanabe T, Morishita Y, Ito K, Ishida T, Kanegae Y, et al. Ligand-independent signaling by overexpressed CD30 drives NF-kappaB activation in Hodgkin-Reed-Sternberg cells. Oncogene. 2002;21:2493-503.

106. Kilger E, Kieser A, Baumann M, Hammerschmidt W. Epstein-Barr virus-mediated B-cell proliferation is dependent upon latent membrane protein 1, which simulates an activated CD40 receptor. EMBO J. 1998;17:1700-9.

107. Baus D, Pfitzner E. Specific function of STAT3, SOCS1, and SOCS3 in the regulation of proliferation and survival of classical Hodgkin lymphoma cells. Int J Cancer. 2006;118:1404-13.

108. Kube D, Holtick U, Vockerodt M, Ahmadi T, Behrmann I, Heinrich PC, et al. STAT3 is constitutively activated in Hodgkin cell lines. Blood. 2001;98:762-70.

109. Skinnider BF, Elia AJ, Gascoyne RD, Patterson B, Trümper L, Kapp U, et al. Signal transducer and activator of transcription 6 is frequently activated in Hodgkin and Reed-Sternberg cells of Hodgkin lymphoma. Blood. 2002; 99:618-26.

110. Kapp U, Yeh WC, Patterson B, Elia AJ, Kagi D, Ho A, et al. Interleukin 13 is secreted by and stimulates the growth of Hodgkin and Reed-Sternberg cells. J Exp Med. 1999;189:1939-46.

111. Skinnider BF, Elia AJ, Gascoyne RD, Trumper LH, von Bonin F, Kapp U, et al. Interleukin 13 and interleukin 13 receptor are frequently expressed by Hodgkin and Reed-Sternberg cells of Hodgkin lymphoma. Blood. 2001;97:250-5.

112. Hinz M, Lemke P, Anagnostopoulos I, Hacker C, Krappmann D, Mathas S, et al. Nuclear factor kappaB-dependent gene expression profiling of Hodgkin's disease tumor cells, pathogenetic significance, and link to constitutive signal transducer and activator of transcription 5a activity. J Exp Med. 2002;196:605-17.

113. Lamprecht B, Kreher S, Anagnostopoulos I, Johrens K, Monteleone G, Jundt F, et al. Aberrant expression of the Th2 cytokine IL-21 in Hodgkin lymphoma cells regulates STAT3 signaling and attracts Treg cells via regulation of MIP-3{alpha}. Blood. 2008;112:3339-47.

114. Blume-Jensen P, Hunter T. Oncogenic kinase signalling. Nature. 2001;411:355-65.

115. Renné C, Willenbrock K, Küppers R, Hansmann M-L, Bräuninger A. Autocrine and paracrine activated receptor tyrosine kinases in classical Hodgkin lymphoma. Blood. 2005;105:4051-9.

116. Teofili L, Di Febo AL, Pierconti F, Maggiano N, Bendandi M, Rutella S, et al. Expression of the c-met proto-oncogene and its ligand, hepatocyte growth factor, in Hodgkin disease. Blood. 2001;97:1063-9.

117. Renné C, Willenbrock K, Martin-Subero JI, Hinsch N, Döring C, Tiacci E, et al. High expression of several tyrosine kinases and activation of the PI3K/AKT pathway in mediastinal large B cell lymphoma reveals further similarities to Hodgkin lymphoma. Leukemia. 2007;21:780-7.

118. Renné C, Hinsch N, Willenbrock K, Fuchs M, Klapper W, Engert A, et al. The aberrant coexpression of several receptor tyrosine kinases is largely restricted to EBV-negative cases of classical Hodgkin's lymphoma. Int J Cancer. 2007;120:2504-9.

119. Renne C, Minner S, Küppers R, Hansmann ML, Bräuninger A. Autocrine NGFbeta/TRKA signalling is an important survival factor for Hodgkin lymphoma derived cell lines. Leuk Res. 2008;32:163-7.

120. Nagel S, Burek C, Venturini L, Scherr M, Quentmeier H, Meyer C, et al. Comprehensive analysis of homeobox genes in Hodgkin lymphoma cell lines identifies dysregulated expression of HOXB9 mediated via ERK5 signaling and BMI1. Blood. 2007;109:3015-23.

121. Zheng B, Fiumara P, Li YV, Georgakis G, Snell V, Younes M, et al. MEK/ERK pathway is aberrantly active in Hodgkin disease: a signaling pathway shared by CD30, CD40, and RANK that regulates cell proliferation and survival. Blood. 2003;102:1019-27.

122. Mathas S, Hinz M, Anagnostopoulos I, Krappmann D, Lietz A, Jundt F, et al. Aberrantly expressed c-Jun and JunB are a hallmark of Hodgkin lymphoma cells, stimulate proliferation and synergize with NF-kappa B. EMBO J. 2002;21: 4104-13.

123. Juszczynski P, Ouyang J, Monti S, Rodig SJ, Takeyama K, Abramson J, et al. The AP1-dependent secretion of galectin-1 by Reed Sternberg cells fosters immune privilege in classical Hodgkin lymphoma. Proc Natl Acad Sci USA. 2007;104:13134-9.

124. Watanabe M, Ogawa Y, Ito K, Higashihara M, Kadin ME, Abraham LJ, et al. AP-1 mediated relief of repressive activity of the CD30 promoter microsatellite in Hodgkin and Reed-Sternberg cells. Am J Pathol. 2003;163:633-41.

125. Dutton A, Reynolds GM, Dawson CW, Young LS, Murray PG. Constitutive activation of phosphatidyl-inositide 3 kinase contributes to the survival of Hodgkin's lymphoma cells through a mechanism involving Akt kinase and mTOR. J Pathol. 2005;205:498-506.

126. Georgakis GV, Li Y, Rassidakis GZ, Medeiros LJ, Mills GB, Younes A. Inhibition of the phosphatidylinositol-3 kinase/Akt promotes G1 cell cycle arrest and apoptosis in Hodgkin lymphoma. Br J Haematol. 2006;132:503-11.

127. Dutton A, O'Neil JD, Milner AE, Reynolds GM, Starczynski J, Crocker J, et al. Expression of the cellular FLICE-inhibitory protein (c-FLIP) protects Hodgkin's lymphoma cells from autonomous Fas-mediated death. Proc Natl Acad Sci USA. 2004;101:6611-6.

128. Mathas S, Lietz A, Anagnostopoulos I, Hummel F, Wiesner B, Janz M, et al. c-FLIP mediates resistance of Hodgkin/Reed-Sternberg cells to death receptor-induced apoptosis. J Exp Med. 2004;199:1041-52.

129. Re D, Hofmann A, Wolf J, Diehl V, Staratschek-Jox A. Cultivated H-RS cells are resistant to CD95L-mediated apoptosis despite expression of wild-type CD95. Exp Hematol. 2000;28:31-5.

130. Chu WS, Aguilera NS, Wei MQ, Abbondanzo SL. Antiapoptotic marker Bcl-X(L), expression on Reed-Sternberg cells of Hodgkin's disease using a novel monoclonal marker, YTH-2H12. Hum Pathol. 1999; 30:1065-70.

131. Kashkar H, Haefs C, Shin H, Hamilton-Dutoit SJ, Salvesen GS, Krönke M, et al. XIAP-mediated caspase inhibition in Hodgkin's lymphoma-derived B cells. J Exp Med. 2003; 198:341-7.

132. Kashkar H, Seeger JM, Hombach A, Deggerich A, Yazdanpanah B, Utermohlen O, et al. XIAP targeting sensitizes Hodgkin lymphoma cells for cytolytic T-cell attack. Blood. 2006;108:3434-40.

133. Sanchez-Beato M, Piris MA, Martinez-Montero JC, Garcia JF, Villuendas R, Garcia FJ, et al. MDM2 and p21WAF1/CIP1, wild-type p53-induced proteins, are regularly expressed by Sternberg-Reed cells in Hodgkin's disease. J Pathol. 1996;180:58-64.

134. Drakos E, Thomaides A, Medeiros LJ, Li J, Leventaki V, Konopleva M, et al. Inhibition of p53-murine double minute 2 interaction by nutlin-3A stabilizes p53 and induces cell cycle arrest and apoptosis in Hodgkin lymphoma. Clin Cancer Res. 2007;13:3380-7.

135. Janz M, Stuhmer T, Vassilev LT, Bargou RC. Pharmacologic activation of p53-dependent and p53-independent apoptotic pathways in Hodgkin/Reed-Sternberg cells. Leukemia. 2007;21:772-9.

# Microenvironment, Cross-Talk, and Immune Escape Mechanisms

**4**

Lydia Visser, Anke van den Berg, Sibrand Poppema, and Arjan Diepstra

## Contents

L. Visser, A. van den Berg, S. Poppema,
and A. Diepstra (✉)
Department of Pathology and Medical Biology, University
Medical Center Groningen, University of Groningen,
Groningen, The Netherlands
e-mail: a.diepstra@path.umcg.nl

## 4.1 Microenvironment

### 4.1.1 Hodgkin Lymphoma Subtypes

When discussing the microenvironment in Hodgkin lymphoma (HL), it is important to recognize the different HL subtypes described by the WHO classification [1, 2]. In fact, the classical HL (cHL) subtypes are defined in large part by the composition of the reactive infiltrate (Table 4.1). The most prevalent subtype is the nodular sclerosis type that consists of a nodular background with thick fibrotic bands, usually with a thickened lymph node capsule. In addition to the lacunar type of Hodgkin/Reed–Sternberg (HRS) cells there is a microenvironment consisting of T cells, eosinophils, and histiocytes, with a variable admixture of neutrophils, plasma cells, fibroblasts, and mast cells. The second most common subtype is mixed cellularity, which is defined by the presence of typical HRS cells and a diffuse infiltrate of T cells, eosinophils, histiocytes, and plasma cells, sometimes with the formation of granuloma-like clusters or granulomas (Fig. 4.1). Lymphocyte-rich cHL also comprises typical HRS cells in a nodular or diffuse microenvironment and small B and/or T lymphocytes dominating the background, sometimes with admixture of histiocytes. Granulocytes are not a component in this subtype. The rare lymphocyte depleted subtype harbors a high percentage of HRS cells in a background consisting of fibroblasts and a low number of T cells. Nodular lymphocyte predominance (NLP) HL is considered a separate entity. The morphology may closely resemble that of the nodular variant of the classical lymphocyte rich subtype, both involving follicular areas with many small B cells. However, the nature of the tumor cells and the T cells is different. In the cHL subtypes, the

A. Engert and S.J. Horning (eds.), *Hodgkin Lymphoma*,
DOI: 10.1007/978-3-642-12780-9_4, © Springer-Verlag Berlin Heidelberg 2011

**Table 4.1** Composition of the microenvironment in different Hodgkin lymphoma (HL) subtypes

| Subtype | EBV (%) | Background | T cells | Other cells |
| --- | --- | --- | --- | --- |
| Nodular sclerosis | 10–40 | Nodular + fibrosis | CD4 > CD8, Th2, Treg > Th1 | Eosinophils, histiocytes, fibroblasts, B cells, mast cells, (neutrophils) |
| Mixed cellularity | 75 | Diffuse | CD4 > CD8, Th2,Treg > Th1 | Eosinophils, histiocytes, plasma cells, B cells |
| Lymphocyte rich | 40–80 | Nodular or diffuse | CD4 > CD8 | Histiocytes |
| Lymphocyte depleted (including HIV+) | 80–100 | Diffuse | – | Fibroblasts |
| Nodular lymphocyte predominant | 0 | Nodular (+diffuse) | Th2, CD57+ Treg, CD4+/8+ | Histiocytes, B cells |

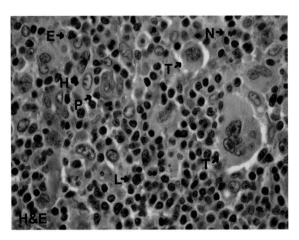

**Fig. 4.1** The microenvironment in classical Hodgkin lymphoma (HL). Histology of a classical HL (mixed cellularity subtype). *T* tumor cell; *L* (T–)lymphocyte; *H* histiocyte; *E* eosinophil; *N* neutrophil; *P* plasma cell. Hematoxylin and eosin staining

HRS cells are transformed B cells with an aberrant postgerminal center cell phenotype, while in LPHL the lymphocyte predominant (LP) cells are transformed B cells with a germinal center cell phenotype. Likewise, the T cells in cHL have features of paracortical T cells, while those in LPHL are similar to germinal center T cells [3, 4].

### 4.1.2 Epstein–Barr Virus

The presence of latent Epstein–Barr virus (EBV) genomes in HRS cells appears to influence the composition of the microenvironment. Positive EBV status is strongly associated with the mixed cellularity subtype (~75% EBV+) and by definition is absent in LPHL.

Depending on the geographic locale, EBV is present in the HRS cells in 10–40% in nodular sclerosis cases. The percentage of EBV+ classical lymphocyte rich cases is not very clear, but probably between 40 and 80%. EBV infects more than 90% of the world population and establishes a lifelong latent infection in B cells in its host. Potent cytotoxic immune responses keep the number of EBV infected B cells at approximately 1/100,000 B cells and usually prevents EBV-driven malignant transformation in immunocompetent individuals. Accordingly, EBV-associated cHL cases contain slightly more CD8+ cytotoxic T cells in the reactive background compared to non-EBV-associated cHL cases [5].

### 4.1.3 T Cell Subsets in cHL

A unifying feature of the reactive infiltrate in virtually all cHL subtypes is the presence of large amounts of CD4+ T cells. Besides being widely distributed in the background, these CD4+ T cells form a tight rosette around the tumor cells. T cells within these rosettes often have a distinct phenotype, different from the phenotype of the T cells that are located further away from the cHL tumor cells (Fig. 4.2).

In general, CD4+ T cells can be divided into naïve (CD45RA+) and memory (CD45RO+) subsets depending on whether they have previously been stimulated by antigen. A large subset of CD4+ T cells consists of the so-called helper T (Th) cells; these cells play an important role in helping other cells to induce an effective immune response. Th cells can be further divided into Th0 (naive), Th1 (cellular response), Th2 (humoral

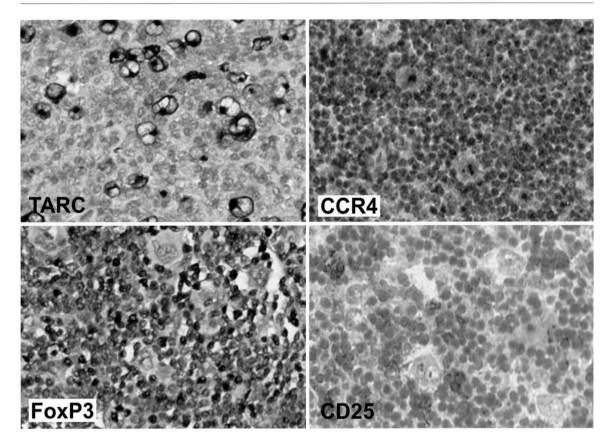

**Fig. 4.2** Shaping the microenvironment in classical Hodgkin lymphoma (HL). Immunohistochemistry of classical HL cases. In the *upper panel left*, strong and specific staining of Hodgkin/Reed–Sternberg (HRS) cells for chemokine CCL17 (TARC). This chemokine attracts CCR4+ lymphocytes (*upper panel right*). A large proportion of reactive T cells are Treg cells, as shown by positive staining for transcription factor FoxP3 (*lower panel left*) and activation marker CD25 (*lower panel right*)

response), Th17 (IL-17 producing), and Treg (regulating other responses) cells. The Treg cells can be further divided into Th3 (transforming growth factor-β (TGF-β)-producing), Tr1 (IL-10-producing), and CD4+CD25+ Treg (originating from the thymus) subpopulations. Some, but not all, Treg cells express the transcription factor FoxP3.

The T cells in cHL consist mainly of CD4+ T cells that have a memory phenotype (CD45RO+) and express several activation markers including CD28, CD38, CD69, CD71, CD25, and HLA-DR, as well as markers like CD28, CTLA-4, PD-1, and CD40L. However, these T cells lack expression of CD26 [6]. This lack of CD26 expression is most striking in the areas surrounding the tumor cells. CD26, dipeptidyl peptidase IV, regulates proteolytic processing of several chemokines, e.g., CCL5 (Rantes), CCL11 (Eotaxin), CCL22 (MDC)

[7]. CD26 is also associated with adenosine deaminase (ADA) and with CD45RO and when interacting with anti-CD26 antibodies leads to enhancement of T cell activation through the T cell receptor [8]. CD26 is preferentially expressed on CD4+CD45RO+ cells and is normally upregulated after activation. However, CD26 cannot be upregulated on the CD26-negative cells from cHL lesions. In general, a high CD26 expression level correlates with a Th1 subtype of cells.

The transcription factor expression pattern indicates that the CD4+ T cells in cHL are predominantly Th2 (c-Maf) and Treg (FoxP3) [3, 9]. The CD4+CD26– T cell subset in cHL has reduced mRNA levels of Th1- and Th2-associated cytokines in comparison to the CD4+CD26+ T cells from cHL and CD4+ T cells (both CD26– and CD26+) in reactive lymph nodes [10]. Based on much higher mRNA expression levels of

IL-2RA (CD25), CCR4, FoxP3, CTLA4, TNFRSF4 (OX-40), and TNFRSF18 (GITR) observed in the CD4+CD26− T cells from cHL, it has been postulated that these cells have a Treg phenotype (Fig. 4.2). In addition, mildly enhanced IL-17 levels can be observed both in CD4+CD26− and CD4+CD26+ T cells from cHL in comparison to the T cells from tonsil. Upon stimulation, the CD4+CD26− T cells fail to induce expression of cytokines, suggesting that the T cell population rosetting around the HRS cells or located in the direct vicinity of the HRS cells have an anergic phenotype [10]. Immunohistochemistry for several Treg-associated molecules demonstrates that the rosetting T cells in cHL express GITR, CCR4, and CD25, but not FoxP3. Scattered FoxP3-positive cells are present in the infiltrate but only rarely in the direct vicinity of the HRS cells, and CTLA-4 shows a more diffuse presence [10]. Likewise, a small number of scattered IL-17-positive cells can be found in the reactive infiltrate. Anergy in T cells is normally induced by lack of costimulation through CD80/CD86, activation by superantigens, or the effect of cytokines like TGF-β and IL-10. The anergic state in cHL is probably not caused by the lack of costimulatory molecules since CD80 and CD86 as well as several other costimulatory molecules are highly expressed on the HRS cells [11, 75]. However, the surrounding lymphocytes express CTLA-4 as well as CD28, where as TGF-β and IL-10 are frequently produced by HRS cells and may cause anergy of the surrounding T cells.

### 4.1.4 T Cell Subsets in LPHL

The CD4+ T cells in LPHL resemble the CD4+ T cells in cHL, regarding the expression of CD45RO, CD69, CTLA4, CD28, PD-1, and lack of CD26. However, these T cells do not express CD40L and a significant proportion of the cells that immediately surround the LP cells express CD57. Similar to the Th2 cells in cHL, the rosetting cells in LPHL strongly express the Th2-associated transcription factor c-Maf (Fig. 4.3; [3]).

Characterization of the CD4+CD57+ T cell subset shows lack of IL-2 and IL-4 mRNA, but elevated interferon-γ (IFN-γ) mRNA levels in comparison to CD57+ T cells from tonsil. Stimulation of these cells fails to induce upregulation of IL-2 and IL-4 mRNA levels [12], which is similar to the lack of cytokine induction upon stimulation of the CD26− T cells in cHL. The normal counterpart of CD4+CD57+ T cells is found almost exclusively in the light zone of reactive germinal centers. These CD57+ T cells also lack CD40L expression. CD57 is known as an activation marker but it has also been demonstrated to be a marker for senescent cells. Senescence is the phenomenon by which normal diploid cells lose the ability to divide, normally after about 50 cell divisions.

In LPHL, a population of CD4+CD8+ T cells has been reported in more than 50% of patients. The function of these cells in LPHL is currently unknown, but in other settings these cells play immunoregulatory roles [13].

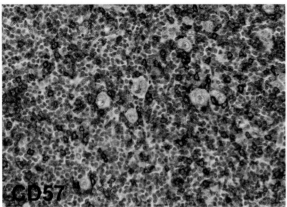 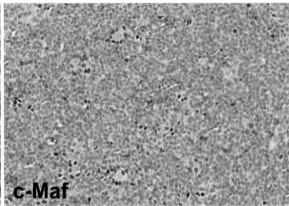

**Fig. 4.3** T cells in nodular lymphocyte predominant Hodgkin lymphoma (HL). Immunohistochemistry of a case of nonclassical nodular lymphocyte predominant HL. A variable but usually high amount of reactive T cells express CD57 and as in this case these cells can encircle the tumor cells (*panel left*). The CD57+ T cells also express transcription factor c-Maf, indicating a Th2-type nature (*panel right*)

## 4.1.5 Fibrosis and Sclerosis

The presence of bands of collagen surrounding nodules and blood vessels are typical of the nodular sclerosis subtype. Several factors can induce the activation of fibroblasts and the subsequent deposition of extracellular matrix proteins. The Th2 cells in cHL might provide a profibrogenic microenvironment by the production of the Th2 cytokine IL-13. IL-13 is expressed at a higher level in nodular sclerosis than in mixed cellularity cHL. Moreover, also the percentage of IL-13 receptor positive fibroblasts is increased in nodular sclerosis cHL cases [14]. IL-13 stimulates collagen synthesis in vitro and also stimulates the production of TGF-β, another potent stimulator of fibrosis. TGF-β can interact with basic fibroblast growth factor (bFGF) to cause fibrosis in cHL. In a mouse model for fibrosis, the simultaneous application of TGF-β and bFGF causes persistent fibrosis [15]. Since both TGF-β and bFGF are produced by the HRS cells as well as the reactive background [16, 17], this can cause fibrosis in cHL. TGF-β and bFGF are both produced more prominently in nodular sclerosis than in mixed cellularity cHL [18], which is consistent with this concept. The third factor that stimulates fibroblasts in cHL is the engagement of CD40. CD40, a member of the tumor necrosis factor receptor (TNFR) superfamily, can be upregulated on fibroblasts by IFN-γ, and its ligand CD40L is present on activated T cells, mast cells, and eosinophils present in the cHL microenvironment.

## 4.1.6 Eosinophils, Plasma Cells, and Mast Cells

Presence of eosinophils in the reactive infiltrate can be promoted by both IL-5, produced by Th2 cells, and by IL-9. In cHL patients with eosinophilia in the peripheral blood, IL-5 and IL-9 have been reported to be expressed by the HRS cells [19]. In addition, eosinophils are attracted to cHL tissues by the production of the chemokine CCL11, especially in nodular sclerosis cHL. CCL11 levels can be enhanced by the production of tumor necrosis factor-α (TNF-α) by the HRS cells, which in turn can induce CCL11 production in fibroblasts. This process is specific for cHL since other lymphomas with tissue eosinophilia show no expression of CCL11 [20]. HRS cells also produce CCL28 (MEC), and expression of CCL28 correlates with the presence of eosinophils and plasma cells in cHL. CCL28 attracts eosinophils by signaling through the chemokine receptor CCR3 and attracts plasma cells through CCR10 [21]. CCL5 is produced at high levels by the reactive infiltrate in cHL and can attract eosinophils as well as mast cells. CCL5 and IL-9 may both contribute to the attraction of mast cells in cHL [22]. The stimulation and recruitment of eosinophils in cHL can be illustrated in staging bone marrow biopsies that often show reactive enhancement of granulopoiesis with many eosinophils, although there are no HRS cells present in the bone marrow. Finally, IL-6 has been shown to be produced by HRS cells in some cases of cHL, and this may explain the presence of variable amounts of plasma cells [23]

## 4.2 Cross-Talk Between HRS Cells and Microenvironment (Fig. 4.4)

## 4.2.1 Clinical Findings

HRS cells shape their environment by attracting specific T cell populations that provide growth supporting factors and by suppressing an effective antitumor response of the immune system. In patients with an impaired immune response, cHL occurs more frequently. After solid organ transplantation, there is a small increase in the incidence of cHL that can largely be attributed to EBV-positive cHL. HIV-infected individuals have an approximate 10 times increased risk of developing cHL [24]. In comparison to non-HIV-associated cHL, these tumors are more often EBV-associated, mixed cellularity, and lymphocyte depletion subtypes and usually contain more tumor cells. This indicates a functional defect in the immune response, in particular to EBV, presumably caused by the impairment of CD4+ T cells by HIV. On the other hand, the importance of CD4+ T cells for supporting the growth of HRS cells is also illustrated in HIV-positive patients, because an increase in HIV-associated cHL incidence has been observed after the introduction of highly active antiretroviral therapy (HAART) [25] (Fig. 4.4).

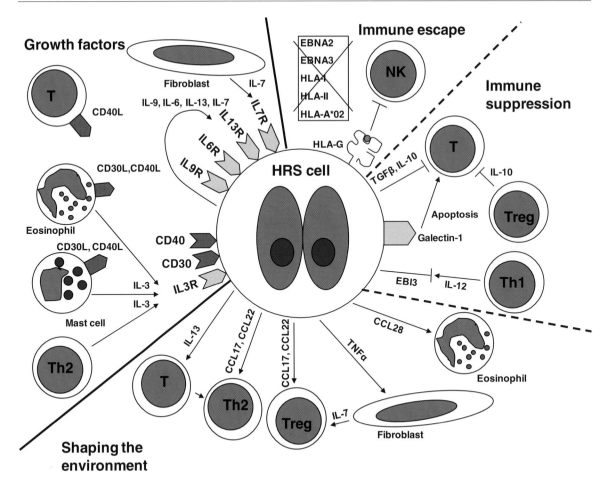

**Fig. 4.4** Schematic overview of the cross-talk between Hodgkin Reed–Sternberg (HRS) cells and the microenvironment. Hodgkin lymphoma tumor cells attract specific cell subsets by chemokines, are dependent on growth factors, and use mechanisms of immune suppression and immune escape. *Arrows* indicate stimulating effects; the other lines indicate inhibitory effects

## 4.2.2 Factors Supporting Tumor Growth

It is likely that HL tumor cells originate from a precursor B cell that has become addicted to activating and growth-supporting stimuli during a deregulated immune response. Many additional events are needed to account for the highly deregulated malignant phenotype of HRS and LP cells. Although the tumor cells attain multiple alternative mechanisms to circumvent the dependence on growth-stimulating signals from the reactive infiltrate, they usually are not self-sufficient at the time of diagnosis. This is reflected by the inability to grow cell lines from primary HL cell suspensions.

IL-3 can function as a growth factor for B cells and is produced by activated Th2 cells, mast cells, and eosinophils. Its functions include protection against apoptosis and stimulation of proliferation. Most HRS cells in cHL cases express the IL-3 receptor, and exogenous IL-3 promotes cell growth in cHL cell lines. Costimulation of IL-3 with IL-9 results in further enhancement of cell growth [26]. There is no evidence for the production of IL-3 by HRS cells themselves, so this signaling pathway depends on the reactive infiltrate. IL-7 is most likely an autocrine as well as a paracrine growth factor for HRS cells, since HRS cells express both the IL-7 receptor and produce IL-7 [27]. Moreover, fibroblasts isolated from cHL tissue are also able to produce IL-7 [28]. cHL cell lines produce very little IL-7 themselves, but anti-IL-7 has some effect on cell growth. Addition of IL-7 results in an increase in proliferation and protection against apoptosis. Other growth factors important for HRS cells are IL-9, IL-13, and, possibly, IL-6. IL-9 is expressed by the tumor cells and not in the infiltrate, and the IL-9 receptor is expressed on the tumor cells and mast cells. IL-9 supports tumor growth in cell lines and is an autocrine factor in cHL tissue [22]. IL-13 produced by HRS cells as well as the surrounding T cells drives proliferation and is mostly autocrine [29]. IL-6 is mainly produced by the HRS cells and occasionally in the infiltrate [23]. In general, IL-6 is found at higher levels in EBV+ cases [30]. IL-6 might have an autocrine effect although neutralizing antibodies have no effect on the growth of the cHL cell lines.

HRS cells express several members of the TNFR superfamily including CD30, which has been used as a marker for cHL since the early 1980s. The CD30 ligand (CD30L) is expressed on eosinophils [31] and mast cells [32] that are present in the cHL infiltrate. Circulating eosinophils in cHL patients also have increased expression levels of CD30L [31]. Binding of CD30L to CD30 causes enhanced secretion of IL-6, TNFα, lymphotoxin-α, increased expression of ICAM-1 and B7, and, possibly, increased clonogenic growth and protection against apoptosis [33]. Another TNFR expressed on HRS cells is CD40. CD40 is generally found on B cells, and B cells can be activated through CD40. In vitro rosetting of activated CD4+ lymphocytes around HRS cells is mediated through the CD40L adhesion pathway [34]. Engagement of CD40 is important for the prevention of apoptosis. Similar to stimulation of CD30, stimulation of HRS cell lines with CD40L causes enhanced secretion of several cytokines and upregulation of costimulatory molecules [33].

### 4.2.3 Shaping the Environment

In addition to the production of several growth factors, HRS cells also produce large amounts of chemokines to attract specific beneficial or nonreacting cells. The lack of CD26 on the T cells surrounding the HRS cells may result in an incapability to cleave the chemokines and thereby modulate the chemotactic effects exerted by the HRS cells. The attraction of a specific population of cells is an important immune escape mechanism exerted by the tumor cells.

The most abundant and cHL-specific chemokine is CCL17 (TARC); it binds to CCR4 and CCR8 on Th2 cells, Treg cells, basophils, and monocytes. CCL17 is highly expressed by HRS cells in the vast majority of cHL patients and not in LPHL or non-Hodgkin lymphomas [35, 36]. CCL17 levels can be measured in serum and are a sensitive and specific marker reflecting cHL tumor burden [37, 38]. High expression levels of CCL17 might explain the influx of lymphocytes with a Th2- and Treg-like phenotype, and CCL17-positive cases are indeed associated with a higher percentage of CCR4-positive cells (Fig. 4.2; [36, 39]). In turn, Th2-type cytokines (IL-4, IL-13) can induce the production of CCL17 by HRS cells. CCR4-positive lymphocytes are found especially in the rosettes immediately surrounding the HRS cells [10, 40]. CCL22 is another chemokine that has a similar function as CCL17. High CCL22 protein expression levels were found in the cytoplasm of HRS cells in 90–100% of cHL patients and also in tumor cells in the majority of LPHL and non-HL patients [41–44]. CCL22 production can also be stimulated by Th2 cytokines, IL-4 and IL-13, and may serve to reinforce the attraction of Th2 and Treg lymphocytes, initiated by CCL17. Stimulation of the IL-21 receptor on HRS by IL-21 activates STAT3, which can induce CCL20 (MIP3α) production. CCL20 in turn attracts memory T cells and Treg cells [45]. HRS cells express both IL-21 and the IL-21 receptor, indicating presence of an autocrine signaling loop. The expression of some chemokines is more pronounced in EBV+ cHL (i.e., CXCL9 and CXCL10), and perhaps as a result the composition of the reactive background is somewhat different from that in EBV− cHL, with a slightly higher proportion of CD8+ T cells in EBV+ cases.

In addition to attracting specific cell subsets by chemotaxis, HRS cells also shape their environment by inducing differentiation of specific T cell subsets that are favorable for HRS cell survival and growth. The expression of IL-13 by the HRS cells stimulates differentiation of naïve T cells to Th2 cells [29]. The production of IL-7 by HRS cells and fibroblasts can induce proliferation of Tregs [28]. Also, cHL cell lines with antigen-presenting functions like KMH2 and L428 have been shown to promote the differentiation of Treg like cells in vitro (expressing CD4, CD25, FoxP3, CTLA4 and GITR and producing large amounts of IL-10). Interestingly, these cell lines can also induce the formation of CD4+ cytotoxic cells (expressing granzyme B and TIA-1) that can kill tumor cells directly, suggesting that CD4+ CTLs have the potential to attack tumor cells in vivo [46].

### 4.2.4 Immune Suppression

Because normal B cells are professional antigen-presenting cells, HRS cells are expected to present antigens to the immune system, at least early in disease pathogenesis. Indeed, most components of the HLA class I and HLA class II antigen-presenting pathways have been detected in the HRS cells at the time of diagnosis. However, at that time Th1 cells are not actively attracted by the HRS cells and CD8+ CTLs are relatively scarce. Moreover, HRS cells have gained the capacity to prevent CTLs from attacking by producing high amounts of the strongly immunosuppressive cytokines TGF-β and IL-10. TGF-β is produced by HRS cells in nodular sclerosis cHL [16, 17] whereas IL-10 is more frequently found in EBV+ (mixed cellularity) cHL [47, 48]. In normal cells, TGF-β is produced in an inactive form, which can be activated by acidification. TGF-β produced by cHL cell line L428 is active at a physiological pH and has a high molecular weight [49]. The same high molecular weight form of TGF-β can also be found in the urine of cHL patients [50] indicating that in patients HRS cells are able to produce the active TGF-β form.

The Tregs that are present in the microenvironment of cHL are highly immunosuppressive and contain Tr1 (IL-10 producing Tregs) as well as CD4+CD25+ Tregs. IL-10, cell–cell contact, and CTLA4 play a main role in executing their immunosuppressive function [51]. In addition, HRS cells express galectin-1, an animal lectin, which can cause apoptosis in activated T cells, and contributes to the elimination of an effective antitumor response in cHL [52]. HRS cells also express FAS and the FAS ligand. There are some mechanisms protecting the HRS cells from apoptosis induction, such as FAS mutations in a small proportion of cases and c-FLIP overexpression in all cases [53]. On the other hand, activated Th1 and CD8 cells expressing FAS would be driven to apoptosis by the FAS ligand expression on the HRS cells. Also, HRS cells were found to express PD-1 ligand whereas the rosetting lymphocytes are PD-1 positive [54]. In EBV+ cHL, the Th1-inducing cytokine IL-12 is expressed in T cells surrounding the HRS cells, and its presence suggests that these T cells have the potential to induce antitumor activity [55]. However, an EBV-induced IL-12-related cytokine called EBI3 can block this Th1 response and is produced by HRS cells [56]. Another immune suppressive mechanism in EBV+ cHL might be the release of anergy-inducing exosomes containing the EBV latent membrane protein 1 (LMP1), galectin-9, and HLA class II. These exosomes have been shown in EBV-associated lymphoblastoid and nasopharyngeal carcinoma cell lines; however, it is unknown whether they are also secreted in EBV+ cHL [57].

## 4.3 Immune Escape Mechanisms (Fig. 4.4)

### 4.3.1 Antigen Presentation

The importance of antigen presentation in the pathogenesis of cHL has been suggested by the association of specific HLA subtypes with increased cHL incidence. cHL is more common in Caucasians as compared to Asians and about 4.5% of cHL cases occur in families [58, 59]. A three to sevenfold increased risk has been observed in first degree relatives and siblings. In monozygotic twins, the cotwin has an approximate 100-fold increased risk of developing cHL compared to dizygotic twins [60]. From the 1970s, a number of serological HLA types have been associated with the occurrence of cHL. More recently, a genetic screen of the entire HLA region showed a strong association between the *HLA-A* gene and EBV+ cHL. This association was not present in EBV− cHL [61, 62]. It can be hypothesized that this association is related to insufficient presentation of EBV antigenic peptides. These antigenic peptides most likely are derived from the latency type II genes that are expressed in cHL, i.e., LMP1, LMP2, and EBV-related nuclear antigen 1 (EBNA1). EBV partially escapes cytotoxic immune responses by downregulating immunodominant latent genes (*EBNA2* and *EBNA3*). In addition, the glycine–alanine repeat in EBNA1 largely prevents its presentation by HLA class I by blocking its degradation into antigenic peptides through the proteasome [63]. However, subdominant immune responses to LMP2 and to a lesser extent LMP1 are present in the healthy EBV-infected population [64]. In fact, adoptive immunotherapy in relapsed EBV-associated cHL has been used in some small studies with success, although limited. In these studies, peripheral blood from cHL patients was used to create EBV-specific cytotoxic T cell lines in vitro and these were reinfused. Some objective responses were observed (3/11 and 5/6), with better responses if the CTLs were specifically targeted to LMP2 [65, 66] (Fig. 4.4).

Interestingly, the genetic association of the *HLA-A* gene with EBV+ cHL is attributed to the presence of the HLA-A*01 type and absence of the HLA-A*02 type [67]. HLA-A*01 is known to have a low affinity for LMP2- and LMP1-derived antigenic peptides, while HLA-A*02 can present these peptides very well. This suggests that EBV+ cHL is more likely to occur after primary EBV infection if an individual's set of HLA class I molecules cannot properly present LMP2 and LMP1 to the immune system. In fact, the HLA polymorphisms associated with EBV+ cHL have also been shown to be related to the occurrence of infectious mononucleosis [68]. Individuals who have had infectious mononucleosis have a three times increased risk of developing EBV+ cHL [69]. It is unknown to what extent the HLA-A*01-associated increased risk is due to an increase in latently EBV-infected B cells (HRS cell "precursors") or to decreased effectiveness of antitumor cell immune responses.

## 4.3.2  HLA Expression

Paradoxically, HLA class I and class II expression by HRS cells is usually retained in EBV+ cHL patients, whereas in EBV− cHL patients these molecules are frequently downregulated. Defects in the antigen-presenting pathways are very common in solid malignancies (HLA class I), as well as in many B cell lymphomas (HLA class I and class II) and are an obvious mechanism to escape from antitumor immune responses. Especially downregulation of HLA class I is a common immune escape mechanism in EBV− cHL, with less than 20% of cases still expressing cell surface HLA class I on the HRS cells at the time of diagnosis [70]. Different mechanisms are involved in this downregulation because immunohistochemistry has shown complete absence of HLA class I or retention of HLA class I heavy chains within the cytoplasm. This retention in the cytoplasm is usually accompanied by an absence of β2-microglobulin expression, which is necessary for HLA class I assembly and transport to the

cell surface. The different mechanisms may indicate that downregulation of HLA class I is based on clonal selection by continuous cytotoxic immune responses. This may be related to the presence of antigenic peptides that are related to malignant transformation or disease progression. However, downregulation of HLA class I generally induces activation of natural killer (NK) cells. These cells contain HLA class I specific inhibitory receptors and are sparse in the reactive infiltrate of cHL. The inhibitory receptors can also be engaged by a nonclassical HLA class I like molecule known as HLA-G. In about two thirds of HLA class I negative cHL cases, the HRS cells indeed express HLA-G [76]. Besides NK cell inhibition, HLA-G might also induce Treg cells and inhibit cytotoxic T cell responses.

### 4.3.2.1  HLA Class I Expression

In contrast to EBV− cHL, 70–80% of EBV+ cHL patients show cell surface expression of HLA class I and β2-microglobulin at the time of diagnosis. This expression is usually particularly strong in mixed cellularity subtype cases [5, 70]. Upregulation of HLA class I and HLA class II expression has been attributed to LMP1, but the function of this upregulation is enigmatic, since it should make latent EBV-infected B cells more susceptible to immune recognition. In fact, in primary lytic EBV infection, HLA class I and HLA class II antigen-presenting pathways are strongly inhibited by EBV proteins. BNFL2a prevents peptide loading of HLA class I molecules by inhibiting the transporter of antigenic peptides (TAP). Viral IL-10 also downregulates the expression of TAP1. In addition, viral IL-10 downregulates the low molecular protein bli/LMP2, which is a subunit of the immunoproteasome (not to be mistaken for the EBV LMP2 protein). BGLF5 inhibits the synthesis of new HLA class I molecules and BILF1 downregulates HLA class I at the cell surface by inducing its endocytosis and subsequent lysosomal degradation. HLA class II function is inhibited by gp42/gH/gL, BGLF5, and viral IL-10 [71]. When the virus goes into latent infection, these immune escape mechanisms are no longer available. As the lytic gene products are switched off, the expression and function of HLA class I and class II are restored. Importantly, the cHL-associated EBV latent gene products LMP1,

LMP2, and EBNA1 are necessary for EBV-infected B cells to go through the germinal center reaction. At that time HLA class I and class II antigen-presenting functions might also be essential for B cell survival. It is generally accepted that HRS cells derive from germinal center B cells and in EBV+ cHL it is likely that the tumor cell precursor expresses LMP1, LMP2, EBNA1, HLA class I, and HLA class II.

### 4.3.2.2 HLA Class II Expression

HLA class II cell surface expression on HRS cells is lost in approximately 40% of all cHL patients. This absence is weakly related to extranodal disease, EBV-negative status, and absence of HLA class I cell surface expression. Lack of HLA class II expression has been associated with adverse failure free survival and relative survival, and is independent of other prognostic factors [70]. It can be hypothesized that antigen presentation in the context of HLA class II is involved in recruitment and activation of CD4+ T cells early in cHL pathogenesis. Under the influence of immunomodulating mechanisms, these T cells are important in providing trophic factors for HRS cells and also have a role in inhibiting Th1 responses. In the initial stages of cHL pathogenesis, HRS cells are probably highly dependent on the reactive infiltrate and expression of HLA class II, but as the lymphoma develops this dependency may weaken because of alternative trophic and immunosuppressive strategies. Thus, downregulation of HLA class II without loss of viability of HRS cells might occur when the HRS cells have grown less dependent on the reactive infiltrate. This is supported by the association of downregulation of HLA class II with extranodal disease [70].

## 4.4 Prognostic Impact of the Microenvironment

Several research groups studied the cHL reactive infiltrate in relation to prognosis. Patients with a higher degree of mast cell infiltration or with tissue eosinophilia have an adverse failure free survival, probably because the CD30L expression by these cell types is advantageous to the HRS cells [31, 32].

Large numbers of Th2 cells in the microenvironment, as determined by c-Maf expression, correlates with improved disease free survival [9]. Also, increased numbers of infiltrating Treg cells seem to correlate with improved survival as this effect was observed in two out of three studies [9, 72, 73]. Accordingly, a high percentage of activated CTLs (CD8+/granzyme B+ T cells) is a strong indicator of unfavorable clinical outcome [74]. A high ratio of FoxP3 to CTL markers, granzyme B [73] or Tia-1 [72], gives the best predictive value for a good prognosis. These results are unexpected since in other malignancies the presence of Tregs and the absence of CTLs is associated with adverse prognosis. One explanation might be that HRS cells are expected to behave more aggressively as they develop a stronger independency from the reactive infiltrate. In this situation a hostile microenvironment is allowed because the HRS cells have acquired alternative immunoevasive strategies. This theory fits with the adverse prognostic impact of absence of HLA class II expression.

## 4.5 Conclusion

The microenvironment is a fundamental component of the tumor mass and an essential pathogenetic factor in cHL and LPHL. It supplies the tumor cells with growth factors and inhibits antitumor immune responses. In fact, it could be stated that "the infiltrate consists not of 'innocent bystanders' but of 'guilty opportunists'" [22]. As the tumor cells and the reactive infiltrate grow up together, there is an extensive cross-talk between these two components. The tumor cells actively attract and shape their environment for their own benefit and make use of a number of mechanisms to fend off antitumor immune responses.

## References

1. Poppema S, Delsol G, Pileri SA, et al. Nodular lymphocyte predominant Hodgkin lymphoma. In: Swerdlow SH, Campo E, Harris NL, et al., editors. WHO classification of tumours of haematopoietic and lymphoid tissues. Lyon: IARC; 2008.
2. Stein H, Delsol G, Pileri SA, et al. Classical Hodgkin lymphoma, introduction. In: Swerdlow SH, Campo E, Harris NL, et al., editors. WHO classification of tumours of haematopoietic and lymphoid tissues. Lyon: IARC; 2008.

3. Atayar C, van den Berg A, Blokzijl T, et al. Hodgkin lymphoma associated T-cells exhibit a transcription factor profile consistent with distinct lymphoid compartments. J Clin Pathol. 2007;60:1092–7.

4. Carbone A, Gloghini A, Cabras A, et al. Differentiating germinal center-derived lymphomas through their cellular microenvironment. Am J Hematol. 2009;84:435–8.

5. Oudejans JJ, Jiwa NM, Kummer JA, et al. Analysis of major histocompatibility complex class I expression on Reed-Sterberg cells in relation to the cytotoxic T-cell response in Epstein–Barr virus-positive and -negative Hodgkin's disease. Blood. 1996;87:3844–51.

6. Poppema S. Immunology of Hodgkin's disease. Ballieres Clin Haematol. 1996;9:447–57.

7. Wolf M, Albrecht S, Marki C. Proteolytic processing of chemokines: implications in physiological and pathological conditions. Int J Biochem Cell Biol. 2008;40:1185–98.

8. Von Bonin A, Huhn J, Fleischer B. Dipeptidyl-peptidase IV/CD26 on T cells: analysis of an alternative T-cell activation pathway. Immunol Rev. 1998;161:43–53.

9. Schreck S, Friebel D, Buettner M, et al. Prognostic impact of tumour-infiltrating Th2 and regulatory cells in classical Hodgkin lymphoma. Hematol Oncol. 2009;27:31–9.

10. Ma Y, Visser L, Blokzijl T, et al. The CD4+CD26- T-cell population in classical Hodgkin's lymphoma displays a distinctive regulatory T-cell profile. Lab Invest. 2008;88:482–90.

11. Munro JM, Freedman AS, Aster JC, et al. In vivo expression of the B7 costimulatory molecule by subsets of antigen-presenting cells and the malignant cells of Hodgkin's disease. Blood. 1994;83:793–8.

12. Atayar C, Poppema S, Visser L, et al. Cytokine gene expression profile distinguishes CD4+/CD57+ T-cells of nodular lymphocyte predominance type of Hodgkin lymphoma from their tonsillar counterparts. J Pathol. 2006;208:423–30.

13. Rahemtullah A, Harris NL, Dorn ME, et al. Beyond the lymphocyte predominant cell: CD4+CD8+ T-cells in nodular lymphocyte predominant Hodgkin lymphoma. Leuk Lymphoma. 2008;49:1870–8.

14. Ohshima K, Akaiwa M, Umeshita R, et al. Interleukin-13 and interleukin-13 receptor in Hodgkin's disease: possible autocrine mechanism and involvement in fibrosis. Histopathology. 2001;38:368–75.

15. Shinozaki M, Kawara S, Hayashi N, et al. Induction of subcutaneous tissue fibrosis in newborn mice by transforming growth factor-b – simultaneous application with basic growth factor causes persistent fibrosis. Biochem Biophys Res Commun. 1997;237:292–6.

16. Kadin M, Butmarc J, Elovic A, et al. Eosinophils are the major source of transforming growth factor-beta 1 in nodular sclerosing Hodgkin's disease. Am J Pathol. 1993;142:11–6.

17. Newcom SR, Gu L. Transforming growth factor beta 1 messenger RNA in Reed–Sternberg cells in nodular sclerosing Hodgkin's disease. J Clin Pathol. 1995;48:160–3.

18. Ohshima K, Sugihara M, Suzumiya J, et al. Basic fibroblast growth factor and fibrosis in Hodgkin's disease. Pathol Res Pract. 1999;195:149–55.

19. Samoszuk M, Nansen L. Detection of interleukin-5 messenger RNA in Reed-Sernberg cells of Hodgkin's disease with eosinophilia. Blood. 1990;75:13–6.

20. Jundt F, Anagnostopoulos I, Bommert K, et al. Hodgkin/Reed–Sternberg cells induce fibroblasts to secrete eotaxin, a potent chemoattractant for T cells and eosinophils. Blood. 1999;94:2065–71.

21. Hanamoto H, Nakayama T, Miyazato H. Expression of CCL28 by Reed–Sternberg cells defines a major subtype of classical Hodgkin's disease with frequent infiltration of eosinophils and/or plasma cells. Am J Pathol. 2004;164:997–1006.

22. Glimelius I, Edstrom A, Amini RM, et al. IL-9 expression contributes to the cellular composition in Hodgkin lymphoma. Eur J Haematol. 2006;76:278–83.

23. Jucker M, Abts H, Li W, et al. Expression of interleukin-6 and interleukin-6 receptor in Hodgkin's disease. Blood. 1991;77:2413–8.

24. Goedert JJ, Cote TR, Virgo P, et al. Spectrum of AIDS-associated malignant disorders. Lancet. 1998;351:1833–9.

25. Biggar RJ, Jaffe ES, Goedert JJ, et al. Hodgkin lymphoma and immunodeficiency in persons with HIV/AIDS. Blood. 2006;108:3786–91.

26. Aldinucci D, Poletto D, Nanni P, et al. Expression of functional interleukin-3 receptors on Hodgkin and Reed–Sternberg cells. Am J Pathol. 2002;160:585–96.

27. Foss HD, Hummel M, Gottstein S, et al. Frequent expression of IL-7 gene transcripts in tumor cells of classical Hodgkin's disease. Am J Pathol. 1995;146:33–9.

28. Cattaruzza L, Gloghini A, Olivo K, et al. Functional coexpression of interleukin (IL)-7 and its receptor (IL-7R) on Hodgkin and Reed–Sternberg cells: involvement of IL-7 in tumor cell growth and microenvironmental interactions of Hodgkin's lymphoma. Int J Cancer. 2009;125:1092–101.

29. Kapp U, Yeh WC, Patterson B, et al. Interleukin 13 is secreted by and stimulates the growth of Hodgkin and Reed–Sternberg cells. J Exp Med. 1999;189:1939–46.

30. Herbst H, Samol J, Foss HD, et al. Modulation of interleukin-6 expression in Hodgkin and Reed–Sternberg cells by Epstein–Barr virus. J Pathol. 1997;182:299–306.

31. Pinto A, Aldinucci D, Gloghini A, et al. Human eosinophils express functional CD30 ligand and stimulate proliferation of a Hodgkin's disease cell line. Blood. 1996;88:3299–305.

32. Molin D, Edstrom A, Glimelius I, et al. Mast cell infiltration correlates with poor prognosis in Hodgkin's lymphoma. Br J Haematol. 2002;119:122–4.

33. Grüss HJ, Ulrich D, Braddy S, et al. Recombinant CD30 ligand and CD40 ligand share common biological activities on Hodgkin and Reed–Sternberg cells. Eur J Immunol. 1995;25:2083–9.

34. Carbone A, Gloghini A, Gattei V, et al. Expression of functional CD40 antigen on Reed–Sternberg cells and Hodgkin's disease cell lines. Blood. 1995;85:780–9.

35. Peh SC, Kim LH, Poppema S. TARC, a CC chemokine, is frequently expressed in classic Hodgkin lymphoma but not in NLP Hodgkin lymphoma, T-cell-rich B-cell lymphoma, and most cases of anaplastic large cell lymphoma. Am J Surg Pathol. 2001;25:925–9.

36. Van Den Berg A, Visser L, Poppema S. High expression of the CC chemokine TARC in Reed–Sternberg cells. A possible explanation for the characteristic T-cell infiltrate in Hodgkin's lymphoma. Am J Pathol. 1999;154:1685–91.

37. Niens M, Visser L, Nolte IM, et al. Serum chemokine levels in Hodgkin lymphoma patients: highly increased levels of CCL17 and CCL22. Br J Haematol. 2008;140:527–36.

38. Weihrauch MR, Manzke O, Beyer M, et al. Elevated levels of CC thymus and activation-related chemokine (TARC) in primary Hodgkin's disease: potential for a prognostic factor. Cancer Res. 2005;65:5516–9.

39. Ohshima K, Tutiya T, Yamaguchi T, et al. Infiltration of Th1 and Th2 lymphocytes around Hodgkin and Reed-Sternberg (H&RS) cells in Hodgkin disease: relation with expression of CXC and CC chemokines on H&RS cells. Int J Cancer. 2002;98:567–72.

40. Ishida T, Ishii T, Inagaki, et al. Specific recruitment of CC chemokine receptor 4-positive regulatory T cells in Hodgkin lymphoma fosters immune privilege. Cancer Res. 2006;66: 5716–22.

41. Andrew DP, Chang MS, McNinch J, et al. STPC-1 (MDC) CC chemokine acts specifically on chronically activated Th2 lymphocytes and is produced by monocytes on stimulation with Th2 cytokines IL-4 and IL-13. J Immunol. 1998;16: 5027–38.

42. Hedvat CV, Jaffe ES, Qin J, et al. Macrophage-derived chemokine expression in classical Hodgkin's lymphoma: application of tissue microarrays. Mod Pathol. 2001;14: 1270–6.

43. Imai T, Chantry D, Raport CJ, et al. Macrophage-derived chemokine is a functional ligand for the CC chemokine receptor 4. J Biol Chem. 1998;273:1764–8.

44. Maggio E, van den Berg A, Visser L, et al. Common and differential chemokine expression patterns in RS cells of NLP, EBV positive and negative classical Hodgkin lymphomas. Int J Cancer. 2002;99:665–72.

45. Lamprecht B, Kreher S, Anagnostopoulos I, et al. Aberrant expression of the Th2 cytokine IL-21 in Hodgkin lymphoma cells regulates STAT3 signaling and attracts Treg cells via regulation of MIP-3alpha. Blood. 2008;112:3339–47.

46. Tanijiri T, Shimizu T, Uehira K, et al. Hodgkin's Reed-Sternberg cell line (KM-H2) promotes a bidirectional differentiation of CD4+CD25+Foxp3+ T cells and CD4+ cytotoxic T lymphocytes from CD4+ naïve T cells. J Leukoc Biol. 2007;82:576–84.

47. Dukers DF, Jaspars LH, Vos W, et al. Quantitative immunohistochemical analysis of cytokine profiles in Epstein–Barr virus-positive and -negative cases of Hodgkin's disease. J Pathol. 2000;190:143–9.

48. Herbst H, Foss HD, Samol J, et al. Frequent expression of interleukin-10 by Epstein–Barr virus-harboring tumor cells of Hodgkin's disease. Blood. 1996;87:2918–29.

49. Newcom SR, Kadin ME, Ansari AA, et al. L-428 nodular sclerosing Hodgkin's cell secretes a unique transforming growth factor-beta active at physiologic pH. J Clin Invest. 1988;82:1915–21.

50. Newcom SR, Tagra KK. High molecular weight transforming growth factor β is excreted in the urine in active nodular sclerosing Hodgkin's disease. Cancer Res. 1992;52:6768–73.

51. Marshall NA, Christie LE, Munro LR, et al. Immunosuppressive regulatory T cells are abundant in the reactive lymphocytes of Hodgkin lymphoma. Blood. 2004;103: 1755–62.

52. Juszczynski P, Ouyang J, Monti S, et al. the AP1-dependent secretion of galectin-1 by Reed–Sternberg cells fosters immune privilege in classical Hodgkin lymphoma. Proc Natl Acad Sci USA. 2007;104:13134–9.

53. Maggio EM, van den Berg A, de Jong D, et al. Low frequency of FAS mutations in Reed–Sternberg cells of Hodgkin's lymphoma. Am J Pathol. 2003;162:29–35.

54. Yamamoto R, Nishikori M, Kitawaki T, et al. PD-1-PD-1 ligand interaction contributes to immunosuppressive microenvironment of Hodgkin lymphoma. Blood. 2008;111: 3220–4.

55. Schwaller J, Tobler A, Niklaus G, et al. Interleukin-12 expression in human lymphomas and nonneoplastic lymphoid disorders. Blood. 1995;85:2182–8.

56. Niedobitek G, Pazolt D, Teichmann M, et al. Frequent expression of the Epstein-Barr virus (EBV)-induced gene, EBI3, an IL-12 p40-related cytokine, in Hodgkin and Reed–Sternberg cells. J Pathol. 2002;198:310–6.

57. Keryer-Bibens C, Pioche-Durieu C, Villemant C, et al. Exosomes released by EBV-infected nasopharyngeal carcinoma cells convey the viral latent membrane protein 1 and the immunomodulatory protein galectin 9. BMC Cancer. 2006;6:283.

58. Ferraris AM, Racchi O, Rapezzi D, et al. Familial Hodgkin's disease: a disease of young adulthood? Ann Hematol. 1997; 74:131–4.

59. Glaser SL, Hsu JL. Hodgkin's disease in Asians: incidence patterns and risk factors in population-based data. Leuk Res. 2002;26:261–9.

60. Mack TM, Cozen W, Shibata DK, et al. Concordance for Hodgkin's disease in identical twins suggesting genetic susceptibility to the young-adult form of the disease. N Engl J Med. 1995;332:413–8.

61. Diepstra A, Niens M, Vellenga E, et al. Association with HLA class I in Epstein–Barr-virus-positive and with HLA class III in Epstein-Barr-virus-negative Hodgkin's lymphoma. Lancet. 2005;365:2216–24.

62. Niens M, van den Berg A, Diepstra A, et al. The human leukocyte antigen class I region is associated with EBV-positive Hodgkin's lymphoma: HLA-A and HLA complex group 9 are putative candidate genes. Cancer Epidemiol Biomarkers Prev. 2006;15:2280–4.

63. Levitskaya J, Coram M, Levitsky V, et al. Inhibition of antigen processing by the internal repeat region of the Epstein–Barr virus nuclear antigen-1. Nature. 1995;375:685–8.

64. Meij P, Leen A, Rickinson AB, et al. Identification and prevalence of CD8(+) T-cell responses directed against Epstein–Barr virus-encoded latent membrane protein 1 and latent membrane protein 2. Int J Cancer. 2002;99:93–9.

65. Bollard CM, Aguilar L, Straathof KC, et al. Cytotoxic T lymphocyte therapy for Epstein-Barr virus+ Hodgkin's disease. J Exp Med. 2004;200:1623–33.

66. Lucas KG, Salzman D, Garcia A, et al. Adoptive immunotherapy with allogeneic Epstein–Barr virus (EBV)-specific cytotoxic T-lymphocytes for recurrent EBV-positive Hodgkin disease. Cancer. 2004;100:1892–901.

67. Niens M, Jarrett RF, Hepkema B, et al. HLA-A*02 is associated with a reduced risk and HLA-A*01 with an increased risk of developing EBV+ Hodgkin lymphoma. Blood. 2007;110:3310–5.

68. McAulay KA, Higgins CD, Macsween KF, et al. HLA class I polymorphisms are associated with development of infectious mononucleosis upon primary EBV infection. J Clin Invest. 2007;117:3042–8.

69. Jarrett RF. Viruses and Hodgkin's lymphoma. Ann Oncol. 2002;13 suppl 1:23–9.
70. Diepstra A, van Imhoff GW, Karim-Kos HE, et al. HLA class II expression by Hodgkin Reed–Sternberg cells is an independent prognostic factor in classical Hodgkin's lymphoma. J Clin Oncol. 2007;25:3101–8.
71. Ressing ME, Horst D, Griffin BD, et al. Epstein-Barr virus evasion of CD8+ and CD4+ T cell immunity via concerted actions of multiple gene products. Semin Cancer Biol. 2008;18:397–408.
72. Alvaro T, Lejeune M, Salvado MT, et al. Outcome in Hodgkin's lymphoma can be predicted from the presence of accompanying cytotoxic and regulatory T cells. Clin Cancer Res. 2005;11:1467–73.
73. Kelley TW, Pohlman B, Elson P, et al. The ratio of Foxp3+ regulatory T cells to Granzyme B+ cytotoxic T/NK cells predicts prognosis in classical Hodgkin lymphoma and is independent of bcl-2 and MAL expression. Am J Clin Pathol. 2007;128:958–65.
74. Oudejans JJ, Jiwa NM, Kummer JA, et al. Activated cytotoxic T cells as prognostic marker in Hodgkin's disease. Blood. 1997;89:1376–82.
75. Delabie J, Chan WC, Weisenburger DD, et al. The antigen-presenting cell function of Reed–Sternberg cells. Leuk Lymphoma. 1995;18:35–40.
76. Diepstra A, Poppema S, Boot M, et al. HLA-G protein expression as a potential immune escape mechanism in classical Hodgkin's lymphoma. Tissue Antigens. 2008;71:219–26.

**Part** **II**

**Diagnosis and Treatment**

# Clinical Evaluation

**5**

Jim Armitage and Christian Gisselbrecht

## Contents

J. Armitage (✉)
University of Nebraska Medical Center, 8th Floor Lied
Transplant Ctr., 987680 Nebraska Med. Ctr., Omaha,
NE 68198-7680, USA
e-mail: joarmita@unmc.edu

C. Gisselbrecht
Service d'Hémato-Oncologie, Hôpital Saint Louis, 1, avenue
Claude Vellefaux, 75010 Paris, France
e-mail: christian.gisselbrecht@sls.aphp.fr

## 5.1 Presenting Manifestations

Hodgkin lymphoma can come to clinical attention in a variety of ways. These include symptoms caused by a growing mass, systemic symptoms that are presumably cytokine induced, and a diagnosis can be made incidentally as part of an evaluation for an unrelated problem. By far the most common presentation of Hodgkin lymphoma is enlargement of lymph nodes that is typically painless and progressive. Although the most common place for lymph nodes to be found is in the neck and supraclavicular region, any lymph node bearing area can be involved. Patients typically find enlarged nodes above the clavicle and seek medical attention when they do not regress, while physicians are relatively more likely to discover lymph nodes in other areas as part of a physical examination. Mediastinal lymphadenopathy is a particularly common finding in young women with Hodgkin lymphoma. This might be found incidentally on a chest X-ray or can be symptomatic. Although unusual, patients with Hodgkin lymphoma can present with superior vena cava syndrome, but chest pain or shortness of breath are more common symptoms caused by a large mediastinal mass. Lymphadenopathy found only below the diaphragm is more common in males and in elderly patients. Mesenteric lymphadenopathy is unusual in Hodgkin lymphoma. Retroperitoneal lymphadenopathy can be painful, but is more commonly asymptomatic and found on a staging evaluation or as part of the investigation to explain system symptoms such as fever, night sweats, or weight loss. Epitrochlear lymph node involvement is unusual in Hodgkin lymphoma.

Hodgkin lymphoma can involve essentially any organ in the body as either a site of presentation or by

A. Engert and S.J. Horning (eds.), *Hodgkin Lymphoma*,
DOI: 10.1007/978-3-642-12780-9_5, © Springer-Verlag Berlin Heidelberg 2011

spread from lymphatic involvement. However, extranodal presentation of Hodgkin lymphoma is unusual. The most common sites to be involved are the spleen, liver, lungs, pleura, and bone marrow, although Hodgkin lymphoma confined to these sites is rare. Hodgkin lymphoma can rarely present in unusual extranodal sites. Primary CNS [1] and cutaneous [2] Hodgkin lymphoma are rare but well described. Perianal presentations are seen more commonly in patients with HIV infection. Gastrointestinal system, bone, genitourinary system, and other unusual sites are extremely rare but have been described. Bone involvement can be seen as an "ivory vertebrae" – i.e., a densely sclerotic vertebrae [3].

By the far the most common systemic symptoms that occur as the presenting manifestations of Hodgkin lymphoma are fevers, night sweats, weight loss, pruritus, and fatigue. These occur in a minority of patients but can present diagnostic challenges. Hodgkin lymphoma is one of the illnesses that can cause fever of unknown origin. Occasionally the fevers of Hodgkin lymphoma occur intermittently with several days of fevers alternating with afebrile periods. This is the Pel–Ebstein fever [4, 5] that is rare but particularly characteristic of Hodgkin lymphoma when it occurs. The fevers of Hodgkin lymphoma typically occur in the evening and often can be prevented with nonsteroidal anti-inflammatory drugs such as naproxyn [6].

The presence of drenching night sweats (i.e., as opposed to dampness of the head and neck) and unexplained weight loss are both characteristic of Hodgkin lymphoma and, along with fever, are associated with a poor prognosis. Pruritus can be the presenting manifestation of Hodgkin lymphoma. Such patients sometimes have severely excoriated skin and sometimes have been diagnosed as having neurodermatitis. Patients who present with refractory pruritus are often grateful to find the explanation of their symptoms which usually disappear with the initiation of therapy. As with other lymphomas, fatigue can be an important, although nonspecific, symptom and also usually improves with therapy. There are many unusual, but well-described, presentations for Hodgkin lymphoma. One rare but very characteristic presentation is alcohol-induced pain [7, 8]. The pain typically begins soon after drinking alcohol and occurs primarily in areas of involvement by lymphoma. The pain can be quite severe and last for variable periods of time. Patients with the symptom have often discontinued alcohol before the diagnosis of Hodgkin lymphoma, and to elicit the symptom often requires specific questioning by the physician.

Patients can present with Hodgkin lymphoma involving the skin, but cutaneous abnormalities are more often paraneoplastic phenomenon. These can include erythema nodosum [9], icthyosiform atrophy [10], acrokeratosis paraneoplastica [11], granulomatous slack skin [12], nonspecific urticarial, vesicular, and bullous lesions [13], and others.

A variety of other unusual presentations of Hodgkin lymphoma have been reported. Patients can present with nephrotic syndrome [14], the symptoms of hypercalcemia [15–17], and jaundice due to cholestasis without involvement of the liver by the lymphoma [18, 19].

Hodgkin lymphoma rarely presents with a primary tumor in the CNS causing the symptoms of a brain tumor characteristic of the site of involvement. Other neurological manifestations that can be present at the diagnosis of Hodgkin lymphoma include a variety of paraneoplastic syndromes. These include paraneoplastic cerebeller degeneration [20], which typically presents with ataxia, dysarthria, nystagmus, and diplopia. The symptoms may precede the diagnosis of Hodgkin lymphoma by many months. Hodgkin lymphoma can, of course, present with spinal cord compression from retroperitoneal and osseous tumors. Other rare manifestations include limbic encephalitis (i.e., which presents with memory loss and amnesia), peripheral neuropathy, and others.

## 5.2 Physical Findings and Laboratory Abnormalities

By far the most common physical findings in Hodgkin lymphoma are enlarged lymph nodes that might be in any lymph node bearing area. The lymph nodes are typically firm (i.e., "rubbery") and vary from barely palpable to large masses. However, almost any aspect of the physical examination can be made abnormal by the presence of Hodgkin lymphoma. This might include icterus, involvement of Waldeyer's ring, findings of superior vena cava syndrome, a sternal or suprasternal mass from tumor growing out of the mediastinum, findings of a pleural effusion or pericardial fusion, an intra-abdominal mass, hepatomegaly or splenomegaly, skin involvement, and, rarely, cutaneous or neurological abnormalities.

Almost any laboratory test can be abnormal at the time of diagnosis of Hodgkin lymphoma, but certain tests are characteristic and should be specifically evaluated. Patients can have leukocytosis or leukopenia. Neutrophilia and lymphopenia are sometimes seen, with the latter having a poor prognosis. Eosinophilia can be found incidentally before the diagnosis of Hodgkin lymphoma, and Hodgkin lymphoma should always be included in the differential diagnosis of unexplained eosinophilia [21]. In some cases, the explanation of the eosinophilia is related to production of interleukin-5 by the tumor cells [22, 23].

The most common hematological manifestation of Hodgkin lymphoma is anemia. The most usual explanation seems to be a normocytic anemia associated with the presence of the tumor that resolves after therapy. However, patients can also have autoimmune hemolytic anemia [24] and a microangiopathic hemolytic anemia as part of the syndrome of thrombotic thrombocytopenic purpura.

Patients can present with thrombocytopenia for a variety of reasons including hypersplenism and bone marrow involvement. However, idiopathic thrombocytopenic purpura can be a presenting manifestation of the disease [25].

Other rare hematological manifestations of Hodgkin lymphoma have included autoimmune neutropenia [26], hemophagocytic syndrome [27], coagulation factor deficiencies [28], and unexplained microcytosis [29], and thrombotic thrombocytopenia purpura has been seen rarely.

Routine chemistry screening should be done in patients with Hodgkin lymphoma and might reveal renal or hepatic dysfunction, protein abnormalities, hypercalcemia, and hyperuracemia.

Elevated erythryocyte sedimentation rate and C-reductive protein are frequently seen and have been associated with a poor prognosis.

## 5.3 Pathologic Diagnosis: The Biopsy

The oncologist must be certain that the Hodgkin lymphoma diagnosis was based on an adequate biopsy specimen that was examined using appropriate morphologic and immunohistochemical criteria. Whole lymph node excision is preferable for pathologic examination. The pathologic diagnosis of Hodgkin lymphoma is fully discussed in Chap. 4.

The site of biopsy must be determined with the radiologist and surgeon. The largest abnormal peripheral lymph node should be excised. However, at certain sites such as the mediastinum, the removal of a bulky lymph node (>5 cm) can lead to major surgery, with a risk of complications or sequelae. Fairly often, only a limited biopsy of the node is performed. On the other hand, too small a lymph node may only be a reactive hyperplasia. If a fluorine-18-deoxyglucose positron emission tomography (FDG-PET-CT) has been performed, the patient should be biopsied in the most avid site to avoid a partially necrotic zone.

If there are only deep node lesions, the following types of biopsy can be proposed.

A thoracoscopic or laparoscopic approach under general anesthesia, with, if necessary, preoperative localization to facilitate resection is now widely used [30].

Image-guided core needle biopsy is increasingly used and has a rising success rate of more than 90% [31–33]. However, the method has the disadvantage of only permitting relatively small biopsies, although progress has been made with automated guns and a coaxial technique. In addition, this type of biopsy is capable of sampling several core specimens with a single biopsy tract. Large-volume cutting needles, ranging from 18 gauge to 14 gauge, yield enough tissue for most immunochemistry stainings and even for RNA extraction from frozen tissue (Fig. 5.1). Moreover, this inexpensive procedure, performed under local anesthesia, can easily be done in a reference center outpatient clinic.

In an experienced center, a multidisciplinary approach with skilled trained radiologists working in conjunction with experienced pathologists should immediately start with image-guided core needle biopsy. In case of failure, video-assisted surgery should be performed. In most situations, open surgery can be avoided as a first diagnosis procedure in the absence of peripheral lymph nodes. Fine needle aspiration cytology should *not* be used for diagnosis of Hodgkin lymphoma, but may help in a screening procedure, before biopsy [34].

A second biopsy can be considered at five stages:

1. At initial diagnosis, when Hodgkin lymphoma is diagnosed from a biopsy of an extranodal site, a node biopsy is desirable to confirm the diagnosis, unless the latter is considered unequivocal

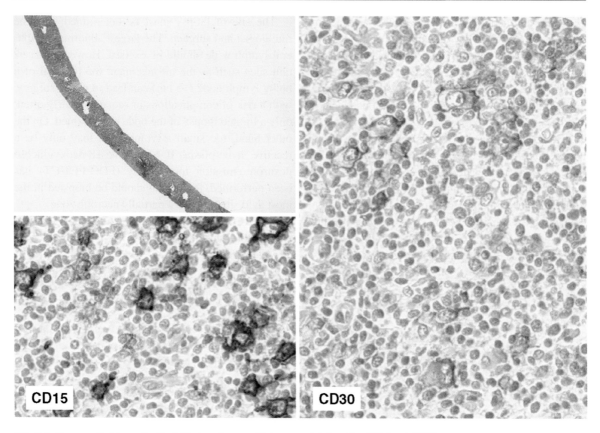

**Fig. 5.1** Core needle biopsy for Hodgkin lymphoma with immunostainings for CD15 and CD30

2. When the amount of tissue is insufficient for adequate immunostaining or molecular biology studies
3. When, after functional imaging with a PET scan, avidity is seen in a noncontiguous lesion, and induces changes in stage and/or therapy
4. When the treatment is evaluated, especially in cases of persistent avidity on PET scan
5. During follow-up, when a new lesion is seen on CT scan, indicating a probable relapse

In case of a second biopsy, the difficulties of sampling artifacts should be taken into account, especially in irradiated areas. In such situations, the anatomic location very often requires a video-assisted surgical approach or an image-guided core biopsy.

These procedures are less aggressive than traditional biopsy methods, and in conjunction with the use of the PET scan, are significantly improving patient management, as they provide more accurate definitions of response and relapse.

Several pathologic pitfalls or differential diagnoses should be kept in mind.

Drugs such as phenytoin or antibiotics may cause histologic changes within lymph nodes that may mimic Hodgkin lymphoma, particularly the mixed cellularity subtype. Other benign conditions like infectious mononucleosis, lymphoid hyperplasia, or Castleman disease may produce lymphadenopathy with histologic features similar to those of Hodgkin lymphoma. In fact, the distinction between different diseases, including certain forms of non-Hodgkin lymphoma (NHL), has been made clearer thanks to a better definition of the entities by the WHO classification. T-cell-rich large B-cell lymphoma is usually included in the differential diagnoses of both nodular lymphocyte-predominant Hodgkin lymphoma and classical Hodgkin lymphoma, while anaplastic CD30-positive NHL may display similar histology to that of classical Hodgkin lymphoma. Nevertheless, molecular studies require adequate material, including frozen tissue in difficult cases, and the role of the clinician is to make sure that the node to be analyzed is given to an experienced network laboratory. If the clinical presentation of disease is not typical for the given pathologic diagnosis, then a review of the pathology by an expert hematopathologist should be considered, or even a second biopsy.

## 5.4 Staging Systems for Hodgkin Lymphoma

The initial clinical evaluation and staging of patients with Hodgkin lymphoma serve to confirm the Hodgkin lymphoma diagnosis, determine the extent and distribution of disease, evaluate the patient's fitness for standard treatments, and provide prognostic information (Table 5.1).

Several staging systems were developed very early and modified according to the progress made in the knowledge, imaging, and treatment of the disease. The Ann Arbor Staging of Hodgkin disease was developed in the 1970s, when radiotherapy was the main curative treatment option, and was based on the tendency of Hodgkin lymphoma to spread to contiguous lymph nodes [35].

Since the Ann Arbor staging, several significant changes in the management of Hodgkin lymphoma have taken place.

**Table 5.1** Recommended studies for initial evaluation of Hodgkin lymphoma

| Mandatory for the Cotswolds classification | Histology and immunophenotyping Individual and familial history, clinical examination as per Cotswolds recommendations Blood counts and routine workup: ESR, LDH, alkaline phosphatase, albumin, liver function, β2-microglobulin, virology Chest radiograms: CT of chest, abdomen, and pelvis; bone marrow biopsy if indicated |
|---|---|
| Recommended for disease assessment | FDG-PET-CT |
| Recommended for toxicity assessment | Heart: ECG, MUGA, or echocardiogram Pulmonary: lung function tests Thyroid and gonadal functions: FSH, LH, and TSH (semen analysis and sperm storage) Psychosocial adaptation |

The Cotswolds modification of the Ann Arbor staging system was introduced in 1989, to approve the use of CT scanning for the detection of intra-abdominal disease, to formalize a definition of disease bulk, and to provide guidelines for evaluating the response to treatment (Table 5.2) [36]. This staging classification provides a basis for selecting the initial treatment and has been widely adopted by most clinical trial groups. Additional factors have been recognized (e.g., tumor bulk and the number of sites of disease) that adversely affect the prognosis of patients with a localized stage treated by radiation alone. A prognostic factor score for advanced Hodgkin lymphoma treated by chemotherapy has been worked out, based mostly on biological parameters, including serum albumin <4 g/dL, hemoglobin <10.5 g/dL, male sex, stage IV disease, age >45 year, white cell count >15,000/mm$^3$, and lymphocyte count <600/mm$^3$ [37].

These prognostic factors are used to define risk-adapted therapy. However, as combined modality treatment with modern chemotherapy has become standard procedure for patients with early-stage disease, the risk

**Table 5.2** Cotswolds modifications of the Ann Arbor staging system

| Stage | Definitions |
|---|---|
| I | Involvement of a single lymph node region or lymphoid structure (e.g., spleen, thymus, Waldeyer ring) |
| II | Involvement of two or more lymph node regions on the same side of the diaphragm (the mediastinum is a single site; hilar lymph nodes are lateralized); the number of anatomic sites should be indicated by a suffix (e.g., II3) |
| III | Involvement of lymph node regions or structures on both sides of the diaphragm |
| III$_1$ | With or without splenic, hilar, celiac, or portal nodes |
| III$_2$ | With para-aortic, iliac, and/or mesenteric nodes |
| IV | Involvement of extranodal site(s) beyond that designated E |

Annotation:
A, no B-symptoms
B, fever, drenching sweats, or weight loss
X, bulky disease, >1/3 mediastinal widening at T5-6, or >10 cm maximum dimension of nodal mass
E, involvement of a single extranodal site, contiguous or proximal to a known nodal site
CS clinical stage; PS pathologic stage
Reprinted from [36] with permission

**Table 5.3** Summary of the new Cheson guidelines for positron emission tomography/computed tomography

| Response | IWG [46] | New Cheson criteria including PET [47], PET positive if uptake >mediastinum (lesions >2 cm), >local background (lesions <2 cm) |
|---|---|---|
| CR | Disappearance of all detectable disease<br><br>LN >1.5 cm must decrease to ≤1.5 cm | CR, CRu, PR, or SD by IWG criteria and PET completely negative; BMB negative |
| CRu | LN >1.5 cm<br>SPD decrease >75%<br>Indeterminate bone marrow | No longer exists |
| PR | SPD regressed >50% | CR, CRu, PR by IWG criteria, and PET positive in at least one previously affected site |
| SD | SPD decrease ≤50% but no progressive disease | SD by IWG criteria and PET positive in previously affected sites |
| PD/relapse | New lesion<br>SPD increase >50% from nadir of any LN | PD by IWG criteria and PET should be positive on the new or increased lesion if >1.5 cm |

*BMB* bone marrow biopsy; *CR* complete response; *CRu* unconfirmed complete response; *CT* computed tomography; *IWG* international working group; *LN* lymph nodes or nodal masses; *PD* progressive disease; *PET* positron emission tomography; *PR* partial response; *SD* stable disease; *SPD* sum of the products of the greatest diameters

distinguish between a viable tumor, and necrosis or fibrosis in residual disease [49]. In this connection, a retrospective study carried out by Juweid et al. demonstrated that the integration of PET into the IWG criteria increased the number of confirmed complete responses (CRs), thus eliminating the need for the CRu category [50]. That is why, the revised criteria state that in routinely FDG-avid lymphomas such as diffuse large B-cell lymphoma and Hodgkin lymphoma, all patients with a negative PET are classified as CR, regardless of the presence of a residual mass on CT. In cases where PET shows the presence of residual disease (i.e., in PET-positive patients), the patient is considered to exhibit a partial response, stable disease, or progressive disease on the basis of the response shown by CT, and the CRu category is eliminated (Table 5.1) [47].

In patients with advanced-stage disease who are treated by chemotherapy alone, the response should be assessed 1 month after the completion of treatment, on the basis of clinical findings and of the same imaging investigations as those that gave abnormal results at presentation (typically CT and PET). However, as false-positive PET scans may occur shortly after RT, repeat imaging should be done later for patients treated by combined therapies, provided they are clinically well. If there is any doubt about the response to treatment, they should be re-evaluated. Note that after the completion of treatment, regression of disease may be

slow, and a residual fibrotic mass may still be visible on a chest radiograph or CT images.

## 5.8 Complete Remission

The patient has no clinical, radiologic, or other evidence of Hodgkin lymphoma. Changes due to the effects of previous therapy (i.e., radiation fibrosis) may, however, be present.

The category (CRu) has been eliminated from the updated response criteria and now denotes patients whose remission status is unclear, because they display no clinical evidence of Hodgkin lymphoma, but some radiologic abnormality that persists at a site of previous disease. In this respect, it is generally recognized that imaging abnormalities may persist following treatment, and do not necessarily signify active disease [51].

This definition of unconfirmed or uncertain remission is still helpful in the absence of FDG-PET, when reviewing a clinical case. However, it must be borne in mind that after mediastinal RT, thymic rebound, reactive lymph node hyperplasia, or subclinical radiation pneumonitis may lead to abnormalities on FDG-PET [52]. To avoid false-positive interpretations, some authors recommend that FDG-PET re-evaluation should be delayed until 3 months after the completion of mediastinal RT, although the characteristic appearance of post-RT lung changes occurring before 3 months can usually be distinguished from lymphoma by experienced nuclear radiographers [53].

The inclusion of PET in the new response criteria and the removal of CRu have simplified the management of lymphoma patients by removing some of the limiting factors of CT, which include the size of lymph nodes that indicates involvement, the differentiation of unopacified bowel from lesions in the abdomen and pelvis, inability to distinguish viable tumor from necrotic/fibrotic lesions after therapy, and the characterization of small lesions. However, even though PET has eliminated many of the limitations attributed to CT, it has several disadvantages, including limited resolution, inaccurate localization of the abnormalities, and physiologic variations in FDG distribution. PET and CT are therefore complementary, and consequently a combined PET/CT examination, when available, should become part of clinical practice, rather than choosing either PET or CT separately [54].

## 5.9 Partial Remission

Partial remission is defined as a decrease of at least 50% in the sum of the products of the largest perpendicular diameters of all the measurable lesions. This would include patients with an abnormal but improved PET scan. Other manifestations of disease (e.g., B-symptoms) should also improve. As described above, re-imaging and/or re-biopsy to detect persistent active disease should be aggressively undertaken if the results can be expected to have a marked effect on treatment decisions (e.g., if the patient is a candidate for aggressive salvage therapy).

## 5.10 Progressive Disease

Progressive disease is defined as an increase of 25% or more in the size of a least one measurable lesion, the appearance of a new lesion, or the recurrence of B-symptoms that cannot be otherwise explained.

Most lymphoma patients will become PET negative after two to three cycles of standard chemotherapy, and response assessments based on the new Cheson criteria are proving to be robust and highly predictive of outcome [55, 56]. However, false-positive lesions occur more frequently at earlier time, particularly with intensified treatment schedules, and preliminary results indicate that the accuracy of PET differs, depending on the treatment given.

## 5.11 Follow-Up Management

The manner in which patients are evaluated after completing treatment may vary according to whether treatment was administered in a clinical trial or clinical practice, or whether it was delivered with curative or palliative intent. In a clinical trial, uniformity of reassessment is necessary to ensure comparability among studies with respect to the major end points of event-free survival, disease-free survival, and progression-free survival. Good clinical judgment, careful recording of history, and thorough physical examination are the most important components of patient monitoring after treatment. To obtain the necessary clinical indications, additional testing at follow-up visits should include blood count and serum chemistry, including measurement of lactate dehydrogenase and other blood parameters, and imaging studies. Persistent elevation of the sedimentation rate, while not a diagnostic criterion of active Hodgkin lymphoma, indicates the need for very close surveillance [57].

There is no evidence to support the need for regular surveillance CT scans, because the patient or physician identifies the relapse in more than 80% of cases without imaging studies [58].

Once therapy, restaging, and response assessment have all been completed, follow-up guidelines vary, but most of them recommend that patients be seen at intervals of about 3 months during the first and second years after therapy, 4-month intervals in the third year, 6-month intervals in the fourth and fifth years, and annually thereafter. Few Hodgkin lymphoma recurrences occur after 5 years. The frequency and type of radiologic imaging during follow-up should primarily be based on the initial sites of disease and the risk of relapse [59].

Although some clinicians perform routine CT re-imaging in asymptomatic patients, the results of three studies suggest that the yield of routine imaging in asymptomatic patients is low [60–62].

FDG-PET has also been suggested as a potential tool for the detection of relapse. In a prospective study of 36 Hodgkin lymphoma patients, the authors found that routine FDG-PET correctly identified all the five relapses that occurred following treatment [63]. However, the false-positive rate was 55%, 6/11 patients with abnormal FDG-PET did not have their relapse confirmed, and 2/5 of the relapsed patients developed symptoms shortly after relapse detection by FDG-PET, so that the benefit of this imaging was unclear.

## 5.12 Conclusion

The careful and accurate clinical evaluation of patients with Hodgkin lymphoma from presentation to follow-up in remission has a significant impact on treatment outcome. The ability to perform an excellent history and physical, and knowledge regarding when, where, and how to perform laboratory evaluations, images, and biopsies are necessary for excellent care.

## References

1. Gerstner ER, Abrey LE, Schiff D, Ferreri AJ, Lister A, Montoto S, et al. CNS Hodgkin lymphoma. Blood. 2008;112(5):1658–61.
2. Tassies D, Sierra J, Montserrat E, Marti R, Estrach T, Rozman C. Specific cutaneous involvement in Hodgkin's disease. Hematol Oncol. 1992;10(2):75–9.
3. Granger W, Whitaker R. Hodgkin's disease in bone, with special reference to periosteal reaction. Br J Radiol. 1967;40(480):939–48.
4. Pel PK. Pseudoleukämie oder chronisches Rückfallsfieber? Zur Symptomatologie der sogenannten Pseudoleukämie II 1887:644.
5. Ebstein W. Das chronische Rückfallsfieber, eine neue Infectionskrankheit. Berl Klin Wochenschr. 1887;24:565.
6. Chang JC, Gross HM. Neoplastic fever responds to the treatment of an adequate dose of naproxen. J Clin Oncol. 1985;3(4):552–8.
7. Bichel J. The alcohol-intolerance syndrome in Hodgkin's disease. Acta Med Scand. 1959;164(2):105–12.
8. James AH. Hodgkin's disease with and without alcohol-induced pain. A clinical and histological comparison. Q J Med. 1960;29:47–66.
9. Simon S, Azevedo SJ, Byrnes JJ. Erythema nodosum heralding recurrent Hodgkin's disease. Cancer. 1985;56(6):1470–2.
10. Ronchese F, Gates DC. Ichthyosiform atrophy of the skin in Hodgkin's disease. N Engl J Med. 1956;255(6):287–9.
11. Lucker GP, Steijlen PM. Acrokeratosis paraneoplastica (Bazex syndrome) occurring with acquired ichthyosis in Hodgkin's disease. Br J Dermatol. 1995;133(2):322–5.
12. Noto G, Pravata G, Miceli S, Arico M. Granulomatous slack skin: report of a case associated with Hodgkin's disease and a review of the literature. Br J Dermatol. 1994;131(2):275–9.
13. Milionis HJ, Elisaf MS. Psoriasiform lesions as paraneoplastic manifestation in Hodgkin's disease. Ann Oncol. 1998;9(4):449–52.
14. Dabbs DJ, Striker LM, Mignon F, Striker G. Glomerular lesions in lymphomas and leukemias. Am J Med. 1986;80(1):63–70.
15. Rieke JW, Donaldson SS, Horning SJ. Hypercalcemia and vitamin D metabolism in Hodgkin's disease. Is there an underlying immunoregulatory relationship? Cancer. 1989;63(9):1700–7.
16. Seymour JF, Gagel RF. Calcitriol: the major humoral mediator of hypercalcemia in Hodgkin's disease and non-Hodgkin's lymphomas. Blood. 1993;82(5):1383–94.
17. Laforga JB, Vierna J, Aranda FI. Hypercalcaemia in Hodgkin's disease related to prostaglandin synthesis. J Clin Pathol. 1994;47(6):567–8.
18. Lieberman DA. Intrahepatic cholestasis due to Hodgkin's disease. An elusive diagnosis. J Clin Gastroenterol. 1986;8(3 Pt 1):304–7.
19. Hubscher SG, Lumley MA, Elias E. Vanishing bile duct syndrome: a possible mechanism for intrahepatic cholestasis in Hodgkin's lymphoma. Hepatology. 1993;17(1):70–7.
20. Hammack J, Kotanides H, Rosenblum MK, Posner JB. Paraneoplastic cerebellar degeneration. II. Clinical and immunologic findings in 21 patients with Hodgkin's disease. Neurology. 1992;42(10):1938–43.
21. Reid III TJ, Mullaney M, Burrell LM, Redmond III J, Mangan KF. Pure red cell aplasia after chemotherapy for Hodgkin's lymphoma: in vitro evidence for T cell mediated suppression of erythropoiesis and response to sequential cyclosporin and erythropoietin. Am J Hematol. 1994;46(1):48–53.
22. Samoszuk M, Nansen L. Detection of interleukin-5 messenger RNA in Reed-Sternberg cells of Hodgkin's disease with eosinophilia. Blood. 1990;75(1):13–6.
23. Di Biagio E, Sanchez-Borges M, Desenne JJ, Suarez-Chacon R, Somoza R, Acquatella G. Eosinophilia in Hodgkin's disease: a role for interleukin 5. Int Arch Allergy Immunol. 1996;110(3):244–51.
24. Bjorkholm M, Holm G, Merk K. Cyclic autoimmune hemolytic anemia as a presenting manifestation of splenic Hodgkin's disease. Cancer. 1982;49(8):1702–4.
25. Kirshner JJ, Zamkoff KW, Gottlieb AJ. Idiopathic thrombocytopenic purpura and Hodgkin's disease: report of two cases and a review of the literature. Am J Med Sci. 1980;280(1):21–8.
26. Heyman MR, Walsh TJ. Autoimmune neutropenia and Hodgkin's disease. Cancer. 1987;59(11):1903–5.
27. Kojima H, Takei N, Mukai Y, Hasegawa Y, Suzukawa K, Nagata M, et al. Hemophagocytic syndrome as the primary clinical symptom of Hodgkin's disease. Ann Hematol. 2003;82(1):53–6.
28. Slease RB, Schumacher HR. Deficiency of coagulation factors VII and XII in a patient with Hodgkin's disease. Arch Intern Med. 1977;137(11):1633–5.
29. Shoho AR, Go RS, Tefferi A. 22-year-old woman with severe microcytic anemia. Mayo Clin Proc. 2000;75(8):861–4.

30. De Kerviler E, Gossot D, Frija J. Localization techniques for the thoracoscopic resection of pulmonary nodules. Int Surg. 1996;81(3):241–4.

31. de Kerviler E, Guermazi A, Zagdanski AM, Meignin V, Gossot D, Oksenhendler E, et al. Image-guided core-needle biopsy in patients with suspected or recurrent lymphomas. Cancer. 2000;89(3):647–52.

32. Picardi M, Gennarelli N, Ciancia R, De Renzo A, Gargiulo G, Ciancia G, et al. Randomized comparison of power Doppler ultrasound-directed excisional biopsy with standard excisional biopsy for the characterization of lymphadenopathies in patients with suspected lymphoma. J Clin Oncol. 2004; 22(18):3733–40.

33. Agid R, Sklair-Levy M, Bloom AI, Lieberman S, Polliack A, Ben-Yehuda D, et al. CT-guided biopsy with cutting-edge needle for the diagnosis of malignant lymphoma: experience of 267 biopsies. Clin Radiol. 2003;58(2):143–7.

34. Landgren O, Porwit MacDonald A, Tani E, Czader M, Grimfors G, Skoog L, et al. A prospective comparison of fine-needle aspiration cytology and histopathology in the diagnosis and classification of lymphomas. Hematol J. 2004;5(1):69–76.

35. Rosenberg SA, Boiron M, DeVita Jr VT, Johnson RE, Lee BJ, Ultmann JE, et al. Report of the committee on Hodgkin's disease staging procedures. Cancer Res. 1971;31(11): 1862–3.

36. Lister TA, Crowther D, Sutcliffe SB, Glatstein E, Canellos GP, Young RC, et al. Report of a committee convened to discuss the evaluation and staging of patients with Hodgkin's disease: Cotswolds meeting. J Clin Oncol. 1989;7(11):1630–6.

37. Hasenclever D, Diehl V. A prognostic score for advanced Hodgkin's disease. International Prognostic Factors Project on Advanced Hodgkin's Disease. N Engl J Med. 1998; 339(21):1506–14.

38. Armitage JO. Staging non-Hodgkin lymphoma. CA Cancer J Clin. 2005;55(6):368–76.

39. Kwee TC, Kwee RM, Nievelstein RA. Imaging in staging of malignant lymphoma: a systematic review. Blood. 2008; 111(2):504–16.

40. Blodgett TM, Meltzer CC, Townsend DW. PET/CT: form and function. Radiology. 2007;242(2):360–85.

41. von Schulthess GK, Steinert HC, Hany TF. Integrated PET/ CT: current applications and future directions. Radiology. 2006;238(2):405–22.

42. Connors JM, Klimo P. Is it an E lesion or stage IV? An unsettled issue in Hodgkin's disease staging. J Clin Oncol. 1984;2(12):1421–3.

43. Laskar S, Gupta T, Vimal S, Muckaden MA, Saikia TK, Pai SK, et al. Consolidation radiation after complete remission in Hodgkin's disease following six cycles of doxorubicin, bleomycin, vinblastine, and dacarbazine chemotherapy: is there a need? J Clin Oncol. 2004;22(1):62–8.

44. Terasawa T, Lau J, Bardet S, Couturier O, Hotta T, Hutchings M, et al. Fluorine-18-fluorodeoxyglucose positron emission tomography for interim response assessment of advanced-stage Hodgkin's lymphoma and diffuse large B-cell lymphoma: a systematic review. J Clin Oncol. 2009;27(11):1906–14.

45. Hutchings M, Loft A, Hansen M, Pedersen LM, Buhl T, Jurlander J, et al. FDG-PET after two cycles of chemotherapy predicts treatment failure and progression-free survival in Hodgkin lymphoma. Blood. 2006;107(1):52–9.

46. Cheson BD, Horning SJ, Coiffier B, Shipp MA, Fisher RI, Connors JM, et al. NCI Sponsored International Working Group. Report of an international workshop to standardize response criteria for non-Hodgkin's lymphomas. J Clin Oncol. 1999;17(4):1244.

47. Cheson BD, Pfistner B, Juweid ME, Gascoyne RD, Specht L, Horning SJ, et al. Revised response criteria for malignant lymphoma. J Clin Oncol. 2007;25(5):579–86.

48. Juweid ME, Stroobants S, Hoekstra OS, Mottaghy FM, Dietlein M, Guermazi A, et al. Use of positron emission tomography for response assessment of lymphoma: consensus of the Imaging Subcommittee of International Harmonization Project in Lymphoma. J Clin Oncol. 2007;25(5):571–8.

49. Zinzani PL, Fanti S, Battista G, Tani M, Castellucci P, Stefoni V, et al. Predictive role of positron emission tomography (PET) in the outcome of lymphoma patients. Br J Cancer. 2004;91(5):850–4.

50. Juweid ME, Wiseman GA, Vose JM, Ritchie JM, Menda Y, Wooldridge JE, et al. Response assessment of aggressive non-Hodgkin's lymphoma by integrated International Workshop Criteria and fluorine-18-fluorodeoxyglucose positron emission tomography. J Clin Oncol. 2005;23(21): 4652–61.

51. Radford JA, Cowan RA, Flanagan M, Dunn G, Crowther D, Johnson RJ, et al. The significance of residual mediastinal abnormality on the chest radiograph following treatment for Hodgkin's disease. J Clin Oncol. 1988;6(6):940–6.

52. Kazama T, Faria SC, Varavithya V, Phongkitkarun S, Ito H, Macapinlac HA. FDG PET in the evaluation of treatment for lymphoma: clinical usefulness and pitfalls. Radiographics. 2005;25(1):191–207.

53. Jerusalem G, Hustinx R, Beguin Y, Fillet G. Positron emission tomography imaging for lymphoma. Curr Opin Oncol. 2005;17(5):441–5.

54. Hillner BE, Siegel BA, Liu D, Shields AF, Gareen IF, Hanna L, et al. Impact of positron emission tomography/computed tomography and positron emission tomography (PET) alone on expected management of patients with cancer: initial results from the National Oncologic PET Registry. J Clin Oncol. 2008;26(13):2155–61.

55. Gallamini A, Hutchings M, Rigacci L, Specht L, Merli F, Hansen M, et al. Early interim 2-[18F]fluoro-2-deoxy-D-glucose positron emission tomography is prognostically superior to international prognostic score in advanced-stage Hodgkin's lymphoma: a report from a joint Italian-Danish study. J Clin Oncol. 2007;25(24):3746–52.

56. Brepoels L, Stroobants S. Is [(18)F]fluorodeoxyglucose positron emission tomography the ultimate tool for response and prognosis assessment? Hematol Oncol Clin North Am. 2007;21(5):855–69.

57. Henry-Amar M, Friedman S, Hayat M, Somers R, Meerwaldt JH, Carde P, et al. The EORTC Lymphoma Cooperative Group. Erythrocyte sedimentation rate predicts early relapse and survival in early-stage Hodgkin disease. Ann Intern Med 1991;114(5):361–5.

58. Guadagnolo BA, Punglia RS, Kuntz KM, Mauch PM, Ng AK. Cost-effectiveness analysis of computerized tomography in the routine follow-up of patients after primary treatment for Hodgkin's disease. J Clin Oncol. 2006;24(25):4116–22.

59. Hoppe RT, Advani RH, Bierman PJ, Bloomfield CD, Buadi F, Djulgegovic B, et al. Hodgkin disease/lymphoma. Clinical

practice guidelines in oncology. J Natl Compr Canc Netw. 2006;4(3):210–30.

60. Radford JA, Eardley A, Woodman C, Crowther D. Follow up policy after treatment for Hodgkin's disease: too many clinic visits and routine tests? A review of hospital records. BMJ. 1997;314(7077):343–6.

61. Dryver ET, Jernstrom H, Tompkins K, Buckstein R, Imrie KR. Follow-up of patients with Hodgkin's disease following curative treatment: the routine CT scan is of little value. Br J Cancer. 2003;89(3):482–6.

62. Torrey MJ, Poen JC, Hoppe RT. Detection of relapse in early-stage Hodgkin's disease: role of routine follow-up studies. J Clin Oncol. 1997;15(3):1123–30.

63. Jerusalem G, Beguin Y, Fassotte MF, Belhocine T, Hustinx R, Rigo P, et al. Early detection of relapse by whole-body positron emission tomography in the follow-up of patients with Hodgkin's disease. Ann Oncol. 2003;14(1):123–30.

# Functional Imaging

**6**

Martin Hutchings and Andrea Gallamini

## Contents

M. Hutchings (✉)
Department of Oncology, Copenhagen University Hospital,
Blegdamsvej 9, 2100, Copenhagen, Denmark
e-mail: hutchings@dadlnet.dk

A. Gallamini
Hematology Department, Azienda Ospedaliera S. Croce e
Carle, Via M. Coppino 26, 12100, Cuneo, Italy

## 6.1 Introduction

Hodgkin lymphoma (HL) is a highly curable disease, with more than 90% of patients still alive and 80% considered cured 6 years after treatment [1]. These rewarding results have been obtained by a combination of factors influencing treatment outcome in different ways. These can be briefly summarised: (a) an increasing accuracy of staging procedures; (b) different treatment strategies tailored to well-defined categories of patients with a different risk of treatment failure; (c) a peculiar neoplastic tissue architecture, different from the one of more frequent lymphoma subtypes such as diffuse large B-cell lymphoma (DLCBL) or follicular lymphoma (FL); and (d) a high chemosensitivity and radiosensitivity of the tumour.

Perhaps no other haematologic tumour has been the object of such accurate staging definitions as HL, using a wide array of radiology, nuclear medicine or even surgical procedures, ranging from chest X-ray to staging laparotomy [2]. Computerised tomography (CT) is the cornerstone procedure for staging and response assessment. However, as CT uses size criteria to distinguish between normal and malignant tissue, it cannot detect involved nodes under a certain size. Moreover, response assessment with CT uses changes in tumour size as the main criterion. But tumour shrinkage takes time, and since a residual HL mass can take years after treatment to disappear, CT does not provide an early assessment of therapy response [3]. This challenge is met by functional imaging, which is dependent on tumour metabolism rather than anatomy.

HL is considered one of the most chemosensitive haematological neoplasms, but the biological mechanism for this phenomenon is unclear. A possible explanation could be found in the peculiar neoplastic

A. Engert and S.J. Horning (eds.), *Hodgkin Lymphoma*,
DOI: 10.1007/978-3-642-12780-9_6, © Springer-Verlag Berlin Heidelberg 2011

architecture of the tumour: only a few scattered neoplastic cells (Hodgkin and Reed-Sternberg cells), accounting for less than 1% of the total cell count of the neoplastic tissue, are surrounded by a population of seemingly non-neoplastic mononuclear bystander cells [4]. The production of chemokines by tumour cells is possibly responsible for this organisation of the neoplastic architecture. The Hodgkin and Reed–Stenberg (HRS) cells produce the chemokines thymus and activation-regulated chemokines (TARC-CCL7) and macrophage-derived chemokines that selectively recruit CCR4-expressing cell subsets, including eosinophils, histiocytes, macrophages, plasma cells, and Th2 and Treg lymphocytes, which are all readily detected at tumour sites. There is convincing evidence that forced expression of CCR4 in these cells provides them with the capacity to migrate towards a TARC gradient, so that the functionality of this receptor is not restricted to the subset of T cells in which it is physiologically expressed [5]. These cells are metabolically very active and are in turn responsible for the production of chemokines that enables them to recruit accessory cells and ensure HRS cell immortalisation. Chemotherapy can switch off the chemokine production of HRS cells, and preliminary observations have shown that serum TARC levels predict therapy response in HL patients [6]. Positron emission tomography (PET) using [18F]-fluoro-2-deoxy-D-glucose (FDG) has emerged as a reliable tool to assess chemosensitivity when performed very early during standard-dose adriamycin, bleomycin, vinblastine and dacarbazine (ABVD) treatment in HL patients [7]. FDG-PET detects the metabolic silencing of the neoplastic tissue induced by chemotherapy, and likewise the persistence of a small chemoresistant clone with a high metabolic activity. Such early assessment of treatment response makes new therapeutic options possible, with treatment tailored to the individual patient that may potentially lead to higher cure rates with less overall toxicity. Several clinical trials exploring the role of early PET-response-adapted therapy have been initiated worldwide [8].

Functional imaging includes a large number of nuclear medicine procedures as well as certain applications of magnetic resonance imaging (MRI). However, apart from relatively rare exceptions (bone scintigraphy, leukocyte scintigraphy in infected patients, lung scintigraphy), only gallium-67 scans and FDG-PET had a clearly defined role in the management of HL.

## 6.2 Gallium Scan

### 6.2.1 Staging

In 1969, Edwards and Hayes first proposed the potential use of gallium-67 ($^{67}$Ga) citrate as a tumour tracer for HL [9]. Johnston studied 248 HL patients staged at baseline with gallium-67 scan and conventional radiological methods such as CT scan and lymphangiography [10]. Overall positive, negative and equivocal results were found in 56, 35 and 9% of the 1,308 nodal sites. Moreover, the accuracy of gallium scan and lymphangiography was evaluated in a subset of 149 patients undergoing staging laparotomy. Sensitivity and specificity were 45 and 83%, respectively; positive and negative predictive values (PPV and NPV) were 70 and 63%, respectively. A lower sensitivity was found in lymphocyte predominant disease than in classical HL. Andrews and Hagemeister, both using planar scintigraphy, evaluated the sensitivity in different affected nodal areas: overall, sensitivity was higher for superficial and mediastinal lesions (48–91%), and lower for abdominal nodes (47 and 48%) [11, 12]. Later on, several studies have investigated the role of high-dose gallium scan and the role of single-photon emission computed tomography (SPECT) as an imaging technique. However, moving from 3–5 mCi (50 µCi/kg) to 7–10 mCi (120 µCi/kg) did not increase specificity (98 and 98%, respectively) nor sensitivity (64 and 66%, respectively) [12]. SPECT imaging slightly improved sensitivity from 78 to 85%, leaving the specificity unchanged (97 and 98%, respectively) [13]. However, in another study, sensitivity increased from 66 to 96% due to a higher detection of mediastinal and retroperitoneal nodes [14].

### 6.2.2 Chemotherapy Response

For post-treatment evaluation with gallium scans, high doses of Gallium-67 citrate (8–10 mCi) and the use of SPECT are essential [13]. Two crucial aspects of chemotherapy response have been studied: (1) the assessment of a residual mass and (2) the prediction of disease-free survival (DFS) and overall survival (OS). It is well known that up to 64–80% of the patients have a residual mass after treatment of a bulky HL, despite a good response to therapy as shown by conventional restaging modalities [15]. Gallium scintigraphy should be performed at least 3 weeks after the end of treatment, to reduce both false-positive and false-negative results. Gallium-67 is a viability tracer and is taken up by viable tumour masses after therapy, as proven by biopsy [16]. The persistence of gallium uptake in a residual mass has been proven to predict both DFS and OS, with a specificity of 95% and sensitivity of 60–96%, depending on the region of persisting disease [17]. Treatment outcome has been efficiently predicted in HL by end-treatment gallium scan: for DFS the NPV was 84% and the PPV 80% (Front 1992). Similar results have been obtained by King in a cohort of 33 HL patients: NPV 92% and PPV 90% [18]. However, when the NPV post-therapy gallium scan was calculated according to stage, it was 92.4% for patients with stage I–II disease and 64.5% for patients with stage III–IV disease [19].

### 6.2.3 Chemosensitivity Assessment

In the beginning of the 1980s, in the pre-CT scan era, the early therapy response assessment with Gallium scans after three cycles of MOPP chemotherapy was already considered an important prognostic tool [20, 21]. A decade later, Front demonstrated that gallium scans, performed after a single cycle of chemotherapy, predicted final treatment outcome accurately in a cohort of HL patients [22]. The NPV was very high; 22/24 patients with a negative scan remained in sustained complete response. The PPV was 57%; however, only seven patients had a positive interim scan. Chemosensitivity assessment with gallium scans has been done also in patients with relapsing HL for whom salvage treatment with high-dose chemotherapy and autologous stem cell transplantation (ASCT) is planned. In a cohort of 174 patients with recurrent/refractory HL, gallium scan has been done after salvage chemotherapy with ESHAP (etoposide, methylprednisolone, cytarabine, and cisplatin) or ASHAP (doxorubicin,

methylprednisolone, cytarabine, and cisplatin) just before ASCT. Thirty two of forty three (74%) patients with a positive gallium scan and 36/131 (24%) with a negative scan showed treatment failure [23].

### 6.2.4 Follow-Up

Early diagnosis of HL recurrence is a very difficult task. So far only physical examination has shown an adequate sensitivity (80%), but unfortunately this method is limited to the superficial nodes [24]. Very few reports have been published on the role of surveillance gallium scan in the follow-up of HL patients. In a mixed cohort of 68 patients affected by aggressive B-cell lymphoma and HL, Front et al. evaluated the overall accuracy of gallium scan for detecting residual disease, when the scan was performed after an average of 8.7 months from diagnosis. The sensitivity and specificity were 95 and 89%, respectively [25]. In this cohort of patients, scintigraphy anticipated the diagnosis of recurrence by a median of 6.7 months. The authors stressed the role of gallium scan in detecting occult disease in the abdomen in 10 patients where physical findings, ultrasonography and CT scans were negative.

Despite its clinical usefulness in certain situations, gallium scanning is a laborious and time-consuming procedure, with relatively high radiation doses. Gallium scans have largely been replaced by FDG-PET, as they have no clear advantages over this method.

## 6.3 FDG-PET in Clinical Management of Lymphoma

### 6.3.1 Basic Principles of PET

PET is a functional imaging modality based on measurements of events related to the decay of positron-emitting radioactive nuclides. These nuclides have excess protons which transform to neutrons under the emission of positrons ($\beta^+$-decay). The positron randomly travels 2–3 mm in the tissue before it annihilates via collision with an electron and hereby emits two photons (each 511 keV) at an angle of almost 180°. The photons are registered by the ring of scintillation detectors in the PET scanner. Two 511 keV photons registered simultaneously (or within a very narrow time frame) by two opposing detectors are considered a coincidence event originating from positron annihilation. A PET scanner holds several thousands of scintillation detectors organised in detector rings. The detector rings are often separated by leaded ring collimators (2D mode) in order to limit sources of noise in the PET images. Data acquisition can be either static or dynamic, and the data generated provide both quantitative information and images. The spatial resolution of PET is typically around 5 mm, limited by the number of detectors and by the random travel of the positron [26]. The unstable positron-emitting isotopes used in PET are produced by fusion of stable nuclei with other particles. This is possible in a cyclotron, in which the electrical repulsion between particles is overcome by accelerating particles up to 30% of the speed of light with a beam towards the target [27]. A radiochemistry laboratory is needed to attach the isotopes to relevant tracer molecules. The most common PET isotopes molecules are $^{15}O$, $^{13}N$, $^{11}C$ and $^{18}F$ [28]. PET tracers of relevance to oncology target glucose metabolism, hypoxia, blood flow, proliferation, amino acid transport, protein synthesis, DNA synthesis, apoptosis and specific receptors.

Fusion PET/CT scanners incorporate the hardware of high-resolution CT and PET into one scanner, so that PET and CT as well as fusion images are obtained in one scanning session. PET/CT scanners have been available commercially since the late 1990s and very few single-modality PET scanners are sold now. PET/CT has obvious advantages over PET, including better anatomical localisation as well as easier distinction between pathological findings and normal physiological uptake [29].

### 6.3.2 The FDG Tracer

The glucose analogue 2-[18F]fluoro-2-deoxyglucose (FDG) is the most versatile and widely used PET tracer, and it is estimated that FDG-PET accounts for 90% of all clinical PET studies. The use of FDG in tumour imaging is based on Warburg's finding that cancer cells show accelerated glucose metabolism [30]. FDG is

transported into the cell via glucose transporter molecules (GLUT 1–5), which are overexpressed in cancer cells [31–33]. In the cell, FDG is phosphorylated by hexokinase to FDG-6-phosphate, which does not cross the cell membrane. Due to the low levels of glucose-6-phosphatase in cancer cells and the inability of FDG-6-phosphate to enter glycolysis, the tracer is retained in the cancer cells [34]. Generally, the uptake of FDG is related to the number of viable tumour cells [35, 36], but dependent on a number of physiological factors including regional blood flow, blood glucose level, and tissue oxygenation [37, 38]. FDG uptake is very high in HL, but since the HRS cells only make up a small fraction of the tumour volume, the surrounding cells are probably accountable for the increased FDG metabolism. FDG is far from tumour-specific and accumulates in a range of non-malignant tissues, such as brain, heart and kidneys. Furthermore, activated inflammatory cells take up FDG, which can cause false-positive results in cancer imaging studies [39, 40]. This is obviously important since HL patients frequently experience infections, but also because chemotherapy and radiotherapy induce inflammatory responses in the tumour cells and the surrounding tissue. An increased tracer uptake is seen in response to the early phase with very low uptake shortly after therapy [41, 42]. FDG is administered by intravenous injection.

### 6.3.3 Staging

Early reports on FDG-PET for lymphoma imaging were published more than 20 years ago [43]. Since most lymphomas showed FDG avidity, a number of studies have followed, investigating the properties of FDG-PET in the primary staging of both HL and NHL. As it would be unethical and laborious to biopsy every suspected focus, the lesions were generally not validated by histopathological analysis. Discrepancies between CT and FDG-PET were later assessed at follow-up, considering all available clinical data and allowing the clinical course to eventually determine a standard of reference for analysis of diagnostic accuracy. Such a reference standard is far from optimal, but probably the best that can be achieved. Especially the early studies of FDG-PET for staging of malignant lymphomas were performed in a retrospective fashion involving mixed lymphoma populations who were scanned at different times during the course of treatment. The general impression from these investigations, regardless of technical differences in scanning protocols and experimental approach, was that FDG-PET had a very high diagnostic sensitivity [44–54]. In both HL and aggressive NHL, FDG-PET detects more disease sites, nodal as well as extranodal, than conventional imaging methods, resulting in a higher sensitivity, and leading to significant upwards stage migration [44–66]. FDG-PET seems to be at least as sensitive as blind bone marrow biopsy [46, 66–68]. Later studies have focused on individual lymphoma subtypes, thus respecting the very variable nature of this heterogeneous group of diseases.

Studies focused on HL have found a very high sensitivity for nodal staging, especially for the detection of peripheral and thoracic lymph nodes. The increased sensitivity apparently does not come at the expense of a significantly decreased specificity. FDG-PET also detects extranodal disease more sensitively than conventional methods, both in the bone marrow and in other organs (Fig. 6.1).

FDG-PET has a consistent, large influence on the staging in HL, with upstaging of approximately 15–25% of patients, and downstaging in only a small minority of patients. This leads to a shift to a more advanced treatment group in approximately 10% of patients [55–66]. The tendency towards upwards stage migration is important, as HL is a disease where early and advanced stages are treated very differently. However, early stage HL patients have an excellent prognosis and are at the same time at high risk of serious treatment-related late morbidity and mortality. With this in mind, the use of FDG-PET for staging of HL should be accompanied by steps to reduce the intensity of therapy to early stage patients in general, and such steps should be taken in the setting of clinical trials.

Almost 100% of all newly sold PET scanners are integrated PET/CT scanners and the dual-modality scanner is rapidly replacing single-modality scanners in most centres. A few studies have looked specifically at the value of FDG-PET/CT as compared with CT and/or FDG-PET in the lymphoma staging. FDG-PET/CT is found to be more accurate for staging than both FDG-PET and CT, with an equal sensitivity and a better specificity. FDG-PET/CT has less of a tendency towards upstaging of patients than PET alone; in fact FDG-PET/CT correctly downstages a number of patients compared with both CT and FDG-PET. FDG-PET/CT has fewer false-positive findings than FDG-PET alone, especially in the deep nodal regions of the abdomen and the mediastinum, a fact probably owed to the improved distinction between malignant and non-malignant FDG uptake (intestinal uptake, brown fat, muscle uptake, etc.) [64, 69].

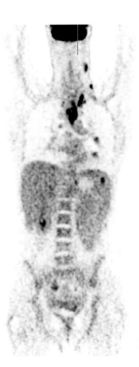

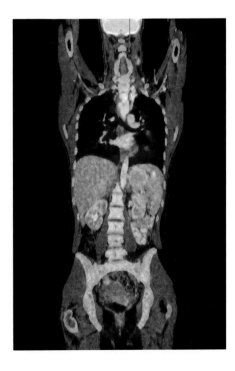

**Fig. 6.1** Example of upstaging due to FDG-PET. This patient had only supradiaphragmal disease visible on CT, but the PET clearly revealed a splenic lesion that disappeared after the first chemotherapy cycle

### 6.3.4 Early Assessment of Chemosensitivity

Seventy to eighty percent of the HL patients show normalisation of the FDG-PET scan after two courses of ABVD [3, 70]. However, very similar findings have been reported as early as after one single cycle [71], or even 7 days after the very first chemotherapy administration [72]. Non-neoplastic cells show an impressive FDG avidity, resulting in a positive baseline scan in 100% of the HL cases, but their metabolic activity and chemokine production are apparently shut down after two courses of chemotherapy. This phenomenon occurs in normal-size but also bulky nodes, in spite of a persisting mass, as tumour shrinkage takes time and depends on several factors in the host. The paradoxical phenomenon of a persisting mass without evidence of a viable neoplastic tissue has been called "metabolic complete remission" [73, 74], and accounts for the high overall accuracy of interim-PET scan in predicting treatment outcome in HL patients. Non-neoplastic micro-environment cells are metabolically very active at baseline. They are shut down in chemotherapy-responsive patients, but they are responsible for the persisting FDG uptake in chemoresistant refractory disease [75]. This situation is quite different in DLBCL. In DLBCL, neoplastic cells make up 85–99% of the nucleate cells. Their proliferative fraction is very high, sometimes up to 90%. The persisting FGD uptake could be the balance between cell kill by chemotherapy and cell re-growth [76].

Interim FDG-PET scan performed very early during treatment has shown a high overall accuracy as it predicts treatment outcome in more than 90% of the patients. In a retrospective analysis of 88 patients scanned after two or three cycles of ABVD-like chemotherapy for HL, Hutchings et al. found a 5-year PFS of 39% in the PET-positive group compared with 92% in the PET-negative group [77]. These results were later confirmed in prospective studies by Hutchings et al. [3], Zinzani et al. [78] and Gallamini et al. [70], the latter study focusing on advanced HL patients alone. In all three studies, almost all (94–100%) of the patients who were PET-positive after two cycles of ABVD had refractory disease or relapsed within two years, while all the early PET-negative patients entered a good remission and very few later relapsed (~6%). More recently, Terasawa et al. systematically reviewed all the studies so far published on this issue and reported

a sensitivity for HL patients ranging between 43 and 100% and a specificity ranging between 67 and 100% [7]. In all reviewed studies, the authors confirmed the prognostic role of early FDG-PET in predicting treatment outcome and concluded that it is useful and reliable for assessment of the treatment response. In a joint Italian and Danish study, the 2-year progression-free survival for early PET-negative and -positive patients was 95 and 12%, respectively. Early interim FDG-PET emerged as the only independent prognostic factor for prediction of treatment outcome, thus eliminating the importance of the pre-therapeutic risk index, the international prognostic score (IPS) [79] (Fig. 6.2).

Recent studies have raised concerns that the PPV of early FDG-PET may be lower in patients treated with the more dose-intensive BEACOPPesc regimen (bleomycin, etoposide, doxorubicin, cyclophosphamide, vincristine, procarbazine, prednisone) than in patients treated with ABVD [80–82].

Eight to ten percent of the patients who undergo early interim FDG-PET show a persisting, faint FDG uptake, most often in a site where a bulky tumour was recorded at baseline. This area of persisting FDG uptake, labelled minimal residual uptake (MRU), was defined as low-grade uptake of FDG, just above background, in an area of previously noted disease [77]. The significance MRU is unknown, but it is probably a consequence of the inflammatory tissue reaction to the

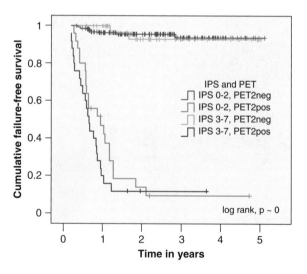

**Fig. 6.2** Kaplan–Meier plot showing the progression-free survival according to the International Prognostic Score (IPS) Group and positron emission tomography results after two cycles of ABVD. (From [80] with permission)

cytolytic effect of the chemotherapy, with an unspecific FDG uptake by inflammatory cells infiltrating the neoplastic lesion [42]. The prognosis of MRU+ patients seems to be similar to the one observed in patients with an early negative scan, and for these reasons it has been proposed that MRU+ patients should be considered as early PET negative.

Two questions concerning the ideal time for early interim FDG-PET scanning are still unanswered: (1) What is the ideal timing of FDG-PET after chemotherapy administration? (2) What is the ideal number of chemotherapy cycles before the early interim FDG-PET scan? In mice undergoing FDG-PET, the FDG uptake by reactive inflammatory macrophages was minimal 14 days after chemotherapy administration [42]. In a review of the published experience of interim FDG-PET early during treatment, Kasamon et al. [83] concluded

that the optimal time for performing interim PET during chemotherapy ranged between 7 and 14 days after chemotherapy. The answer to question (2) could depend on the aggressiveness of the tumour and the efficacy of the chemotherapy. Hutchings et al. found no prognostic difference between FDG-PET performed after two and four cycles of chemotherapy for HL [3]. In a small cohort of 20 HL and NHL patients, Iagaru et al. [84] found that FDG-PET obtained at two and four cycles both correlated well with end-of-treatment response. Furthermore, standardised uptake value (SUV) reduction from the baseline value did not differ significantly in scans performed at two and four cycles. In HL, there is most evidence for the use of FDG-PET after two courses of chemotherapy, but promising preliminary reports point towards an equally high predictive value as early as after one cycle [71] (Fig. 6.3).

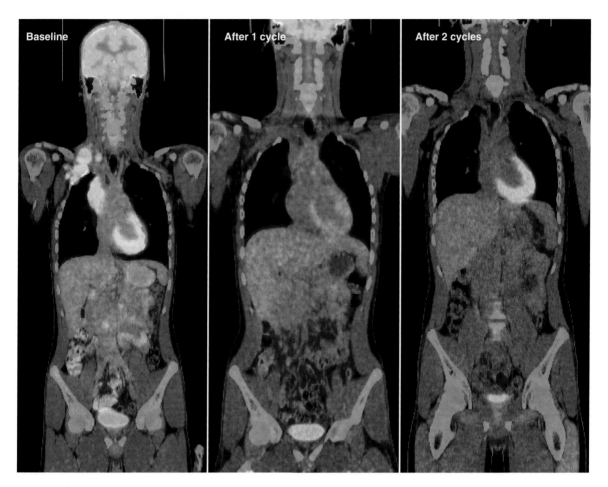

**Fig. 6.3** Early PET-response to ABVD chemotherapy. This patient with stage IIA disease has marked FDG uptake at baseline. After both one and two cycles of therapy, FDG distribution is normal although there is only a partial remission on CT

### 6.3.5 Treatment Response Assessment

From 1999 to 2001, several reports in the literature demonstrated the high sensitivity and specificity of FDG-PET in tumour response assessment. In a recent accurate meta-analysis from 13 studies on 408 HL patients, upon exclusion of other studies not fulfilling the minimal requirements for review (full ring of CT-PET, adequate follow-up, definition of the reference test), Zijlstra and colleagues [85] were able to demonstrate a pooled sensitivity and specificity of PET in defining treatment outcomes of 84 and 90%, respectively (Fig. 6.4).

As a consequence, FDG-PET was proposed as a determining tool for the definition of treatment response, and it has been integrated into the most recent definitions of CR, PR, stable or progressive disease by the International Workshop Criteria on treatment response in lymphomas [86]. Recent publications report on the clinical consequences of these new criteria. The concept of CRu has been abandoned,

and patients defined in CR or CRu at the end of treatment had an identical outcome; patients in PR had a progression-free survival similar to the ones in stable or progressive disease [87]. Therefore, the number of false-negative results obtained with the new response criteria is much smaller than the number of false-positive results obtained with the old ones, thus sparing a significant number of patients from unnecessary treatment.

Despite the good response to therapy, treatment of HL results in residual mass in up to 64–80% of the patients, as shown by conventional restaging modalities [15, 88]. Since the study by Jerusalem et al. [89], many reports focused on the role of FDG-PET for post-treatment evaluation of a residual mass in lymphoma. Quite recently, Terasawa et al. [90] systematically reviewed all the studies published so far on this issue, and reported a sensitivity for HL patients ranging between 43 and 100%, and a specificity ranging between 67 and 100%. FDG-PET has been proposed as determinant for the decision to deliver consolidation radiotherapy in cases of single residual

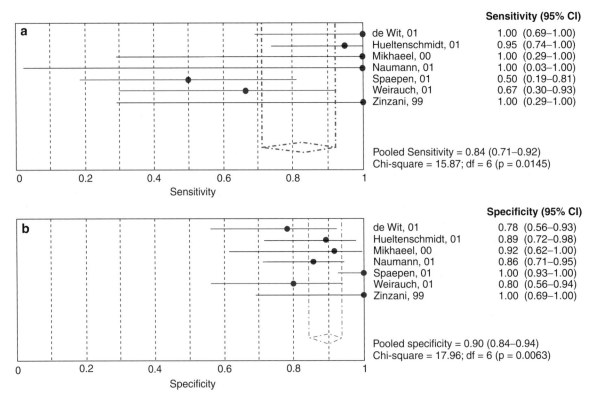

**Fig. 6.4** (a) Sensitivities and 95% confidence intervals for studies assessing the diagnostic accuracy of FDG-PET in patients with Hodgkin lymphoma. (b) Specificity and 95% confidence intervals for studies assessing the diagnostic accuracy of FDG-PET in patients with HD. The *diamond* represents the 95% CI of the pooled estimate. (From [85] with permission)

mass persistence at the end of chemotherapy, and its role has been proven essential [91, 92].

## 6.3.6 PET in Radiotherapy Planning

In the treatment of HL, radiotherapy is used in a combined modality setting. Extended fields developed for single-modality treatment have been replaced by more and more conformal fields designed for combined modality treatment, encompassing the initially macroscopically involved tissue volumes in early stage disease and bulky masses and/or residual masses after chemotherapy in advanced disease [93–96]. These changes have led to dramatic reductions in the volume of normal tissue being irradiated and similar reductions in the risk of serious late effects of radiotherapy. But such modern therapy also demands a higher accuracy of the imaging procedures used for treatment planning. As FDG-PET has been shown to be more accurate for staging of HL, it is by implication also more precise in defining the initially involved regions which are intended to be irradiated in patients with early stage disease. No diagnostic modality has 100% sensitivity and specificity, so the delineation of the lymphoma volume must be based on a combination of all the diagnostic information available of both anatomy and physiology of the disease [97, 98]. Therefore, treatment planning using a combined FDG-PET/CT scan is preferable [99].

In the primary treatment of early stage HL, chemotherapy is most often the initial treatment followed by radiotherapy. In this situation the initial lymphoma volume seen on the pre-chemotherapy FDG-PET/CT scan must be contoured on a planning CT scan done after chemotherapy. Image fusion may then be employed later on to allow pre-chemotherapy images to be combined with the post-chemotherapy planning CT, thus aiding the accurate delineation of the initially involved volume on the planning CT. If PET is to be used to its full potential in this situation, pre-chemotherapy PET/CT should be acquired with the patient in the same position as the position which will later be used for radiotherapy. In advanced disease, radiotherapy is used less frequently and usually only to residual disease. In this situation, FDG-PET/CT may help in discriminating between a residual mass with viable lymphoma cells and a residual mass consisting only of fibrotic tissue. However, FDG-PET cannot detect microscopic

disease, and it is not clear whether the target volume for irradiation in this situation should be only PET-positive lesions or whether it should also include CT positive but PET-negative areas.

Relatively limited clinical data are available on the role of FDG-PET in target definition for the planning of radiotherapy for HL [100, 101]. Where extended field irradiation is still used, the impact of FDG-PET is not expected to be very large since additional involvement found on FDG-PET will often be included in the large treatment fields anyway [102, 103]. But with modern, more conformal radiotherapy, changes due to FDG-PET are significant [104–106].

A likely future development is respiratory gated PET/CT-guided radiotherapy (Fig. 6.5). This technique makes mediastinal masses appear smaller and better defined. When radiotherapy is delivered with a similar respiratory gated technique, the technique can be used to

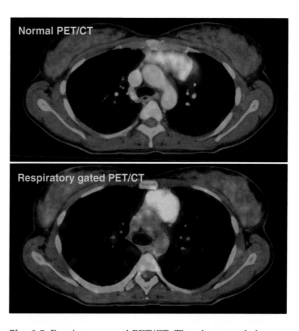

**Fig. 6.5** Respiratory gated PET/CT. The *above* panel shows a cross-sectional conventional PET/CT image of a female patient with mediastinal disease. The CT images are acquired at a random point during the respiratory cycle, and the PET images are acquired over 3–5 min and thus represent a summation of many breath cycles. The *below* panel shows the respiratory gated PET/CT images, acquired during maximum inspiration using a voice-guided, laser-controlled breath hold technique. The mediastinal mass appears smaller and better defined while the lungs are more inflated than in the normal PET/CT situation . (Courtesy of Loft and Pedersen, Copenhagen University Hospital)

refine and reduce radiotherapy fields and margins, and to minimise the damage to the lungs.

### 6.3.7 PET for Response Prediction Before High-Dose Salvage Therapy

Standard or high-dose second-line chemotherapy followed by ASCT is considered the standard treatment for relapsing or primary resistant HL [107, 108]. The only significant prognostic factors were the duration of response to first-line chemotherapy and the status of the disease at transplant or, in other words, the chemo-sensitivity assessment before ASCT. A review of the published literature points towards a high predictive value of pre-transplant FDG-PET [109]. Some reports include a mixture of NHL and HL patients, while others focus exclusively on HL. In general, the predictive value is higher in HL than in NHL, and the PPV is higher than the NPV [110–115] (Table 6.1).

In particular the PPV ranges between 91 and 43%, while the NPV between 90 and 46%. These wide-range fluctuations are mainly due to the presence of a wide array of NHL subtypes that, as already known, display different FDG avidity [116, 117]. The role of FDG-PET in this setting is unclear, and there is no evidence to support a less than curative strategy in patients who achieve a suboptimal metabolic response to induction therapy.

### 6.3.8 PET for Follow-Up

The value of surveillance procedures during follow-up in lymphoma patients achieving a CR after treatment is still a matter of debate. Generally, HL tends to recur in sites of disease at baseline, with a preference for bulky tumour sites [118]. By contrast, aggressive B-cell lymphomas tend to recur both in sites involved at baseline and in new sites [24]. As mentioned above, gallium scintigraphy has shown a high accuracy in detecting disease recurrence in HL [13]. Dittmann et al. [119] retrospectively studied 21 HL patients and found that FDG-PET and CT were equally sensitive in detecting relapsing patients before the occurrence of symptoms. Jerusalem et al. performed FDG-PET every 4–6 months for 3 years in 36 HL patients in CR after ABVD therapy. Six false-positive studies, and no false-negative studies were found out of 119 performed scans. In five positive studies, FDG-PET preceded the relapse after a median of 3.5 (1–9) months [120]. In the largest study so far, Zinzani et al. [121] investigated the role of surveillance FDG-PET performed every 6 months for 4 years after CR entry in a cohort of 160 HL patients. Results were given as positive, negative and inconclusive. Inconclusive results were regarded as positive if clinical or radiological evidence pointed towards an impending relapse. Overall, 778 scans were evaluated in HL. In 11/778 scans (1.4%), PET results were classified as inconclusive/positive, mostly in the first 18 months after CR. All these patients underwent a confirmatory biopsy and 6/11 were proven true positive. According to the authors, the major finding was the capability of FDG-PET to identify unsuspected relapse in 74% of the high risk and 20% of the low-risk HL patients. However, nobody knows if this translates into a clinical benefit for this patient subset.

For the moment, surveillance FDG-PET cannot be recommended as a routine follow-up procedure for HL patients. Early FDG-PET detection will probably allow a number of patients to enter salvage therapy with minimal disease rather than overt relapse, but is doubtful if this carries a survival benefit, and if so, one that justifies

**Table 6.1** Prognostic value of FDG-PET prior to ASCT

| Reference | Number of patients | Histology | Indication | PPV (%) | NPV (%) | 2-year PFS (PET responders) (%) | 2-year PFS (PET non-responders) (%) |
|---|---|---|---|---|---|---|---|
| Jabbour et al. [110] | 68 | HL | Rel/Pro | 72 | 76 | 76 | 27 |
| Schot et al. [111] | 117 | NHL/HL | Rel/Pro | 73 | 67 | 73 | 25 |
| Spaepen et al. [112] | 60 | NHL/HL | Rel/Pro | 87 | 90 | 100 | 24 |
| Filmont et al. [113] | 20 | NHL/HL | Rel/Pro | 91 | 87 | 87 | 7 |
| Svoboda et al. [114] | 50 | NHL/HL | Rel/Pro;3-line | 94 | 46 | 50 | 12 |
| Crocchiolo et al. [115] | 53 | NHL/HL | Rel/Pro | 43 | 72 | 90 | 55 |

the large number of scans needed. A possible exception could be the follow-up of high-risk patients, e.g. those with positive interim-PET during first-line treatment; however further studies are warranted to investigate the cost-effectiveness of such procedures.

## 6.4 PET-Response-Adapted Therapy

### 6.4.1 Ongoing Trials

While early FDG-PET quite precisely identifies responders and non-responders, there is yet no evidence that HL patients benefit from having treatment adapted according to the results of early FDG-PET. Seeing that a large fraction of early stage HL patients are subject to some amount of over-treatment, there is potential benefit in identifying good-risk early stage patients eligible for less intensive treatment. A number of trials investigate such PET-response-adapted therapy in early stage HL (Table 6.2).

The UK National Cancer Research Institute (NCRI) Lymphoma Group RAPID trial for early stage patients as well as the German Hodgkin Study Group (GHSG) HD16 protocol investigate the non-inferiority of reducing treatment intensity by omitting radiotherapy to interim PET-negative early stage patients [122, 123]. The experimental arms of EORTC/GELA/IIL[1] H10 protocol also omits radiotherapy for PET-negative patients while escalating to BEACOPPesc followed by radiotherapy in PET-positive patients. So this trial tests the non-inferiority of a less toxic treatment for good-risk patients, while at the same time attempting treatment intensification for patients regarded as having a high risk of failure based on a positive interim FDG-PET [124].

In advanced-stage HL, patients who fail to reach remission or relapse early after first-line therapy have a

---

[1]EORTC: European Organisation for the Research and Treatment of Cancer, GELA: Groupe des Etudes des Lymphomes de l'Adulte, IIL: Intergruppo Italiano dei Linfomi.

**Table 6.2** Ongoing HL trials using early PET-response-adapted therapies

| Study title/description | Study group | Patients | Main PET-driven intervention | Study type |
|---|---|---|---|---|
| HD16 for early stage Hodgkin lymphoma (HL) | German Hodgkin Study Group [122] | Early stage HL | No radiotherapy in experimental arm if PET-negative after 2 × ABVD | Phase III |
| RAPID trial | UK NCRI Lymphoma Group [123] | Early stage HL | If PET-negative after 3 × ABVD randomization to RT vs. no RT | Phase III |
| FDG-PET guided therapy or standard therapy in stage I–II HL (H10 trial) | EORTC/GELA/IIL [124] | Early stage HL | No radiotherapy in experimental arm if PET-negative after 2 × ABVD | Phase III |
| PET-adapted chemotherapy in advanced HL | GITIL [127] | Advanced HL | Intensification to BEACOPPesc if PET-positive after 2 × ABVD | Phase II |
| FDG-PET-response-adapted therapy in advanced-stage HL | UK NCRI lymphoma group [128] | Advanced HL | Intensification to BEACOPP if PET-positive after 2 × ABVD | Phase III[a] |
| HD + ASCT in patients PET-positive after 2 × ABVD and RT vs. no RT in PET-negative patients (HD0801) | IIL [129] | Advanced HL | Salvage regimen if PET-negative after 2 × ABVD | Phase III[a] |
| HD18 for advanced-stage HL | German Hodgkin Study Group [131] | Advanced HL | 4 vs. 8 × BEACOPPesc in experimental arm if PET-negative after two cycles | Phase III |

*ABVD* doxorubicin, bleomycin, vinblastin, dacarbazine; *UK NCRI* United Kingdom National Cancer Research Institute; *GELA* Groupe d'Etudes des Lymphomes de l'Adulte; *EORTC* European Organisation for the Research and Treatment of Cancer; *IIL* Intergruppo Italiano dei Linfomi; *GITIL* Gruppo Italiano Terapie Innovative nei Linfomi
[a]No randomization regarding PET-response-adapted therapy

much worse prognosis and need to be identified as early as possible to lower their risk of treatment failure, avoid unnecessary toxicity and increase the chance of long-term survival [125]. Around 70% of patients are cured with a prolonged course of ABVD with or without consolidation radiotherapy, which is first-line therapy in most centres. The more intensive BEACOPPesc cures 85–90% of patients if given upfront, but also gives reason for serious concerns regarding acute toxicity and second malignancies [126]. A number of trials investigating PET-response-adapted HL therapy have been launched. Most trials use early treatment intensification with BEACOPPesc (Italian GITIL trial and the European RATHL trial)[2] [127, 128] or even ASCT (Italian IIL trial) [129] in patients who are still PET-positive after two cycles of ABVD. Quite recently the Italian GITIL group reported its experience in a cohort of 164 advanced-stage, ABVD-treated HL patients in which treatment was intensified with escalated BEACOPP only in the small subset of patients showing an interim-PET positive after two ABVD courses, with an overall 2-year progression free for the entire cohort of patients of 88% [130]. This is contrary to the BEACOPPesc based GHSG HD18 trial, where advanced-stage HL patients in the experimental arm will be randomised to an abbreviated treatment course if PET-negative after two cycles of BEACOPPesc [131].

### 6.4.2 Interpretation Criteria

As stated above, MRU was first defined as low-grade uptake of FDG (just above background) in a focus within an area of previously noted disease reported by the nuclear medicine physicians as not likely to represent malignancy [77]. Since the prognosis of MRU+ patients is similar to that of early PET-negative patients, it has been proposed that MRU+ patients be considered PET negative. In 2007, MRU was defined by Gallamini et al. [79] as a weak persisting FDG uptake with an intensity equal or slightly superior to the mediastinal blood pool structures. Finally, in 2008, expert nuclear medicine physicians from the PET Centre at Guy's and St. Thomas Hospital, London, proposed a definition of MRU as a residual FDG uptake with an intensity lower or equal to

the one recorded in the liver [132]. This evolution has resulted in a widened definition of MRU, thus increasing the specificity and reducing the number of false-positive interim-PET scans [75]. These different MRU definitions, however, have been used for interim-PET interpretation in the different ongoing PET-response-adapted HL trials (Fig. 6.6).

Moreover, the same criteria are not necessarily adequate for HL and DLCBL, and for therapies with different dose-intensity such as ABVD or BEACOPP. For this reason, and in order to increase reproducibility, the first international meeting on interim-PET interpretation in lymphoma took place in Deauville, France during the annual GELA meeting in April 2009. This meeting followed two previous international workshops in London (2007) and Lugano (2008). The aim of this workshop was to propose simple, reproducible criteria for interim-PET interpretation and to launch one or more international validation studies to validate these rules. The results of this consensus meeting were recently published [76]. Briefly, the criteria for interim-PET interpretation in HL were contained in three major statements: (i) visual assessment is preferred, but SUV determination can assist visual assessment in some cases; (ii) interim-PET interpretation should always be made by comparing the single foci of FDG uptake to the ones recorded in the baseline study; (iii) the intensity of FDG uptake should be graded according to a five-point scale in which the liver and the mediastinal background are used as references to define different grades of FDG uptake. Two international validation studies are underway to validate these criteria; one for advanced-stage ABVD-treated HL and one for R-CHOP-treated DLCBL. A consequence of the absence of validated criteria for interim-PET reporting is the need for a central review panel for PET interpretation in the ongoing prospective trials incorporating a PET-response-adapted strategy [133]

## 6.5 Other PET Tracers

FDG is a glucose analogue and FDG uptake reflects the level of glucose metabolism in the tissue. However, like other cancers, lymphoma is characterised by deregulated cell cycle progression, and most anticancer drugs are designed to inhibit cell proliferation. So a tracer enabling imaging of cell proliferation could

---

[2]GITIL: Gruppo Italiano Therapie Innovative nei Linfomi,
RATHL: Response-Adapted Therapy in Hodgkin Lymphoma.

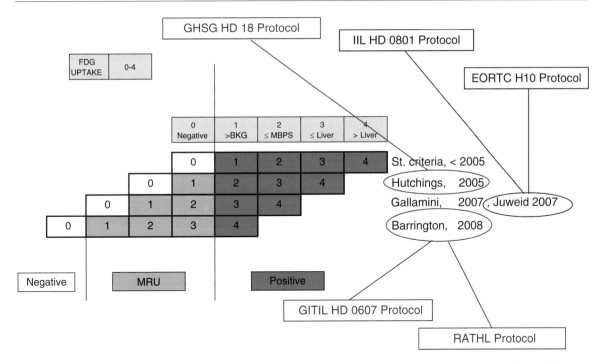

**Fig. 6.6** Different proposed criteria for minimal residual uptake (MRU) definitions. The broadening of the area of MRU in advanced-stage HL has been proposed in order to reduce false-positive results and increase the specificity of interim-PET scan in predicting treatment outcome. (From [109] with permission)

be useful for both initial characterization and treatment monitoring of the disease. FDG uptake is correlated with cell proliferation, but this correlation is weakened by a number of factors, including FDG uptake in non-malignant lesions [134–136]. The nucleoside [$^{11}$C]thymidine was the first PET tracer to specifically address cell proliferation. Early studies showed that [$^{11}$C]thymidine could determine both disease extent and early response to chemotherapy in aggressive NHL patients [137, 138]. However, the short 20 min half-life of $^{11}$C along with rapid in vivo metabolism has limited the clinical application of [$^{11}$C]thymidine. The thymidine analogue 3'-deoxy-3'-[$^{18}$F]fluorothymidine (FLT) offers a more suitable half-life of 110 min and is stable in vivo [139]. More recent studies have shown that FLT-PET can sensitively identify lymphoma sites [140]. FLT uptake is highly correlated with proliferation rate and may thus be able to distinguish between high- and low-grade lymphomas [141, 142]. And furthermore, recent studies have shown a potential of FLT for imaging early response to treatment in lymphoma [143, 144]. Amino acid metabolism of cancer cells is influenced by catabolic processes favouring tumour growth [145]. It has

been shown that increased uptake of amino acids reflects the increased transport and protein synthesis of malignant tissue [146, 147]. This is the background for PET imaging of amino acid metabolism with the labelled amino acids L-[methyl-$^{11}$C]methionine (MET) and O-2-[$^{18}$F]fluoroethyl)-L-tyrosine. Nuutinen et al. studied 32 lymphoma patients and found MET-PET highly sensitive for the detection of disease sites although there was no correlation between MET uptake and patient outcome. While these results are encouraging, it should be noted that no studies have shown the usefulness or cost-effectiveness of amino acid or nucleoside tracers in large patient cohorts. Furthermore, high physiological tracer uptake in the abdomen limits the usefulness of these tracers for imaging of abdominal and pelvic lymphomas.

## 6.6 Future Perspectives

Ongoing and upcoming clinical trials will hopefully identify patients who can benefit from early treatment adaptations based on early FDG-PET-response monitoring. However, this approach is still response-adapted and not risk-adapted. Further insight into the natural history of lymphomas on a molecular level will result in more precise pre-treatment prognostic and predictive markers. Hopefully, such markers will, in due time, help us offer more refined therapy upfront, tailored to the individual patient's risk profile and responsiveness and thus reduce the importance of treatment monitoring. New imaging techniques such as diffusion NMR have been developed, aimed to assess the microscopic mobility of water within the neoplastic tissue at diagnosis and after treatment. They have shown, in preliminary studies, high accuracy in lymphoma staging [148], and treatment response [143]. More recently, ultrasonography with tissue harmonic compound technology and intravenous microsphere-based microvasculature studies (named angiosonography) improves ultrasound accuracy [149–151]. Angiosonography has recently been reported to be more sensitive than CT or FDG-PET for detecting nodular infiltration in the spleen of patients with newly diagnosed HL [152]. Modern radiotherapy is evolving rapidly, and PET/CT plays an increasingly important role in both the selection of patients and in the radiotherapy planning. Other PET tracers are likely to emerge, including radiosensitivity tracers and perhaps tracers directly targeting HL-specific cell surface molecules. The most predictable evolution is the ongoing technical development, involving image acquisition and image processing/reconstruction, brought about by advances in hardware development and increased computing power. Integrated PET/MRI systems are being introduced into clinical practice and are likely to prove useful for evaluation of bone marrow involvement and other forms of extranodal disease.

## 6.7 General Recommendations

The value of adding FDG-PET/CT to conventional HL staging procedures is well established. Although no studies show better outcomes in cohorts staged with FDG-PET/CT, the method is recommended as a standard procedure. FDG-PET/CT has a general tendency to upstage the patients, so the method should be accompanied by steps to reduce the overall amount of treatment. FDG-PET and FDG-PET/CT are operational in the revised response criteria for post-treatment evaluation of aggressive lymphomas. The benefit for the patients of FDG-PET in this setting remains to be clearly shown, but a number of ongoing trials address the issue. There is insufficient evidence for routine use of FDG-PET in the follow-up setting. While the prognostic value of early interim FDG-PET is well established in HL, there is still no evidence that it improves patient outcomes. For this reason, it is highly recommended that the use of FDG-PET for early response monitoring takes place in the setting of clinical investigations, including the early PET-response-adapted trials. With the abundance of early PET-response-adapted clinical trials, there is an urgent need for uniform, evidence-based interpretation criteria and reporting guidelines for early interim FDG-PET/CT. A number of novel PET tracers are promising, but their use is still experimental.

## References

1. Diehl V, Stein H, Hummel M, Zollinger R, Connors JM. Hodgkin's lymphoma: biology and treatment strategies for primary, refractory, and relapsed disease. Hematology Am Soc Hematol Educ Program. 2003;2003:225–47.
2. Gospodarowicz MK. Hodgkin's lymphoma – patient's assessment and staging. Cancer J. 2009;15(2):138–42.
3. Hutchings M, Loft A, Hansen M, Pedersen LM, Buhl T, Jurlander J, et al. FDG-PET after two cycles of chemotherapy predicts treatment failure and progression-free survival in Hodgkin lymphoma. Blood. 2006;107(1):52–9.
4. Canellos GP. Residual mass in lymphoma may not be residual disease. J Clin Oncol. 1988;6(6):931–3.
5. Di Stasi A, De Angelis B, Rooney CM, Zhang L, Mahendravada A, Foster AE, et al. T lymphocytes coexpressing CCR4 and a chimeric antigen receptor targeting CD30 have improved homing and antitumor activity in a Hodgkin tumor model. Blood. 2009;113(25):6392–402.
6. Weihrauch MR, Manzke O, Beyer M, Haverkamp H, Diehl V, Bohlen H, et al. Elevated serum levels of CC thymus and activation-related chemokine (TARC) in primary Hodgkin's disease: potential for a prognostic factor. Cancer Res. 2005;65(13):5516–9.
7. Terasawa T, Lau J, Bardet S, Couturier O, Hotta T, Hutchings M, et al. Fluorine-18-fluorodeoxyglucose positron emission tomography for interim response assessment of advanced-stage Hodgkin's lymphoma and diffuse large B-cell lymphoma: a systematic review. J Clin Oncol. 2009;27(11):1906–14.
8. Hutchings M, Barrington SF. PET/CT for therapy response assessment in lymphoma. J Nucl Med. 2009;50 suppl 1:21S–30.

9. Edwards CL, Hayes RL. Tumor scanning with gallium-67 citrate. J Nucl Med. 1969;10:103–5.

10. Johnston GS, Go MF, Benua RS, Larson SM, Andrews AG, Karl F, et al. Gallium-67 citrate imaging in Hodgkin's disease: final report of cooperative group. J Nucl Med. 1977; 18:692–8.

11. Andrews GA, Hubner KF, Greenlawf RH. Ga-67 citrate imaging in malignant lymphoma: final report of cooperative group. J Nucl Med. 1978;19:1013–9.

12. Hagemeister FB, Fesus SM, Lamki LM, Haynie TP. Role of the gallium scan in Hodgkin's disease. Cancer. 1990;65: 1090–6.

13. Front D, Israel O, Epelbaum R, Ben Haim S, Even Sapir E, Jerushalmi J, et al. Ga-67 SPECT before and after treatment of lymphoma. Radiology. 1990;175:515–9.

14. Front D, Israel O. Present state and future role of gallium-67 scintigraphy in lymphoma. J Nucl Med. 1996;37(3):530–2.

15. Radford JA, Cowan RA, Flanagan M, Dunn G, Crowther D, Johnson RJ, et al. The significance of residual mediastinal abnormality on the chest radiograph following treatment for Hodgkin's disease. J Clin Oncol. 1988;6:940–6.

16. Kostakoglu L, Yeh SDJ, Portlock C, Heelan R, Yao TJ, Niedzwiecki D, et al. Validation of Gallium-67-Citrate single-photon emission computed tomography in biopsy-confirmed residual Hodgkin's disease in the mediastinum. J NuclMed. 1992;33:345–50.

17. Israel O, Front D, Lam M, Ben Aim S, Kleinhaus U, Ben-Shachat M, et al. Gallium 67 imaging in monitoring lymphoma response to treatment. Cancer. 1988;61:2439–43.

18. King SC, Reiman RJ, Prosnitz LR. Prognostic Importance of restaging gallium scans following induction chemotherapy for advanced Hodgkin's Disease. J Clin Oncol. 1994;12: 306–11.

19. Salloum E, Schwab Brandt D, Caride VJ, Cornelius E, Zelterman D, Schubert W, et al. Gallium scans in the management of patients with Hodgkin's disease: a study of 101 patients. J Clin Oncol. 1997;15:518–27.

20. Kuentz M, Reyes F, Brun B, Lebourgeois JP, Bierling P, Farcet JP, et al. Early response to chemotherapy as a prognostic factor in Hodgkin's disease. Cancer. 1983;52:780–5.

21. Levis A, Vitolo U, Ciocca Vasino MA, Cametti G, Urgesi A, Bertini M, et al. Predictive value of the early response to chemotherapy in high-risk stages II and III Hodgkin's disease. Cancer. 1987;73:1713–9.

22. Front D, Bar-Shalom R, Mor M, Haim N, Epelbaum R, Frenkel A, et al. Hodgkin disease: prediction of outcome with 67Ga scintigraphy after one cycle of chemotherapy. Radiology. 1999;210(2):487–91.

23. Jabbour E, Hosing C, Ayers G, Nunez R, Anderlini P, Pro B, et al. Pretransplant positive positron emission tomography/ gallium scans predict poor outcome in patients with recurrent/refractory Hodgkin lymphoma. Cancer. 2007;109(12): 2481–9.

24. Weeks JC, Yeap BY, Canellos GP, Shipp MA. Value of follow-up procedures in patients with large-cell lymphoma who achieve a complete remission. J Clin Oncol. 1991;9(7): 1196–203.

25. Front D, Bar-Shalom R, Epelbaum R, Haim N, Ben Arush MW, Ben Shahar M, et al. Early detection of lymphoma recurrence with gallium-67 scintigraphy. J Nucl Med. 1993; 34(12):2101–4.

26. Thompson CJ. Instrumentation. In: Wahl RL, editor. Principles and Practice of Positron Emission Tomography. Philadelphia: Lippincott Williams & Wilkins; 2002. p. 48–64.

27. Finn RD, Schlyer DJ. Production of radionuclides for PET. In: Wahl RL, editor. Principles and Practice of Positron Emission Tomography. Philadelphia: Lippincott Williams & Wilkins; 2002. p. 1–15.

28. Fowler JS, Ding Y. Chemistry. In: Wahl RL, editor. Principles and Practice of Positron Emission Tomography. Philadelphia: Lippincott Williams & Wilkins; 2002. p. 16–47.

29. Ell PJ, von Schulthess GK. PET/CT: a new road map. Eur J Nucl Med Mol Imaging. 2002;29(6):719–20.

30. Warburg O. Über den Stoffwechsel der Tumoren: arbeiten aus dem Kaiser Wilhelm-Institut für Biologie, Berlin-Dahlem. Berlin: Springer; 1926.

31. Yamamoto T, Seino Y, Fukumoto H, Koh G, Yano H, Inagaki N, et al. Over-expression of facilitative glucose transporter genes in human cancer. Biochem Biophys Res Commun. 1990;170(1):223–30.

32. Brown RS, Wahl RL. Overexpression of Glut-1 glucose transporter in human breast cancer. An immunohistochemical study. Cancer. 1993;72(10):2979–85.

33. Au KK, Liong E, Li JY, Li PS, Liew CC, Kwok TT, et al. Increases in mRNA levels of glucose transporters types 1 and 3 in Ehrlich ascites tumor cells during tumor development. J Cell Biochem. 1997;67(1):131–5.

34. Aloj L, Caraco C, Jagoda E, Eckelman WC, Neumann RD. Glut-1 and hexokinase expression: relationship with 2-fluoro-2-deoxy-D-glucose uptake in A431 and T47D cells in culture. Cancer Res. 1999;59(18):4709–14.

35. Higashi K, Clavo AC, Wahl RL. Does FDG uptake measure proliferative activity of human cancer cells? In vitro comparison with DNA flow cytometry and tritiated thymidine uptake. J Nucl Med. 1993;34(3):414–9.

36. Brown RS, Leung JY, Fisher SJ, Frey KA, Ethier SP, Wahl RL. Intratumoral distribution of tritiated-FDG in breast carcinoma: correlation between Glut-1 expression and FDG uptake. J Nucl Med. 1996;37(6):1042–7.

37. Wahl RL, Henry CA, Ethier SP. Serum glucose: effects on tumor and normal tissue accumulation of 2-[F-18]-fluoro-2-deoxy-D-glucose in rodents with mammary carcinoma. Radiology. 1992;183(3):643–7.

38. Clavo AC, Brown RS, Wahl RL. Fluorodeoxyglucose uptake in human cancer cell lines is increased by hypoxia. J Nucl Med. 1995;36(9):1625–32.

39. Kubota R, Yamada S, Kubota K, Ishiwata K, Tamahashi N, Ido T. Intratumoral distribution of fluorine-18-fluorodeoxyglucose in vivo: high accumulation in macrophages and granulation tissues studied by microautoradiography. J Nucl Med. 1992;33(11):1972–80.

40. Brown RS, Leung JY, Fisher SJ, Frey KA, Ethier SP, Wahl RL. Intratumoral distribution of tritiated fluorodeoxyglucose in breast carcinoma: I. Are inflammatory cells important? J Nucl Med. 1995;36(10):1854–61.

41. Higashi K, Clavo AC, Wahl RL. In vitro assessment of 2-fluoro-2-deoxy-D-glucose, L-methionine and thymidine as agents to monitor the early response of a human adenocarcinoma cell line to radiotherapy. J Nucl Med. 1993;34(5): 773–9.

42. Spaepen K, Stroobants S, Dupont P, Bormans G, Balzarini J, Verhoef G, et al. [(18)F]FDG PET monitoring of tumour

response to chemotherapy: does [(18)F]FDG uptake correlate with the viable tumour cell fraction? Eur J Nucl Med Mol Imaging. 2003;30(5):682–8.

43. Paul R. Comparison of fluorine-18-2-fluorodeoxyglucose and gallium-67 citrate imaging for detection of lymphoma. J Nucl Med. 1987;28(3):288–92.

44. Moog F, Bangerter M, Diederichs CG, Guhlmann A, Kotzerke J, Merkle E, et al. Lymphoma: role of whole-body 2-deoxy-2-[F-18]fluoro-D-glucose (FDG) PET in nodal staging. Radiology. 1997;203(3):795–800.

45. Bangerter M, Kotzerke J, Griesshammer M, Elsner K, Reske SN, Bergmann L. Positron emission tomography with 18-fluorodeoxyglucose in the staging and follow-up of lymphoma in the chest. Acta Oncol. 1999;38(6): 799–804.

46. Buchmann I, Reinhardt M, Elsner K, Bunjes D, Altehoefer C, Finke J, et al. 2-(fluorine-18)fluoro-2-deoxy-D-glucose positron emission tomography in the detection and staging of malignant lymphoma. A bicenter trial. Cancer. 2001; 91(5):889–99.

47. Schoder H, Meta J, Yap C, Ariannejad M, Rao J, Phelps ME, et al. Effect of whole-body (18)F-FDG PET imaging on clinical staging and management of patients with malignant lymphoma. J Nucl Med. 2001;42(8):1139–43.

48. Sasaki M, Kuwabara Y, Koga H, Nakagawa M, Chen T, Kaneko K, et al. Clinical impact of whole body FDG-PET on the staging and therapeutic decision making for malignant lymphoma. Ann Nucl Med. 2002;16(5):337–45.

49. Delbeke D, Martin WH, Morgan DS, Kinney MC, Feurer I, Kovalsky E, et al. 2-deoxy-2-[F-18]fluoro-D-glucose imaging with positron emission tomography for initial staging of Hodgkin's disease and lymphoma. Mol Imaging Biol. 2002; 4(1):105–14.

50. Moog F, Bangerter M, Diederichs CG, Guhlmann A, Merkle E, Frickhofen N, et al. Extranodal malignant lymphoma: detection with FDG PET versus CT. Radiology. 1998; 206(2):475–81.

51. Stumpe KD, Urbinelli M, Steinert HC, Glanzmann C, Buck A, von Schulthess GK. Whole-body positron emission tomography using fluorodeoxyglucose for staging of lymphoma: effectiveness and comparison with computed tomography. Eur J Nucl Med. 1998;25(7):721–8.

52. Hoh CK, Glaspy J, Rosen P, Dahlbom M, Lee SJ, Kunkel L, et al. Whole-body FDG-PET imaging for staging of Hodgkin's disease and lymphoma. J Nucl Med. 1997; 38(3):343–8.

53. Jerusalem G, Warland V, Najjar F, Paulus P, Fassotte MF, Fillet G, et al. Whole-body 18F-FDG PET for the evaluation of patients with Hodgkin's disease and non-Hodgkin's lymphoma. Nucl Med Commun. 1999;20(1):13–20.

54. Shah N, Hoskin P, McMillan A, Gibson P, Lowe J, Wong WL. The impact of FDG positron emission tomography imaging on the management of lymphomas. Br J Radiol. 2000;73(869):482–7.

55. Wiedmann E, Baican B, Hertel A, Baum RP, Chow KU, Knupp B, et al. Positron emission tomography (PET) for staging and evaluation of response to treatment in patients with Hodgkin's disease. Leuk Lymphoma. 1999;34(5–6): 545–51.

56. Partridge S, Timothy A, O'Doherty MJ, Hain SF, Rankin S, Mikhaeel G. 2-Fluorine-18-fluoro-2-deoxy-D glucose positron emission tomography in the pretreatment staging of Hodgkin's disease: influence on patient management in a single institution. Ann Oncol. 2000;11(10):1273–9.

57. Hueltenschmidt B, Sautter-Bihl ML, Lang O, Maul FD, Fischer J, Mergenthaler HG, et al. Whole body positron emission tomography in the treatment of Hodgkin disease. Cancer. 2001;91(2):302–10.

58. Jerusalem G, Beguin Y, Fassotte MF, Najjar F, Paulus P, Rigo P, et al. Whole-body positron emission tomography using 18F-fluorodeoxyglucose compared to standard procedures for staging patients with Hodgkin's disease. Haematologica. 2001;86(3):266–73.

59. Menzel C, Dobert N, Mitrou P, Mose S, Diehl M, Berner U, et al. Positron emission tomography for the staging of Hodgkin's lymphoma – increasing the body of evidence in favor of the method. Acta Oncol. 2002;41(5):430–6.

60. Weihrauch MR, Re D, Bischoff S, Dietlein M, Scheidhauer K, Krug B, et al. Whole-body positron emission tomography using 18F-fluorodeoxyglucose for initial staging of patients with Hodgkin's disease. Ann Hematol. 2002; 81(1):20–5.

61. Cohade C, Wahl RL. Applications of positron emission tomography/computed tomography image fusion in clinical positron emission tomography–clinical use, interpretation methods, diagnostic improvements. Semin Nucl Med. 2003; 33(3):228–37.

62. Naumann R, Beuthien-Baumann B, Reiss A, Schulze J, Hanel A, Bredow J, et al. Substantial impact of FDG PET imaging on the therapy decision in patients with early-stage Hodgkin's lymphoma. Br J Cancer. 2004;90(3):620–5.

63. Munker R, Glass J, Griffeth LK, Sattar T, Zamani R, Heldmann M, et al. Contribution of PET imaging to the initial staging and prognosis of patients with Hodgkin's disease. Ann Oncol. 2004;15(11):1699–704.

64. Hutchings M, Loft A, Hansen M, Pedersen LM, Berthelsen AK, Keiding S, et al. Position emission tomography with or without computed tomography in the primary staging of Hodgkin's lymphoma. Haematologica. 2006;91(4):482–9.

65. Rigacci L, Vitolo U, Nassi L, Merli F, Gallamini A, Pregno P, et al. Positron emission tomography in the staging of patients with Hodgkin's lymphoma. A prospective multicentric study by the Intergruppo Italiano Linfomi. Ann Hematol. 2007; 86(12):897–903.

66. Bangerter M, Moog F, Buchmann I, Kotzerke J, Griesshammer M, Hafner M, et al. Whole-body 2-[18F]-fluoro-2-deoxy-D-glucose positron emission tomography (FDG-PET) for accurate staging of Hodgkin's disease. Ann Oncol. 1998;9(10): 1117–22.

67. Carr R, Barrington SF, Madan B, O'Doherty MJ, Saunders CA, van der WJ, et al. Detection of lymphoma in bone marrow by whole-body positron emission tomography. Blood 1998;91(9):3340–46.

68. Pakos EE, Fotopoulos AD, Ioannidis JP. 18F-FDG PET for evaluation of bone marrow infiltration in staging of lymphoma: a meta-analysis. J Nucl Med. 2005;46(6):958–63.

69. Allen-Auerbach M, Quon A, Weber WA, Obrzut S, Crawford T, Silverman DH, et al. Comparison between 2-deoxy-2-[18F]fluoro-D-glucose positron emission tomography and positron emission tomography/computed tomography hardware fusion for staging of patients with lymphoma. Mol Imaging Biol. 2004;6(6):411–6.

70. Gallamini A, Rigacci L, Merli F, Nassi L, Bosi A, Capodanno I, et al. The predictive value of positron emission tomography scanning performed after two courses of standard therapy on treatment outcome in advanced stage Hodgkin's disease. Haematologica. 2006;91(4):475–81.

71. Kostakoglu L, Goldsmith SJ, Leonard JP, Christos P, Furman RR, Atasever T, et al. FDG-PET after 1 cycle of therapy predicts outcome in diffuse large cell lymphoma and classic Hodgkin disease. Cancer. 2006;107(11):2678–87.

72. Romer W, Hanauske AR, Ziegler S, Thodtmann R, Weber W, Fuchs C, et al. Positron emission tomography in non-Hodgkin's lymphoma: assessment of chemotherapy with fluorodeoxyglucose. Blood. 1998;91(12):4464–71.

73. MacManus MP, Seymour J, Hicks RJ. Overview of early response assessment in lymphoma with FDG-PET. Cancer Imaging. 2007;7:10–8.

74. Kostakoglu L. Early prediction of response to therapy: the clinical implications in Hodgkin's and non-Hodgkin's lymphoma. Eur J Nucl MedMol Imaging. 2008;35:1413–20.

75. Gallamini A, Fiore F, Sorasio R, Meignan M. Interim positron emission tomography scan in Hodgkin lymphoma: definitions, interpretation rules, and clinical validation. Leuk Lymophoma. 2009;50:1761–4.

76. Meignan M, Itti E, Gallamini A, Haioun C. Interim 18F-fluorodeoxyglucose positron emission tomography in diffuse large B-cell lymphoma: qualitative or quantitative interpretation – where do we stand? Leuk Lymphoma. 2009; 50:1753–6.

77. Hutchings M, Mikhaeel NG, Fields PA, Nunan T, Timothy AR. Prognostic value of interim FDG-PET after two or three cycles of chemotherapy in Hodgkin lymphoma. Ann Oncol. 2005;16(7):1160–8.

78. Zinzani PL, Tani M, Fanti S, Alinari L, Musuraca G, Marchi E, et al. Early positron emission tomography (PET) restaging: a predictive final response in Hodgkin's disease patients. Ann Oncol. 2006;17(8):1296–300.

79. Gallamini A, Hutchings M, Rigacci L, Specht L, Merli F, Hansen M, et al. Early interim 2-[18F]fluoro-2-deoxy-D-glucose positron emission tomography is prognostically superior to international prognostic score in advanced-stage Hodgkin's lymphoma: a report from a joint Italian-Danish study. J Clin Oncol. 2007;25(24):3746–52.

80. Gallamini A, Viviani S, Bonfante V, Levis A, Di Raimondo F, Merli F, et al. Early interim FDG-PET during intensified BEACOPP therapy shows a lower predictive value than during conventional ABVD chemotherapy. Haematologica. 2007;92(s5):71.

81. Avigdor A, Bulvik S, Dann EJ, Levi I, Perez-Avraham G, Shemtov N, et al. Combined ESCBEACOPP-ABVD therapy for advanced Hodgkin's lymphoma patients with high IPS score: an effective regimen and low positive predictive value of early FDG-PET/CT. Haematologica. 2007;92(s5):66.

82. Markova J, Kobe C, Skopalova M, Klaskova K, Dedeckova K, Plütschow A, et al. FDG–PET for assessment of early treatment response after four cycles of chemotherapy in patients with advanced-stage Hodgkin's lymphoma has a high negative predictive value. Ann Oncol. 2009;20(7): 1270–4.

83. Kasamon YL, Jones RJ, Wahl RL. Integrating PET and PET/CT into the risk-adapted therapy of lymphoma. J Nucl Med. 2007;48:19S–27.

84. Iagaru A, Wang Y, Mari C, Quon A, Goris ML, Horning S, et al. (18)F-FDG-PET/CT evaluation of response to treatment in lymphoma: when is the optimal time for the first re-evaluation scan? Hell J Nucl Med. 2008;11(3):153–6.

85. Zijlstra JM, Lindauer-van der Werf G, Hoekstra OS, Hooft L, Riphagen II, Huijgens PC. 18F-fluoro-deoxyglucose positron emission tomography for post-treatment evaluation of malignant lymphoma: a systematic review. Haematologica. 2006;91(4):522–9

86. Cheson BD, Pfistner B, Juweid ME, Gascoyne RD, Specht L, Horning SJ, et al. Revised response criteria for malignant lymphoma. J Clin Oncol. 2007;25(5):579–86.

87. Brepoels L, Stroobants S, De Wever W, Spaepen K, Vandenberghe P, Thomas J, et al. Hodgkin lymphoma: response assessment by revised International Workshop Criteria. Leuk Lymphoma. 2007;48(8):1539–47.

88. Naumann R, Vaic A, Beuthien-Baumann B, Bredow J, Kropp J, Kittner T, et al. Prognostic value of positron emission tomography in the evaluation of post-treatment residual mass in patients with Hodgkin's disease and non-Hodgkin's lymphoma. Br J Haematol. 2001;115:793–800.

89. Jerusalem G, Beguin Y, Fassotte MF, Najjar F, Paulus P, Rigo P, et al. Whole-body positron emission tomography using 18F-fluorodeoxyglucose for posttreatment evaluation in Hodgkin's disease and non-Hodgkin's lymphoma has higher diagnostic and prognostic value than classical computed tomography scan imaging. Blood. 1999;94(2): 429–33.

90. Terasawa T, Nihashi T, Hotta T, Nagai H. 18F-FDG PET for posttherapy assessment of Hodgkin's disease and aggressive non-Hodgkin's lymphoma: a systematic review. J Nucl Med. 2008;49(1):13–21.

91. Kobe C, Dietlein M, Franklin J, Markova J, Lohri A, Amthauer H, et al. Positron emission tomography has a high negative predictive value for progression or early relapse for patients with residual disease after first-line chemotherapy in advanced-stage Hodgkin lymphoma. Blood. 2008;112: 3989–94.

92. Sher DJ, Mauch PM, Van Den Abbeele A, LaCasce AS, Czerminski J, Ng AK. Prognostic significance of mid- and post-ABVD PET imaging in Hodgkin's lymphoma: the importance of involved-field radiotherapy. Ann Oncol. 2009;20(11): 1848–53.

93. Girinsky T, Pichenot C, Beaudre A, Ghalibafian M, Lefkopoulos D. Is intensity-modulated radiotherapy better than conventional radiation treatment and three-dimensional conformal radiotherapy for mediastinal masses in patients with Hodgkin's disease, and is there a role for beam orientation optimization and dose constraints assigned to virtual volumes? Int J Radiat Oncol Biol Phys. 2006; 64(1):218–26.

94. Girinsky T, van der Maazen R, Specht L, Aleman B, Poortmans P, Lievens Y, et al. Involved-node radiotherapy (INRT) in patients with early Hodgkin lymphoma: concepts and guidelines. Radiother Oncol. 2006;79(3):270–7.

95. Specht L, Gray RG, Clarke MJ, Peto R. Influence of more extensive radiotherapy and adjuvant chemotherapy on long-term outcome of early-stage Hodgkin's disease: a meta-analysis of 23 randomized trials involving 3,888 patients. International Hodgkin's Disease Collaborative Group. J Clin Oncol. 1998;16(3):830–43.

96. Yahalom J. Transformation in the use of radiation therapy of Hodgkin lymphoma: new concepts and indications lead to modern field design and are assisted by PET imaging and intensity modulated radiation therapy (IMRT). Eur J Haematol Suppl. 2005;66:90–7.

97. Gregoire V. Is there any future in radiotherapy planning without the use of PET: unraveling the myth. Radiother Oncol. 2004;73(3):261–3.

98. Jarritt PH, Carson KJ, Hounsell AR, Visvikis D. The role of PET/CT scanning in radiotherapy planning. Br J Radiol. 2006;79(spec no 1):S27–35.

99. Berthelsen AK, Dobbs J, Kjellén E, Landberg T, Möller T, Nilsson P, et al. What's new in target volume definitions for radiologists in ICRU Report 71? How can the ICRU volume definitions be integrated in clinical practice? Cancer Imaging. 2006;7:104–16.

100. Specht L. 2-[18F]fluoro-2-deoxyglucose positron-emission tomography in staging, response evaluation, and treatment planning of lymphomas. Semin Radiat Oncol. 2007;17(3): 190–7.

101. Van Baardwijk A, Baumert BG, Bosmans G, van Kroonenburgh M, Stroobants S, Gregoire V, et al. The current status of FDG-PET in tumour volume definition in radiotherapy treatment planning. Cancer Treat Rev. 2006; 32(4):245–60.

102. Dizendorf EV, Baumert BG, von Schulthess GK, Lutolf UM, Steinert HC. Impact of whole-body 18F-FDG PET on staging and managing patients for radiation therapy. J Nucl Med. 2003;44(1):24–9.

103. Lee YK, Cook G, Flower MA, Rowbottom C, Shahidi M, Sharma B, et al. Addition of 18F-FDG-PET scans to radiotherapy planning of thoracic lymphoma. Radiother Oncol. 2004;73(3):277–83.

104. Girinsky T, Ghalibafian M, Bonniaud G, Bayla A, Magne N, Ferreira I, et al. Is FDG-PET scan in patients with early stage Hodgkin lymphoma of any value in the implementation of the involved-node radiotherapy concept and dose painting? Radiother Oncol. 2007;85(2):178–86.

105. Hutchings M, Berthelsen AK, Loft A, Hansen M, Specht L. Clinical impact of FDG-PET/CT in the planning of radiotherapy for early stage Hodgkin lymphoma. Eur J Haematol. 2006;78(3):206–12.

106. Krasin MJ, Hudson MM, Kaste SC. Positron emission tomography in pediatric radiation oncology: integration in the treatment-planning process. Pediatr Radiol. 2004;34(3):214–21.

107. Schmitz N, Pfistner B, Sextro M, Sieber M, Carella AM, Haenel M, et al. Aggressive conventional chemotherapy compared with high-dose chemotherapy with autologous haemopoietic stem-cell transplantation for relapsed chemosensitive Hodgkin's disease: a randomised trial. Lancet. 2002;359(9323):2065–71.

108. Tarella C, Cuttica A, Vitolo U, Liberati M, Di Nicola M, Cortelazzo S, et al. High-dose sequential chemotherapy and peripheral blood progenitor cell autografting in patients with refractory and/or recurrent Hodgkin lymphoma. Cancer. 2003;97:2748–59.

109. Gallamini A. The prognostic role of positron emission tomography scan in Hodgkin's lymphoma. The education program for the annual congress of the European Hematology Association. Haematologica. 2009;3:144–50.

110. Jabbour E, Hosing C, Ayers G, et al. Pretransplant positive positron emission tomography/gallium scans predict poor outcome in patients with recurrent/refractory Hodgkin lymphoma. Cancer. 2007;109:2481–9.

111. Schot BW, Zijlstra JM, Sluiter WJ, et al. Early FDG-PET assessment in combination with clinical risk scores determines prognosis in recurring lymphoma. Blood. 2007;109: 486–91.

112. Spaepen K, Stroobants S, Dupont P, et al. Prognostic value of pretransplantation positron emission tomography using fluorine 18-fluorodeoxyglucose in patients with aggressive lymphoma treated with high-dose chemotherapy and stem cell transplantation. Blood. 2003;102: 53–9.

113. Filmont JE, Czernin J, Yap C, et al. Value of F-18 fluorodeoxyglucose positron emission tomography for predicting the clinical outcome of patients with aggressive lymphoma prior to and after autologous stem-cell transplantation. Chest. 2003;124:608–13.

114. Svoboda J, Andreadis C, Elstrom R, et al. Prognostic value of FDG-PET scan imaging in lymphoma patients undergoing autologous stem cell transplantation. Bone Marrow Transplant. 2006;38:211–6.

115. Crocchiolo R, Canevari C, Assanelli A, et al. Pre-transplant 18FDG-PET predicts outcome in lymphoma patients treated with high-dose sequential chemotherapy followed by autologous stem cell transplantation. Leuk Lymphoma. 2008;49:727–33.

116. Elstrom R, Guan L, Baker G, Nakhoda K, Vergilio JA, Zhuang H, et al. Utility of FDG-PET scanning in lymphoma by WHO classification. Blood. 2003;101:3875–6.

117. Tsukamoto N, Kojima M, Hasegawa M, Oriuchi N, Matsushima T, Yokohama A, et al. The usefulness of 18F-fluorodeoxyglucose positron emission tomography (18F-FDG-PET) and a comparison of 18F-FDG-PET with 67Gallium scintigraphy in the evaluation of lymphoma. Cancer. 2007;110:652–9.

118. Young RC, Canellos GP, Chabner BA, Hubbard SM, DeVita Jr VT. Patterns of relapse in advanced Hodgkin's disease treated with combination chemotherapy. Cancer. 1978;42(2 suppl):1001–7.

119. Dittmann H, Sokler M, Kollmannsberger C, Dohmen BM, Baumann C, Kopp A, et al. Comparison of 18FDG-PET with CT scans in the evaluation of patients with residual and recurrent Hodgkin's lymphoma. Oncol Rep. 2001;8(6): 1393–9.

120. Jerusalem G, Beguin Y, Fassotte MF, Belhocine T, Hustinx R, Rigo P, et al. Early detection of relapse by whole-body positron emission tomography in the follow-up of patients with Hodgkin's disease. Ann Oncol. 2003;14(1):123–30.

121. Zinzani PL, Stefoni V, Tani M, Fanti S, Musuraca G, Castellucci P, et al. Role of [18F]Fluorodeoxyglucose positron emission tomography scan in the follow-up of lymphoma. J Clin Oncol. 2009;27(11):1781–7.

122. HD16 for early stage Hodgkin lymphoma. Available from: http://www.clinicaltrials.gov/ct2/show/NCT00736320.

123. PET scan in planning treatment in patients undergoing combination chemotherapy for stage IA or stage IIA Hodgkin lymphoma. Available from: http://www.clinicaltrials.gov/ct2/show/NCT00943423.

124. Fluorodeoxyglucose F18 PETscan guided therapy or standard therapy in treating patients with previously untreated stage I or stage II Hodgkin's lymphoma. Available from: http://www.clinicaltrials.gov/ct2/show/NCT00433433.

125. Oza AM, Ganesan TS, Leahy M, Gregory W, Lim J, Dadiotis L, et al. Patterns of survival in patients with Hodgkin's disease: long follow up in a single centre. Ann Oncol. 1993;4(5):385–92.

126. Diehl V, Franklin J, Pfreundschuh M, Lathan B, Paulus U, Hasenclever D, et al. Standard and increased-dose BEACOPP chemotherapy compared with COPP-ABVD for advanced Hodgkin's disease. N Engl J Med. 2003; 348(24):2386–95.

127. Positron emission tomography (PET)-adapted chemotherapy in advanced Hodgkin lymphoma (HL). Available from: http://www.clinicaltrials.gov/ct2/show/NCT00795613.

128. Fludeoxyglucose F 18-PET/CT imaging in assessing response to chemotherapy in patients with newly diagnosed stage II, stage III, or stage IV Hodgkin lymphoma. Available from: http://www.clinicaltrials.gov/ct2/show/NCT00678327.

129. High-dose chemotherapy and stem cell transplantation, in patients PET-2 positive, after 2 courses of ABVD and comparison of RT versus no RT in PET-2 negative patients (HD0801). Available from: http://www.clinicaltrials.gov/ct2/show/NCT00784537.

130. Gallamini A, Fiore F, Sorasio F, Rambaldi A, Patti C, Stelitano C, Viviani S,Di Raimondo F, et al. Early chemotherapy intensification with BEACOPP in high-risk, interim PET-positive, advanced-stage Hodgkin lymphoma improves the overall treatment outcome of ABVD: a GITIL multicenter clinical study. Haematologica 2009;94(suppl 2):204 (abs. 0502).

131. HD18 for advanced stages in Hodgkins lymphoma. Available from: http://www.clinicaltrials.gov/ct2/show/NCT00515554.

132. Barrington SF, Qian W, Somer EJ, et al. (2009) Concordance between four European Centres of PET reporting criteria designed for use in multicentre trials in Hodgkin lymphoma. [Abstract]. 22nd annual EANM meeting. Barcelona, 10 October 2009. Abstract no. S-347

133. Meignan M, Itti E, Bardet S, Lumbroso J, Edeline V, Olivier P, et al. Development and application of a real-time on-line blinded independent central review of interim PET scans to determine treatment allocation in lymphoma trials. J Clin Oncol. 2009;27:2739–41.

134. Buck AK, Halter G, Schirrmeister H, Kotzerke J, Wurziger I, Glatting G, et al. Imaging proliferation in lung tumors with PET: 18F-FLT versus 18F-FDG. J Nucl Med. 2003; 44(9):1426–31.

135. Kazama T, Faria SC, Varavithya V, Phongkitkarun S, Ito H, Macapinlac HA. FDG PET in the evaluation of treatment for lymphoma: clinical usefulness and pitfalls. Radiographics. 2005;25(1):191–207.

136. Sandherr M, von Schilling C, Link T, Stock K, von Bubnoff N, Peschel C, et al. Pitfalls in imaging Hodgkin's disease with computed tomography and positron emission tomography using fluorine-18-fluorodeoxyglucose. Ann Oncol. 2001;12(5):719–22.

137. Martiat P, Ferrant A, Labar D, Cogneau M, Bol A, Michel C, et al. In vivo measurement of carbon-11 thymidine

138. Shields AF, Mankoff DA, Link JM, Graham MM, Eary JF, Kozawa SM, et al. Carbon-11-thymidine and FDG to measure therapy response. J Nucl Med. 1998;39(10):1757–62.

139. Shields AF, Grierson JR, Dohmen BM, Machulla HJ, Stayanoff JC, Lawhorn-Crews JM, et al. Imaging proliferation in vivo with [F-18]FLT and positron emission tomography. Nat Med. 1998;4(11):1334–6.

140. Buchmann I, Neumaier B, Schreckenberger M, Reske S. [18F]3'-deoxy-3'-fluorothymidine-PET in NHL patients: whole-body biodistribution and imaging of lymphoma manifestations – a pilot study. Cancer Biother Radiopharm. 2004;19(4):436–42.

141. Buck AK, Bommer M, Stilgenbauer S, Juweid M, Glatting G, Schirrmeister H, et al. Molecular imaging of proliferation in malignant lymphoma. Cancer Res. 2006;66(22): 11055–61.

142. Kasper B, Egerer G, Gronkowski M, Haufe S, Lehnert T, Eisenhut M, et al. Functional diagnosis of residual lymphomas after radiochemotherapy with positron emission tomography comparing FDG- and FLT-PET. Leuk Lymphoma. 2007;48(4):746–53.

143. Buck AK, Kratochwil C, Glatting G, Juweid M, Bommer M, Tepsic D, et al. Early assessment of therapy response in malignant lymphoma with the thymidine analogue [18F] FLT. Eur J Nucl Med Mol Imaging. 2007;34(11):1775–82.

144. Graf N, Herrmann K, den Hollander J, Fend F, Schuster T, Wester HJ, et al. Imaging proliferation to monitor early response of lymphoma to cytotoxic treatment. Mol Imaging Biol. 2008;10(6):349–55.

145. Hoffman RM. Altered methionine metabolism. DNA methylation and oncogene expression in carcinogenesis. A review and synthesis. Biochim Biophys Acta. 1984;738(1–2):49–87.

146. Stern PH, Wallace CD, Hoffman RM. Altered methionine metabolism occurs in all members of a set of diverse human tumor cell lines. J Cell Physiol. 1984;119(1):29–34.

147. Wheatley DN. On the problem of linear incorporation of amino acids into cell protein. Experientia. 1982;38(7):818–20.

148. King AD, Ahuja AT, Yeung DKW, Fong DKY, Lee YYP, Kenny IK, et al. Malignant cervical lymphadenopathy: diagnostic accuracy of diffusion-weighted MR imaging. Radiology. 2007;245:806–13.

149. Padhani AR, Liu G, Mu-Koh D, Chenevert TL, Thoeny HC, Takahara T, et al. Diffusion-weighted magnetic resonance imaging as a cancer biomarker: consensus and recommendations. Neoplasia. 2009;11:102–25.

150. Lencioni R, Cioni D, Bertolazzi C. Tissue harmonic and contrast-specific imaging: back to grey scale in ultrasound. Eur Radiol. 2002;12:151–65.

151. Oktar SO, Yucel C, Ozdemir H, Uluturk A, Isik S. Comparison of conventional sonography, real-time compound sonography, tissue harmonic compound sonography of abdominal and pelvic lesions. Am J Roentgenol. 2003;181:1341–7.

152. Picardi M, Soricelli A, Pane F, Zeppa P, Nicolai E, De Laurentis M, et al. Contrast-enhanced harmonic compound US of the spleen to increase staging accuracy in patients with Hodgkin lymphoma: a prospective study. Radiology. 2009;251:574–82.

# Prognostic Factors

## 7

Lena Specht and Dirk Hasenclever

## Contents

L. Specht (✉)
Department of Oncology, Section 5073,
The Finsen Centre, Rigshospitalet, University of Copenhagen,
Blegdamsvej 9, 2100 Copenhagen, Denmark
e-mail: lena.specht@rh.regionh.dk

D. Hasenclever
Institut für Medizinische Informatik, Statistik & Epidemiologie (IMISE), Universität Leipzig, Härtelstrasse 16-18,
04107 Leipzig, Germany

## Abbreviations

| | |
|---|---|
| ABVD | Adriamycin, bleomycin, vinblastine, dacarbazine |
| BEACOPPesc | Bleomycin, etoposide, adriamycin, cyclophosphamide, vincristine, procarbazine, prednisolone, escalated |
| BNLI | British National Lymphoma Investigation |
| CALGB | Cancer and Leukemia Group B |
| ECOG | Eastern Cooperative Oncology Group |
| EORTC | European Organisation for Research and Treatment of Cancer |
| ESR | Erythrocyte sedimentation rate |
| FDG | 2-[18F]fluoro-2-deoxy-D-glucose |
| GELA | Groupe d'Etudes des Lymphomes de l'Adulte |
| GHSG | German Hodgkin Study Group |
| IPS | International Prognostic Score |
| LDH | Lactic dehydrogenase |
| MOPP | Mechlorethamine, vincristine, procarbazine, prednisolone |
| NCI-C | National Cancer Institute of Canada |
| NCI-US | National Cancer Institute of the United States |
| PET | Positron emission tomography |
| SWOG | Southwest Oncology Group |

## 7.1 Historical Perspective

The concept that Hodgkin lymphoma (initially called Hodgkin's disease) passes through successive clinical stages with increasing spread of the disease and

A. Engert and S.J. Horning (eds.), *Hodgkin Lymphoma*,
DOI: 10.1007/978-3-642-12780-9_7, © Springer-Verlag Berlin Heidelberg 2011

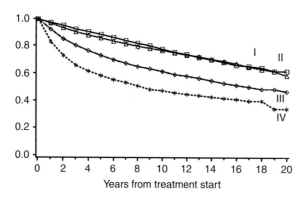

**Fig. 7.1** Overall survival according to clinical Ann Arbor stage for 14,037 patients in the International Database on Hodgkin's Disease treated over the past 25 years. (Reprinted from [14] with permission)

progressive worsening of prognosis was developed early on [1]. Different staging classifications were proposed based on the anatomic extent of disease [2–8]. A consensus was reached at the Workshop on the Staging of Hodgkin's Disease at Ann Arbor in 1971 [9], and the Ann Arbor staging classification was universally adopted. It remains the basis for the evaluation of patients with Hodgkin lymphoma, and its prognostic significance has been documented in numerous studies of patients treated with different treatment modalities [10–17]. Survival curves according to the Ann Arbor stages for more than 14,000 patients in the International Database on Hodgkin's Disease are shown in Fig. 7.1 [14].

However, the extent of disease varies within the Ann Arbor stages leading to variations in prognosis. A modification of the Ann Arbor classification was proposed at the Cotswold meeting, incorporating a designation for number of sites and bulk [18]. This modification has not been universally adopted. Numerous other prognostic factors for different Ann Arbor stages, disease presentations, treatments, and outcomes have been introduced, and varying combinations of these factors are being used by different centers and groups.

## 7.2 Prognostic Factors

### 7.2.1 Definition and Use

Prognostic factors are variables measured in individual patients that offer a partial explanation of the

heterogeneity in the outcome of a given disease [19]. They are important in clinical practice for distinguishing patients into different risk groups, for selection of treatment strategy, and as an aid in patient counseling [20]. However, it is important to realize that prediction is very uncertain for the individual patient. Statements of probability can be made, but even these will be more accurate for groups of patients than for individuals [21]. Prognostic factors can also be used in the design of clinical trials to define eligibility criteria and strata to ensure comparability of treatment groups [19–22]. However, prognostic factors are rarely sufficiently explanatory to justify the comparison of treatments by use of nonrandomized data [23, 24].

### 7.2.2 Types of Prognostic Factors

Prognostic factors are divided into tumor-related factors, host-related factors, and environment-related factors [20]. Tumor-related factors include those directly related to the presence of the tumor or its effect on the host, reflecting tumor pathology, anatomic extent, or tumor biology. Host-related factors include factors that are not directly related to the tumor but which may significantly influence outcome, such as demographic characteristics and comorbidity. Environment-related factors include factors outside the patient, such as socioeconomic status, and access to and quality of health care.

The values of prognostic factors are generally assumed to be known from the outset, before the start of treatment, so-called fixed covariates. However, other important prognostic variables may only be known later, such as time to response, toxicity of treatment, and the value of presumed markers. These are time-dependent covariates. They may be important for answering biological questions, but they should not be applied for adjustment for treatment comparison, as they are themselves affected by treatment [19–21].

### 7.2.3 Different Endpoints

Different outcomes may be of interest in analyses of prognostic factors. Overall survival and progression-free survival are usually analyzed, but others may be relevant, e.g., disease-free survival for early stage patients as virtually all patients achieve remission. For each endpoint, there must be clear information on the point in time from which it is measured, and the clinical characteristics of events and censoring. International guidelines have recently been published [25].

## 7.2.4 Types and Analyses of Prognostic Studies

Three different study phases of prognostic factors have been proposed, beginning with Phase I early exploratory analyses to identify potential markers and generate hypotheses for further investigation. Phase II studies are exploratory studies attempting to use values of a proposed prognostic factor to discriminate between high and low risk patients. Phase III studies are large, confirmatory studies based on prespecified hypotheses involving one or a few new factors, and the purpose of these studies is to determine how much the new factor adds to the predictive power of already accepted factors [22, 26].

A useful prognostic factor must be significant, independent, and clinically important [27]. Many variables may be prognostic in univariate analysis. However, different variables are likely to be interrelated. The important question is whether a particular variable adds useful information to what is already known. Multiple regression analysis is commonly employed to determine whether a variable has independent significance when other known variables are taken into account. This kind of analysis may form the basis for the development of a prognostic model and a risk score or risk groups [26]. The Cox proportional hazards regression model is most commonly used when time-to-event outcomes are of interest [28]. The selection of variables for the final model is usually done by stepwise selection. By play of chance, different factors may be selected in different studies. An important additional analysis for a new marker is therefore to determine its prognostic ability in a model including all previously defined prognostic factors [26, 29]. Differences may also be due to small sample size, different assay techniques, different cut points for variables, inclusion of different subsets of patients, and different study endpoints.

## 7.3 Prognostic Factors in Early Stage Disease

In the past when patients were still treated with radiotherapy alone, those with stage I or II disease were staged with laparotomy and splenectomy to select patients suited for radiotherapy alone [30, 31]. In these patients the information on the extent and anatomic distribution of disease was very accurate, and numerous studies of prognostic factors showed that the anatomic extent of disease, measured as the number of involved lymph node regions and the volume of disease in individual regions, in particular the mediastinum, were prognostically important [32–38]. An estimate of the total tumor burden, based on a combination of the number of involved regions and the volume of disease in individual regions, was shown to be by far the most important prognostic factor of all [39–41]. Prognosis seemed to be determined by the bulk of disease rather than the precise localization in the body [34, 42–48]. The prognostic significance of E-lesions, localized extralymphatic lesions, is controversial, partly because of disagreement regarding the distinction between E-lesions and stage IV disease [32, 49–51]. Today, patients are no longer staged with laparotomy. Consequently, information on extent and distribution of the disease is less accurate in the individual patient. Therefore, additional factors become important: usually factors providing an indirect measure of the total tumor burden and possibly also the growth characteristics of the tumor.

Today, very few patients are treated with radiotherapy alone, except for patients with lymphocyte predominant histology. From early studies it is evident that the number of involved regions and size of mediastinal disease, B-symptoms, histological subtype, age, gender, ESR, hemoglobin, and serum albumin are prognostically significant [14, 47, 52–58].

Most patients with early stage disease are today treated with a combination of chemotherapy and radiotherapy. A meta-analysis showed that combined modality therapy improves progression-free survival compared with radiotherapy alone, but that it does not improve the chance of being cured of Hodgkin lymphoma (although with very long follow-up survival is superior with combined modality treatment due to an excess mortality from long-term complications in patients who relapse) [59–61]. In the meta-analysis, the size of the reduction in the risk of failure in patients separated by stage, B-symptoms, gender, and age was remarkably similar. Therefore, prognostic factors in patients treated with combined modality therapy do not seem to differ from the factors in patients treated with radiotherapy alone. Treatment of early stage patients is now often tailored according to prognostic subgroups. Hence, in many publications patients are selected, making the detection of prognostic factors difficult. However, a number of studies have confirmed the significance of the prognostic factors mentioned above also for patients treated with combined modality [62–65].

Most of the important prognostic factors are correlated and provide indirect measures of the patient's total tumor burden [40, 41, 47]. Modern imaging with CT scans and FDG-PET scans makes it possible to directly quantify the total tumor volume in each individual patient. Studies using these techniques have confirmed the pivotal prognostic role of the total tumor burden [66–69]. Figure 7.2 shows time to treatment failure for patients with stage I and II disease according to whether their mean tumor burden normalized to body surface area was below or above the mean value for each stage [66].

Functional imaging with FDG-PET has recently become an important part of staging and treatment evaluation of lymphomas. An early interim FDG-PET

scan after one or two cycles of chemotherapy has been shown to be highly predictive of outcome after combined modality treatment [70–72]. Figure 7.3 shows progression-free survival curves for early stage and advanced disease according to the result of an FDG-PET scan after two cycles of chemotherapy with ABVD [70]. The data are, in fact, rather sparse with regard to early stage disease, and the prediction of disease recurrence and inferior survival in patients with a positive early interim FDG-PET scan is largely based on data from patients with advanced disease. In a recent study of mid-treatment FDG-PET in early stage patients, most of the patients with interim PET positivity were cured with combined modality therapy, yielding a positive predictive value of only 15% [73]. However, the negative predictive value is very high in early stage disease. The early interim FDG-PET scan may be regarded as an in vivo test of the chemosensitivity of the disease. As the result of the scan is not known at the outset there is a methodological problem with this test. Strictly speaking, outcome according to the result of an early interim FDG-PET scan should only be measured from the time when it is available, and it should be regarded more as a predictive factor indicating the sensitivity to a particular treatment rather than as a usual prognostic factor.

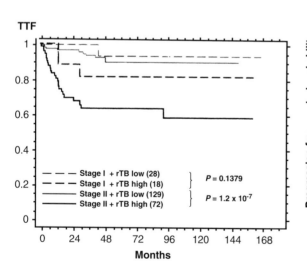

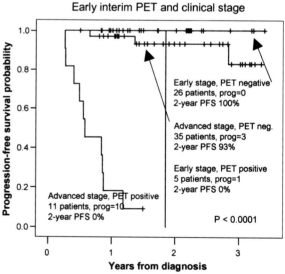

**Fig. 7.2** Time to treatment failure curves for 46 patients with stage I and 201 patients with stage II disease divided according to whether their mean tumor burden normalized to body surface area (rTB) was below or above the mean value for each stage. (Reprinted from [66] with permission)

**Fig. 7.3** Progression-free survival in 31 patients with early stage and 46 patients with advanced stage disease divided according to the result of an early interim FDG-PET scan (after two cycles of chemotherapy). (Reprinted from [70] with permission)

**Table 7.1** Prognostic factors in early stage Hodgkin lymphoma

| |
| --- |
| Number of involved lymph node regions |
| Large tumor mass, particularly mediastinal |
| Tumor burden |
| B-symptoms |
| Histological subtype |
| Age |
| Gender |
| Erythrocyte sedimentation rate (ESR) |
| Hemoglobin |
| Serum albumin |
| Early interim FDG-PET scan |

Table 7.1 lists the established prognostic factors in early stage Hodgkin lymphoma. Today, early stage patients are commonly divided into favorable and unfavorable groups, depending on various combinations of these factors.

Recently, chemotherapy alone has been used in early stage patients. Relapse-free survival is poorer than with combined modality therapy, and a recent meta-analysis has shown that overall survival is also poorer for patients treated with chemotherapy alone [74]. Prognostic factors in this group of patients have not been analyzed as large cohorts of patients with reasonable follow-up are not yet available.

## 7.4 Prognostic Factors in Advanced Disease

Advanced stage patients, although this term is not sharply defined, are those requiring full systemic treatment. Stages IIIB and IV certainly form the core group. Most study groups also include stage IIIA and possibly selected stage I or II patients with multiple adverse prognostic factors.

The role of radiotherapy added to full systemic treatment in advanced stages is limited [75]. Thus, these treatment variants can be considered together in prognostic factors analysis.

Large data sets are important to reliably assess the independent contributions of single routinely documented prognostic factors, which tend to be small to moderate (5–10% in tumor control) [76]. Two very large data sets resulted from international cooperation: The International Database on Hodgkin's Disease was set up in 1989, combining more than 14,000 individual patient data in all stages from 20 study groups in the MOPP era [14]. In 1995, the International Prognostic Factors Project on advanced Hodgkin disease combined data of 5,141 advanced stage patients mainly treated with doxorubicin-containing regimen [76].

### 7.4.1 Patients Treated with Conventional Chemotherapy with or Without Additional Radiotherapy

Important prognostic factors are shown in Table 7.2. The most important patient-related prognostic factor for overall survival in advanced Hodgkin disease is age [77–84]. Elderly patients (>60–65 years) are often excluded from general adult study populations and treated in separate studies [85]. Prevalence of comorbidity increases with age, and the risk of treatment-related mortality and toxicity-associated treatment reductions are increased [86, 87]. In patients up to 65 years of age,

**Table 7.2** Prognostic factors in advanced Hodgkin lymphoma

| |
| --- |
| Age |
| Gender |
| Histology |
| Stage IV disease |
| Tumor burden |
| Inguinal involvement |
| Very large mediastinal mass |
| B-symptoms |
| Anemia |
| Low serum albumin |
| High ESR |
| High serum alkaline phosphatase |
| Leukocytosis |
| Lymphocytopenia |
| High serum lactic dehydrogenase (LDH) |
| High serum β2-microglobulin |
| Early interim FDG-PET scan |

age (e.g., >45 years) is an independent prognostic factor for freedom from progression. This may be related to tumor biology as unfavorable histological subtypes are more frequent in the elderly [14]. The impact of age is more pronounced on overall survival due to compromised results of salvage treatment in elderly relapsed patients: 5-year survival rates after progression/relapse decrease with advancing age from about 40% in the patients up to 35 years to less than 5% in patients with 55–65 years of age at diagnosis [76].

About two-thirds of advanced stage patients are men [14, 76]. Male gender is an independent, although quantitatively moderate, adverse prognostic factor within advanced stages [14, 76, 83, 88, 89].

The histological subtype plays a minor role among the tumor-related prognostic factors. Some studies report mixed cellularity or lymphocyte depletion subtypes as unfavorable prognostic factors [12, 14, 90], whereas several other studies do not confirm these findings [76, 77, 82, 83, 91]. The prognostic relevance of grading the nodular sclerosis subtype remains controversial [92–96]. Unfavorable subtypes are correlated with male gender, age, lack of mediastinal involvement, stage, systemic symptoms, and related abnormal blood parameters [14, 57]. Histology subtyping does not lend itself to prognostication, at least in multicenter settings because of a relatively high reclassification rate under expert pathological review [92].

The principle that tumor burden is the main determinant of prognosis also holds for advanced disease [66, 82, 83]. Tumor burden can be quantified directly from imaging [67, 97]. Unfortunately, this is not done routinely. Moreover information on the number of involved areas [82, 91], the amount of tumor in the spleen [98–101], and the subdivision of stage III [98, 99, 102–104] are all surrogates for tumor burden which were established as prognostic in the era of pathological staging and radiotherapy alone. Regional inguinal involvement may be seen as a surrogate marker for maximal nodal spread and was reported as an independent prognostic factor [84].

Very large mediastinal bulk (e.g., >0.45 of the thoracic aperture) is relatively rare (i.e., <10% of advanced disease), but has been reported as an adverse prognostic factor in some studies [84, 105], but not in others [106]. Large, but not very large (e.g., 0.33–0.45 of the thoracic aperture), mediastinal mass (e.g., 0.33–0.45 of the thoracic aperture) is not related to prognosis in advanced Hodgkin disease treated with modern chemotherapy [76].

Several hematological and biochemical laboratory parameters form a cluster of interrelated prognostic indicators that mirror both tumor burden as well as inflammatory processes [53]. Decreased serum albumin [76, 79, 107, 108] and hemoglobin levels [14, 76, 78, 81] (or hematocrit [84]) as well as an elevated ESR [57, 109] or alkaline phosphatase [109–111] are correlated [14, 57, 76, 112] with one another as well as with the presence of B-symptoms [14, 113] and tumor burden [66]. Serum albumin [76, 107] (see Fig. 7.4) and hemoglobin level [76] (see Fig. 7.5) show a remarkably monotone relation to prognosis over their full range of variation and singles both out as the most informative prognostic factors in advanced Hodgkin lymphoma. Given hemoglobin and serum albumin, the other

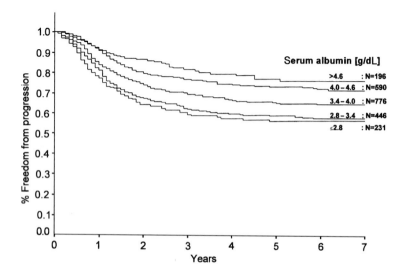

**Fig. 7.4** Freedom from progression according to albumin levels for 2,239 patients with advanced disease in the International Prognostic Factors Project. (Reprinted from [76] with permission)

**Fig. 7.5** Freedom from progression according to hemoglobin levels for 4,314 patients with advanced disease in the International Prognostic Factors Project. (Reprinted from [76] with permission)

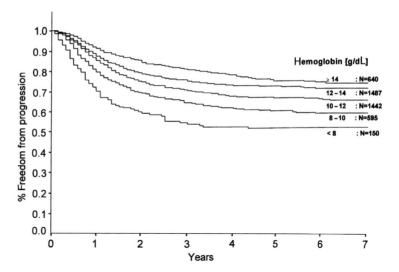

members of this cluster, in particular B-symptoms, lose their independent prognostic impact [76].

Stage IV marks dissemination of the disease to extranodal sites and has independent prognostic value within advanced disease [14, 76, 90]. It remains controversial whether a specific organ involvement site carries a particularly bad prognosis within stage IV. Bone marrow involvement was an adverse factor in some studies [83, 84, 114], but not in others [115, 116]. Pleura, lung, or liver involvement have been reported as prognostically unfavorable [114, 115, 117, 118], but not in other studies [83, 84, 119]. The number of involved extranodal sites has been reported to be independently prognostic [78, 120, 121], but this could not be confirmed in the International Prognostic Factors Project [76].

Leukocyte and lymphocyte counts form a second correlation cluster of laboratory parameters. Analyzing the joint distribution of leukocyte and lymphocyte counts in advanced Hodgkin lymphoma, there is a simultaneous shift away from the normal pattern toward both leukocytosis [76] and lymphocytopenia [78, 79, 81, 83] that carries independent prognostic impact [76]. These relatively unspecific measurements may indirectly capture dysregulation of hematopoiesis due to cytokine release by Hodgkin lymphoma cells.

Serum LDH plays a lesser role in Hodgkin lymphoma than in aggressive non-Hodgkin lymphoma. Elevated serum LDH was found by some groups [78, 84], but was not confirmed in large data sets [14, 76]. The relevance of elevated $\beta_2$-microglobulin is controversial [122, 123]. Table 7.3 summarizes the prognostic factors in advanced disease.

**Table 7.3** Adverse prognostic factors incorporated in the International Prognostic Factors Project score for freedom from progression in advanced Hodgkin disease

| |
|---|
| Age ≥45 years |
| Male gender |
| Stage IV disease |
| Hemoglobin <10.5 g/dL |
| Serum albumin <4.0 g/dL |
| Leukocytosis ≥15 × 10⁹/L |
| Lymphocytopenia <0.6 × 10⁹/L or <8% of white blood cell count |

A plethora of biological parameters such as levels of cytokines released by Hodgkin and Reed–Sternberg cells, soluble forms of membrane-derived antigens, and molecular markers have been investigated for prognostic value. Many of these studies have been done in rather small data sets (N from 40 to 300). The soluble form of the CD30 molecule is released by Hodgkin and Reed–Sternberg cells and is detectable in the serum of virtually all untreated patients [124–127]. It maintains independent prognostic significance in multivariate analysis in moderately sized data sets [126, 128–130]. The relevance of cytokine levels requires further investigation [129] and results for further biologic parameters are mostly still immature or controversial.

An early interim FDG-PET scan after one or two cycles of chemotherapy has been shown to be highly

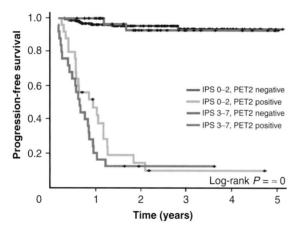

**Fig. 7.6** Progression-free survival in 260 patients with advanced disease according to International Prognostic Score (IPS) and PET results after two cycles of ABVD. (Reprinted from [133] with permission)

predictive of clinical outcomes in advanced Hodgkin lymphoma [70, 71, 131, 132]. In a large study of patients treated with ABVD, the prognostic value of an early PET scan completely overshadowed the role of the International Prognostic Score (IPS) (see below) [133]. Figure 7.6 shows progression-free survival according to the IPS and the result of an early PET scan. However, an early FDG-PET scan is a marker for chemosensitivity, and it is therefore dependent on the specific given treatment. Concerns have been raised that the positive predictive value may be lower in patients treated with more aggressive regimens such as BEACOPPesc [134].

### 7.4.2　Prognostic Indices or Scores in Advanced Hodgkin Lymphoma

Prognostic indices or scores for advanced Hodgkin lymphoma are clinically important to tailor treatment to patients: to select patients who may be overtreated and in whom treatment reduction may be considered, or to select patients in whom standard treatment is likely to fail to eliminate the disease and for whom experimental approaches may be indicated.

Several trial groups developed prognostic indices or scores based on a few hundred cases and defined high risk groups. Wagstaff et al. [135] defined risk groups based on age >45, male gender, absolute lymphocyte

count $<0.75 \times 10^9/L$, and stage IV [111, 135]. Straus et al. proposed a five-factor score including age >45, elevated serum LDH, low hematocrit, regional inguinal involvement, and mediastinal mass >0.45 of the thoracic aperture [84]. Proctor et al. developed a numerical index to predict overall survival based on age, stage, hemoglobin level, absolute lymphocyte count, and bulky disease (>10 cm) [81, 105]. Gobbi et al. set up a predictive equation based on age, sex, stage, histology, B-symptoms, mediastinal mass, ESR, hemoglobin, and serum albumin [12, 136]. Low et al. defined a score based on age ≥45, serum albumin <35 g/L, and lymphocyte count <1.5 g/L and validated the score in a large historic BNLI data set [79, 137]. However, none of these indices have received general acceptance.

Gobbi et al. developed a parametrical model to derive numerical estimates of expected survival in all stages [88]. Seven factors were incorporated: stage, age, histology, B-symptoms, serum albumin, sex, and involved area distribution (infradiaphragmatic disease or more than three supradiaphragmatic areas). This work was based on 5,023 patients in both early and advanced stages from the International Database on Hodgkin's Disease [14]. They were treated heterogeneously with radiotherapy alone or mainly MOPP-type chemotherapy with or without radiotherapy. All these models used overall survival as the main endpoint.

The International Prognostic Factors Project on advanced Hodgkin disease focused on freedom from progression [76]. Individual patient data were collected from 23 centers or study groups on 5,141 patients diagnosed as having advanced stage Hodgkin disease and treated with (mainly) doxorubicin-containing chemotherapy with and without radiotherapy according to a defined protocol. A prognostic score was developed from this data set in patients up to 65 years of age. The score is the simple count of how many of seven binary adverse prognostic factors (summarized in Table 7.3) of approximately similar prognostic impact are present: age ≥45, male gender, stage IV, albumin <4.0 g/dL, hemoglobin <10.5 g/dL, leukocytosis $>15 \times 10^9/L$, and lymphocytopenia (lymphocyte count $<0.6 \times 10^9/L$, or <8% of leukocytes, or both).

The IPS predicts 5-year tumor control rates in the range of 45–80%. Each additional factor reduces the prognosis by about 8%. Figure 7.7 shows freedom from progression according to the number of adverse prognostic factors for 1,618 patients in the International Prognostic Factors Project on advanced Hodgkin disease.

**Fig. 7.7** Freedom from progression according to the number of adverse prognostic factors (see Table 7.3) for 1,618 patients with advanced disease in the International Prognostic Factors Project. (Reprinted from [76] with permission)

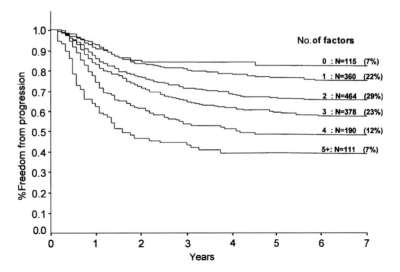

Since its publication, the IPS has performed reasonably well in independent data sets [138–142]. With intensified BEACOPP chemotherapy outcome uniformly improved in all IPS groups [138]. Differences persisted, but were quantitatively reduced.

Two publications compared several prognostic models [78, 140]. None of the models including the IPS is able to select neither a very low risk group (e.g., <10% failure rate) or a substantial very high risk group (>50%). The prognostic models only discriminate between relatively low risk and relatively high risk patients (e.g., IPS≤2 vs. IPS>2). Until new powerful, biologically more specific prognostic markers emerge, the IPS remains a workable method of choice and is currently used in intergroup trials to select higher-risk advanced stage patient for treatment intensification.

Several authors tried to extend the IPS beyond advanced stages, and according to some literature the IPS works nicely to predict outcome after autologous hemapoietic stem cell transplantation [143]. It appears to be moderately predictive in early and intermediate stages, extending the factor stage IV to include any extranodal disease [52, 144].

## 7.5 Prognostic Factors for Outcome After Relapse

Relapses of Hodgkin lymphoma after radiotherapy alone are qualitatively different from relapses after chemotherapy alone or combined modality therapy.

Both freedom from second relapse and overall survival are considerably better for patients relapsing after radiotherapy alone than for the others [61, 145, 146]. However, today patients are rarely treated with radiotherapy alone except for patients with lymphocyte predominance subtype. Hence, it is now very rare for patients to relapse after radiotherapy alone.

### 7.5.1 Patients Treated for Relapse with Conventional Treatment

Patients relapsing after initial treatment with chemotherapy or combined modality therapy, whether for early stage or advanced disease, have a poor prognosis with conventional chemotherapy. Durable remissions are obtained in only 10–30% of cases [147–154]. The extent and duration of the initial remission is the most important prognostic factor for outcome after relapse. Patients who never achieve a complete remission have an extremely poor prognosis, patients who relapse within 12 months of complete remission have an intermediate prognosis, and patients who relapse more than 12 months after achieving complete remission have the best prognosis [147–151, 154, 155]. But even for the latter, long-term outlook is poor with conventional chemotherapy. Figure 7.8 shows survival curves for patients relapsing after initial chemotherapy divided into these three prognostic groups [156]. Patients in second or higher relapse have a dismal prognosis [153, 157, 158].

**Fig. 7.8** Overall survival of patients with primary progressive, early relapse, or late relapse of Hodgkin lymphoma, treated in the German Hodgkin Study Group from 1988 to 1999, primarily with conventional salvage. (Reprinted from [156] with permission)

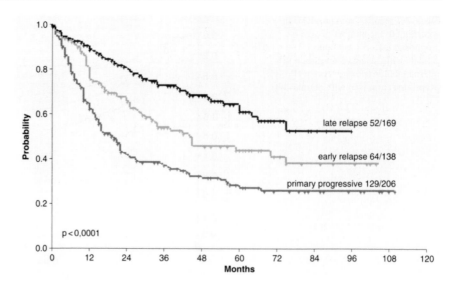

The extent of disease at relapse is also independently significant for prognosis. Advanced stage, extranodal disease, and more than three involved sites at relapse are adverse prognostic factors [147, 148, 154, 159]. Age, performance status, histology other than nodular sclerosis, B-symptoms at relapse, and a low hemoglobin have also been shown to be significant [147, 150, 151, 154, 155, 159]. Prognostic factors that have been shown to be independently significant for outcome after relapse following primary chemotherapy or combined modality therapy are summarized in Table 7.4.

A subgroup of patients relapsing after chemotherapy have anatomically limited relapse in nodal sites alone. For selected patients in this subgroup, radiotherapy with or without additional chemotherapy offers some chance of durable remission [151, 160–165]. Prognostic

factor analyses indicate that patients suitable for this kind of relapse treatment are those relapsing exclusively in supradiaphragmatic nodal sites, with no B-symptoms at relapse, with favorable histology (lymphocyte predominance or nodular sclerosis), and after a disease-free interval of 12 months or more [160, 161, 164, 166]. In patients with these favorable characteristics durable remission with radiotherapy may be achieved in up to 50% of cases.

### 7.5.2 Patients Treated for Relapse with High-Dose Chemotherapy and Stem Cell Transplantation

High-dose chemotherapy with stem cell transplantation is superior to conventional chemotherapy in patients relapsing after chemotherapy or combined modality treatment [167, 168]. It is the preferred treatment in patients able to tolerate intensive treatment. A number of prognostic factors are independently significant for therapeutic outcomes in this situation. The chemosensitivity of the disease is extremely important. Hence, the response to initial or salvage therapy, the duration of initial remission, and the number of prior failed regimens have been shown to be important for outcome [169–178].

The disease burden before transplantation is another important prognostic factor, and measures

**Table 7.4** Prognostic factors for outcome after relapse treated with conventional salvage treatment

| |
|---|
| Extent and durability of first remission |
| Extent of disease at relapse (relapse stage, extranodal relapse, ≥3 sites of relapse) |
| B-symptoms at relapse |
| Hemoglobin at relapse |
| Histology |
| Age |
| Performance status |

reflecting tumor burden such as stage of disease, and bulky or extranodal disease at salvage have been shown to be independently significant [155, 169, 170, 176, 179, 180]. B-symptoms, low hemoglobin, and an elevated serum LDH at relapse are also significant [170, 172, 174, 175, 181]. A poor performance status is an important adverse prognostic feature [169, 171, 173], whereas age has not been significant in most series, probably due to the fact that most patients are relatively young at transplantation [182–186]. Pediatric patients have, however, the same outcome as adults [187].

The seven factors included in the IPS for advanced Hodgkin lymphoma have been examined [143]. Only low serum albumin, anemia, age ≥45, and lymphocytopenia were independently significant. A simplified prognostic score including these four factors has been proposed, but it has not yet been tested in analyses including chemosensitivity and extent of prior therapy.

A number of studies have shown that an FDG-PET scan performed after two cycles of induction therapy before stem cell transplantation can predict which patients are likely to achieve long-term remission after the salvage regimen [188–193]. In most of the studies patients with different types of lymphoma are analyzed together, and Hodgkin patients are only a minority. Nevertheless, the result of an early PET scan in this setting is promising, but further research is needed.

The prognostic factors known to be independently significant for outcome after high-dose chemotherapy and stem cell transplantation are shown in Table 7.5.

**Table 7.5** Prognostic factors for outcome after high-dose chemotherapy and stem cell transplantation for refractory or recurrent disease

| |
| --- |
| Chemosensitivity of the disease |
|     Response to initial or salvage therapy |
|     Duration of initial remission |
|     Number of failed prior regimens |
|     Early interim FDG-PET scan |
| Disease burden before salvage |
|     Stage of disease at salvage |
|     Bulky disease at salvage |
|     Extranodal relapse |
| B-symptoms at relapse |
| Hemoglobin at relapse |
| Serum LDH at relapse |

## 7.6 Use of Prognostic Factors in Clinical Trials

Optimizing the treatment strategy for Hodgkin lymphoma is an attempt to make all prognostic factors disappear [194]. Ideally, when the amount and aggressiveness of therapy is adequately tailored to the patient's risk and disease burden nearly all patients should have the same excellent prognosis. For example, in data of the German Hodgkin's Lymphoma Study Group, early, intermediate, and advanced stage patients have nearly the same failure-free survival curve with the advanced stage curve in the middle, but many patients are probably overtreated [194]. Thus, with therapeutic progress prognostic factors should be expected to lose their prognostic value and become mere "disease burden" indicators.

As such, prognostic factors help to stratify the patient population into more homogeneous groups which are then treated with disease burden adapted treatment options. Together with strategies of response adaptation, this hopefully will lead to increasingly individualized and more adequate treatment.

### 7.6.1 Prognostic Factor Combinations Currently Used by Major Trial Groups

In clinical trials, prognostic factors are primarily used in the definition of the study population (entry and exclusion criteria). Further uses include description of study population and adjustment for prognostic imbalances in the final analysis.

Inclusion criteria that are currently used differ by trial and study group. The Hodgkin lymphoma patients' population does not fall into naturally defined groups. Instead, prognosis varies on a continuum scale from low-risk minimal disease to high-risk maximally advanced disease. The delineation of study populations depends on the prognosis, the respective therapeutic approach, and study group history.

The classical Ann Arbor [9] or Cotswold [18] staging systems are based on the anatomic distribution of the disease. The Ann Arbor staging system is well established and universally accepted and still forms the reference system for most definitions of study entry criteria. Most study groups currently use hybrid systems to define their study entry criteria, basically using stage and in addition presence or absence of unfavorable prognostic factors (also called risk factors in this context).

Most study groups divide Hodgkin lymphoma patient population into two (early vs. advanced stages) or three (early vs. intermediate vs. advanced stages) separate trials or treatment groups. Attempts to use a fourth "very favorable" early stage group with minimal treatment have been abandoned by the EORTC [195]. Tables 7.6 and 7.7 describe inclusion criteria currently or recently used by study groups in early stage and advanced disease respectively.

Early stages comprise patients in whom full systemic treatment is considered overtreatment. As the prognosis in this group is excellent, study questions focus on curative intent with minimal toxicity or cost. Table 7.6 illustrates that early stages are typically defined as stage I or II without risk factors, with lists

of unfavorable prognostic factors that vary by study group.

Studies in advanced stage Hodgkin lymphoma include patients from the unfavorable end of the prognostic scale in which full systemic treatment is required. Clinical trials either focus on improving results in high-risk advanced stages or minimizing side effects of treatments felt to be satisfactory. Most study groups have stages IIIB/IV as the core group of advanced disease (Table 7.7). Studies differ in whether they include all stage IIIA patients, none, or only selected stage IIIA patients with unfavorable prognostic factors. Some groups also include stages I and II with "systemic" risk factors.

Stages I and II with risk factors and stage IIIA form what may be called "intermediate stages." "Intermediate stage" essentially denotes a gray zone between early and advanced disease. Study aims and the treatment modalities therefore overlap.

**Table 7.6** Eligibility criteria of recent or current studies in early stages. "Early stage" disease is typically defined by stage I or II and the absence of certain unfavorable prognostic factors

| Study group | "Early stage" vs. "intermediate stage/advanced disease" (Early stage = stages I or II without any of the listed risk factors) |
|---|---|
| EORTC (H7 study, H8 study, H9 study) | Age >50<br>4+ involved nodal sites<br>ESR >50 mm/h or B-symptoms and ESR >30 mm/h<br>Bulky mediastinum (mediastinal thoracic ratio ≥0.35)<br>(Infradiaphragmatic disease) |
| Cancer Research UK FDG-PET | B-symptoms<br>Infradiaphragmal disease<br>Large mediastinal mass (>0.33 of the thoracic aperture) |
| GHSG (HD7 study, HD10 study, HD13 study) | Large mediastinal mass (>0.33 of the thoracic aperture)<br>Massive spleen involvement<br>E-lesions<br>ESR >50 mm/h or B-symptoms and ESR >30 mm/h<br>3+ involved lymph-node areas |
| SWOG (9133) CALGB (9391) | B-symptoms<br>Mediastinal mass ≥1/3 maximum thoracic diameter<br>Infradiaphragmatic presentation |
| NCI-C | B-symptoms<br>Mixed cellularity or lymphocyte depletion<br>Age >40 years<br>ESR >50 mm/h<br>4+ disease sites |
| Stanford (G1 study ,G5 study) | Constitutional (B) symptoms present at diagnosis<br>Mediastinal mass equal to or greater than one-third the maximum intrathoracic diameter on a standing posteroanterior chest X-ray<br>Any lymph node mass >10 cm in greatest transaxial diameter<br>Two or more extranodal sites of disease |

*EORTC* European Organization for Research and Treatment of Cancer; *GHSG* German Hodgkin's Lymphoma Study Group; *SWOG* Southwest Oncology Group; *CALGB* Cancer and Leukemia Group B; *NCI-C* National Cancer Institute of Canada

**Table 7.7** Eligibility criteria of recent or current studies in advanced disease

| Study group | Eligibility criteria for trials in advanced disease |
|---|---|
| EORTC (H34 study) | III/IV |
| BNLI<br>Stanford V protocol | Stage IB, IIB, IIIA, IIIB, or IV or<br>Stage IA or IIA with locally extensive disease (e.g., bulky mediastinal disease (e.g., greater than 0.33 of the maximum transthoracic diameter on routine chest X-ray or at least two extranodal sites of disease) or "other poor risk features") |
| Manchester Lymphoma Group (VAPEC-B study) | I/II with B-symptoms or bulk, III, IV |
| GHSG (HD9 study, HD12 study, HD 15 study) | IIB with bulk, massive spleen, or E-lesion<br>PS IIIA S<br>PS IIIA,N with bulk, E-lesion or elevated ESR<br>CS IIIA bulk, massive spleen, E-lesions, elevated ESR or ≥3 lymph node areas<br>IIIB/IV |
| Milano (MAMA study) | IB, IIA bulk, IIB, III, IV |
| GELA (H89 study) | IIIB,IV |
| Stanford V study<br>ECOG-2496<br>NCT00003389,<br>CALGB-59905,<br>CAN-NCIC-HD7,<br>SWOG-E2496 Stanford | Stage I–IIA/B with massive mediastinal adenopathy<br>Stage III or IV |
| BEACOPP intergroup study<br>EORTC-20012<br>NCT00049595, ALLG-HD04, BNLI-EORTC-20012, CAN-NCIC-EORTC-20012, GELA-EORTC-20012, GELCAB-EORTC-20012, NORDICLG-EORTC-20012 | Only higher risk advanced stages:<br>III, IV with International Prognostic Score >2 |

*EORTC* European Organization for Research and Treatment of Cancer; *BNLI* British National Lymphoma Investigation; *GHSG* German Hodgkin's Lymphoma Study Group; *GELA* Groupe d'Etudes des Lymphomes de l'Adulte; *NCI-US* National Cancer Institute of the United States; *SWOG* Southwest Oncology Group; *CALGB* Cancer and Leukemia Group B; *ECOG* Eastern Cooperative Oncology Group; *NCI-C* National Cancer Institute of Canada

## 7.7 Conclusion and Future Aspects

As demonstrated above, a large number of variables have been shown to possess prognostic significance in Hodgkin lymphoma, both at presentation and in the relapse situation. Today, treatment is tailored to prognostic factors, with the aim of decreasing treatment intensity for patients with favorable characteristics in order to reduce toxicity, and increasing treatment intensity for patients with unfavorable characteristics with the aim of increasing cure rates. Different centers and groups use slightly differing criteria for treatment selection, which may make direct comparisons problematic, thus making some form of international harmonization desirable. The introduction of functional imaging with FDG-PET very early in the treatment as a prognostic marker opens up new possibilities for tailoring treatment, but further research is needed before it is implemented for routine use to determine treatment intensity.

## References

1. Reed DM. On the pathological changes in Hodgkin's disease, with especial reference to its relation to tuberculosis. Johns Hopkins Hosp Rep. 1902;10:133–96.
2. Banfi A, Bonadonna G, Buraggi G, et al. Proposta di classificazione e terapia della malattia di Hodgkin. Tumori. 1965; 51:97–112.
3. Easson EC, Russell MH. The cure of Hodgkin's disease. BMJ. 1963;1963:1704–7.
4. Jelliffe AM, Thomson AD. The prognosis in Hodgkin's disease. Br J Cancer. 1955;9:21–36.
5. Kaplan HS. On the natural history, treatment and prognosis of Hodgkin's disease. In: Harvey lectures 1968–1969. New York: Academic; 1970.

6. Musshoff K, Stamm H, Lummel G, et al. Zur prognose der lymphogranulomatose. Klinisches bild un strahlentherapie. Freiburger Krankengut 1938-1958. In: Keiderling W, editor. Beiträge zur Inneren Medizin. Stuttgart: FK Schattauer; 1964.

7. Peters MV. A study of survivals in Hodgkin's disease treated radiologically. Am J Roentgenol. 1950;63:299–311.

8. Rosenberg SA. Report of the Committee on the Staging of Hodgkin's Disease. Cancer Res. 1966;26:1310.

9. Carbone PP, Kaplan HS, Musshoff K, et al. Report of the Committee on Hodgkin's disease staging classification. Cancer Res. 1971;31:1860–1.

10. Aisenberg AC, Qazi R. Improved survival in Hodgkin's disease. Cancer. 1976;37:2423–9.

11. Davis S, Dahlberg S, Myers MH, et al. Hodgkin's disease in the United States: a comparison of patient characteristics and survival in the Centralized Cancer Patient Data System and the Surveillance, Epidemiology, and End Results Program. J Natl Cancer Inst. 1987;78:471–8.

12. Gobbi PG, Cavalli C, Federico M, et al. Hodgkin's disease prognosis: a directly predictive equation. Lancet. 1988;1: 675–9.

13. Hancock BW, Aitken M, Martin JF, et al. Hodgkin's disease in Sheffield (1971–76) (with computer analysis of variables). Clin Oncol. 1979;5:283–97.

14. Henry-Amar M, Aeppli DM, Anderson J, et al. Workshop statistical report. In: Somers R, Henry-Amar M, Meerwaldt JH, et al., editors. Treatment strategy in Hodgkin's disease. INSERM/John Libbey Eurotext: London; 1990.

15. Kaplan HS. Survival and relapse rates in Hodgkin's disease: Stanford experience, 1961-71. Monogr Natl Cancer Inst. 1973;36:487–96.

16. Musshoff K, Hartmann C, Niklaus B, et al. Results of therapy in Hodgkin's disease: Freiburg i. Br. 1964-1971. In: Musshoff K, editor. Diagnosis and therapy of malignant lymphoma. Berlin: Springer; 1974.

17. Sutcliffe SB, Gospodarowicz MK, Bergsagel DE, et al. Prognostic groups for management of localized Hodgkin's disease. J Clin Oncol. 1985;3:393–401.

18. Lister TA, Crowther D, Sutcliffe SB, et al. Report of a committee convened to discuss the evaluation and staging of patients with Hodgkin's disease: Cotswolds meeting. J Clin Oncol. 1989;7:1630–6.

19. George SL. Identification and assessment of prognostic factors. Semin Oncol. 1988;15:462–71.

20. Gospodarowicz MK, O'Sullivan B, Koh ES. Prognostic factors: principles and applications. In: Gospodarowicz MK, O'Sullivan B, Sobin LH, editors. Prognostic factors in cancer. 3rd ed. Hoboken, NJ: Wiley-Liss; 2006.

21. Byar DP. Identification of prognostic factors. In: Buyse ME, Staquet MJ, Sylvester RJ, editors. Cancer clinical trials. Methods and practice. Oxford: Oxford University Press; 1988.

22. Riley RD, Sauerbrei W, Altman DG. Prognostic markers in cancer: the evolution of evidence from single studies to meta-analysis, and beyond. Br J Cancer. 2009;100:1219–29.

23. Byar DP. Problems with using observational databases to compare treatments. Stat Med. 1991;10:663–6.

24. Simon R. Importance of prognostic factors in cancer clinical trials. Cancer Treat Rep. 1984;68:185–92.

25. Cheson BD, Pfistner B, Juweid ME, et al. Revised response criteria for malignant lymphoma. J Clin Oncol. 2007;25: 579–86.

26. Altman DG. Studies investigating prognostic factors: conduct and evaluation. In: Gospodarowicz MK, O'Sullivan B, Sobin LH, editors. Prognostic factors in cancer. 3rd ed. Hoboken, NJ: Wiley-Liss; 2006.

27. Burke HB, Henson DE. The American Joint Committee on Cancer. Criteria for prognostic factors and for an enhanced prognostic system. Cancer. 1993;72:3131–5.

28. Cox DR. Regression models and life-tables. J R Stat Soc B. 1972;34:187–220.

29. Simon R. Evaluating prognostic factor studies. In: Gospodarowicz MK, Henson DE, Hutter RVP, et al., editors. Prognostic factors in cancer. 2nd ed. New York: Wiley-Liss; 2001.

30. Kaplan HS, Dorfman RF, Nelsen TS, et al. Staging laparotomy and splenectomy in Hodgkin's disease: analysis of indications and patterns of involvement in 285 consecutive, unselected patients. Natl Cancer Inst Monogr. 1973;36:291–301.

31. Piro AJ, Hellman S, Moloney WC. The influence of laparotomy on management decisions in Hodgkin's disease. Arch Intern Med. 1972;130:844–8.

32. Hoppe RT, Coleman CN, Cox RS, et al. The management of stage I–II Hodgkin's disease with irradiation alone or combined modality therapy: the Stanford experience. Blood. 1982;59:455–65.

33. Horwich A, Easton D, Nogueira-Costa R, et al. An analysis of prognostic factors in early stage Hodgkin's disease. Radiother Oncol. 1986;7:95–106.

34. Lee CK, Bloomfield CD, Goldman AI, et al. Prognostic significance of mediastinal involvement in Hodgkin's disease treated with curative radiotherapy. Cancer. 1980;46:2403–9.

35. Mauch P, Tarbell N, Weinstein H, et al. Stage IA and IIA supradiaphragmatic Hodgkin's disease: prognostic factors in surgically staged patients treated with mantle and paraaortic irradiation. J Clin Oncol. 1988;6:1576–83.

36. Mendenhall NP, Cantor AB, Barre DM, et al. The role of prognostic factors in treatment selection for early-stage Hodgkin's disease. Am J Clin Oncol. 1994;17:189–95.

37. Tubiana M, Henry-Amar M, Hayat M, et al. Prognostic significance of the number of involved areas in the early stages of Hodgkin's disease. Cancer. 1984;54:885–94.

38. Willett CG, Linggood RM, Leong JC, et al. Stage IA to IIB mediastinal Hodgkin's disease: three-dimensional volumetric assessment of response to treatment. J Clin Oncol. 1988;6:819–24.

39. Enblad G. Hodgkin's disease in young and elderly patients. Clinical and pathological studies. Minireview based on a doctoral thesis. Ups J Med Sci. 1994;99:1–38.

40. Specht L. Tumor burden as the main indicator of prognosis in Hodgkin's disease. Eur J Cancer. 1992;28A:1982–5.

41. Specht L, Nordentoft AM, Cold S, et al. Tumor burden as the most important prognostic factor in early stage Hodgkin's disease. Relations to other prognostic factors and implications for choice of treatment. Cancer. 1988;61:1719–27.

42. Enrici RM, Osti MF, Anselmo AP, et al. Hodgkin's disease stage I and II with exclusive subdiaphragmatic presentation. The experience of the Departments of Radiation Oncology and Hematology, University "La Sapienza" of Rome. Tumori. 1996;82:48–52.

43. Hagemeister FB, Fuller LM, Velasquez WS, et al. Stage I and II Hodgkin's disease: involved-field radiotherapy versus extended-field radiotherapy versus involved-field radiotherapy

followed by six cycles of MOPP. Cancer Treat Rep. 1982;66: 789–98.

44. Hoppe RT, Horning SJ, Rosenberg SA. The concept, evolution and preliminary results of the current Stanford clinical trials for Hodgkin's disease. Cancer Surv. 1985;4:459–75.

45. Mauch P, Gorshein D, Cunningham J, et al. Influence of mediastinal adenopathy on site and frequency of relapse in patients with Hodgkin's disease. Cancer Treat Rep. 1982;66: 809–17.

46. Prosnitz LR, Curtis AM, Knowlton AH, et al. Supradiaphragmatic Hodgkin's disease: significance of large mediastinal masses. Int J Radiat Oncol Biol Phys. 1980;6:809–13.

47. Specht L. Prognostic factors in Hodgkin's disease. Cancer Treat Rev. 1991;18:21–53.

48. Tarbell NJ, Thompson L, Mauch P. Thoracic irradiation in Hodgkin's disease: disease control and long-term complications. Int J Radiat Oncol Biol Phys. 1990;18:275–81.

49. Connors JM, Klimo P. Is it an E lesion or stage IV? An unsettled issue in Hodgkin's disease staging. J Clin Oncol. 1984;2:1421–3.

50. Levi JA, Wiernik PH. Limited extranodal Hodgkin's disease. Unfavorable prognosis and therapeutic implications. Am J Med. 1977;63:365–72.

51. Prosnitz LR. The Ann Arbor staging system for Hodgkin's disease: does E stand for error? Int J Radiat Oncol Biol Phys. 1977;2:1039.

52. Franklin J, Paulus U, Lieberz D, et al. Is the international prognostic score for advanced stage Hodgkin's disease applicable to early stage patients? German Hodgkin Lymphoma Study Group. Ann Oncol. 2000;11:617–23.

53. Gobbi PG, Gendarini A, Crema A, et al. Serum albumin in Hodgkin's disease. Cancer. 1985;55:389–93.

54. Gospodarowicz MK, Sutcliffe SB, Clark RM, et al. Analysis of supradiaphragmatic clinical stage I and II Hodgkin's disease treated with radiation alone. Int J Radiat Oncol Biol Phys. 1992;22:859–65.

55. Haybittle JL, Hayhoe FG, Easterling MJ, et al. Review of British National Lymphoma Investigation studies of Hodgkin's disease and development of prognostic index. Lancet. 1985; 1:967–72.

56. Tubiana M, Henry-Amar M, Werf-Messing B, et al. A multivariate analysis of prognostic factors in early stage Hodgkin's disease. Int J Radiat Oncol Biol Phys. 1985;11:23–30.

57. Vaughan HB, MacLennan KA, Bennett MH, et al. Systemic disturbance in Hodgkin's disease and its relation to histopathology and prognosis (BNLI report No. 30). Clin Radiol. 1987;38:257–61.

58. Vaughan HB, MacLennan KA, Easterling MJ, et al. The prognostic significance of age in Hodgkin's disease: examination of 1500 patients (BNLI report no. 23). Clin Radiol. 1983;34:503–6.

59. Franklin J, Pluetschow A, Paus M, et al. Second malignancy risk associated with treatment of Hodgkin's lymphoma: meta-analysis of the randomised trials. Ann Oncol. 2006; 17:1749–60.

60. Specht L. Very long-term follow-up of the Danish National Hodgkin Study Group's randomized trial of radiotherapy (RT) alone vs. combined modality treatment (CMT) for early stage Hodgkin lymphoma, with special reference to second tumors and overall survival. Blood. 2003; 102:637A.

61. Specht L, Gray RG, Clarke MJ, et al. Influence of more extensive radiotherapy and adjuvant chemotherapy on long-term outcome of early-stage Hodgkin's disease: a meta-analysis of 23 randomized trials involving 3,888 patients. International Hodgkin's Disease Collaborative Group. J Clin Oncol. 1998;16:830–43.

62. Bonfante V, Santoro A, Viviani S, et al. Early stage Hodgkin's disease: ten-year results of a non-randomised study with radiotherapy alone or combined with MOPP. Eur J Cancer. 1993;29A:24–9.

63. Glimelius I, Molin D, Amini RM, et al. Bulky disease is the most important prognostic factor in Hodgkin lymphoma stage IIB. Eur J Haematol. 2003;71:327–33.

64. Pavlovsky S, Maschio M, Santarelli MT, et al. Randomized trial of chemotherapy versus chemotherapy plus radiotherapy for stage I-II Hodgkin's disease. J Natl Cancer Inst. 1988;80:1466–73.

65. Tubiana M, Henry-Amar M, Carde P, et al. Toward comprehensive management tailored to prognostic factors of patients with clinical stages I and II in Hodgkin's disease. The EORTC Lymphoma Group controlled clinical trials: 1964-1987. Blood. 1989;73:47–56.

66. Gobbi PG, Broglia C, Di Giulio G, et al. The clinical value of tumor burden at diagnosis in Hodgkin lymphoma. Cancer. 2004;101:1824–34.

67. Gobbi PG, Ghirardelli ML, Solcia M, et al. Image-aided estimate of tumor burden in Hodgkin's disease: evidence of its primary prognostic importance. J Clin Oncol. 2001;19: 1388–94.

68. Grow A, Quon A, Graves EE, et al. Metabolic tumor volume as an independent prognostic factor in lymphoma. J Clin Oncol. 2005;23 Suppl:583S.

69. Hutchings M, Berthelsen AK, Jakobsen AL, et al. Volume of abnormal tumor tissue on FDG-PET – a predictor of progression-free survival in Hodgkin lymphoma? Int J Radiat Oncol Biol Phys. 2005;63:S45.

70. Hutchings M, Loft A, Hansen M, et al. FDG-PET after two cycles of chemotherapy predicts treatment failure and progression-free survival in Hodgkin lymphoma. Blood. 2006; 107:52–9.

71. Hutchings M, Mikhaeel NG, Fields PA, et al. Prognostic value of interim FDG-PET after two or three cycles of chemotherapy in Hodgkin lymphoma. Ann Oncol. 2005; 16:1160–8.

72. Kostakoglu L, Coleman M, Leonard JP, et al. PET predicts prognosis after 1 cycle of chemotherapy in aggressive lymphoma and Hodgkin's disease. J Nucl Med. 2002;43: 1018–27.

73. Sher DJ, Mauch PM, Van Den AA, et al. Prognostic significance of mid- and post-ABVD PET imaging in Hodgkin's lymphoma: the importance of involved-field radiotherapy. Ann Oncol. 2009;20(11):1848–53.

74. Herbst C, Rehan FA, Brillant C, et al. Combined modality treatment improves tumor control and overall survival in patients with early stage Hodgkin lymphoma: a systematic review. Haematologica. 2010;95:494–500

75. Loeffler M, Brosteanu O, Hasenclever D, et al. Meta-analysis of chemotherapy versus combined modality treatment trials in Hodgkin's disease. International Database on Hodgkin's Disease Overview Study Group. J Clin Oncol. 1998;16: 818–29.

76. Hasenclever D, Diehl V. A prognostic score for advanced Hodgkin's disease. International Prognostic Factors Project on Advanced Hodgkin's Disease. N Engl J Med. 1998;339: 1506–14.

77. Canellos GP, Anderson JR, Propert KJ, et al. Chemotherapy of advanced Hodgkin's disease with MOPP, ABVD, or MOPP alternating with ABVD. N Engl J Med. 1992;327: 1478–84.

78. Ferme C, Bastion Y, Brice P, et al. Prognosis of patients with advanced Hodgkin's disease: evaluation of four prognostic models using 344 patients included in the Group d'Etudes des Lymphomes de l'Adulte Study. Cancer. 1997;80:1124–33.

79. Low SE, Horsman JM, Walters SJ, et al. Risk-adjusted prognostic models for Hodgkin's disease (HD) and grade II non-Hodgkin's lymphoma (NHL II): validation on 6728 British National Lymphoma Investigation patients. Br J Haematol. 2003;120:277–80.

80. Peterson BA, Pajak TF, Cooper MR, et al. Effect of age on therapeutic response and survival in advanced Hodgkin's disease. Cancer Treat Rep. 1982;66:889–98.

81. Proctor SJ, Taylor P, Donnan P, et al. A numerical prognostic index for clinical use in identification of poor-risk patients with Hodgkin's disease at diagnosis. Scotland and Newcastle Lymphoma Group (SNLG) Therapy Working Party. Eur J Cancer. 1991;27:624–9.

82. Specht L, Nissen NI. Prognostic factors in Hodgkin's disease stage III with special reference to tumor burden. Eur J Haematol. 1988;41:80–7.

83. Specht L, Nissen NI. Prognostic factors in Hodgkin's disease stage IV. Eur J Haematol. 1988;41:359–67.

84. Straus DJ, Gaynor JJ, Myers J, et al. Prognostic factors among 185 adults with newly diagnosed advanced Hodgkin's disease treated with alternating potentially noncross-resistant chemotherapy and intermediate-dose radiation therapy. J Clin Oncol. 1990;8:1173–86.

85. Proctor SJ, Rueffer JU, Angus B, et al. Hodgkin's disease in the elderly: current status and future directions. Ann Oncol. 2002;13 Suppl 1:133–7.

86. Engert A, Ballova V, Haverkamp H, et al. Hodgkin's lymphoma in elderly patients: a comprehensive retrospective analysis from the German Hodgkin's Study Group. J Clin Oncol. 2005;23:5052–60.

87. van Spronsen DJ, Janssen-Heijnen ML, Lemmens VE, et al. Independent prognostic effect of co-morbidity in lymphoma patients: results of the population-based Eindhoven Cancer Registry. Eur J Cancer. 2005;41:1051–7.

88. Gobbi PG, Comelli M, Grignani GE, et al. Estimate of expected survival at diagnosis in Hodgkin's disease: a means of weighting prognostic factors and a tool for treatment choice and clinical research. A report from the International Database on Hodgkin's Disease (IDHD). Haematologica. 1994;79:241–55.

89. Klimm B, Reineke T, Haverkamp H, et al. Role of hematotoxicity and sex in patients with Hodgkin's lymphoma: an analysis from the German Hodgkin Study Group. J Clin Oncol. 2005;23:8003–11.

90. Ranson MR, Radford JA, Swindell R, et al. An analysis of prognostic factors in stage III and IV Hodgkin's disease treated at a single centre with MVPP. Ann Oncol. 1991;2:423–9.

91. Somers R, Carde P, Henry-Amar M, et al. A randomized study in stage IIIB and IV Hodgkin's disease comparing eight courses of MOPP versus an alteration of MOPP with ABVD: a European Organization for Research and Treatment of Cancer Lymphoma Cooperative Group and Groupe Pierre-et-Marie-Curie controlled clinical trial. J Clin Oncol. 1994;12:279–87.

92. Georgii A, Fischer R, Hubner K, et al. Classification of Hodgkin's disease biopsies by a panel of four histopathologists. Report of 1,140 patients from the German National Trial. Leuk Lymphoma. 1993;9:365–70.

93. Hess JL, Bodis S, Pinkus G, et al. Histopathologic grading of nodular sclerosis Hodgkin's disease. Lack of prognostic significance in 254 surgically staged patients. Cancer. 1994; 74:708–14.

94. MacLennan KA, Bennett MH, Tu A, et al. Relationship of histopathologic features to survival and relapse in nodular sclerosing Hodgkin's disease. A study of 1659 patients. Cancer. 1989;64:1686–93.

95. Masih AS, Weisenburger DD, Vose JM, et al. Histologic grade does not predict prognosis in optimally treated, advanced-stage nodular sclerosing Hodgkin's disease. Cancer. 1992;69:228–32.

96. van Spronsen DJ, Vrints LW, Hofstra G, et al. Disappearance of prognostic significance of histopathological grading of nodular sclerosing Hodgkin's disease for unselected patients, 1972-92. Br J Haematol. 1997;96:322–7.

97. Torricelli P, Grimaldi PL, Fiocchi F, et al. Hodgkin's disease: a quantitative evaluation by computed tomography of tumor burden. Clin Imaging. 2004;28:239–44.

98. Hoppe RT, Cox RS, Rosenberg SA, et al. Prognostic factors in pathologic stage III Hodgkin's disease. Cancer Treat Rep. 1982;66:743–9.

99. Mauch P, Goffman T, Rosenthal DS, et al. Stage III Hodgkin's disease: improved survival with combined modality therapy as compared with radiation therapy alone. J Clin Oncol. 1985;3:1166–73.

100. Powlis WD, Mauch P, Goffman T, et al. Treatment of patients with "minimal" stage IIIA Hodgkin's disease. Int J Radiat Oncol Biol Phys. 1987;13:1437–42.

101. Stein RS, Golomb HM, Wiernik PH, et al. Anatomic substages of stage IIIA Hodgkin's disease: followup of a collaborative study. Cancer Treat Rep. 1982;66:733–41.

102. Brada M, Ashley S, Nicholls J, et al. Stage III Hodgkin's disease–long-term results following chemotherapy, radiotherapy and combined modality therapy. Radiother Oncol. 1989;14:185–98.

103. Desser RK, Golomb HM, Ultmann JE, et al. Prognostic classification of Hodgkin disease in pathologic stage III, based on anatomic considerations. Blood. 1977;49:883–93.

104. Golomb HM, Sweet DL, Ultmann JE, et al. Importance of substaging of stage III Hodgkin's disease. Semin Oncol. 1980;7:136–43.

105. Proctor SJ, Taylor P, Mackie MJ, et al. A numerical prognostic index for clinical use in identification of poor-risk patients with Hodgkin's disease at diagnosis. The Scotland and Newcastle Lymphoma Group (SNLG) Therapy Working Party. Leuk Lymphoma. 1992;7 Suppl:17–20.

106. Hasenclever D, Schmitz N, Diehl V. Is there a rationale for high-dose chemotherapy as first line treatment of advanced Hodgkin's disease? German Hodgkin's Lymphoma Study Group (GHSG). Leuk Lymphoma. 1995;15 Suppl 1: 47–9.

107. Gobbi PG, Cavalli C, Gendarini A, et al. Prognostic significance of serum albumin in Hodgkin's disease. Haematologica. 1986;71:95–102.

108. Straus DJ. High-risk Hodgkin's disease prognostic factors. Leuk Lymphoma. 1995;15 Suppl 1:41–2.

109. Loeffler M, Pfreundschuh M, Hasenclever D, et al. Prognostic risk factors in advanced Hodgkin's lymphoma. Report of the German Hodgkin Study Group. Blut. 1988; 56:273–81.

110. Aviles A, Talavera A, Garcia EL, et al. La fosfatasa alcalina como factor pronóstico en enfermedad de Hodgkin (Alkaline phosphatase as a prognostic factor in Hodgkin's disease). Rev Gastroenterol Mex. 1990;55:211–4.

111. Wagstaff J, Gregory WM, Swindell R, et al. Prognostic factors for survival in stage IIIB and IV Hodgkin's disease: a multivariate analysis comparing two specialist treatment centres. Br J Cancer. 1988;58:487–92.

112. MacLennan KA, Vaughan HB, Easterling MJ, et al. The presentation haemoglobin level in 1103 patients with Hodgkin's disease (BNLI report no. 21). Clin Radiol. 1983;34:491–5.

113. Brusamolino E, Orlandi E, Morra E, et al. Analysis of long-term results and prognostic factors among 138 patients with advanced Hodgkin's disease treated with the alternating MOPP/ABVD chemotherapy. Ann Oncol. 1994;5 Suppl 2:53–7.

114. Carde P, MacKintosh FR, Rosenberg SA. A dose and time response analysis of the treatment of Hodgkin's disease with MOPP chemotherapy. J Clin Oncol. 1983;1:146–53.

115. DeVita Jr VT, Simon RM, Hubbard SM, et al. Curability of advanced Hodgkin's disease with chemotherapy. Long-term follow-up of MOPP-treated patients at the National Cancer Institute. Ann Intern Med. 1980;92:587–95.

116. Munker R, Hasenclever D, Brosteanu O, et al. Bone marrow involvement in Hodgkin's disease: an analysis of 135 consecutive cases. German Hodgkin's Lymphoma Study Group. J Clin Oncol. 1995;13:403–9.

117. Bonadonna G, Valagussa P, Santoro A. Alternating non-cross-resistant combination chemotherapy or MOPP in stage IV Hodgkin's disease. A report of 8-year results. Ann Intern Med. 1986;104:739–46.

118. Longo DL, Young RC, Wesley M, et al. Twenty years of MOPP therapy for Hodgkin's disease. J Clin Oncol. 1986; 4:1295–306.

119. Selby P, Patel P, Milan S, et al. ChlVPP combination chemotherapy for Hodgkin's disease: long-term results. Br J Cancer. 1990;62:279–85.

120. Jaffe HS, Cadman EC, Farber LR, et al. Pretreatment hematocrit as an independent prognostic variable in Hodgkin's disease. Blood. 1986;68:562–4.

121. Pillai GN, Hagemeister FB, Velasquez WS, et al. Prognostic factors for Stage IV Hodgkin's disease treated with MOPP, with or without bleomycin. Cancer. 1985;55:691–7.

122. Dimopoulos MA, Cabanillas F, Lee JJ, et al. Prognostic role of serum beta 2-microglobulin in Hodgkin's disease. J Clin Oncol. 1993;11:1108–11.

123. Vassilakopoulos TP, Nadali G, Angelopoulou MK, et al. The prognostic significance of beta(2)-microglobulin in patients with Hodgkin's lymphoma. Haematologica. 2002; 87:701–8.

124. Gause A, Jung W, Keymis S, et al. The clinical significance of cytokines and soluble forms of membrane-derived acti-

vation antigens in the serum of patients with Hodgkin's disease. Leuk Lymphoma. 1992;7:439–47.

125. Gause A, Jung W, Schmits R, et al. Soluble CD8, CD25 and CD30 antigens as prognostic markers in patients with untreated Hodgkin's lymphoma. Ann Oncol. 1992;3 Suppl 4:49–52.

126. Nadali G, Vinante F, Ambrosetti A, et al. Serum levels of soluble CD30 are elevated in the majority of untreated patients with Hodgkin's disease and correlate with clinical features and prognosis. J Clin Oncol. 1994;12:793–7.

127. Pizzolo G, Vinante F, Chilosi M, et al. Serum levels of soluble CD30 molecule (Ki-1 antigen) in Hodgkin's disease: relationship with disease activity and clinical stage. Br J Haematol. 1990;75:282–4.

128. Axdorph U, Sjoberg J, Grimfors G, et al. Biological markers may add to prediction of outcome achieved by the International Prognostic Score in Hodgkin's disease. Ann Oncol. 2000;11:1405–11.

129. Casasnovas RO, Mounier N, Brice P, et al. Plasma cytokine and soluble receptor signature predicts outcome of patients with classical Hodgkin's lymphoma: a study from the Groupe d'Etude des Lymphomes de l'Adulte. J Clin Oncol. 2007;25:1732–40.

130. Zanotti R, Trolese A, Ambrosetti A, et al. Serum levels of soluble CD30 improve International Prognostic Score in predicting the outcome of advanced Hodgkin's lymphoma. Ann Oncol. 2002;13:1908–14.

131. Gallamini A, Rigacci L, Merli F, et al. The predictive value of positron emission tomography scanning performed after two courses of standard therapy on treatment outcome in advanced stage Hodgkin's disease. Haematologica. 2006; 91:475–81.

132. Zinzani PL, Tani M, Fanti S, et al. Early positron emission tomography (PET) restaging: a predictive final response in Hodgkin's disease patients. Ann Oncol. 2006;17: 1296–300.

133. Gallamini A, Hutchings M, Rigacci L, et al. Early interim 2-[18F]fluoro-2-deoxy-D-glucose positron emission tomography is prognostically superior to international prognostic score in advanced-stage Hodgkin's lymphoma: a report from a joint Italian-Danish study. J Clin Oncol. 2007;25: 3746–52.

134. Avigdor A, Bulvik S, Levi I, et al. Two cycles of escalated BEACOPP followed by four cycles of ABVD utilizing early-interim PET/CT scan is an effective regimen for advanced high-risk Hodgkin's lymphoma. Ann Oncol. 2009;21(1):126–32.

135. Wagstaff J, Steward W, Jones M, et al. Factors affecting remission and survival in patients with advanced Hodgkin's disease treated with MVPP. Hematol Oncol. 1986;4: 135–47.

136. Gobbi PG, Gobbi PG, Mazza P, et al. Multivariate analysis of Hodgkin's disease prognosis. Fitness and use of a directly predictive equation. Haematologica. 1989;74:29–38.

137. Low SE, Horsman JM, Hancock H, et al. Prognostic markers in malignant lymphoma: an analysis of 1,198 patients treated at a single centre. Int J Oncol. 2001;19:1203–9.

138. Diehl V, Franklin J, Pfreundschuh M, et al. Standard and increased-dose BEACOPP chemotherapy compared with COPP-ABVD for advanced Hodgkin's disease. N Engl J Med. 2003;348:2386–95.

139. Duggan DB, Petroni GR, Johnson JL, et al. Randomized comparison of ABVD and MOPP/ABV hybrid for the treatment of advanced Hodgkin's disease: report of an intergroup trial. J Clin Oncol. 2003;21:607–14.

140. Gobbi PG, Zinzani PL, Broglia C, et al. Comparison of prognostic models in patients with advanced Hodgkin disease. Promising results from integration of the best three systems. Cancer. 2001;91:1467–78.

141. Johnson PW, Radford JA, Cullen MH, et al. Comparison of ABVD and Alternating or Hybrid Multidrug Regimens for the Treatment of Advanced Hodgkin's Lymphoma: results of the United Kingdom Lymphoma Group LY09 Trial (ISRCTN97144519). J Clin Oncol. 2005;23:9208–18.

142. Radford JA, Rohatiner AZ, Ryder WD, et al. ChlVPP/EVA hybrid versus the weekly VAPEC-B regimen for previously untreated Hodgkin's disease. J Clin Oncol. 2002;20: 2988–94.

143. Bierman PJ, Lynch JC, Bociek RG, et al. The International Prognostic Factors Project score for advanced Hodgkin's disease is useful for predicting outcome of autologous hematopoietic stem cell transplantation. Ann Oncol. 2002; 13:1370–7.

144. Gisselbrecht C, Mounier N, Andre M, et al. How to define intermediate stage in Hodgkin's lymphoma? Eur J Haematol Suppl. 2005;(66):111–14.

145. Healey EA, Tarbell NJ, Kalish LA, et al. Prognostic factors for patients with Hodgkin disease in first relapse. Cancer. 1993;71:2613–20.

146. Mauch PM. Controversies in the management of early stage Hodgkin's disease. Blood. 1994;83:318–29.

147. Bonfante V, Santoro A, Viviani S, et al. Outcome of patients with Hodgkin's disease failing after primary MOPP-ABVD. J Clin Oncol. 1997;15:528–34.

148. Brice P, Bastion Y, Divine M, et al. Analysis of prognostic factors after the first relapse of Hodgkin's disease in 187 patients. Cancer. 1996;78:1293–9.

149. Canellos GP, Petroni GR, Barcos M, et al. Etoposide, vinblastine, and doxorubicin: an active regimen for the treatment of Hodgkin's disease in relapse following MOPP. Cancer and Leukemia Group B. J Clin Oncol. 1995; 13:2005–11.

150. Ferme C, Bastion Y, Lepage E, et al. The MINE regimen as intensive salvage chemotherapy for relapsed and refractory Hodgkin's disease. Ann Oncol. 1995;6:543–9.

151. Lohri A, Barnett M, Fairey RN, et al. Outcome of treatment of first relapse of Hodgkin's disease after primary chemotherapy: identification of risk factors from the British Columbia experience 1970 to 1988. Blood. 1991;77: 2292–8.

152. Longo DL, Duffey PL, Young RC, et al. Conventional-dose salvage combination chemotherapy in patients relapsing with Hodgkin's disease after combination chemotherapy: the low probability for cure. J Clin Oncol. 1992;10:210–8.

153. Straus DJ, Myers J, Koziner B, et al. Combination chemotherapy for the treatment of Hodgkin's disease in relapse. Results with lomustine (CCNU), melphalan (Alkeran), and vindesine (DVA) alone (CAD) and in alternation with MOPP and doxorubicin (Adriamycin), bleomycin, and vinblastine (ABV). Cancer Chemother Pharmacol. 1983; 11:80–5.

154. Viviani S, Santoro A, Negretti E, et al. Salvage chemotherapy in Hodgkin's disease. Results in patients relapsing more than twelve months after first complete remission. Ann Oncol. 1990;1:123–7.

155. Josting A, Franklin J, May M, et al. New prognostic score based on treatment outcome of patients with relapsed Hodgkin's lymphoma registered in the database of the German Hodgkin's Lymphoma Study Group. J Clin Oncol. 2001;20:221–30.

156. Josting A, Schmitz N. Insights into 25 years of clinical trials of the GHSG: relapsed and refractory Hodgkin's disease. In: Diehl V, Josting A, editors. 25 years German Hodgkin Study Group. Munich: Urban & Vogel; 2004.

157. Hagemeister FB, Tannir N, McLaughlin P, et al. MIME chemotherapy (methyl-GAG, ifosfamide, methotrexate, etoposide) as treatment for recurrent Hodgkin's disease. J Clin Oncol. 1987;5:556–61.

158. Perren TJ, Selby PJ, Milan S, et al. Etoposide and adriamycin containing combination chemotherapy (HOPE-Bleo) for relapsed Hodgkin's disease. Br J Cancer. 1990;61: 919–23.

159. Salvagno L, Soraru M, Aversa SM, et al. Late relapses in Hodgkin's disease: outcome of patients relapsing more than twelve months after primary chemotherapy. Ann Oncol. 1993;4:657–62.

160. Brada M, Eeles R, Ashley S, et al. Salvage radiotherapy in recurrent Hodgkin's disease. Ann Oncol. 1992;3:131–5.

161. Josting A, Nogova L, Franklin J, et al. Salvage radiotherapy in patients with relapsed and refractory Hodgkin's lymphoma: a retrospective analysis from the German Hodgkin Lymphoma Study Group. J Clin Oncol. 2005;23:1522–9.

162. Leigh BR, Fox KA, Mack CF, et al. Radiation therapy salvage of Hodgkin's disease following chemotherapy failure. Int J Radiat Oncol Biol Phys. 1993;27:855–62.

163. Mauch P, Tarbell N, Skarin A, et al. Wide-field radiation therapy alone or with chemotherapy for Hodgkin's disease in relapse from combination chemotherapy. J Clin Oncol. 1987;5:544–9.

164. O'Brien PC, Parnis FX. Salvage radiotherapy following chemotherapy failure in Hodgkin's disease – what is its role? Acta Oncol. 1995;34:99–104.

165. Roach III M, Kapp DS, Rosenberg SA, et al. Radiotherapy with curative intent: an option in selected patients relapsing after chemotherapy for advanced Hodgkin's disease. J Clin Oncol. 1987;5:550–5.

166. Wirth A, Corry J, Laidlaw C, et al. Salvage radiotherapy for Hodgkin's disease following chemotherapy failure. Int J Radiat Oncol Biol Phys. 1997;39:599–607.

167. Linch DC, Winfield D, Goldstone AH, et al. Dose intensification with autologous bone-marrow transplantation in relapsed and resistant Hodgkin's disease: results of a BNLI randomised trial. Lancet. 1993;341:1051–4.

168. Schmitz N, Pfistner B, Sextro M, et al. Aggressive conventional chemotherapy compared with high-dose chemotherapy with autologous haemopoietic stem-cell transplantation for relapsed chemosensitive Hodgkin's disease: a randomised trial. Lancet. 2002;359:2065–71.

169. Anderson JE, Litzow MR, Appelbaum FR, et al. Allogeneic, syngeneic, and autologous marrow transplantation for Hodgkin's disease: the 21-year Seattle experience. J Clin Oncol. 1993;11:2342–50.

170. Argiris A, Seropian S, Cooper DL. High-dose BEAM chemotherapy with autologous peripheral blood progenitor-cell transplantation for unselected patients with primary

refractory or relapsed Hodgkin's disease. Ann Oncol. 2000;11:665–72.

171. Bierman PJ, Anderson JR, Freeman MB, et al. High-dose chemotherapy followed by autologous hematopoietic rescue for Hodgkin's disease patients following first relapse after chemotherapy. Ann Oncol. 1996;7:151–6.

172. Ferme C, Mounier N, Divine M, et al. Intensive salvage therapy with high-dose chemotherapy for patients with advanced Hodgkin's disease in relapse or failure after initial chemotherapy: results of the Groupe d'Etudes des Lymphomes de l'Adulte H89 Trial. J Clin Oncol. 2002;20: 467–75.

173. Hahn T, Benekli M, Wong C, et al. A prognostic model for prolonged event-free survival after autologous or allogeneic blood or marrow transplantation for relapsed and refractory Hodgkin's disease. Bone Marrow Transplant. 2005;35:557–66.

174. Josting A, Rudolph C, Mapara M, et al. Cologne high-dose sequential chemotherapy in relapsed and refractory Hodgkin lymphoma: results of a large multicenter study of the German Hodgkin Lymphoma Study Group (GHSG). Ann Oncol. 2005;16:116–23.

175. Lazarus HM, Loberiza Jr FR, Zhang MJ, et al. Autotransplants for Hodgkin's disease in first relapse or second remission: a report from the autologous blood and marrow transplant registry (ABMTR). Bone Marrow Transplant. 2001;27:387–96.

176. Poen JC, Hoppe RT, Horning SJ. High-dose therapy and autologous bone marrow transplantation for relapsed/ refractory Hodgkin's disease: the impact of involved field radiotherapy on patterns of failure and survival. Int J Radiat Oncol Biol Phys. 1996;36:3–12.

177. Sureda A, Constans M, Iriondo A, et al. Prognostic factors affecting long-term outcome after stem cell transplantation in Hodgkin's lymphoma autografted after a first relapse. Ann Oncol. 2005;16:625–33.

178. Yahalom J, Gulati SC, Toia M, et al. Accelerated hyperfractionated total-lymphoid irradiation, high-dose chemotherapy, and autologous bone marrow transplantation for refractory and relapsing patients with Hodgkin's disease. J Clin Oncol. 1993;11:1062–70.

179. Popat U, Hosing C, Saliba RM, et al. Prognostic factors for disease progression after high-dose chemotherapy and autologous hematopoietic stem cell transplantation for recurrent or refractory Hodgkin's lymphoma. Bone Marrow Transplant. 2004;33:1015–23.

180. Stewart DA, Guo D, Gluck S, et al. Double high-dose therapy for Hodgkin's disease with dose-intensive cyclophosphamide, etoposide, and cisplatin (DICEP) prior to high-dose melphalan and autologous stem cell transplantation. Bone Marrow Transplant. 2000;26:383–8.

181. Lumley MA, Milligan DW, Knechtli CJ, et al. High lactate dehydrogenase level is associated with an adverse outlook in autografting for Hodgkin's disease. Bone Marrow Transplant. 1996;17:383–8.

182. Bierman PJ, Bagin RG, Jagannath S, et al. High dose chemotherapy followed by autologous hematopoietic rescue in Hodgkin's disease: long-term follow-up in 128 patients. Ann Oncol. 1993;4:767–73.

183. Brice P, Bouabdallah R, Moreau P, et al. Prognostic factors for survival after high-dose therapy and autologous stem cell transplantation for patients with relapsing Hodgkin's disease: analysis of 280 patients from the French registry. Societe Francaise de Greffe de Moelle. Bone Marrow Transplant. 1997;20:21–6.

184. Chopra R, McMillan AK, Linch DC, et al. The place of high-dose BEAM therapy and autologous bone marrow transplantation in poor-risk Hodgkin's disease. A single-center eight-year study of 155 patients. Blood. 1993;81: 1137–45.

185. Horning SJ, Chao NJ, Negrin RS, et al. High-dose therapy and autologous hematopoietic progenitor cell transplantation for recurrent or refractory Hodgkin's disease: analysis of the Stanford University results and prognostic indices. Blood. 1997;89:801–13.

186. Wheeler C, Eickhoff C, Elias A, et al. High-dose cyclophosphamide, carmustine, and etoposide with autologous transplantation in Hodgkin's disease: a prognostic model for treatment outcomes. Biol Blood Marrow Transplant. 1997;3:98–106.

187. Williams CD, Goldstone AH, Pearce R, et al. Autologous bone marrow transplantation for pediatric Hodgkin's disease: a case-matched comparison with adult patients by the European Bone Marrow Transplant Group Lymphoma Registry. J Clin Oncol. 1993;11:2243–9.

188. Becherer A, Mitterbauer M, Jaeger U, et al. Positron emission tomography with [18F]2-fluoro-D-2-deoxyglucose (FDG-PET) predicts relapse of malignant lymphoma after high-dose therapy with stem cell transplantation. Leukemia. 2002;16:260–7.

189. Filmont JE, Gisselbrecht C, Cuenca X, et al. The impact of pre- and post-transplantation positron emission tomography using 18-fluorodeoxyglucose on poor-prognosis lymphoma patients undergoing autologous stem cell transplantation. Cancer. 2007;110:1361–9.

190. Jabbour E, Hosing C, Ayers G, et al. Pretransplant positive positron emission tomography/gallium scans predict poor outcome in patients with recurrent/refractory Hodgkin lymphoma. Cancer. 2007;109:2481–9.

191. Schot BW, Pruim J, van Imhoff GW, et al. The role of serial pre-transplantation positron emission tomography in predicting progressive disease in relapsed lymphoma. Haematologica. 2006;91:490–5.

192. Spaepen K, Stroobants S, Dupont P, et al. Prognostic value of pretransplantation positron emission tomography using fluorine 18-fluorodeoxyglucose in patients with aggressive lymphoma treated with high-dose chemotherapy and stem cell transplantation. Blood. 2003;102:53–9.

193. Svoboda J, Andreadis C, Elstrom R, et al. Prognostic value of FDG-PET scan imaging in lymphoma patients undergoing autologous stem cell transplantation. Bone Marrow Transplant. 2006;38:211–6.

194. Hasenclever D. The disappearance of prognostic factors in Hodgkin's disease. Ann Oncol. 2002;13 Suppl 1:75–8.

195. Cosset JM, Mauch PM. The role of radiotherapy for early stage Hodgkin's disease: limitations and perspectives. Ann Oncol. 1998;9 Suppl 5:S57–62.

# Principles of Radiation Techniques in Hodgkin Lymphoma

**8**

Joachim Yahalom and Richard T. Hoppe

## Contents

J. Yahalom (✉)
Department of Radiation Oncology, Memorial Sloan-Kettering Cancer Center, 1275 York Avenue, New York, NY 10065, USA
e-mail: yahalomj@mskcc.org

R.T. Hoppe
Department of Radiation Oncology,
Stanford University Medical Center,
1000 Welch Road, Palo Alto, CA 94304-1808,
USA

## Abbreviations

| 3DCRT | Three-dimensional conformal radiotherapy |
|---|---|
| ABVD | Adriamycin (doxorubicin), bleomycin, vinblastine, and dacarbazine |
| AP-PA | Opposed anterior and posterior fields |
| ASCT | Autologous stem cell transplantation |
| CR | Complete response |
| CT | Computed tomography |
| CTV | Clinical treated |
| EBVP | Epirubicine, bleomycin, vinblastine, and dacarbazine |
| EFS | Event-free survival |
| EORTC | European Organization for Research and Treatment of Cancer |

A. Engert and S.J. Horning (eds.), *Hodgkin Lymphoma*,
DOI: 10.1007/978-3-642-12780-9_8, © Springer-Verlag Berlin Heidelberg 2011

FFTF        Freedom from treatment failure
GELA        Groupe d'Études des Lymphomes Adultes
GHSG        German Hodgkin Study Group
HL          Hodgkin lymphoma
IFRT        Involved-field radiation therapy
IMRT        Intensity-modulated radiotherapy
INRT        Involved node radiation therapy
LPHL        Lymphocye predominance HL
MOP-BAP     Mechlorethamine, Oncovin [vincristine], prednisone, bleomycin, Adriamycin (doxorubicin), and procarbazine
MOPP        Mustargen, Oncovin, procarbazine, prednisone
MSKCC       Memorial Sloan Kettering Cancer Center
NCCN        National Comprehensive Cancer Network
OS          Overall survival
PET         Positron emission tomography
PTV         Planned treatment volume
RT          Radiation therapy
STLI        Subtotal lymphoid irradiation
TLI         Total lymphoid irradiation
TSH         Thyroid-stimulating hormone

## 8.1  Principles of Radiation Therapy of Hodgkin Lymphoma

Radiation therapy (RT) is a major component of the current successful treatment of Hodgkin lymphoma (HL). For decades, radiation was used alone to cure the majority of patients with HL; RT is still the most effective single agent in the the oncologic armamentarium for this disease, and it remains the treatment of choice for patients with early-stage lymphocye predominance HL (LPHL) and for selected patients with classic HL who have contraindications to chemotherapy [1]. Currently, most patients with HL are treated with combined modality programs in which RT is given as consolidation after chemotherapy. As the role of RT has transformed over the years from a single modality into a component of combined modality therapy, the classic principles of RT fields, dose, and technique have fundamentally changed.

The following principles guide the current strategy of using RT in HL:

1. RT as a part of a combined modality program is radically different from the large-field, high-dose RT that was used in the past. The volume and doses that are required following chemotherapy are significantly less than when RT is used alone. In addition, the planning and delivery of RT has improved considerably over the last two decades.
2. Adding RT to chemotherapy improves disease control and allows the administration of shorter and less toxic chemotherapy programs for all stages of HL.
3. The new "mini-radiotherapy" for HL is well tolerated and results in a decreased risk for long-term morbidities that were associated with large-field, high-dose RT in the past [2].

## 8.2  The Evolution of Radiotherapy for HL

RT has been used in the management of HL since shortly after the discovery of X-rays [3, 4]. Initially it was used for local palliation, but careful study by pioneers in the field including Rene Gilbert and Vera Peters demonstrated that more aggressive treatment with higher doses and larger fields resulted in the cure of many patients, especially those who presented with limited disease [5, 6]. At Stanford, Henry Kaplan, advantaged by access to the medical linear accelerator, refined the RT concepts and together with Saul Rosenberg advocated strongly for the curative potential of RT [7]. RT remained the standard therapy for patients until effective chemotherapy was developed in the second half of the twentieth century. The success of chemotherapy and appreciation of adverse late events linked to RT such as secondary solid tumors and cardiac disease led to a decrease in the use of RT, but the eventual realization that its judicious application in lower doses and more tailored fields could enhance curability and allow decrease in chemotherapy doses led to the development of programs of refined combined modality therapy.

This refinement includes the use of involved field RT techniques that improve conformality and dose homogeneity. These field reductions require detailed clinical information to delineate the target accurately. Pre- and postchemotherapy imaging is required to define the tumor volume. The integration of computed tomography (CT) and positron emission tomography (PET)/CT treatment planning reduces the variability in treatment field design. A margin of safety to address subclinical disease, and random and systematic error, is still necessary in field setup, but techniques to minimize inaccuracies in treatment planning and delivery continue to improve. The tailoring of the radiation field to the initially involved lymph nodes has been termed involved node radiation therapy (INRT). The volumes for INRT are designed to be smaller than the classic IFRT that encompasses entire predefined anatomical regions. Recommendations for INRT design have been established and INRT is increasingly implemented in combined modality programs, particularly in Europe [8].

## 8.3   Indications for Radiation Therapy in HL

It is important to distinguish between classical HL and nodular lymphocyte-predominant HL (LPHL). The management of each entity is different. Most patients with LPHL may be treated with radiation alone, with curative intent, whereas combined modality therapy is the standard approach for the majority of patients with classical HL.

### 8.3.1   Lymphocyte-Predominant HL

Most (>75%) patients with LPHL present with stage IA or IIA disease; the disease is commonly limited to one peripheral site (neck, axilla, or groin) and involvement of the mediastinum is extremely rare. The American National Comprehensive Cancer Network (NCCN) guidelines [9], the German Hodgkin Lymphoma Study Group (GHSG), and the European Organization for Research and Treatment of Cancer (EORTC) currently recommend *involved-field radiation alone* as the treatment of choice for early-stage LPHL. Since the mediastinum is rarely involved, it need not be treated, thus avoiding the site most responsible for radiation-related short- and long-term side effects. In a recent retrospective study of 131 patients with stage IA disease, 98% of patients obtained a complete response (CR), 98% after extended-field RT alone, 100% after involved-field RT alone, and 95% after combined modality therapy [10]. With a median follow-up of 43 months only 5% of patients relapsed and only three patients died. Toxicity of treatment was

generally mild and was the greatest in association with combined modality therapy. Two other studies, one from the Peter MacCallum in Australia [11], and another from the Dana Farber in Boston, supported the adequacy of limited-field RT for LPHL and suggested a reduced risk of second tumors compared to extended-field RT [12].

Although there has not been a prospective study comparing extended-field RT (commonly used in the past) with involved field RT, retrospective data suggest that the involved field is adequate [10, 13]. The radiation dose recommended is 30–36 Gy with an optional additional boost of 4 Gy to a (rare) bulky site.

### 8.3.2   Classical Hodgkin: Early Stage

Over the last two decades, the treatment of stage I–II classical HL has changed markedly. Combined modality therapy consisting of short-course chemotherapy (most often ABVD) followed by reduced-dose radiation carefully directed only to the involved lymph node(s) site has replaced radiation alone as the treatment of choice. Combined modality is the standard treatment for favorable and unfavorable presentations of early-stage disease in Europe, including the EORTC/GELA (Groupe d'Études des Lymphomes Adultes) and GHSG. In the United States, chemotherapy followed by involved-field radiation therapy (IFRT) is the preferred treatment recommended by the NCCN guidelines [9].

Several randomized studies have demonstrated that excellent results in stage I–II may be obtained with combined modality treatment that includes only IFRT – more extensive fields of total or subtotal lymphoid irradiation (STLI and TLI) are not required.

The strategy to reduce the number of chemotherapy cycles and/or the radiation dose was tested by two large-scale randomized studies conducted by the GHSG. In the HD10 study, 1,370 patients with early favorable HL were randomly assigned in a 2×2 factorial design to receive either four or two cycles of ABVD followed by 30 or 20 Gy IFRT. The 8-year freedom from treatment failure (FFTF) and overall survival (OS) for all patients were 87 and 95%, respectively. Most importantly, there were no significant differences between patients receiving the minimal treatment of ABVDX2 followed by IFRT of only 20 Gy and patients receiving more chemotherapy and/or more RT [14].

Patients with unfavorable early-stage HL ($n = 1,395$) were randomized on the GHSG HD-11 to receive either four cycles of ABVD or four cycles of baseline BEACOPP, followed by IFRT of either 30 or 20 Gy. Five-year FFTF and OS for all patients were 85 and 94.5%, respectively. There was no difference in FFTF when BEACOPPX4 was followed by either 30 or 20 Gy and similar excellent results were obtained with ABVDX4 and IFRT of 30 Gy. Patients who received ABVDX4 and only 20 Gy had FFTF that was lower by 4%. OS was similar in all treatment groups [15].

These large trials of the GHSG, as well as studies of the EORTC, have established combined modality therapy with limited RT as the treatment of choice for patients with stage I–II disease. Although there have been small reports using chemotherapy alone for patients with stage I–IIA disease, this approach is suitable for only a small proportion of patients and has been associated with a greater risk for relapse. Recently a meta-analysis by the Cochrane group pooled together all the randomized studies comparing chemotherapy alone to combined modality showed a statistically significant advantage for combined modality over chemotherapy alone in both tumor control and overall survival [16].

### 8.3.3 Advanced-Stage HL

Although the role of consolidative RT after induction chemotherapy in stage III–IV remains controversial, irradiation is often added in patients who present with bulky disease or remain in uncertain complete remission after chemotherapy [17]. Retrospective studies have demonstrated that adding low-dose radiotherapy to all initial disease sites following chemotherapy decreases the relapse rate by ~25% and significantly improves overall survival. The results of prospective studies testing the concept have been conflicting [18, 19]. A Southwest Oncology Group (SWOG) randomized study of 278 patients with stage III–IV HL suggested that the addition of low-dose irradiation to all sites of initial disease after a CR to MOP-BAP (mechlorethamine, Oncovin [vincristine], prednisone, bleomycin, Adriamycin [doxorubicin], and procarbazine) chemotherapy improves remission duration [20]. An intention-to-treat analysis showed that the advantage of combined modality therapy was limited to patients with nodular sclerosis. No survival differences were

observed. A meta-analysis of several randomized studies demonstrated that the addition of radiotherapy to chemotherapy reduces the rate of relapse but did not show survival benefit for combined modality compared to chemotherapy alone [21].

The EORTC reported the results of a randomized study that evaluated the role of IFRT in patients with stage III–IV Hodgkin disease who obtained a CR after MOPP/ABV [22]. Patients received six or eight cycles of MOPP/ABV chemotherapy (number of cycles depended upon the response). Patients who did not achieve a CR (40%) were not randomized, but were assigned to receive IFRT. Among the 333 randomized patients, the 5-year overall survival rates were 91% (no RT) and 85% (RT) ($p = 0.07$). The authors concluded that IFRT did not improve outcome for patients with stage III–IV HL who achieved a CR after six to eight courses of MOPP/ABV chemotherapy. The data indicated more cases of leukemia among patients who achieved a CR and were treated with RT, compared to those treated with chemotherapy alone, but surprisingly this was not in the case for the large group of patients who did not achieve a CR with chemotherapy, all of whom received RT. This suggests that the increased mortality on the randomized RT arm was a statistical aberration resulting from small number of events. Interestingly, among the partial responders after six cycles of MOPP/ABV, the addition of IFRT yielded overall survival and event-free survival rates that were similar to those obtained among patients who achieved a CR to chemotherapy. There are other limitations of the EORTC study that affect its applicability. A relatively small proportion of patients achieved a CR and were eligible for randomization. The MOPP/ABV regimen is quite toxic and has been abandoned for use in North America [23]. Relatively few patients with bulky disease were randomized on the trial, making interpretation of results in this important subgroup challenging. Lastly, the purported increase for secondary malignancy following combined modality therapy was not evident in the PR patients, all of whom received even higher doses of RT to initially involved sites.

Another randomized study that evaluated the role of consolidation RT after CR to chemotherapy used ABVDX6 (the most common regimen currently used for advance-stage HL). This trial was conducted at the Tata medical center in India [24]. It included patients of all stages, but almost half were stage III–IV. A subgroup analysis of the advanced-stage patients showed a statistically significant improvement of both 8-year event-free survival (EFS) and 8-year overall survival with added RT compared to ABVD alone (EFS 78 vs. 59%; $p < 0.03$ and OS 100 vs. 80%; $p < 0.006$).

When advanced-stage HL is treated with the new highly effective and less toxic treatment program of Stanford V, it is imperative to follow the brief chemotherapy program with involved field radiotherapy to sites originally larger than 5 cm or to a clinically involved spleen [25]. When these RT guidelines were not followed and RT was completely or partially omitted, the results were inferior [26].

In summary, patients in CR after full dose chemotherapy program like MOPP/ABV may not need RT consolidation. Yet, patients with bulky disease, incomplete or uncertain CR or patients treated on brief chemotherapy programs will benefit from involved field RT to originally bulky or residual disease.

### 8.3.4 RT in Salvage Programs for Refractory and Relapsed HL

High-dose therapy supported by autologous stem cell transplantation (ASCT) has become a standard salvage treatment for patients who relapsed or remained refractory to primary therapy. Many of these patients have not received prior radiotherapy or have relapsed at sites outside the original radiation field. These patients could benefit from integrating radiotherapy into the salvage regimen.

Poen and colleagues from Stanford analyzed the efficacy and toxicity of adding cytoreductive or consolidative RT to 24 of 100 patients receiving high-dose therapy [27]. When involved sites were irradiated in conjunction with transplantation, no in-field failures occurred. While only a trend in favor of IF-RT could be shown for the entire group of transplanted patients, analysis restricted to patients who had no prior RT or those with relapse stage I–III demonstrated significant improvement in freedom from relapse. Fatal toxicity in this series was not influenced significantly by IF-RT.

At Memorial Sloan Kettering Cancer Center (MSKCC), a program that integrated RT into the high-dose regimen for salvage therapy was developed and included accelerated hyperfractionated irradiation (b.i.d. fractions of 1.8 Gy each) to start after the completion of reinduction chemotherapy and stem cell collection and prior to the high-dose chemotherapy and stem cell transplantation. Patients who have not been previously irradiated received involved field RT (18 Gy in 5 days) to sites of initially bulky (>5 cm) disease and/or residual clinical abnormalities, followed by total lymphoid irradiation (TLI) of 18 Gy (1.8 Gy per fraction, b.i.d.) during an additional 5 days. Patients who had prior RT received only involved-field RT (when feasible) to a maximal dose of 36 Gy. This treatment strategy has been in place since 1985 with over 350 patients treated thus far. The first generation program demonstrated an EFS of 47% [28]. The recent report of the second generation two-step high-dose chemoradiotherapy program indicated that after a median follow-up of 34 months the intent-to-treat event-free survival and overall survival were 58 and 88%, respectively. For patients who underwent transplantation, the EFS was 68% [29]. Treatment-related mortality was 3% with no treatment-related mortality over the last 10 years. The results of this treatment program in refractory patients were similar to those of relapsed patients [30]. Both groups showed favorable EFS and overall survival compared to most recently reported series. Recent report on quality of life and treatment-related complications of long-tem survivors of the MSKCC program disclosed only a small number of late complications and is highly encouraging [31].

### 8.4 Radiation Fields: Principles and Design

In the past, radiation-fields design attempted to include multiple involved and uninvolved lymph node sites. The large fields known as *mantle*, *inverted Y*, and *TLI* were synonymous with the radiation treatment of HL. These fields are now only rarely used. *IFRT* encompasses a significantly smaller but adequate volume when radiotherapy is used as consolidation after chemotherapy in HL. Even when radiation is used as primary management for LPHL, the field should be limited to the involved site or to the involved sites and immediately adjacent lymph node groups. Extending this concept further, even more limited radiation fields termed INRT have been introduced into investigational combined modality programs, primarily in Europe [8].

The terminologies that define radiation fields may be confusing and create difficulties in comparing treatment programs. However, general definitions and guidelines are available and should be followed.

The following are definitions of types of radiation fields used in HL.

### 8.4.1 Involved Field

This field is limited to the clinically involved lymph node *region*. For extra-nodal sites, the field includes the organ alone (if no evidence for lymph node involvement). The "grouping" of lymph nodes is not clearly defined, and involved field borders for common presentation of HL are noted below (Fig. 8.1a–c).

### 8.4.2 Extended Field

This field includes the involved lymph node group field *plus* the adjacent clinically uninvolved region(s). For extra nodal disease, it includes the involved organ plus the clinically uninvolved lymph nodes region (Fig. 8.2).

It was common during the era of treatment with RT alone to treat large fields encompassing multiple lymph node regions, both involved and uninvolved. The field design that includes all of the supradiaphragmatic lymph node regions was referred to as the *mantle* field. The field that includes all lymph nodes sites below the diaphragm (with or without the spleen and called after its shape) is the *inverted Y* (Figs. 8.3 and 8.4).

When radiation treatment includes all lymph nodes on both sides of the diaphragm, mantle plus inverted Y, the resulting field is called *TLI* or *total nodal irradiation (TNI)*, if the pelvic lymph nodes are excluded the field is called *STLI* (Fig. 8.5).

### 8.4.3 Involved Node(s) Field

This is the most limited radiation field that has just recently been introduced [8]. The clinical treated volume (CTV) includes only the originally involved lymph node(s) volume (prechemotherapy) with the addition of 1 cm margin to create planned treatment

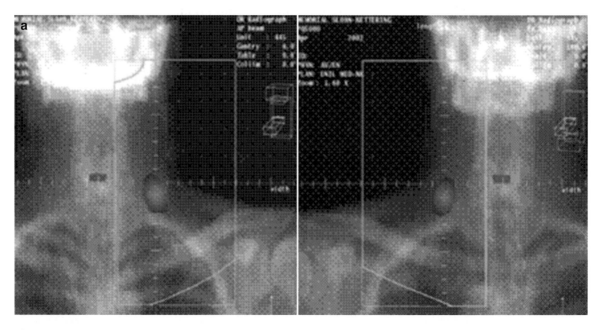

**Fig. 8.1** Involved-field radiation therapy. (**a**) Stage I HL involving the right neck. (**b**) Stage II HL involvement of the right neck and the left lower neck. (**c**) Stage IIX HL with involvement of the right neck, bulky mediastinum, right hilum, and right cardio-phrenic area. *Top*: CT scan display of the mediastinum; *bottom left*: FDG-PET mapping of disease involvement; *bottom right*: involved field covering the right neck, left supraclavicular area, mediastinum, and right costophrenic area

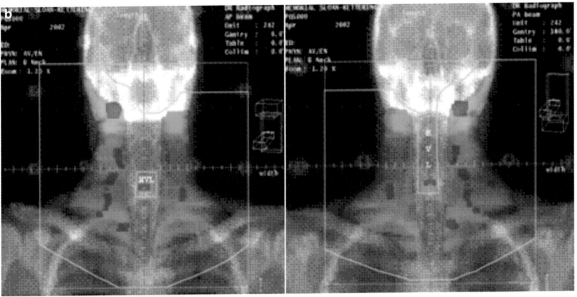

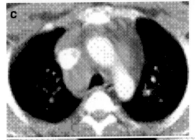

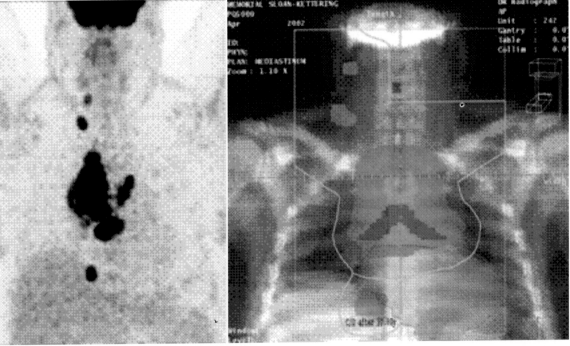

Fig. 8.1 (continued)

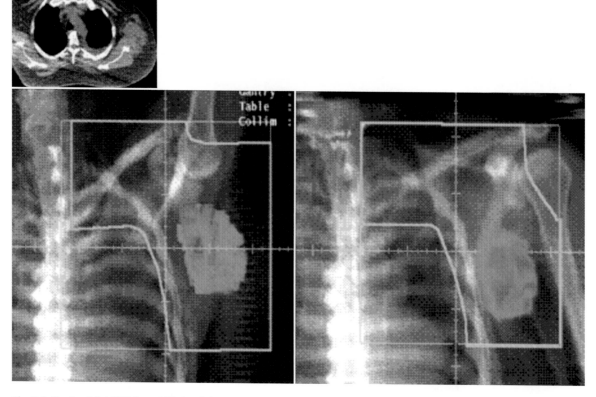

**Fig. 8.2** Regional field RT. Stage I HL involving the left axilla. *Top*: CT scan display; *bottom left*: treatment with the arm up; *bottom right*: treatment with the arm akimbo

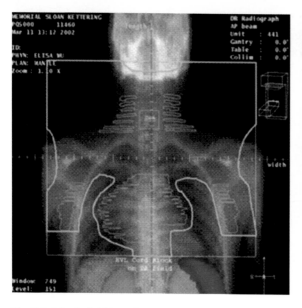

**Fig. 8.3** Mantle field (anterior aspect)

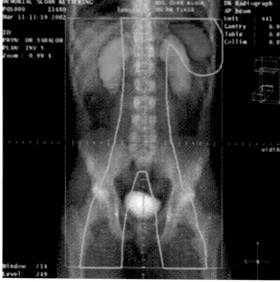

**Fig. 8.4** Inverted Y field (anterior aspect)

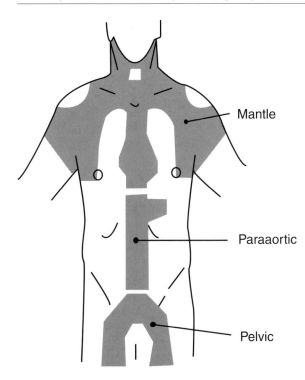

**Fig. 8.5** Subtotal and total lymphoid irradiation (STLI and TLI) fields. Subtotal lymphoid irradiation will include the mantle and paraaortic fields; if the pelvic field is also included, the field is called total lymphoid irradiation. In this diagram, the spleen was resected and only the splenic pedicle is irradiated. If the spleen remains intact, it is included in the paraaortic–splenic field

volume (PTV) (Figs. 8.6 and 8.7). Several groups have begun to evaluate the potential advantages and risks of this minimal RT volume approach, but only short outcome data are available, and treatment techniques and guidelines are still evolving. At present, IFRT, as described in more detail below, remains the usual treatment field in combined modality programs, although further reductions in field extent are often incorporated based on availability of adequate imaging, prechemotherapy clinical information, and clinical judgment.

## 8.5 Guidelines for Delineating the Involved Fields [32]

1. IFRT is treatment of a region, not of an individual lymph node.
2. The main involved-field nodal regions are neck (unilateral), mediastinum (including the hilar regions bilaterally), axilla (usually including the supraclavicular and infraclavicular lymph nodes), spleen, paraaortic lymph nodes, and inguinal (including the femoral and iliac) nodes.
3. In general, the fields include the involved prechemotherapy sites and volume, with an important

**Fig. 8.6** Involved lymph nodes field. Single lymph node in the left lower neck prior to chemotherapy (*left*) and following chemotherapy (*right*). The border of the field encompass the original volume of the node and not of the whole unilateral neck (as in IFRT approach). (Courtesy of Dr. Theodore Girinsky from Institute Goustave-Roussy)

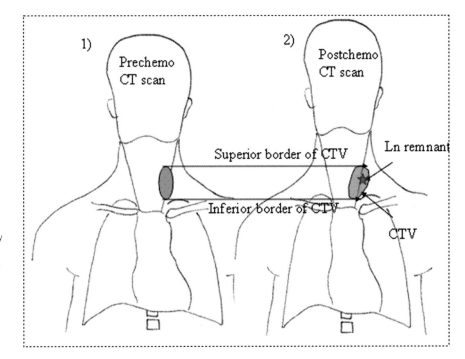

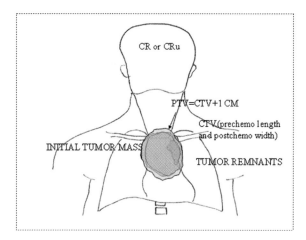

**Fig. 8.7** Involved lymph node field in the mediastinum. *Note:* The length of the treated area is determined by original longitudinal tumor diameter on CT scan while the width considers the decrease in transverse diameter following chemotherapy as determined by CT scan. (Courtesy of Dr. Theodore Girinsky from Institute Goustave-Roussy)

exception being the transverse diameter of the mediastinal and paraaortic lymph nodes. For the field width of these sites, it is recommended to use the reduced postchemotherapy diameter (width). In these areas, the regression of the lymph nodes is easily depicted by CT and/or PET imaging, and the critical normal tissues are saved by reducing the irradiated volume.

4. The supraclavicular lymph nodes are considered part of the cervical region and if involved along with other cervical nodes, the entire ipsilateral neck is treated. However, if the supraclavicular involvement is an extension of mediastinal disease and other areas of the neck are not involved (based on PET–CT imaging), the upper neck (above the larynx) is spared. This is to spare irradiation of the salivary glands.

5. If 3D treatment planning is employed and pre-chemotherapy PET–CT imaging is fused to the treatment planning CT, involved field treatment should generally extend 2–5 cm proximal and distal to involved nodes and adequate medial and lateral margins to ensure coverage of the lymph node chains. Although using a dedicated CT simulator for designing involved fields is highly recommended, the anatomic borders for conventional treatment fields are easy to outline (most are bony landmarks) and plan on a 2D standard simulation unit. However, CT data are preferred for outlining the mediastinal and paraaortic region and will also help in designing the axillary field.

6. Prechemotherapy and postchemotherapy information (both CT and PET) regarding lymph node localization and size is critical and should be available at the time of planning the field.

## 8.6 Involved Field Guidelines for Common Nodal Sites

### 8.6.1 Unilateral Cervical/ Supraclavicular Region

Involvement at any cervical level with or without involvement of the supraclavicular (SCL) nodes (Fig. 8.1a).

Arm position: akimbo or at sides. *Upper border:* 1–2 cm above the lower tip of the mastoid process and midpoint through the chin. *Lower border:* 2 cm below the bottom of the clavicle. *Lateral border:* To include the medial 2/3 of the clavicle. *Medial border:* (a) If the supraclavicular nodes are not involved, the border is placed at the ipsilateral edge of the vertebral body or ipsilateral transverse processes, except when medial nodes close to the vertebral bodies are seen on the initial staging neck CT scan. When medial nodes are involved, the entire vertebral body is included. (b) When the supraclavicular nodes are involved, the border should be placed at the contra-lateral traverse processes. For patients with stage I disease, the larynx and vertebral bodies above the larynx can be blocked (assuming no medial cervical nodes). *Blocks:* A posterior cervical cord block is required only if the calculated cord dose exceeds 40 Gy. Midneck calculations should be performed to determine the maximum cord dose, especially when the central axis is in the mediastinum. A laryngeal block should be used, unless lymph nodes are present in that location. In that case the block should be added at 20 Gy.

### 8.6.2 Bilateral Cervical/ Supraclavicular Region

Both cervical and supraclavicular regions should be treated as described above regardless of the extent of disease on each side. Posterior cervical cord and larynx blocks should be used as described above. Use a posterior mouth block if treating the patient supine (preferably with an extended travel couch at greater than 100 cm FSD) to block the upper field divergence through the mouth (Fig. 8.1b).

### 8.6.3 Mediastinum

Involvement of the mediastinum and/or the hilar nodes: In HL, this field includes also the medial SCL nodes even if not clinically involved.

Arms position: akimbo or at sides. The arms up position is optional if the axillary nodes are involved. *Upper border*: C5–C6 interspace. If supraclavicular nodes were also involved, the upper border should be placed at the top of the larynx and the lateral border should be adjusted as described in the section on treating neck nodes. *Lower border*: The lower of (a) 5 cm below the carina or (b) 2 cm below the *prechemotherapy* inferior border. *Lateral border*: The *postchemotherapy* volume with 1.5 cm margin. *Hilar area*: To be included with 1 cm margin unless initially involved where as the margin should be 1.5 cm.

If paracardiac lymph nodes are involved, they should be treated either as an extension of the mediastinal field or if significantly lower than the mediastinal field as a separate targeted involved lymph node area. Irradiation of the whole heart (for even a lower dose) is not recommended in most cases (Fig. 8.1c).

### 8.6.4 Mediastinum with Involvement of the Cervical Nodes

When both cervical regions are involved, the field is a mantle, without the axilla, using the guidelines described above. If only one cervical chain is involved the vertebral bodies, contralateral upper neck, and larynx can be blocked as previously described. Because of the increased dose to the neck (the isocenter is in the upper mediastinum), unless compensators or wedges are employed, the neck above the lower border of the larynx should be shielded at ~30 Gy.

### 8.6.5 Axillary Region

The ipsilateral axillary, infraclavicular, and supraclavicular areas are generally treated when the axilla is involved.

Whenever possible, use CT-based planning for this region. Arms position: akimbo or arms up. *Upper border*: C5–C6 interspace. *Lower border*: The lower of the two: (a) the tip of the scapula or (b) 2 cm below the lowest axillary node. *Medial border*: Ipsilateral cervical transverse process. Include the vertebral bodies only if the supraclavicular nodes are involved. *Lateral border*: Flash axilla (Fig. 8.2).

### 8.6.6 Spleen

The spleen is treated only if abnormal imaging was suggestive of involvement. The *postchemotherapy* volume is treated with 1.5 cm margins, preferably utilizing respiratory gating.

### 8.6.7 Abdomen (Paraaortic Nodes)

*Upper border*: Top of T11 and at least 2 cm above prechemotherapy volume. *Lower border*: Bottom of L4 and at least 2 cm below prechemotherapy volume. *Lateral borders:* The edge of the transverse processes and at least 2 cm from the postchemotherapy volume. A case illustration is shown in Fig. 8.8a, b.

### 8.6.8 Inguinal/Femoral/External Iliac Region

These ipsilateral lymph node groups are treated together if any of the nodes are involved (Fig. 8.9a, b).

*Upper border*: Middle of the sacro-iliac joint. *Lower border*: 5 cm below the lesser trochanter *Lateral border*: The greater trochanter and 2 cm lateral to initially involved nodes. *Medial border*: Medial border of the obturator foramen with at least 2 cm medial to involved nodes. If common iliac nodes are involved the field should extend to the L4–L5 interspace and at least 2 cm above the initially involved nodal border.

### 8.6.9 Involved Field Radiotherapy of Extranodal Sites

In most cases, the whole involved organ is the target and draining lymph nodes are not included unless

**Fig. 8.8** (**a**) Paraaortic and pelvic involvement. *Top*: CT illustrates massive paraaortic involvement with extension into the left kidney; *bottom right*: FDG-PET uptake; *bottom left*: renal scan demonstrating left kidney loss of function. (**b**) Treatment plan for the patient in Fig. 8.8a

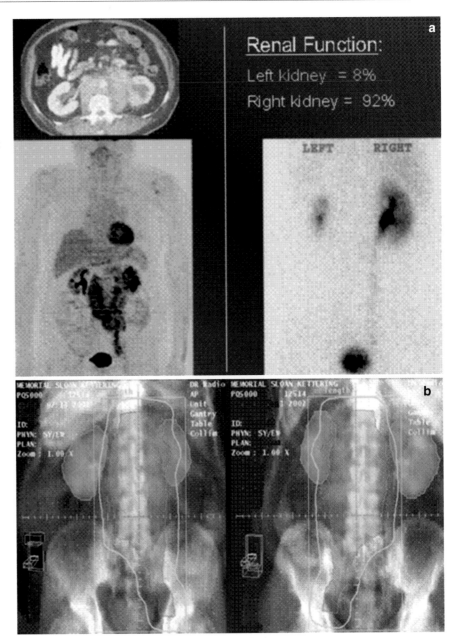

involved. The optimal plan is 3D-conformal and CT-simulation based. The margins for the PTV depend on the quality of imaging and reliability of immobilization, and most importantly, should account for organ motion during respiration. Typically, areas of extranodal extension in the head and neck require margins of 1 cm and areas in the mediastinum, abdomen, and pelvis require margins of 2 cm.

## 8.7 Technical Aspects of Radiotherapy for HL

### 8.7.1 Choice of Equipment

The linear accelerator is the machine of choice for radiotherapy of HL. The desired energy is 6 megavoltage

Fig. 8.9 (a) Involvement of the right pelvic lymph nodes. *Right*: CT scan at the level of mid-pelvis; *left*: FDG-PET uptake. (b) Treatment volume for patient illustrated in Fig. 8.9a

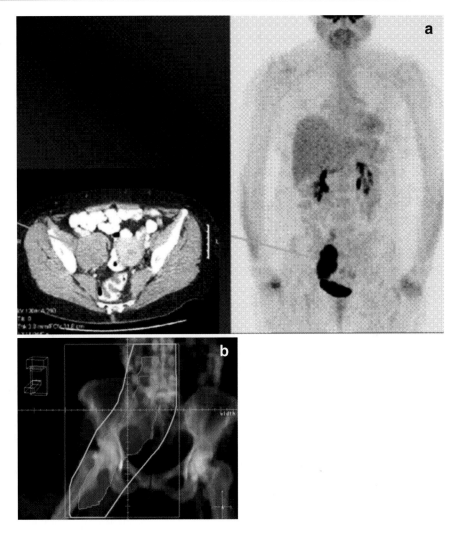

(MV) for treatment of peripheral nodal sites but higher energies such as 10 or 15 MV may be used for abdominal and thoracic tumors, depending on anatomy and choice of treatment plan. If high energies are used and superficial nodes require radiation, a "beam spoiler" or bolus should be used. A 6 MV beam is sufficiently penetrating to produce good dose homogeneity throughout most treatment fields. The maximum dose point of a 6 MV is close enough to the skin surface to avoid underdosing superficially located lymph nodes, such as the cervical or inguinal nodes. The dose inhomogeneity measured in fields treated with 6 MV beam may be as high as 10%, due primarily to differences in patient separation within the field and to large separations in big patients. For patients with large nodes right at the skin,

tissue equivalent bolus may be needed to increase the subcutaneous dose.

### 8.7.2 Positioning and Immobilization and Simulation

For most anatomical sites selected for IFRT as primary or complementary treatment of HL, CT simulation will provide essential information for determining treatment volume and optimal plan. This is particularly important as the recommended RT fields have become smaller. In current practice, most radiation oncologists will incorporate indirectly acquired or direct CT-simulation information into the treatment planning process. In selective cases, FDG-PET imaging and/or MRI performed in the same treatment position with fiduciary markers is also incorporated into the simulation and treatment planning process.

One of the important lessons learned from 3D treatment planning is that radiotherapy accuracy during a course of fractionated radiation is only as good as the immobilization of the patient. With Cerrobend© blocks attached to a standard machine block-holding tray or automated multileaf collimator blocks, very small changes in patient position may result in considerable field variations. Accurate positioning requires reproducible neck and arm positioning, and reproducible alignment and rotation of the torso and pelvis. Reproducible knee and foot positioning may also be required under certain circumstances.

An upper body mold is useful for the treatment of lower neck and thoracic fields.

Wall-mounted lasers in the simulation and treatment rooms can aid in reproducing torso and pelvic alignment and rotation. Leveling tattoos, one pair of lateral tattoos on each side of the central axis, will aid in lining up with the side lasers.

### 8.7.3 Shielding of Reproductive Organs

Of the normal tissues, the testes are the most sensitive to low-dose fractionated radiation. A total dose of 3–3.5 Gy may result in sterility in over 50% of patients. Thus, the 3% received from the primary beam through the block may significantly add to the scattered dose and bring the total dose into this range. This is of importance in patients receiving external iliac, inguinal, and femoral irradiation where the testes are within the radiation field borders but under the block. One way to reduce the primary beam dose to the testes is to utilize both the templated blocks and the multileaf collimators. This should provide 10 half layers of protection and reduce the primary dose component to 0.01% of the total dose.

The testicles may be shielded from internally scattered radiation by using a special clamshell-like testicular shield [33]. It is important that the testicles are positioned behind the front wall of the shield. These shields will provide a three- to tenfold reduction in scatter dose to the testes. Loss of fertility is also significantly reduced by limiting the radiation field to one side of the pelvis. With bilateral pelvic nodal irradiation, the internal scatter component increases greatly. Monitoring testicular radiation dose during treatment using a thermoluminescent dosimeter (TLD) is possible and patients at risk should be counseled and encouraged to undergo sperm banking prior to radiation and preferably prior to starting chemotherapy.

Normally, the ovaries lie just medial to the external iliac nodes and would be within a standard pelvic radiation field. The tolerance of the ovaries to radiation is well below the doses employed for lymphoma. If preservation of ovarian function, including fertility, is desired, the ovaries must be transposed to a location outside the primary radiation beam, or to a location over which sufficient secondary shielding can be provided to prevent ovarian ablation. Surgical transposition or oophoropexy may be accomplished through a laparoscopic procedure. Careful coordination between surgeon and radiation oncologist is required so that the surgeon understands exactly where the ovaries must be placed, marks them with radio-opaque clips, and takes radiographs at the time of surgery on the operating room table to ensure that the placement is correct. With unilateral pelvic irradiation, one ovary should remain outside of the field and should have normal function. In many patients with lymphoma, the age at onset is beyond childbearing age. In the young patient receiving whole pelvic irradiation, transposition of the ovaries is the only way to preserve hormonal function and fertility.

Ovarian dose is affected by scattered radiation generated within the treatment field as well as primary transmission through the block. A number of technical factors can affect the dose delivered to the ovaries including the field size and distance of the ovaries from the edge of the field. Combined modality therapy can be used to reduce the treatment field size so that involved field radiation may be considered.

### 8.7.4 Treatment Verification and Documentation

A number of studies have documented difficulty with accurate daily delivery of treatment [34, 35]. With the frequent use of imaging films, which document the volume of tissue actually exposed to radiation during a treatment, it is clear that both systematic errors and random errors may occur. Systematic errors result from a flawed simulation, perhaps because the patient was tense and later relaxed on the actual treatment table or because the initial simulation position was uncomfortable and not sustainable [34]. Typically, systematic errors can be identified with an imaging film on the first day of treatment. Random errors are related to poor positioning of the patient or shielding blocks in daily treatment setups. The use of better positioning tools such as immobilization devices and lasers have aided in securing more accurate setups, and the use of frequent imaging films has focused attention on accuracy and identified systematic problems [35].

## 8.7.5 Quality Control

Quality control and assurance is critical to the interpretation of clinical trial results and ensuring uniformly optimal patient care. The quality of radiation treatment depends on the successful completion of each of the following steps.

1. Identification of sites of involvement and sites at significant risk for microscopic disease. This requires an ability to perform an accurate and complete physical examination, to interpret the diagnostic images used in staging, and to understand the regions at risk and patterns of spread of HL.
2. Selection and design of treatment fields that will adequately cover all areas requiring treatment and adequately spare normal tissues.
3. Prescription of the optimal dose for disease control and normal tissue preservation.
4. Meticulous delivery of the treatment plan.

Proper execution of each these steps is important in ensuring the quality and success of overall treatment. Quality control programs for radiation treatment in HL have been established by European cooperative groups. In the EORTC H8 protocol, a quality control program for verification of radiation technical files was implemented. Among 161 files reviewed, major deviations in radiation volumes and dose were observed in 13.6 and 39.7% of the cases, respectively [22]. The number of major deviations was felt to justify such a radiation quality control program. In the GHSG HD4 trial [36], all planning and verification films as well as dose charts were prospectively reviewed. Cases with protocol violations were found to have a significantly lower

5-year FFTF (70 vs. 82%, $p<0.04$), illustrating the importance of quality assurance. Ongoing cooperative trials on non-Hodgkin lymphoma treatment may provide an opportunity to collect similar data. The GHSG has established a special central pretreatment review mechanism to ensure adequate field selection to improve the quality of RT in the large number of centers participating in the group studies.

The Patterns of Care Studies in the United States have reported extensively on Hodgkin disease. The results demonstrated that patients with adequate portal margins had significantly fewer in-field or marginal recurrences, or relapses of any type [37, 38]. Furthermore, the experience of the treating radiation oncologists, use of a dedicated simulator, performance of routine port films to ensure set-up accuracies, use of individually shaped blocks, linear accelerators and extended-field treatments were all associated with an improved treatment outcome [37–39].

## 8.8 Dose Considerations and Recommendations

Although doses in the range of 40–44 Gy were at one time recommended for the definitive treatment of patients with HL, these recommendations have been modified over time, especially in the context of combined modality therapy or the treatment of patients with LPHL.

Clinical factors likely to impact disease control include tumor size, use of chemotherapy, disease extent, and technical considerations related to field design, and accuracy of patient setup. The radiation dose is typically delivered in 1.8–2.0 Gy fractions. If significant portions of lung or heart are included, the dose per fraction can be reduced to 1.5 Gy. The available data indicate that the choice of fractionation is not critical for tumor control, and that a schedule with minimal risk of damage to normal structures should be selected [40].

The GHSG evaluated dose in patients with stage IA to IIB disease without risk factors in a randomized trial of 40 Gy extended-field radiation alone vs. 30 Gy extended-field radiation with a boost of 10 Gy to the involved site of disease [36, 41]. There was no significant difference in outcome between the two arms of the study indicating that 30 Gy is sufficient for clinically uninvolved areas when RT is used alone. The optimum dose for clinically involved sites of disease with radiotherapy alone has not been tested in a randomized trial.

More relevant to current practice is the determination of the adequate radiation dose after treatment with chemotherapy. In many early studies, radiation doses were kept at ~40 Gy even after achieving a CR to chemotherapy; others reduced the dose in the combined modality setting to 20–24 Gy with excellent overall results [42]. Studies of combined modality in advanced stage also used reduced doses of RT for patients who achieved a CR to chemotherapy and higher doses (~30 Gy) for patients in PR [22].The pediatric groups addressing the concern of radiation effects on skeletal and muscular development also effectively reduced the dose of RT after combination chemotherapy to 21–24 Gy [43].

Several recent studies addressed the adequacy of low IFRT dose following chemotherapy. A study conducted by the EORTC/GELA [44] randomized patients with favorable early-stage HL to 36, 20, or 0 Gy IFRT after achieving a CR to six cycles of EBVP. Because an excessive number of relapses occurred in the no-RT arm, this arm was closed early. There was no difference in EFS at 4 years between patients receiving IFRT 36 (87%) vs. 20 Gy (84%).

A recent GHSG randomized study (HD 10) addressed the radiation dose question after short-course chemotherapy. Patients with favorable stage I–II were randomized to receive either 4 or only 2 cycles of ABVD followed by either IFRT of 30 or 20 Gy. At a median follow-up of 7 years, there was no difference in FFTF between the four arms. FFTF at 5 years was 93.4% in patients treated with 30 Gy (91.0–95.2%) and 92.9% in those receiving 20 Gy (90.4–94.8%). These results, taken together with the better tolerability and the lack of inferiority in secondary efficacy endpoints, lead to the conclusion that 20 Gy IFRT, when combined with even only two cycles of ABVD, is equally effective to 30 Gy IFRT in this very favorable group of patients [14]. The GHSG HD11 study targeted patients with unfavorable early-stage and randomized them to either ABVDX4 or BEACOPPX4, either program was followed by either 20 or 30 Gy to the involved field. Five-year FFTF and OS for all patients were 85 and 94.5%, respectively. There was no difference in FFTF when BEACOPPX4 was followed by either 30 or 20 Gy and similar excellent results were obtained with ABVDX4 and IFRT of 30 Gy. Patients who received ABVDX4 and only 20 Gy had FFTF that was lower by 4%. OS was similar in all

treatment groups [15]. These results suggest that 30 Gy should remain the standard IFRT dose following ABVD in unfavorable early-stage HL [15].

## 8.8.1 The Significance of Reducing the Radiation Dose

Recent studies clearly indicate that the risk of secondary solid tumor induction is radiation dose-related. This was carefully analyzed for secondary breast and lung cancers as well as for other tumors [45–49]. While it will take more years of careful follow-up of patients in randomized studies to display the full magnitude of risk tapering by current reduction of radiation field and dose, recent data suggest that this likely to be the case. In a recent Duke University study, two groups of patients with early-stage HL were treated with different radiation approaches over the same period. One group received radiotherapy alone, given to extended fields with a median dose of 38 Gy; the second group received chemotherapy followed by involved-field low-dose (median of 25 Gy) radiotherapy. While 12 patients developed second tumors in the first group and 8 of them died, no second tumors were detected in the second group. The median follow-up was 11.7 and 8.1 years, respectively [50] Similar observations with an even longer follow-up were made by the Yale group [51]. In a study that used data-based radiobiological modeling to predict the radiation-induced second cancer risk, lowering the dose from 35 to 20 Gy and reducing the extended field to IFRT reduced lung cancer risk and breast cancer risk by 57 and 77%, respectively [45].

## 8.8.2 Dose Recommendations

Radiation alone (as primary treatment for LPHL)
   Clinically involved sites: 30–36 Gy
   Clinically uninvolved sites: 30 Gy
Radiation alone (as primary treatment for cHL [uncommon])
   Clinically involved sites: 36–40 Gy
   Clinically uninvolved sites: 30 Gy
Radiation following chemotherapy in a combined modality program

Patients in CR after chemotherapy: 20–30 Gy

Most guidelines recommend 30 Gy (for adults) until lower dose (20 Gy) data mature

For pediatric or adolescent patients: 21–24 Gy

In some programs of short chemotherapy for bulky or advanced-stage disease (e.g., Stanford V), the recommended RT dose is 36 Gy

Patients in PR after chemotherapy: 30–40 Gy

## 8.9 New Aspects of Radiation Field Design and Delivery

The abandonment of large-field irradiation for most patients with HL permits the use of more conformal RT fields and introduction of other innovative RT techniques.

The change in the lymphoma radiotherapy paradigm coincided with substantial improvement in imaging and treatment planning technology that have revolutionized the field of radiotherapy. The integration of fast high-resolution computerized tomography into the simulation and planning systems of radiation oncology has changed how treatment volumes and relationship to normal critical structures are determined and planned. In the recent past, tumor volume determinations were made with fluoroscopy-based simulators that produced often poor quality imaging requiring wide "safety margins" that detracted from accuracy and sparing of critical organs. Most modern simulators are in fact high-resolution CT scanners with software programs that allow accurate conformal treatment planning and provide detailed information on the dose volume delivered to normal structures within the treatment field and the homogeneity of dose delivered to the target. More recently, these simulators are integrated also with a PET scanner that provides additional tumor volume information for consideration during radiation planning.

Intensity-modulated radiotherapy (IMRT) is the most advanced planning and radiation delivery mode and is mainly used for small volume cancers that require high radiation doses (e.g., prostate and head neck cancers) or are adjacent to critical organs. IMRT allows for accurately enveloping the tumor with either a homogenous radiation dose ("sculpting") or delivering higher doses to predetermined areas in the tumor volume ("painting"). The end result of this new modality is highly accurate treatment with maximal sparing of normal tissues. In the

radiotherapy of lymphoma, there are several clinical situations where IMRT provides a benefit: treatment of very large or complicated tumor volumes in the mediastinum and abdomen, and head and neck lymphomas. IMRT also allows re-irradiation of sites prior to high-dose salvage programs that otherwise will be prohibited by normal tissue tolerance, particularly of the spinal cord [52] (Figs. 8.10a–d and 8.11a–c).

## 8.10 Common Side Effects and Supportive Care During Radiotherapy

Side effects of radiotherapy depend on the irradiated volume, dose administered, and technique employed. They are also influenced by the extent and type of prior chemotherapy, if any, and by the patient's age. Most of the information that we use today to estimate risk of radiotherapy is derived from strategies that used radiation alone. The field size and configuration, doses, and technology have all drastically changed over the last decade. It is thus misleading to judge current radiotherapy for HL, and inform patients on risks of radiotherapy using information of past radiotherapy that is no longer practiced.

It is of interest that most of the data of long-term complications associated with radiotherapy and particularly second solid tumors and coronary heart disease were reported from databases of patients with HL treated more than 25 years ago. It is also important to note that we have very limited long-term follow-up data on patients with HL who were treated with chemotherapy alone.

### 8.10.1 Acute Effects

Radiation, in general, may cause fatigue and areas of the irradiated skin may develop mild sun-exposure-like dermatitis. The acute side effects of irradiating the full neck include mouth, dryness, change in taste, and pharyngitis. With the doses currently employed in HL, these side effects are usually mild and transient. The main potential side effects of subdiaphragmatic irradiation are loss of appetite, nausea, and

**Fig. 8.10** (**a**) CT–MR fusion for target localization of HL involving the mediastinum and right chest wall. *CTV* clinical treatment volume; *PTV* planning treatment volume. (**b**, **c**) Treatment plans comparing AP/PA, 3D-CRT, and IMRT. *PTV* planning treatment volume; *AP/PA* opposed anterior and posterior fields; *3DCRT* 3-dimensional conformal radiotherapy; *IMRT*: intensity-modulated radiotherapy. (**d**) Comparison of lung complication probability of different plans

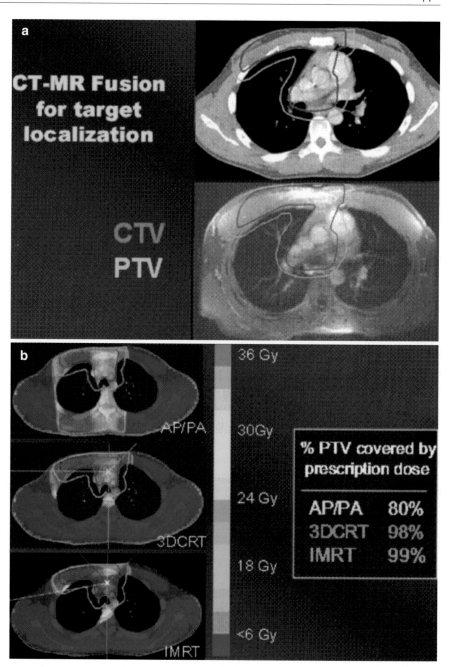

**Fig. 8.10** (continued)

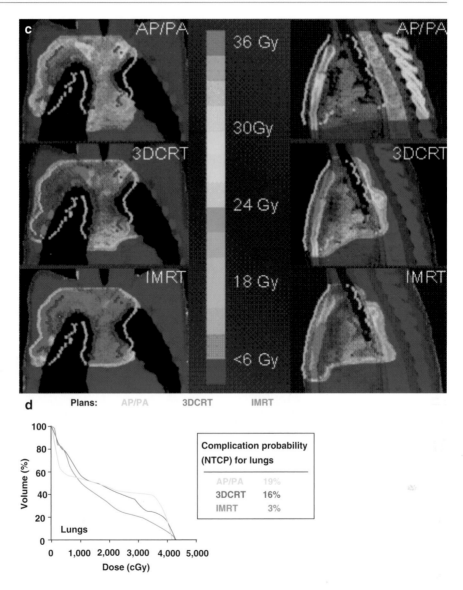

increased bowel movements. These reactions are usually mild and can be minimized with standard antiemetic medications.

Irradiation of more than one field, particularly after chemotherapy, can cause myelosuppression, which may necessitate short treatment interruption and very rarely administration of G-CSF, erythropoietin-type drugs, or platelet transfusion.

### 8.10.2  Early Side Effects

*Lhermitte's sign*: Less than 5% of patients may note an electric shock sensation radiating down the backs of both legs when the head is flexed (Lhermitte's sign) 6 weeks to 3 months after mantle-field radiotherapy. Possibly secondary to transient demyelinization of the spinal cord, Lhermitte's sign resolves spontaneously after a few months and is not associated with late or permanent spinal cord damage.

*Pneumonitis and pericarditis*: During the same period, radiation pneumonitis and/or acute pericarditis may occur in <5% of patients; these side effects occur more often in those who have extensive mediastinal disease. Both inflammatory processes have become rare with modern radiation techniques.

The consideration and discussion of radiotherapy and chemotherapy potential late side effects and complications is of prime importance and is detailed in Chap. 20.

Fig. 8.11 (a) Use of IMRT for re-irradiation of a patient relapsing after ABVD and mantle field irradiation to 36 Gy. (b, c) Treatment planning options for re-irradiation. *AP/PA* opposed anterior and posterior fields; *3DCRT* 3-dimensional conformal radiotherapy; *IMRT* intensity-modulated radiotherapy

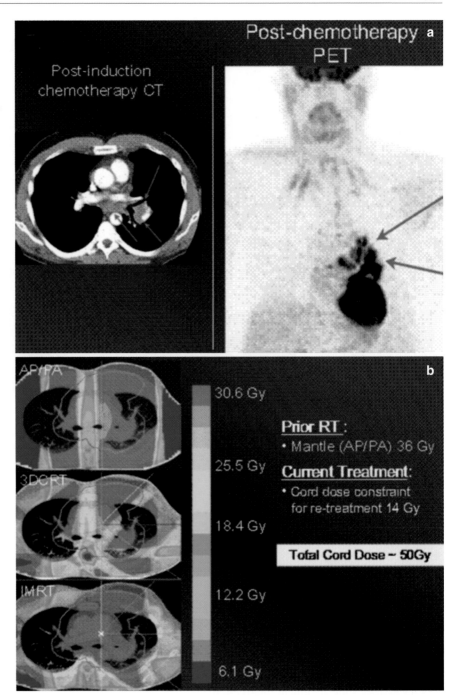

### 8.10.3 Supportive Care During Treatment

It is important to prepare the patient to the potential side effects, and many organizations and cancer centers also provide written patient information regarding radiotherapy of lymphomas. Since some level of mouth dryness is often associated with radiotherapy that involves the upper neck and/or lower mandible and mouth attention to dental care is advised. If dryness is a concern, it is advised to arrange for an expert dental appointment for overall

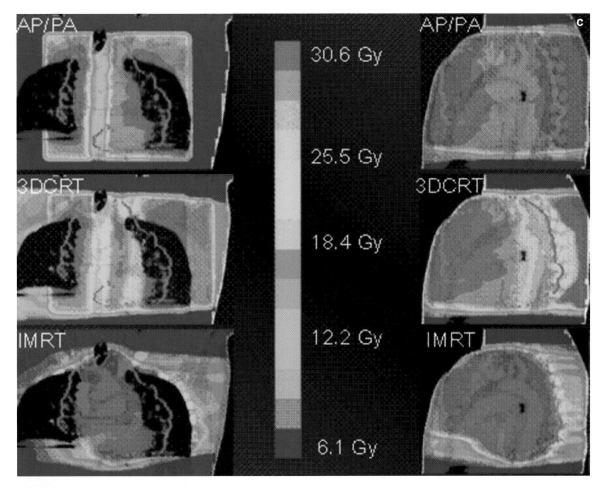

**Fig. 8.11** (continued)

dental evaluation and consideration of mouth guards (from scatter) and/or supplemental fluoride treatment during and after radiotherapy.

Soreness of the throat and mild to moderate difficulty of swallowing solid and dry food may also occur during neck irradiation, with onset at a dose of ~20 Gy. These side effects are almost always mild, self-limited, and subside shortly after completion of radiotherapy. Skin care with and use of sun screen is advised for all patients undergoing radiotherapy. Temporary hair loss is expected in irradiated areas and recovery is observed after several months.

We normally recommend a first post-RT follow-up visit 6 weeks after the end of treatment and obtain post-RT baseline blood count, standard biochemistry tests, as well as TSH levels and lipid profile (if applicable) at that visit. Follow-up imaging studies normally commence 3 months after completion of treatment. Other follow-up studies are included in the NCCN guidelines for HL [9].

# References

1. Hoppe RT, Advani RH, et al. Hodgkin disease/lymphoma. J Natl Compr Canc Netw. 2008;6:594–622.
2. Yahalom J. Role of radiation therapy in Hodgkin's lymphoma. Cancer J. 2009;15:155–60.
3. Pusey W. Cases of sarcoma and of Hodgkin's disease treated by exposures to X-rays: a preliminary report. JAMA. 1902;38:166–9.
4. Senn N. Therapeutical value of rontgen ray in treatment of pseudoleukemia. New York Med J. 1903;77:665–8.
5. Gilbert R. La roentgentherapie de la granulomatose maligne. J Radiol Electrol. 1925;9:509–14.
6. Peters M. A study in survivals in Hodgkin's disease treated radiologically. Am J Roentgenol. 1950;63:299–311.
7. Kaplan H. The radical radiotherapy of Hodgkin's disease. Radiology. 1962;78:553–61.
8. Girinsky T, van der Maazen R, et al. Involved-node radiotherapy (INRT) in patients with early Hodgkin lymphoma: concepts and guidelines. Radiother Oncol. 2006;79:270–7.
9. Hoppe RT, AR H, et al. NCCN physician guidelines: Hodgkin Lymphoma 2010 v.1. www.nccn.org; 2010.
10. Nogova L, Reineke T, et al. Extended field radiotherapy, combined modality treatment or involved field radiotherapy for patients with stage IA lymphocyte-predominant Hodgkin's lymphoma: a retrospective analysis from the German Hodgkin Study Group (GHSG). Ann Oncol. 2005;16:1683–7.
11. Wirth A, Yuen K, et al. Long-term outcome after radiotherapy alone for lymphocyte-predominant Hodgkin lymphoma: a retrospective multicenter study of the Australasian Radiation Oncology Lymphoma Group. Cancer. 2005;104:1221–9.
12. Chen RC, Chin MS, et al. Early-stage, lymphocyte-predominant Hodgkin's lymphoma: patient outcomes from a large, single-institution series with long follow-up. J Clin Oncol. 2010;28:136–41.
13. Schlembach PJ, Wilder RB, et al. Radiotherapy alone for lymphocyte-predominant Hodgkin's disease. Cancer J. 2002;8:377–83.
14. Engert A, Diehl V, et al. Two cycles of ABVD followed by involved field radiotherapy with 20 gray (Gy) is the new standard of care in the treatment of patients with early-stage Hodgkin lymphoma: final analysis of the randomized German Hodgkin Study Group (GHSG) HD10. Study Supported by the Deutsche Krebshilfe and in Part by the Competence Network Malignant Lymphoma. Blood 2009; (ASH 2009 abstract #716).
15. Borchmann P, Diehl V, et al. Combined modality treatment with intensified chemotherapy and dose-reduced involved field radiotherapy in patients with early unfavourable Hodgkin lymphoma (HL): final analysis of the German Hodgkin Study Group (GHSG) HD11 Trial. Blood 2009;114:299 (ASH abstract # 717).
16. Herbst C, Rehan FA, et al. Combined modality treatment improves tumor control and overall survival in patients with early stage Hodgkin lymphoma: a systematic review. Haematologica. 2009;95:494.
17. Prosnitz LR, Wu JJ, et al. The case for adjuvant radiation therapy in advanced Hodgkin's disease. Cancer Investigation. 1996;14:361–70.
18. Brizel DM, Winer EP, et al. Improved survival in advanced Hodgkin's disease with the use of combined modality therapy [see comments]. Int J Radiat Oncol Biol Phys. 1990;19:535–42.
19. Yahalom J, Ryu J, et al. Impact of adjuvant radiation on the patterns and rate of relapse in advanced-stage Hodgkin's disease treated with alternating chemotherapy combinations. J Clin Oncol. 1991;9:2193–201.
20. Fabian C, Mansfield C, et al. Low-dose involved field radiation after chemotherapy in advanced Hodgkin's disease. Ann Intern Med. 1994;120:903–12.
21. Loeffler M, Diehl V, et al. Dose-response relationship of complementary radiotherapy following four cycles of combination chemotherapy in intermediate-stage Hodgkin's disease. J Clin Oncol. 1997;15:2275–87.
22. Aleman BM, Raemaekers JM, et al. Involved-field radiotherapy for advanced Hodgkin's lymphoma. N Engl J Med. 2003;348:2396–406.
23. Duggan DB, Petroni GR, et al. Randomized comparison of ABVD and MOPP/ABV hybrid for the treatment of advanced Hodgkin's disease: report of an intergroup trial. J Clin Oncol. 2003;21:607–14.
24. Laskar S, Gupta T, et al. Consolidation radiation after complete remission in Hodgkin's disease following six cycles of doxorubicin, bleomycin, vinblastine, and dacarbazine chemotherapy: is there a need? J Clin Oncol. 2004;22:62–8.
25. Horning SJ, Hoppe RT, et al. Stanford V and radiotherapy for locally extensive and advanced Hodgkin's disease: mature results of a prospective clinical trial. J Clin Oncol. 2002;20:630–7.
26. Chisesi T, Federico M, et al. ABVD versus stanford V versus MEC in unfavourable Hodgkin's lymphoma: results of a randomised trial. Ann Oncol. 2002;13 Suppl 1:102–6.
27. Poen JC, Hoppe RT, et al. High-dose therapy and autologous bone marrow transplantation for relapsed/refractory Hodgkin's disease: the impact of involved field radiotherapy on patterns of failure and survival [see comments]. Int J Radiat Oncol Biol Phys. 1996;36:3–12.
28. Yahalom J, Gulati SC, et al. Accelerated hyperfractionated total-lymphoid irradiation, high-dose chemotherapy, and autologous bone marrow transplantation for refractory and relapsing patients with Hodgkin's disease. J Clin Oncol. 1993;11:1062–70.
29. Moskowitz CH, Nimer SD, et al. A 2-step comprehensive high-dose chemoradiotherapy second-line program for relapsed and refractory Hodgkin's disease: analysis by intent to treat and development of a prognostic model. Blood. 2001;97:617–23.
30. Moskowitz CH, Kewalramani T, et al. Effectiveness of high dose chemoradiotherapy and autologous stem cell transplantation for patients with biopsy-proven primary refractory Hodgkin's disease. Br J Haematol. 2004;124:645–52.
31. Goodman KA, Riedel E, et al. Long-term effects of high-dose chemotherapy and radiation for relapsed and refractory Hodgkin's lymphoma. J Clin Oncol. 2008;26:5240–7.

32. Yahalom J, Mauch P. The involved field is back: issues in delineating the radiation field in Hodgkin's disease. Ann Oncol. 2002;13 Suppl 1:79–83.

33. Fraass BA, Kinsella TJ, et al. Peripheral dose to the testes: the design and clinical use of a practical and effective gonadal shield. Int J Radiat Oncol Biol Phys. 1985;11:609–15.

34. Hulshof M, Vanuytsel L, et al. Localization errors in mantle-field irradiation for Hodgkin's disease. Int J Radiat Oncol Biol Phys. 1989;17:679–83.

35. Taylor Jr BW, Mendenhall NP, et al. Reproducibility of mantle irradiation with daily imaging films. Int J Radiat Oncol Biol Phys. 1990;19:149–51.

36. Duhmke E, Diehl V, et al. Randomized trial with early-stage Hodgkin's disease testing 30 Gy vs. 40 Gy extended field radiotherapy alone. Int J Radiat Oncol Biol Phys. 1996;36: 305–10.

37. Kinzie JJ, Hanks GE, et al. Patterns of care study: Hodgkin's disease relapse rates and adequacy of portals. Cancer. 1983;52:2223–6.

38. Hanks GE, Kinzie JJ, et al. Patterns of care outcome studies. Results of the national practice in Hodgkin's disease. Cancer. 1983;51:569–73.

39. Hoppe RT, Hanlon AL, et al. Progress in the treatment of Hodgkin's disease in the United States, 1973 versus 1983. The Patterns of Care Study. Cancer. 1994;74:3198–203.

40. Brincker H, Bentzen SM. A re-analysis of available dose-response and time-dose data in Hodgkin's disease. Radiother Oncol. 1994;30:227–30.

41. Duhmke E, Franklin J, et al. Low-dose radiation is sufficient for the noninvolved extended-field treatment in favorable early-stage Hodgkin's disease: long-term results of a randomized trial of radiotherapy alone. J Clin Oncol. 2001;19: 2905–14.

42. Prosnitz LR. Radiation doses following intensive chemotherapy in the treatment of Hodgkin's disease. Int J Radiat Oncol Biol Phys. 1976;1:803–4.

43. Donaldson SS, Link MP. Combined modality treatment with low-dose radiation and MOPP chemotherapy for children with Hodgkin's disease. J Clin Oncol. 1987;5:742–9.

44. Ferme C, Eghbali H, et al. Chemotherapy plus involved-field radiation in early-stage Hodgkin's disease. N Engl J Med. 2007;357:1916–27.

45. Hodgson DC, Koh ES, et al. Individualized estimates of second cancer risks after contemporary radiation therapy for Hodgkin lymphoma. Cancer. 2007;110:2576–86.

46. Kuttesch Jr JF, Wexler LH, et al. Second malignancies after Ewing's sarcoma: radiation dose-dependency of secondary sarcomas. J Clin Oncol. 1996;14:2818–25.

47. Travis LB, Gospodarowicz M, et al. Lung cancer following chemotherapy and radiotherapy for Hodgkin's disease. J Natl Cancer Inst. 2002;94:182–92.

48. Travis LB, Hill D, et al. Breast cancer following radiotherapy and chemotherapy among young women with Hodgkin's disease. JAMA 2003;290:465–475.

49. van Leeuwen FE, Klokman WJ, et al. Effects of radiation dose, chemotherapy, and ovarian hormones on breast cancer risk following Hodgkin's disease. In: Eighth International Conference on Malignant Lymphoma, Lugano, Switzerland; 2002.

50. Koontz B, Kirkpatrick J, et al. Combined modality therapy versus radiotherapy alone for treatment of early stage Hodgkin disease: cure versus complications. J Clin Oncol. 2006;24:605–11.

51. Salloum E, Doria R, et al. Second solid tumors in patients with Hodgkin's disease cured after radiation or chemotherapy plus adjuvant low-dose radiation. J Clin Oncol. 1996;14: 2435–43.

52. Goodman KA, Toner S, et al. Intensity modulated radiation therapy in the treatment of lymphoma involving the mediastinum. Int J Radiat Oncol Biol Phys. 2005;62:198–206.

# Principles of Chemotherapy in Hodgkin Lymphoma

**9**

Patrice Carde and Peter Johnson

## Contents

P. Carde
Institut Gustave Roussy, F-94800 Villejuif
e-mail: Patrice.carde@orange.fr

P. Johnson (✉)
Southampton General Hospital, Southampton, UK
e-mail: johnsonp@southampton.ac.uk

## 9.1 Historical Introduction

Hodgkin lymphoma (HL) was perhaps the disease for which the possibility of cure with combination chemotherapy in the majority of patients was first realized. As such, it has provided a model upon which studies in many other types of malignancy have been based, and it is interesting to follow the trajectory of knowledge from early single-agent work through combinations, combined modalities, increasing complexity, and most recently, selective de-escalation. Patients with advanced disease represent a minority of those affected by HL. However, these patients represent the group in which the development and effects of chemotherapy are most readily appreciated, since the role of radiation therapy is markedly less than in those with localized disease. Historically, chemotherapy and radiotherapy contended for primacy in the management of this illness, a tension which persisted until the mid-1970s.

The first successful treatment for HL was with radiotherapy, at least a decade in advance of chemotherapy in its application. Vera Peters showed the curability of localized HL using fractionated and high-dose radiation therapy [1]. The first cure of a disseminated malignancy

A. Engert and S.J. Horning (eds.), *Hodgkin Lymphoma*,
DOI: 10.1007/978-3-642-12780-9_9, © Springer-Verlag Berlin Heidelberg 2011

was claimed in 1963 for radiotherapy in HL. Easson and Russel reported their cure of a series of patients, including some with advanced disease, with extensive irradiation [2]. This early success gave rise to endeavor across several areas in the succeeding decades, based upon the need for rigorous determination of the anatomy in order to guide the radiotherapy fields. Controlled trials were launched from the early 1960s in the prospect that cure would become possible if the treated areas encompassed not only all nodal and visceral areas known to be involved, but also adjacent fields, free of macroscopic disease, but already with microscopic disease [3].

As early as 1942, four patients with HL were treated with nitrogen mustard by Wilkinson and Fletcher at Manchester Royal Infirmary, although a military embargo prevented the dissemination of this information [4]. Similar considerations applied to the bombing of the ship "USS Liberty" on December 3, 1943 in Bari, and the hematological consequences of a nitrogen mustard gas leak among the survivors. Cornelius Rhoads, an American cancer researcher, was involved in their care and understood from his observations of the effects on the bone marrow that nitrogen mustard derivatives might be effective against lymphoid and hematological malignancies [5, 6]. In 1958, another alkylating agent, cyclophosphamide, proved effective in non-HL [7]. Shortly after this, vinblastine was first shown to be an effective drug in HL, as was vincristine. Although encouraging, the early results of chemotherapy were modest, with most responses short lived after corticosteroids, alkylating, and spindle cell agents [8–10] There was a prevalent view that only extensive irradiation could yield full cures [11, 12].

One of the first modern randomized studies was the EORTC H1 trial, which investigated whether "adjuvant" chemotherapy (weekly vinblastine for 2 years) could improve the results over radiotherapy alone [13]. A durable advantage was seen in the chemotherapy arm for relapse-free survival (at 15 years 60% vs. 38%, $p<0.001$), although more than 50% of patients with mixed cellularity histology developed recurrences [14]. To reduce the relapse rate, irradiation was extended to infradiaphragmatic nodal and spleen areas. Single-agent or doublet chemotherapy was added after radiotherapy, but no immediate attempt was made to use polychemotherapy, based upon the idea that the cure rate would depend upon the adequacy of irradiation [15, 16]. Two factors gradually undermined the dominance of strict pathological delineation and extensive irradiation as the basis of curative

therapy in HL: The advent of accurate cross-sectional imaging by computed tomographic (CT) scanning and the recognition that relapses after irradiation alone had minimal impact on survival owing to the efficacy of salvage chemotherapy [17]. With the development of 4-drug combination therapy, which for the first time resulted in cures for advanced HL without the need for irradiation, the transition to systemic therapy began in earnest.

## 9.2 Chemotherapy Applied to Advanced Stage HL: Theories and Practice

### 9.2.1 Classes of Active Classical Agents in HL

Almost every class of chemotherapy drug has been shown to have some efficacy in HL, with the possible exception of the antimetabolite drugs such as 5-fluorouracil [18]. The original combination treatments were based upon the evidence of single-agent activity among alkylating agents, vinca alkaloids, corticosteroids, and the hydralazine monoamine oxidase inhibitor, procarbazine. All of these produced response rates of over 50% when used singly in patients not previously exposed to multiagent chemotherapy (Table 9.1). Later entrants to this field included the antibiotic drugs doxorubicin and bleomycin, the nitrosoureas and dacarbazine, and the podophyllotoxins, all of which showed appreciable single-agent activity after prior combination regimens. More recently, newer cytotoxics such as gemcitabine have been introduced, often in combination with platinum drugs, and found to produce significant response rates in recurrent disease.

It is clear that HL is broadly sensitive to phase-specific, cycle-specific, and noncycle-specific agents, although it is less clear whether this is a feature of the malignant cells themselves or their associated inflammatory infiltrate, which may be critical to sustaining them. The development of combination therapies has been based mainly upon the use of agents with nonoverlapping toxicity as far as possible, and as cure rates have risen, the emphasis has fallen increasingly upon avoiding long-term side effects. The most important among these are infertility and myelodysplasia (MDS), mainly caused by the alkylating agents; pulmonary fibrosis caused by bleomycin and nitrosoureas, and cardiomyopathy related to

**Table 9.1** Single-agent activity of cytotoxic drugs in Hodgkin lymphoma (HL) [18]

| Drug | Overall response rate (%) | Complete response rate (%) |
|---|---|---|
| **Single agents tested before combination chemotherapy** | | |
| **Alkylating agents** | | |
| Chlorambucil | 61 | 16 |
| Mustine | 63 | 13 |
| Cyclophosphamide | 54 | 12 |
| **Vinca alkaloids** | | |
| Vinblastine | 68 | 30 |
| Vincristine | 60 | 36 |
| **Agents mainly tested after prior multiagent therapy** | | |
| Dacarbazine | 56 | 6 |
| **Nitrosoureas** | | |
| Carmustine | 44 | 5 |
| Lomustine | 48 | 12 |
| **Antibiotics** | | |
| Doxorubicin | 30 | 5 |
| Bleomycin | 38 | 6 |
| **Podophyllotoxin** | | |
| Etoposide | 27 | 6 |
| **Antimetabolite** | | |
| Gemcitabine | 22 | 0 |

anthracyclines, a risk increased by the concomitant use of mediastinal radiotherapy.

## 9.2.2 Polychemotherapy: Models and Comparative Clinical Studies

### 9.2.2.1 The Skipper and Schabel L1210 Model

One of the earliest models to influence the design of chemotherapy treatments was the L1210 leukemia in mice studied by Skipper and Schabel: repeated administrations of a single effective drug result in a proportionally identical tumor cell kill with each treatment, so that if the cells proliferate with a constant tumor doubling time, cure can be obtained and time to cure can be predicted by knowing

the initial tumor burden and the proportion of cells killed for a given dose and interval[19, 20]. Conversely, if death will occur when reaching a specific number of malignant cells, there is a predictable likelihood of death based upon initial cell dose and treatment: "The cardinal rule of chemotherapy, the invariable inverse relationship between cell number and curability." Unfortunately, human tumors are far more complex than the L1210, the model confounded by the presence of resting stem cells, variable growth factors, and apoptosis along the tumor course, together with tumor cell heterogeneity, putting the cure of advanced HL beyond the reach of single chemotherapy agents, with inevitable relapse even after complete remission has been achieved [21, 22].

### 9.2.2.2 MOPP and Derivatives

Combination chemotherapy was first attempted clinically in childhood acute lymphoblastic leukemia by Jean Bernard [23] who designed two doublets of cortisone – methotrexate and prednisone – vincristine, at the same time as pursuing work on chemotherapy for HL. Later at the NCI, Freirich, Frei, and Katon added 6-mercaptopurine into the more effective VAMP regimen [8]. This led on to MOMP (cyclophosphamide, vincristine, methotrexate, and prednisone), and MOPP (mechlorethamine, vincristine, procarbazine, prednisone), developed by DeVita and Carbone at the NCI [24, 25]. Some of the critical features of success were: prolonged treatment (6 months, more than any other regimen at the time), use of each drug at "optimal" dose and schedule with a sliding scale for dose adjustment according to marrow suppression, an interval of 2 weeks for recovery of normal tissue (marrow, GI epithelium), hopefully before HL recovery, and treatment with curative intent rather than palliation. MOPP provided an 80% response rate, and long-term disease-free and overall survival (OS) of almost 50 and 40%, respectively [26]. The results have held up, and the 20-year analysis confirmed among 198 patients a CR rate of 81%, induction failures of 19%, relapses 36%, and deaths 54%. Of the 106 deaths, 30 occurred in patients free of disease; among the 92 patients who survived (46%), only two had persistent HL [27]. These results have been reconfirmed in subsequent trials (Table 9.3) [28–31]. Although the rise in cures from HL can be ascribed to multiple advances and not just the introduction of effective chemotherapy, the 1970 report convinced almost all groups treating HL to accept the inclusion of polychemotherapy (MOPP or MOPP derivatives) in the treatment strategy for localized as well as advanced disease. In almost all instances where a combined treatment was compared to irradiation alone, whether patients were staged or not with laparotomy, an advantage in terms of response, disease- and relapse-free survival was observed when MOPP or a MOPP-derived chemotherapy was used [32].

Analysis of the results with MOPP has proven a fruitful source of information to design and interpret future studies. Thus, complete response was seen to be a prerequisite for sustained remission, and a high percentage of complete responses were correlated with higher survival rates. Capping the vincristine dose at 2 mg may have been detrimental to the results. Patient and initial disease characteristics were good predictors of outcome, with confirmation of the adverse prognostic significance of systemic "B" symptoms. Maintenance treatment with intermittent MOPP or carmustine did not appear beneficial [33]. In patients treated previously by irradiation and chemotherapy, MOPP was less well-tolerated and less effective [34]. Conversely, retreatment in relapsed patients but with initial remission lasting over a year proved efficient again [35]. Chemotherapy has detrimental consequences in terms of carcinogenicity with second acute myeloid leukemia [36, 37]. Chemotherapy is responsible for impaired fertility in both men and women [38]. Immunosuppression related to the treatment, or to the underlying disease, brings risks of different types. (Pneumocystis Pneumonia diagnosed and cured for the first time) [39].

There were many attempts to improve upon the results. The three best known MOPP-derived regimens have been MVPP, with vinblastine instead of vincristine, ChlVPP, and COPP, with an additional substitution of mechlorethamine, replaced by chlorambucil or cyclophosphamide (Tables 9.2 and 9.3). These alternatives have never undergone direct comparison, and historical controls are difficult to interpret. In addition, the proportion of patients who have been irradiated varies considerably among series. For example in the NCI series, 32/198 patients had been irradiated prior to MOPP and 28/198 patients received TNI "to prevent recurrent disease in previously involved nodes" as consolidation after chemotherapy. MVPP, devised in Great Britain, proved easier to handle than MOPP (with less constipation and neurological toxicity), but was slightly more hematotoxic [40–42]. ChlVPP appeared more patient-friendly with minimal nausea/vomiting, constipation or neurologic toxicity, limited hematotoxicity, and the number cycles adapted to the response: a maximum five beyond CR. The 66% OS rate in advanced HL could be compared to mustine-containing regimens, at lower toxic cost, for all of these acute toxicities, except myelosuppression [43, 44]. COPP is less hematotoxic than MOPP and often used in children [45].

### 9.2.2.3 ABVD and Derivatives

The ABVD regimen was built just 10 years after MOPP started, in 1973, on intravenous-only administration at fixed 2-week intervals. Like MOPP, ABVD was a combination of hematotoxic and neurotoxic drugs. Two, doxorubicin and vinblastine, had been shown highly effective in HL. The results with dacarbazine were numerous, but possibly less convincing, and bleomycin was also felt to have considerable potential [13, 21, 46–48]. By comparison to MOPP, hematotoxicity after ABVD was predictable, noncumulative, and milder as a result of the intravenous dosing and short intervals. Further, ABVD was far less neurotoxic. Bonadonna developed ABVD at the Milan NCI with a vision: "to compare the efficacy of ABVD with MOPP, and to demonstrate absence of cross-resistance between the two regimens" [49]. The results of MOPP were well-established and the potential of ABVD in terms of "alternative to MOPP to be used either in MOPP failures or in sequential combination with MOPP" was clearly in the mind of the authors, based on these very early results achieved in 45 patients. No significant cardiac toxicity was seen in this first series, probably because of the relatively small cumulative dose of doxorubicin (6 cycles = 300 mg/m$^2$), the short follow-up, and the small numbers. Conversely, bleomycin pulmonary toxicity was apparent from the outset, while the effects upon fertility were initially overestimated through short observation which did not take into account the reversal of temporary amenorrhoea in some women.

It took a surprisingly long time for ABVD to be accepted as a standard of care and it was initially considered only as a salvage treatment in MOPP failures. However, the Milan group undertook a larger trial, comparing MOPP and ABVD directly in patients with stage IIB, IIIA, and IIIB HL. In 232 patients, a combined

**Table 9.2** Chemotherapy regimens designed for advanced HL

| Drugs | Dose (mg/m²) | Route | Schedule |
|---|---|---|---|
| **4-Drug regimens** | | | |
| MOPP | | | q. 28 d |
| Mechlorethamine | 6 | i.v. | d1 and 8 |
| Vincristine | 1.4 (cap 2 mg) | i.v. | d1 and 8 |
| Procarbazine | 100 | p.o. | d1–14 |
| Prednisolone | 40 | p.o. | d1–14 |
| MVPP | | | q. 42 d |
| Mechlorethamine | 6 | i.v. | d1 and 8 |
| Vinblastine | 6 (cap 10 mg) | i.v. | d1 and 8 |
| Procarbazine | 100 | p.o. | d1–14 |
| Prednisolone | 40 | p.o. | d1–14 |
| ChlVPP | | | q. 28 d |
| Chlorambucil | 6 (cap 10 mg) | p.o. | d1–14 |
| Vinblastine | 6 (cap 10 mg) | i.v. | d1 and 8 |
| Procarbazine | 100 | p.o. | d1–14 |
| Prednisolone | 40 | p.o. | d1–14 |
| COPP | | | q. 28 d |
| Cyclophosphamide | 650 | i.v. | d1 and 8 |
| Vinblastine | 6 | i.v. | d1 and 8 |
| Procarbazine | 100 | p.o. | d1–14 |
| Prednisolone | 40 | p.o. | d1–14 |
| ABVD | | | q. 28d |
| Doxorubicin | 25 | i.v. | d1 and 15 |
| Bleomycin | 10 iu/m² | i.v. | d1 and 15 |
| Vinblastine | 6 | i.v. | d1 and 15 |
| Dacarbazine | 375 | i.v. | d1 and 15 |
| **Hybrid regimens** | | | |
| MOPP/ABV | | | q. 28d |
| Mechlorethamine | 6 | i.v. | d1 |
| Vincristine | 1.4 | i.v. | d1 |
| Procarbazine | 100 | p.o. | d1–7 |
| Prednisolone | 40 | p.o. | d1–14 |
| Doxorubicin | 35 | i.v. | d8 |
| Bleomycin | 10 Iu/m² | i.v. | d8 |
| Vinblastine | 6 | i.v. | d8 |
| ChlVPP/EVA | | | q. 28 d |
| Chlorambucil | 6 (cap 10 mg) | p.o. | d1–7 |
| Vincristine | 1.4 (cap 2 mg) | i.v. | d1 . |
| Procarbazine | 90 | p.o. | d1–7 |
| Etoposide | 75 | p.o. | d1–5 |
| Prednisolone | 50 | p.o. | d1–7 |
| Doxorubicin | 50 | i.v. | d8 |
| Vinblastine | 6 (cap 10 mg) | i.v. | d8 |
| BEACOPP baseline | | | q. 21 d |
| Bleomycin | 10 iu/m² | i.v. | d8 |
| Etoposide | 100 | i.v. | d1–3 |
| Doxorubicin | 25 | i.v. | d1 |
| Cyclophosphamide | 650 | i.v. | d1 |
| Vincristine | 1.4 (cap 2 mg) | i.v. | d8 |
| Procarbazine | 100 | p.o. | d1–7 |
| Prednisolone | 40 | p.o. | d1–14 |
| **Escalated regimens** | | | |
| Escalated BEACOPP | | | q. 28 d |
| Bleomycin | 10 iu/m² | i.v. | d8 |
| Etoposide | 200 | i.v. | d1–3 |
| Doxorubicin | 35 | i.v. | d1 |
| Cyclophosphamide | 1,250 | i.v. | d1 |
| Vincristine | 1.4 (cap 2 mg) | i.v. | d8 |
| Procarbazine | 100 | p.o. | d1–7 |
| Prednisolone | 40 | p.o. | d1–14 |
| G-CSF | | s.c. | d8–14 |
| BEACOPP-14 | | | q. 14 d |
| Bleomycin | 10 iu/m² | i.v. | d8 |
| Etoposide | 100 | i.v. | d1–3 |
| Doxorubicin | 25 | i.v. | d1 |
| Cyclophosphamide | 650 | i.v. | d1 |
| Vincristine | 1.4 (cap 2 mg) | i.v. | d8 |
| Procarbazine | 100 | p.o. | d1–7 |
| Prednisolone | 80 | p.o. | d1–7 |
| G-CSF | | s.c. | d8–13 |
| **Weekly regimens** | | | |
| Stanford V | | | 4-week-cycle |
| Doxorubicin | 25 | i.v. | d1 and 15 |
| Vinblastine | 6 | i.v. | d1 and 15 |
| Mechlorethamine | 6 | i.v. | d1 |
| Vincristine | 1.4 (cap 2 mg) | i.v. | d8 and 22 |
| Bleomycin | 5 iu/m² | i.v. | d8 and 22 |
| Etoposide | 60 | i.v. | d15 and 16 |
| Prednisolone | 40 | p.o. | daily to week 10 then taper |
| VAPEC-B | | | 4-week-cycle |
| Doxorubicin | 35 | i.v. | d1 and 15 |
| Cyclophosphamide | 350 | i.v. | d1 |
| Etoposide | 75–100 | i.v. | d15–20 |
| Vincristine | 1.4 (cap 2 mg) | i.v. | d8 and 22 |
| Bleomycin | 10 | i.v. | d8 and 22 |
| Prednisolone | 50 | p.o. | daily to week 6 then taper |

**Table 9.3** Summary results of combination chemotherapy regimens used in first-line therapy of advanced HL

| Regimen | % CR | % EFS (5 years) | % OS (5 years) | % OS (≥7 years) |
|---|---|---|---|---|
| MOPP [26–29, 51] | 67–81 | 40–60 | 65–73 | 51–70 |
| MVPP [42, 57, 126] | 72–76 | 60 | 65–75 | |
| ChlVPP [43, 127] | 57–74 | 55–60 | 66 | 65 |
| ABVD [28, 59, 60, 77, 78, 85, 86] | 68–92 | 61–80 | 73–90 | 77 |
| MOPP/ABVD alternating [28, 53, 128] | 83–92 | 65–70 | 75–84 | 74 |
| COPP/ABVD alternating [58, 72, 73] | 85 | 69 | 83 | 75 |
| MOPP/ABV hybrid [55, 56, 59, 128] | 80–88 | 66–75 | 76–83 | 72 |
| Stanford V [75–78] | 72–91 | 54–94 | 82–96 | |
| VAPEC-B [79] | 47 | 62 | 79 | |
| ChlVPP/EVA [60, 79] | 67 | 82–84 | 89 | |
| BEACOPP baseline [72, 73] | 88 | 76 | 88 | 80 |
| Escalated BEACOPP [72, 73] | 81–96 | 87 | 91 | 86 |

modality approach of three cycles before and after extensive irradiation yielded an 80.7% CR rate after MOPP/radiotherapy and 92.4% after ABVD/radiotherapy ($p < 0.02$). At 7-year follow-up, ABVD surpassed MOPP for FFP (80.8% vs. 62.8%; $p < 0.002$), RFS (87.7% vs. 77.2%; $p = 0.06$), and OS (77.4% vs. 67.9%; $p = 0.03$). With longer follow-up, the disadvantages of MOPP in terms of fertility damage and second MDS/leukemia were more apparent.

Currently, ABVD is considered by most investigators as the standard chemotherapy for most patients with HL, with the possible exception of high-risk patients with advanced disease and poor prognostic features. Reasons to avoid ABVD relate to previous lung impairment and decreased left ventricular ejection fraction. Hematological toxicity is usually mild and ABVD may be delivered safely at full dose and on schedule, to a nonselected average population of adult patients without the need to modify doses in the presence of neutropenia [50].

### 9.2.2.4 Alternating and Hybrid Regimens

Although the study of drug resistance mechanisms and mathematical modeling was widely pursued during the 1970s, the first alternating regimen emerged from the plan by Bonadonna to use the ABVD regimen together with MOPP as a means to test it in initial therapy [51]. This was based on the observation of a higher salvage rate with ABVD than with MOPP in patients previously treated with MOPP, and the deduction that ABVD could be "non-cross resistant" with MOPP. By contrast with the pragmatic testing of alternating regimens, hybrid regimens had their origins in a more scientific approach, being designed to circumvent innate and acquired mechanisms of resistance as modeled by [52].

### MOPP/ABVD Alternating Therapy

ABVD (with irradiation) had yielded good results when compared to MOPP. Despite the small numbers of patients studied, a study comparing MOPP alone with a monthly alternation of MOPP and ABVD was considered the logical next move. The originators felt no need for a large study, nor a long follow-up, because the first results were quite convincing and appeared rapidly. At 5 years, MOPP-ABVD alternation, compared to MOPP alone, yielded a superior CR rate (92 vs. 71%; $p = 0.02$), FFP (70 vs. 37%; $p < 0.0001$), and disease-free survival (84 vs. 54%; $p < 0.005$) [51–53].

It took more than 20 years to confirm the superiority of MOPP/ABVD over MOPP [28, 54]. There are several reasons for this: the original studies were small and lacked follow-up by comparison to the extensive evidence base for MOPP; ABVD, with bleomycin and without corticosteroids, was considered more toxic than MOPP when combined with irradiation, especially to the mediastinum; and the biological rationale behind the superiority of the alternating regimen was not clearly understood. This critical question was investigated by the CALGB through the addition of a third arm, ABVD alone, and by the SFOP in children. In neither study did the alternating regimen prove superior to ABVD alone, suggesting that it is the superiority of ABVD over MOPP which is the key determinant of outcome, rather than the use of multiple chemotherapy drugs. This hypothesis is supported by the design of the CALGB trial where an unbalanced number of cycles (12 MOPP/ABVD vs. 6 ABVD) should favor the alternating arm. If Bonadonna's initial results demonstrating the superiority of ABVD over MOPP had been widely accepted, despite the small numbers, the next logical trial would have been to test ABVD vs. MOPP/ABVD, which could have saved 20 years of studies. In the event, alternating MOPP and ABVD was considered a good compromise of old and new and served as the regimen to test against MOPP, at least in Europe [31].

## The Goldie and Coldman Model and the "Hybrid" Regimens

Goldie and Coldman described the relationship between tumor drug sensitivity and spontaneous mutation rates. This mathematical model was the rationale for the development of "hybrid" regimens, which introduced many different drugs with different mechanisms of action, early in the course of treatment and with a rapidly cycling schedule, to erase preexisting resistance to one or the other drug [52]. The MOPP/ABV hybrid regimen and the similar ChlVPP/EVA were widely used for over two decades [55–57]. Several features explain this: a high and durable complete response rate, the short duration of the program by comparison to alternating therapies, the overall decrease in the cumulative doses of doxorubicin and mechlorethamine, and less extensive irradiation required for residual disease.

Unfortunately, although theoretically attractive, this concept did not bring any advantage compared to conventional 4-drug or alternating regimens. In the GHSG HD6 trial, HL control was similar with the hybrid COPP/ABV/IMEP and alternating COPP/ABVD, with more toxicity in the hybrid [58]. Two later trials, designed to test the benefit of the early introduction of all drugs in a rotating fashion, actually favored ABVD in that the control of lymphoma was the same, but the

toxicity more severe with the hybrid regimens [59, 60]. Both the intergroup and the UK studies reported similar findings, with a hazard ratio of 10.5 for grade 3/4 mucosal toxicity and 3.94 for grade 3/4 infection in the UK study. In the Intergroup study there was a small, but worrying, increase in the incidence of MDS or acute myelogenous leukemia, with 11 cases in patients randomized to the hybrid arm and two among patients randomized to ABVD ($p=0.011$).

### 9.2.2.5 The Dose/Response Relationship: Norton and Simon Model

Much of the thinking about how to maximize the cure rate in lymphoma has centered upon the relationship between dose and response to cytotoxic therapy. Theories of tumor cell ecology have suggested that as the mass of disease is reduced, the growth fraction may rise. This, together with the assumed selection of resistant subclones, underlies the idea that tumor eradication is dependent upon the delivery of treatment at adequate dose intensity early in a course of treatment. If doses are too small or too infrequent, the fractional cell kill might be expected to decline and allow the emergence of resistance [61].

Three prospective clinical trials have directly addressed the question of dose vs. response using the same chemotherapy drugs in both arms. In the first-line treatment of advanced disease, a critical study was performed by the German Hodgkin study group (HD9), as detailed later on, in which patients were randomized between the baseline BEACOPP regimen and an escalated regimen, with the doses of doxorubicin, cyclophosphamide, and etoposide increased to 140, 185, and 200%, respectively. This resulted in an increase in freedom from treatment failure (FFTF) at 5 years from 76 to 87% ($p<0.01$), which was translated into a small but significant improvement in survival on longer follow-up (80 vs. 86% at 10 years, $p=0.0053$). This was at the cost of an increased risk of MDS and acute leukemia in the escalated arm, but at a frequency too low to reverse the gain in survival from better control of the lymphoma [62].

There are two randomized studies for recurrent disease which have yielded similar data on the dose-response relationship. The UK group compared the myeloablative BEAM regimen to mini-BEAM, which uses the same drugs at nonmyeloablative doses. The high-dose treatment yielded superior progression-free survival ($p = 0.005$), although the trial was closed with only 44 patients recruited and had insufficient power to demonstrate a survival advantage [63]. A study of similar design was conducted by the German group, and this too demonstrated superior FFTF at 3 years (55% for BEAM, 34% for nonmyeloablative dexa-BEAM, $p = 0.019$), although once again no survival difference could be demonstrated [64].

While there is good evidence for an overall dose-response relationship, there are several areas of continuing uncertainty. For example, it is not clear whether the dose of treatment over a whole course is the critical determinant of outcome, or whether initial dose intensity during the first weeks of treatment is more important. From retrospective analyses comparing outcomes to doses administered, it appears that the most influential factor is the total dose of treatment given, with some scope for compensating suboptimal early treatment by later escalation, a finding that may distinguish HL from many other malignancies [65–67].

### Dose/Response Relationships and Treatment Tolerance: An Individual Characteristic?

A dose response for both malignant and normal tissue toxicity is well-recognized, raising the question of whether the efficacy of tumor control can be related to toxic side effects, effectively using each subject as their own pharmacodynamic control. It would be convenient if no such relationship existed as it would allow moderation of drug doses and thereby minimize patient toxicity, but there is evidence to suggest that this would be the wrong approach. The GHSG explored hemato-toxicity as a surrogate for pharmacological and metabolic heterogeneity, in relation to reduced systemic dose and disease control. Patients treated with various regimens in the HD6 trial (validated on two other cohorts) were retrospectively classified as showing WHO grade of leukocytopenia 0–2 and over two, respectively. Patients with a high hematological toxicity had a 5-year FFTF rate of 68 vs. 47% for those with low toxicity, independent of the actual drug doses received [68]. No pretreatment pharmacokinetic parameters could be found to explain these observations; however, recent work from the GELA has explored polymorphisms in a population of HL patients that might determine anticancer agent metabolism. The

UGT1A1 polymorphism has been identified as a possible candidate for influencing the metabolism of several anticancer drugs and patient outcomes [69]. Unfortunately, similar dose-response relationships are also seen for long-term toxicities, for example, infertility and secondary leukaemia [70–73].

### 9.2.2.6 Sustained/Weekly Regimens

Pursuing the idea of increased dose intensity, several groups developed novel, brief duration regimens for the treatment of advanced HL. The underlying rationale for the development of these regimens was, firstly, an increase in the dose intensity of chemotherapy by reduction in the total duration of treatment, but an increase in the number of different agents, and secondly, reduced cumulative doses of drugs responsible for long-term toxic effects, including alkylating agents, doxorubicin, and bleomycin. The PACEBOM, VAPEC-B, and Stanford V regimens were all designed to deliver weekly treatments, alternating between myelosuppressive and nonmyelo-suppressive agents. The preliminary results from single arm studies appeared promising, with high response and survival rates [74]. Unfortunately, the results of randomized trials did not confirm the early promise of these regimens.

The Stanford V program developed from the close collaboration of radiotherapy and chemotherapy, endeavoring to minimize the use of each modality, aiming at improved results with less toxicity. Initial chemotherapy was composed of the standard drugs from the MOPP/ABVD scheme (mechlorethamine, doxorubicin, bleomycin), plus etoposide, with dose intensity increased for better/earlier tumor response while cumulative doses, thought to be responsible for late toxicity (marrow, heart, lung), were reduced. The use of alkylating agents was limited in order to avert gonadal damage. The final scheme was an abbreviated 12-week program with radiotherapy started 2–4 weeks after chemotherapy, restricted to sites at higher risk for relapse (bulky sites), and delivered at 36 Gy, in order to reduce the incidence of late cardio-pulmonary effects, and "mini-mantle" instead of mantle fields sparing the axillae to decrease the risk of second breast carcinoma. The results of the initial "Stanford V" phase 2 were confirmed in the Eastern Cooperative Oncology Group (ECOG) E1492 study in 45 patients, of whom 87% received radiotherapy; FFP was 85% at

5 years, OS 96% with one death from HL, and one from an M5 acute myeloblastic leukemia (AML) [75]. Later analysis confirmed these excellent results and the relative preservation of fertility in both women and men; no case of second MDS/leukemia or NHL had been registered at a 65-month median follow-up [76].

A randomized trial (Italian Lymphoma Group: ILL) compared Stanford V to mechlorethamine, vincristine, procarbazine, prednisone, epidoxirubicin, bleomycin, vinblastine, lomustine, doxorubicin, vindesine (MOPPEBVCAD), and to ABVD as the standard in 355 patients with stage IIB–IV HL. In this trial the Stanford V arm was inferior to the other two arms in terms of 5-year failure-free survival (FFS) (54 vs. 78% for ABVD and 81% for MOPPEBVCAD, respectively ($p < 0.01$ for comparison of Stanford V with the other two regimens)) [77]. However, only 66% of patients in the Stanford V arm received irradiation, against 87% in the ECOG phase 2 study: this is important in a strategy that was originally designed to combine both modalities. The Stanford V program was also compared to ABVD in a large prospective trial run by the UK National Cancer Research Institute Lymphoma Group (NCRI) in 520 patients with stage IIB–IV HL. Results in the Stanford V and in the ABVD arm were similar for 5-year progression-free survival (PFS) and OS rates (76 and 90%, for ABVD; 74 and 92% for Stanford V, with radiotherapy administered in 53 and 73%, respectively) [78]. The relatively extensive use of radiotherapy required to achieve optimum results for weekly regimens makes them a less attractive choice for many patients: in the UK study 73% of patients treated with Stanford V received consolidation radiotherapy, compared to 37% in the previous UK study using ABVD in a similar group of patients. However, the short 12-week duration of the Stanford V regimen, with appropriate radiotherapy, remains an acceptable approach, mainly for patients with low-risk nonbulky disease.

The only other weekly regimen to be compared with a hybrid regimen in a randomized trial was one featuring myelosuppressive (doxorubicin, cyclophosphamide, and etoposide) and relatively nonmyelosuppressive (vincristine and bleomycin) drugs given on an alternating weekly basis for 11 weeks: VAPEC-B. This was compared to a hybrid ChlVPP-EVA schedule for advanced disease, expected to still be significantly more myelosuppressive and to impair fertility, and showed inferior progression-free survival for the weekly regimen in all but the best prognosis subgroup. Event-free survival at 5 years in newly diagnosed patients with advanced disease following the hybrid regimen was 78% vs. 58% for VAPEC-B, which translated into better OS, at 89% vs. 79% [79].

### 9.2.2.7 Escalated-Dose Regimens

In order to spare patients the acute gastrointestinal and hematologic toxicities, the original recommendation of the NCI to follow a "sliding scale" of dose adaptation for MOPP was gradually superceded by fixed doses at well-tolerated levels and intervals. Retrospective studies of MOPP and MVPP suggested that the cumulative dose, as much as frequency of administration or dose intensity, might determine the outcomes [29, 80]. These observations also appear to hold for ABVD [67], although all these are retrospective and need to be confirmed in a prospective study.

The German Hodgkin Study Group has pioneered the exploration of two levels of dose increment, in the conventional dose range, by reducing the length of treatment and adding etoposide to the standard regimen, COPP/ABVD [81]. Further intensification was carried out by increasing the myelosuppressive drug doses, with growth factor support. Both intensified regimens provided higher CR, FFTF and, crucially, statistically higher OS as compared to standard COPP/ABVD [62]. The early effects of dose intensification were maintained in the long-term results at 10 years: FFTF was 64, 70, and 82% with OS rates of 75, 80, and 86% for patients treated with standard COPP/ABVD, BEACOPP baseline, and BEACOPP escalated, respectively ($p < 0.001$)[72]. The higher overall chemotherapy doses, as given in the escalated BEACOPP scheme, appear to provide greater disease control than any of the previous or contemporary regimens. This is supported by the very low number of deaths due to the progression of lymphoma (2.8%). The GHSG has conducted a series of studies, HD12, HD15, HD18, all using escalated BEACOPP in advanced HL patients (under the age of 61) whose preliminary results appear to replicate closely those of the escalated BEACOPP arm in the HD9 study [82–84].

The GHSG reported early on its concerns for the immediate toxicity, especially among patients older than 65, and in younger patients, impaired fertility and risk of MDS or secondary AML. A review of the HD9 results concerning the cumulative incidence of all second tumors at 10 years confirmed that the rate for AML/MDS was lower after COPP/ABVD (0.4%) vs. BEACOPP baseline (2.2%) and BEACOPP escalated (3.2%; log-rank test: $p=0.03$). However, counting all secondary malignancies, there was no difference (5.3% after COPP/ABVD, 7.9% after BEACOPP baseline, and 6.5% after BEACOPP escalated [72].

The immediate and long-term toxic effects of escalated BEACOPP and the reluctance of many specialists to consider COPP/ABVD as a standard comparator have hindered acceptance of escalated BEACOPP as a new standard of care. Two Italian trials, HD2000 and GSM-HD, have demonstrated superior PFS with escalated BEACOPP in comparison to ABVD. In HD2000, BEACOPP resulted in an 81% (95% CI, 70–89%) 5-year PFS vs. 68% (95% CI, 56–78%) for ABVD, but no significant OS difference was observed [85]. Similarly, the GSM-HD trial demonstrated a higher 3-year FFP for escalated plus baseline BEACOPP (4+4) vs. ABVD (87±3% and 71±4%), respectively, but freedom from second progression (FF2P) and OS were alike [86]. ABVD was declared preferable, taking into account the lesser toxicity, including fewer toxic deaths (1 vs. 6).

Despite these reservations, the outstanding results of escalated BEACOPP are appealing, particularly in higher risk patients. A large intergroup trial (NCT00049595), led by the EORTC and GELA, has compared 8 cycles of ABVD to a sequence of 4 escalated and 4 standard dose BEACOPP (4+4), without any radiotherapy, in 550 high-risk patients (IPS≥3). This study closed for entry in early 2010, and the results are pending.(www.cancer.gov).

### 9.2.2.8 High-Dose Treatment and Autologous Stem Cell Transplantation as Part of Initial Therapy

Attempts have been made to improve results by using intensified consolidation and peripheral blood stem cell (PBSC) rescue for patients considered at high risk. Two randomized studies have explored this concept for HL. The Scotland and Newcastle Lymphoma Group HD3 study randomized 65 out of 126 high-risk patients: resulting in a nonsignificant advantage for the conventional arm (TTF 85 vs. 79%, $p=0.35$) [87]. A European study of similar design randomized 163

high-risk patients achieving CR or PR after 4 ABVD or an equivalent regimen to receive HDT plus ASCT (83 patients) or four more courses of conventional chemotherapy (80 patients). There was no evidence of a benefit to the group receiving high-dose therapy: CR 92 vs. 89%, 5-year FFS 75 vs. 82%, and OS 88 vs. 88%, respectively [88].

The Groupe Ouest-Est d'Etude des Leucémies et Autres Maladies du Sang (GOELAMS) undertook a randomized study in 158 high-risk patients, comparing conventional intensive chemotherapy ($n=82$) with vindesine (5 mg/m²), doxorubicin (99 mg/m²), carmustine (140 mg/m²), etoposide (600 mg/m²), and methylprednisolone (600 mg/m²) (VABEM) followed by low-dose lymph node irradiation vs. ($n=76$) 4 cycles of ABVD followed by myeloablative carmustine (300 mg/m²), etoposide (800 mg/m²), cytarabine (1,600 mg/m²), and melphalan (140 mg/m²) and ASCT. The results were remarkably similar for CR (89 vs. 88%), 5-year FFTF (79 vs. 75%), and OS (87 vs. 86%) [89].

In summary, there is no evidence to support the use of high-dose consolidation at first remission in HL at present.

## 9.3 Chemotherapy in Combined Modality Treatment for Advanced Disease

Up to 30% of the patients with advanced HL will relapse, or progress, often in initially involved areas where bulky disease was present [90]. Because of this and the undoubted efficacy of irradiation in controlling localized disease, radiotherapy is widely used in consolidation to improve cure rates in advanced disease. Several retrospective or older studies supported this approach; a metaanalysis of 14 randomized trials in all stages of HL demonstrated improved EFS but not survival, albeit with adverse survival effects when the radiation was extensive [91]. There are, however, concerns regarding the long-term side effects of such irradiation, which necessitate a careful review of the approach. The usefulness of consolidation in general, and of radiation therapy in particular, may be better understood from a more detailed analysis of the key studies.

### 9.3.1 Does Consolidation Radiotherapy Improve Outcomes Compared to Chemotherapy Alone?

The answer here depends to a large extent on the effectiveness of the chemotherapy. Series that demonstrate an EFS advantage for combined chemotherapy-radiotherapy tend to be those with shorter or less intense regimens. For example, if the results of three different studies of the Stanford V regimen are compared, there is a correlation between the EFS and the proportion of patients receiving radiotherapy: in the Italian Lymphoma Group (IIL) study 66% of patients received radiotherapy for a EFS of 73%, while in the UK NCRI trial the figures were 73% irradiated and 75% EFS, and in the series from Stanford, 91% irradiated and 89% EFS [76–78]. The correlation is much less evident for radiation after the more intensive escalated BEACOPP regimen: in the IIL study 45% were irradiated for an EFS of 81%, while in the German HL Study Group a radiotherapy rate of 71% yielded EFS of 87% [62, 85]. The results with ABVD appear to lie somewhere between these two: analysis of the UK NCRI trial results with ABVD showed that patients selected to receive consolidation radiotherapy had superior EFS, despite more adverse baseline prognostic factors such as bulk disease, and a lower proportion being in CR at the end of chemotherapy, a finding which held across all prognostic subgroups [92].

### 9.3.2 For Patients Who Received Induction Chemotherapy, Is Radiotherapy Consolidation More Effective than Additional Chemotherapy?

In adults, two well-designed trials have addressed this question. In the GHSG HD-3 trial, 288 patients received 6 cycles of COPP/ABVD, and 100 patients in radiological CR were randomized to one additional COPP/ABVD or IF RT $20 \pm 20$ Gy. There was no difference in terms of tumor control, but patients who did not receive any consolidation fared poorly [93]. The GELA group conducted a larger trial which gave much the same result: 533 patients with advanced HL were randomized to 6 cycles of MOPP/ABV or doxorubicin, bleomycin, vinblastine, procarbazine, prednisone (ABVPP). Patients in CR or PR $\geq 75\%$ after 6 cycles were randomized between two additional cycles of chemotherapy or subtotal nodal irradiation (STNI). There was some interaction between the randomizations, with the best OS seen after ABVPP alone; however, there was no significant difference overall in the second randomization: the 10-year DFS figures for patients treated with consolidation CT or STNI were 73 and 78%, respectively ($p = 0.07$). Once again, patients who received no consolidation at all had poorer survival [94].

### 9.3.3 If Complete Response is Achieved After Chemotherapy, Does Additional Radiotherapy Provide an Advantage?

Once again the intensity and efficacy of the prior chemotherapy appear to be influential, as does the level of detail at which the response is assessed. Two trials have suggested that radiotherapy may be unnecessary for many patients.

The EORTC conducted a trial in patients with stage III–IV HL who were in CR after 6 or 8 cycles of hybrid MOPP-ABV. 333 of 421 potentially eligible patients were randomized over a 10-year period to receive either no further treatment or IF RT 24 Gy to all initially involved nodal areas and 16–24 Gy to all initially involved extranodal sites. The 5-year EFS was 84% in the no treatment group and 79% in the IF RT group ($p = 0.35$). There was a nonsignificant trend toward inferior survival in the radiated group, a finding ascribed to cardiac toxicity and second malignancies [55].

Chemotherapy or radiotherapy consolidation in CR patients enrolled in the HD-3 trial was shown to be equivalent [93]. Following a series of studies in which consolidation radiotherapy continued to be used, the GHSG HD 12 trial examined the role of consolidation radiotherapy following either 8 escalated BEACOPP or 4 escalated and 4 baseline. Nine hundred and thirty-four patients were randomized between radiotherapy or no radiotherapy, and no difference was seen in FFTF or OS [82].

The findings from the UK NCRI LY09 study are in contrast with patients who received consolidation radiotherapy following complete remission showing a significantly greater EFS, although this was not a randomized comparison. If anything, the irradiated group had less favorable baseline characteristics [92].

The findings in the German HD 15 study offer an interesting perspective on the potential future role of consolidation radiotherapy for advanced HL. In this trial, patients with residual masses over 2.5 cm after BEACOPP chemotherapy which showed positive uptake on a FDG-PET scan underwent radiotherapy to 30 Gy, while those with a PET-negative mass were managed expectantly. The results in the latter group were excellent, with 96% disease-free at 1 year. In the PET-positive group who underwent irradiation, the success rate was also relatively high, with 85% disease-free, suggesting that for residual active disease irradiation can play a valuable role [84].

As a conclusion, there is no need to cure patients twice, and radiotherapy may be avoidable in patients who achieve a true CR after adequate chemotherapy. Patients without evidence of active disease can be expected to have an excellent prognosis without irradiation, while those in whom there is still an abnormality seem likely to require additional therapy, and in this situation, radiotherapy may be effective. It is to be hoped that the controversy surrounding the use of consolidation radiotherapy may finally be resolved with the functional assessment of residual disease.

## 9.4 Chemotherapy for Localized HL: A Radiation/Chemotherapy Balance

From the first combined modality trials up to the present, there has been a progressive shift in the relative roles of radiation and chemotherapy. There have been several factors behind this, including increasing cure rates, better means of determining the extent of disease, better prognostic indices, and most importantly, the increasing recognition of the long-term risks from treatment.

### 9.4.1 Early Favorable Localized Disease

The first trial of ABVD in combination with radiotherapy confirmed that 4 cycles of ABVD with adjuvant IF

RT gave results as good as those seen with STNI [95]. The GHSG HD-7 study used a similar design to show that 2 cycles of ABVD followed by EF RT 30 Gy with a 10 Gy boost were superior to STNI in favorable localized HL [96]. The GHSG HD-10 study compared the number of cycles of ABVD (4 as standard vs. 2) and the dose of IF RT (20 vs. 30 Gy) in the same early favorable group. The results were similar in all four treatment arms, contributing to the proposal that ABVD x2 cycles + IF RT 20 Gy could be the standard approach for favorable early stage localized HL [73].

MOPP/ABV is no longer used in early HL owing to its more severe acute and long-term toxicity when compared to ABVD, with equivalent tumor control. However, the EORTC/GELA H8F trial demonstrated a survival advantage for 3 cycles of MOPP/ABV+ IF RT over STNI in favorable localized HL [97]. This result confirmed an earlier finding obtained by the same group in the H7F trial, where EBVP and IFRT produced clearly superior results to extended radiotherapy [98].

### 9.4.2 Early Unfavorable Localized Disease

The superiority of ABVD over MOPP in combination with mantle RT was demonstrated in the EORTC H6U study, where 3 cycles of ABVD cycles prior and after mantle RT provided the best results seen in an EORTC study for this group of patients. The trial was also designed to monitor short and long-term toxicities and showed the pulmonary hazards associated with bleomycin, as well as the absence of gonadal and cardiac toxicity of the ABVD arm [99].

Similar results were achieved with 4 cycles of ABVD and IF RT in the EORTC/GELA H9U trial. Here, 4 cycles of ABVD followed by 30 Gy IF RT produced results as good as 6 cycles of ABVD or 4 BEACOPP baseline [100].

The results of the GHSG HD-11 trial for unfavorable/intermediate localized HL strike a note of caution regarding the de-escalation of combined modality treatment. This study compared 4 cycles of ABVD with 4 BEACOPP baseline, followed by either 20 or 30 Gy IF RT. Progression-free survival was significantly inferior in the ABVD+20 Gy arm (Hazard ratio 1.49, $p = 0.03$), suggesting once more an interaction between the intensity of chemotherapy and the role of radiation [101].

In young patients, especially females, the Stanford V program has provided excellent results while preserving fertility in most cases. For comparison with the European experience, the Stanford V data in early stage HL have been retrospectively analyzed: Favorable/early patients received 8 weeks of chemotherapy + 20 or 30 Gy IF RT, while unfavorable/intermediate risk patients were treated with 12 weeks of chemotherapy + 36 Gy. By comparison with European (EORTC and GHSG risk factors), this resulted in excellent FFP and OS, although second-line treatment proved less successful in the unfavorable group [102]. Fertility was preserved with 25 live births/pregnancies reported in this group of 120 patients [103, 104].

## 9.4.3 Chemotherapy Regimens Designed to be Combined with Radiotherapy for Early Disease

Several regimens have been devised specifically for use in early HL in combination with radiotherapy. These have generally represented attenuated versions of regimens used in advanced disease, with the intention they would be less toxic, both acutely and in the long term (Table 9.4).

The VBM regimen was specifically designed to avoid cardiac and gonadal toxicities. The results of the initial phase II study in laparotomy-staged patients were unfortunately not confirmed in a clinically staged group when compared to STNI, and this approach has

not been pursued. With an interval of only 2 weeks between the last bleomycin dose and RT, the reported effects on the lung function were moderate [105]. However, more severe pulmonary toxicity was reported in two other studies in the UK and Italy and this approach has not been pursued.

EBVP was adopted by the EORTC in the hope of reducing cardiac toxicity. The regimen was well-tolerated and only required six administrations at 3-week intervals. In a large trial, EORTC H7F for localized favorable clinically staged patients, combined with IF RT, it demonstrated an OS advantage by comparison to STNI [98]. Unfortunately, the same combination proved less effective as a chemotherapy alone option: in the 3-arm H9F trial the EBVP-alone arm was markedly inferior to the two arms where it was combined with IF RT (20 or 30 Gy). Similarly in patients with unfavorable localized HL, FFP, and OS with EBVP, x6 + IF RT were inferior to MOPP/ABV x6 + IF RT [100]. This is a further evidence of the interaction between chemotherapy dose, irradiation, and severity of HL.

Attempts have been made to delete some components of ABVD for combined modality therapy of early HL, with mixed results. The SWOG tested AV, and the study was closed at the second planned interim analysis due to a superior 3-year FFS with the CMT arm (94%) compared with STLI (81%) [106]. The question of which drugs from the original ABVD should be retained remains controversial, but the initial results of GHSG HD-13 trial give some indication. In this study of early favorable HL, a comparison is made between 2 cycles of ABVD, AVB, AVD, and AV, all followed by 30 Gy IFRT. The final result is not available for this trial, but two arms have been closed prematurely: AV and ABV. Removal of dacarbazine appears to have been detrimental in both cases.

**Table 9.4** Chemotherapy regimens specifically designed for localized HL

| Drugs | Dose (mg/m²) | Route | Schedule |
|---|---|---|---|
| AB | | | q. 28d |
| Doxorubicin | 25 | i.v. | d1 and 15 |
| Vinblastine | 6 | i.v. | d1 and 15 |
| EBVP | | | q. 21d |
| Epirubicin | 75 | i.v. | d1 |
| Bleomycin | 6 iu/m² | i.v. | d1 |
| Vinblastine | 6 | i.v. | d1 |
| Prednisone | 40 | p.o. | d1–5 |
| VBM | | | q. 28d |
| Vinblastine | 6 | i.v. | d1 and 8 |
| Bleomycin | 10 iu/m² | i.v. | d1 and 8 |
| Methotrexate | 30 | i.v. | d1 and 8 |

## 9.4.4 Chemotherapy Alone Trials

Attempts to use chemotherapy-only approaches to early stage HL have not met with success to date, perhaps owing to the use of insufficiently intensive or prolonged cytotoxic treatment. In the pediatric and adolescent population, a large Children's Cancer Group (CCG) trial assessed radiotherapy in CR patients (CCG 5942 trial). Initial treatment was with a response-adapted COPP/ABV (4–6 cycles), of which a number of patients received only 4 cycles. Half of 501 patients achieving a CR were allocated to IF RT and half to observation: the observation arm suffered a higher rate of recurrence [107].

In adults with localized favorable and unfavorable HL, ABVD was compared to a radiation therapy containing strategy (HD6 National Cancer Institute of Canada Clinical Trials Group and ECOG) and demonstrated inferior outcomes [108]. Similarly the European H9F trial demonstrated inferior EFS, as already mentioned, resulting in a worsening of OS [100]. The Memorial Sloan Kettering Cancer Center conducted a randomized trial of 6 cycles of ABVD cycles ± RT in favorable localized and stage IIIA HL: no significant difference emerged, although there was once again a trend in favor of the CMT arm [109].

The search continues for an effective and safe method to treat patients with localized disease with minimal or no radiotherapy exposure. One approach may be to reduce the size of the fields using involved node RT, relying upon accurate pretreatment delineation of the disease. For the elimination of radiotherapy altogether in some patients, it is hoped that a response-adapted strategy may provide a solution, using FDG-PET evaluation to determine whether radiation may safely be omitted. The current trials of the UK NCRI Group [110] and others in Europe (EORTC H10, GHSG HD-16) take this approach.

**Table 9.5** Salvage regimens in common use for recurrent/refractory HL

| Drugs | Dose (mg/m$^2$) | Route | Schedule |
|---|---|---|---|
| Dexa-BEAM | | | q. 21d |
|   Dexamethasone | 24 mg daily | p.o. | d1–10 |
|   Carmustine | 60 | i.v. | d2 |
|   Etoposide | 250 | i.v. | d4–7 |
|   Cytarabine | 100 bd | i.v. | d4–7 |
|   Melphalan | 20 | i.v. | d3 |
| DHAP | | | q. 21d |
|   Dexamethasone | 40 mg daily | i.v. | d1–4 |
|   Cytarabine | 2,000 bd | i.v. | d2 |
|   Cisplatin | 100 | i.v. | d1 |
| ESHAP | | | q. 21d |
|   Etoposide | 40 | i.v. | d1–4 |
|   Cytarabine | 2,000 | i.v. | d5 |
|   Cisplatin | 25 | i.v. | d1–4 |
|   Methylprednisolone | 500 mg daily | i.v. | d1–5 |
| ICE | | | q. 21d |
|   Ifosfamide | 5,000 | i.v. | d2 |
|   Carboplatin | AUC 5 | i.v. | d2 |
|   Etoposide | 100 | i.v. | d1–3 |
| GDP | | | q. 21d |
|   Gemcitabine | 1,000 | i.v. | d1 and 8 |
|   Dexamethasone | 40 mg daily | p.o. | d1–4 |
|   Cisplatin | 75 | i.v. | d1 |

## 9.5 Chemotherapy Treatment for Recurrent and Refractory Hodgkin Lymphoma

### 9.5.1 Salvage Chemotherapy Regimens

A variety of agents with activity against HL have permitted the development of many salvage regimens for use in that minority of patients whose lymphoma is not eradicated by first-line therapy. The preference in designing these regimens is to select agents with sufficiently different mechanisms of action to reduce the likelihood of cross-resistance to the prior treatment. In the majority of patients, the aim of second-line therapy is to produce a sufficient response to proceed to high-dose treatment with autologous progenitor cell rescue, as this appears to be the only means to produce long-term remission in more than 50% of patients.

There is currently no accepted standard salvage chemotherapy for HL. The regimens in common use are listed in Table 9.5. Many regimens in wide use contain cisplatin, such as DHAP (dexamethasone, cytosine arabinoside, and cisplatin) [111] and ESHAP (etoposide, methylprednisolone, cytosine arabinoside, and cisplatin) [112], or may use an ifosfamide–etoposide backbone such as ICE (ifosfamide, carboplatin, and etoposide) [113]. There is interest in using gemcitabine following promising single-agent data from its use in refractory disease and in vitro studies showing its ability to circumvent multidrug resistance (MDR) due to increased P-glycoprotein overexpression [114]. Cells expressing MDR often have increased deoxycytidine kinase activity and reduced deoxycytidine deaminase, allowing intracellular accumulation of gemcitabine phospho-derivatives and thereby increasing its cytotoxicity. Combining gemcitabine with DNA-damaging agents such as platinum drugs and other alkylating agents is a logical approach

**Table 9.6**  Published results of salvage regimens used in HL

| Regimen | Number of patients | Responses (%) | | | Grade 3/4 toxicity (%) | | | Toxic deaths (%) |
|---------|-------------------|----|----|-----|------------|-------------------|----------|-----|
| | | CR | PR | ORR | Neutropenia | Thrombo cytopenia | Vomiting | |
| Dexa-BEAM [64] | 144 | 27 | 54 | 81 | NS | NS | NS | 5 |
| Mini-BEAM [63] | 55 | 49 | 33 | 82 | 86 | 60 | NS | 2 |
| ASHAP [129] | 56 | 34 | 36 | 70 | 100 | NS | NS | 0 |
| ESHAP [112] | 22 | 41 | 32 | 73 | 59 | NS | NS | 4 |
| ICE [113] | 65 | 26 | 59 | 85 | NS | NS | NS | 0 |
| DHAP [111] | 102 | 21 | 68 | 89 | 88 | 69 | 26 | 0 |
| GDP [130] | 23 | 17 | 52 | 69 | 9 | 13 | 13 | 0 |

for disease that has recurred after prior treatment with anthracycline and vinca alkaloid drugs. It should be noted, however, that the combination of gemcitabine with bleomycin, while superficially attractive for HL, was accompanied by severe lung toxicity and should be avoided [115] (Table 9.8).

The response rate to salvage regimens is generally high irrespective of the combination chosen, with between 60 and 90% overall response rates and between 20 and 30% complete responses, depending upon the selection of patients. Table 9.6 gives details of the reported response rates and toxicity of a variety of regimens reported in the literature.

### 9.5.2  High-Dose Therapy

The principles of high-dose therapy for HL are similar to those for other chemosensitive malignancies. Combinations are chosen to include agents which are active against the lymphoma, have different mechanisms of action, where possible, from the previous therapy, show a steep dose-response curve, and have hematologic toxicity as their dose-limiting characteristic. The most widely used regimens are based upon alkylating agents and nitrosoureas, often with etoposide. Total body irradiation has been incorporated with some regimens, but is no longer widely used following the demonstration of increased toxicity in several series. Two regimens have dominated the published literature for high-dose therapy and autologous progenitor cell rescue, CBV and BEAM [116]. Details of the most widely used regimens are given in Table 9.7.

**Table 9.7**  High-dose regimens commonly used for HL

| Regimen | Drugs included | Total dose administered (mg/m$^2$) |
|---------|----------------|------------------------------------|
| CBV | Cyclophosphamide | 4,800–7,200 |
| | Carmustine | 300–600 |
| | Etoposide | 750–2,400 |
| BEAM | Carmustine | 300 |
| | Etoposide | 800–1,200 |
| | Cytarabine | 1,600 |
| | Melphalan | 140 |
| BEAC | Carmustine | 200–300 |
| | Etoposide | 600–1,200 |
| | Cytarabine | 800–1,200 |
| | Cyclophosphamide | 6,000 |
| LACE | Lomustine | 200 |
| | Cytarabine | 4,000 |
| | Cyclophosphamide | 1,800 |
| | Etoposide | 1,000 |

The outcomes of treatment with these have been widely reported, with long-term remissions in 30–60% of cases (Table 9.8). The likelihood of durable remission can be estimated from the antecedent features of the lymphoma [117]. Several retrospective studies have identified risk factors that stratify patients based on disease characteristics, such as the presence of B symptoms, extranodal disease, and duration of remission from front-line chemotherapy. The 5-year event-free survival rate for patients with low-risk disease ranges from 65 to 80%, whereas EFS for patients with intermediate or high-risk disease is less than 30%, with the majority of relapses occurring within the first 2 years after high-dose therapy. Even for patients with disease that does not enter remission with first-line therapy, there are some long-term remissions achieved using

**Table 9.8** Published results of treatment with high-dose therapy and autologous progenitor cell rescue in HL

| Regimen | Number of patients | Status of disease | EFS/FFTF (%) | OS | Reference |
|---------|-------------------|-------------------|--------------|-----|-----------|
| CBV | 128 | Relapse/refractory | 25 | 45 | Bierman et al. [119] |
| BEAM | 280 | Relapse | 60 | 66 | Brice, Marolleau et al. 1996 |
| BEAM | 139 | Relapse | 45 | 50 | Sweetenham et al. [116] |
| BEAM | 175 | Primary refractory | 32 | 36 | Sweetenham et al. [118] |
| BEAM | 86 | Primary refractory | 25 | 35 | Andre, Henry-Amar et al. 1999 |
| BEAM | 76 | Primary refractory | 23 | 30 | Ferme, Mounier et al. 2002 |
| LACE | 67 | Relapse/refractory | 64 | 68 | Perz, Giles et al. 2007 |

high-dose treatment, with a retrospective study of the European Bone Marrow Transplant registry reporting a 5-year PFS of 32% among 175 such cases [118].

There has been no formal comparative study to determine the best high-dose regimen, although analyses of transplant registries have been used and suggest a marginal advantage for BEAM over CBV. Raising the doses of the individual drugs within a high-dose regimen has not in general been effective. A study in which the drugs in the CBV regimen were increased yielded significant pulmonary toxicity when the dose of carmustine exceeded 450 mg/m$^2$ [119]. A similar study of increasing etoposide dose in the BEAM regimen resulted in higher transplant-related mortality and gastrointestinal complications at a total dose of 2,400 mg/m$^2$.

### 9.5.3 New Systemic Treatments

There have been relatively few new conventional cytotoxic agents developed recently for HL, but both monoclonal antibodies and small molecule therapeutics targeting specific abnormal pathways in HL have recently started to show some promising results.

Antibody therapies have been directed at relatively specific molecules such as CD30 on the surface of Reed-Sternberg cells, but the results with unconjugated anti-CD30 have been discouraging, probably because it targets only a small proportion of the cells within a mass of lymphoma [120]. Anti-CD20, given with the intention of targeting the infiltrating B-cells and interrupting autocrine growth factor loops, has shown some promise in an early pilot study [121], but awaits confirmatory data from a prospective trial. This approach

may find more application in the treatment of nodular lymphocyte predominant disease, in which CD20 is present on the surface of the malignant cells [122]. Immunotoxin therapy has shown some very promising results, with a response rate of 86% reported using the anti-CD30 – monomethyllauristatin E (SGN-35) for patients with recurrent and refractory disease [123].

Among the small molecule therapies being tested, proteosome inhibitors have been disappointing in HL [124], whereas inhibitors of histone deacetylase (HDACi's) have resulted significant responses in early phase studies, despite significant marrow toxicity [125]. It is not clear whether the principal target of HDACi's is the malignant cell itself or the surrounding inflammatory infiltrate, but further studies using a range of more or less specific agents targeting different members of the HDAC family may yield further information.

### 9.6 Conclusions

A variety of pharmacologic hypotheses have been tested in the course of the last 50 years, and none has been found entirely satisfactory for predicting the outcomes of treatment. The superiority of ABVD over MOPP is established, but the place of the more intensive multiagent regimens such as BEACOPP is still to be conclusively proven, and high-dose therapy as a component of initial treatment was unrewarding. There appears to be a potential trade-off between the intensity of chemotherapy and the value of consolidation radiotherapy in advanced disease: it is not clear whether any chemotherapy is intensive enough for radiation to be dropped altogether, but functional imaging holds promise for lowering the proportion of patients irradiated very significantly.

As treatment has evolved, the balance between toxicity and efficacy has been established, and new approaches using response-adapted therapy hold the promise of identifying the minority of patients for whom early intensification is a necessity, while allowing de-escalation of treatment in those destined to do well. Finally, there are a small number of novel reagents currently undergoing testing against recurrent and refractory disease which appear to hold some promise.

# References

1. Peters MV. A study of survivals in Hodgkin's disease treated radiologically. Am J Roentgenol. 1950;63:299–311.
2. Easson EC, Russel MH. The cure of Hodgkin's disease. Br Med J. 1963;1:1704–7.
3. Kaplan HS. Clinical evaluation and radiotherapeutic management of Hodgkin's disease and the malignant lymphomas. N Engl J Med. 1968;278(16):892–9.
4. Papac RJ. Origins of cancer therapy. Yale J Biol Med. 2001;74:191–8.
5. Goodman LS, Wintrobe MM, et al. Nitrogen mustard therapy. Use of methyl bis (B-chloroethyl) amine hydrochloride and tris (B-chloroethyl) amine hydrochloride for Hodgkin's disease, lymphosarcoma, leukemia, certain allied and miscellaneous disorders. JAMA. 1946;132:126–32.
6. Zubrod CG. Historic milestones in curative chemotherapy. Semin Oncol. 1979;6:490–505.
7. Gross R, Lambers K. Erste erfahrungen in der Behandlung malignen tumoren mit einem neuen N-lost phosphamidester. Dtsch Med Wschr. 1958;83:458–62.
8. Burchenal JH. From wild fowl to stalking horses: alchemy in chemotherapy. Cancer. 1975;35:1121–35.
9. Mathe G, Cattan A, et al. Experimental therapeutic trials of leukemia and hematosarcomas: technologic and philosophic aspects. Ann N Y Acad Sci. 1969;164(3):776–92.
10. Rotolo V. Vincaleukoblastine in the therapy of malignant neoplasms. Friuli Med. 1968;23(1):31–52.
11. Gilman A. The initial clinical trial of nitrogen mustard. Am J Surg. 1963;105(574):578.
12. Wagener DJT. The development of chemotherapy. In: The history of oncology. Berlin: Springer; 2009. p. 145–80.
13. Mathe G, Schweisguth O, et al. Value of vincaleukoblastine in the treatment of Hodgkin's disease and other hematosarcomas and leukemias. Sem Ther. 1964;40(5):320–4.
14. Tubiana M, Henry-Amar M, et al. Long-term results of the E.O.R.T.C. randomized study of irradiation and vinblastine in clinical stages I and II of Hodgkin's disease. Eur J Cancer. 1979;15(5):645–57.
15. Rosenberg SA, Kaplan HS. Evidence for an orderly progression in the spread of Hodgkin's disease. Cancer Res. 1966; 26(6):1225–31.
16. Tubiana M, Hayat M, et al. Five-year results of the E.O.R.T.C. randomized study of splenectomy and spleen irradiation in clinical stages I and II of Hodgkin's disease. Eur J Cancer. 1981;17(3):355–63.
17. Bergsagel DE, Alison RE, et al. Results of treating Hodgkin's disease without a policy of laparotomy staging. Cancer Treat Rep. 1982;66:717–31.
18. Selby P, McElwain TJ, et al. Chemotherapy for Hodgkin's disease. Section I: MOPP and its variants. In: Selby P, McElwain TJ, editors. Hodgkin's disease. Oxford: Blackwell; 1987.
19. DeVita Jr VT et al. Principles of chemotherapy. In: DeVita Jr VT, editor. Cancer: principles and practice of oncology. 3rd ed. Philadelphia: J.B. Lipincott Company; 1989. p. 276–300.
20. Skipper HE, Schabel FM, et al. Experimental evaluation of potential anti-cancer agents. XII. On the criteria and kinetics associated with "curability" of experimental leukemia. Cancer Chemother Rep. 1964;35:1–111.
21. Bonadonna G, Monfardini S, et al. Comparative effects of vinblastine and procarbazine in advanced Hodgkin's disease. Eur J Cancer. 1969;5(4):393–402.
22. Coltman CA. Chemotherapy of advanced Hodgkin's disease. Semin Oncol. 1980;7:155–73.
23. Bernard J. Current general principles of the treatment of Hodgkin's disease, lymphosarcoma and reticulosarcoma. Rev Prat. 1966;16(7):871–9.
24. DeVita Jr VT, Carbone PP. Treatment of Hodgkin's disease. Med Ann Dist Columbia. 1967;36(4):232–4.
25. DeVita VT, Serpick AA, et al. Combination chemotherapy in the treatment of advanced Hodgkin's disease. Ann Intern Med. 1970;73(6):881–95.
26. DeVita VT, Simon RM, et al. Curability of advanced Hodgkin's disease with chemotherapy. Ann Intern Med. 1980;92(5):587–95.
27. Longo DL, Young RC, et al. Twenty years of MOPP therapy for Hodgkin's disease. J Clin Oncol. 1986;4(9):1295–306.
28. Canellos GP, Anderson JR, et al. Chemotherapy of advanced Hodgkin's disease with MOPP, ABVD, or MOPP alternating with ABVD. N Engl J Med. 1992;327(21):1478–84.
29. Carde P, MacKintosh FR, et al. A dose and time response analysis of the treatment of Hodgkin's disease with MOPP chemotherapy. J Clin Oncol. 1983;1(2):146–53.
30. Frei III E, Luce JK, et al. Combination chemotherapy in advanced Hodgkin's disease: induction and maintenance of remission. Ann Intern Med. 1973;79(3):376–82.
31. Somers R, Carde P, et al. A randomized study in stage IIIB and IV Hodgkin's disease comparing eight courses of MOPP versus an alteration of MOPP with ABVD: a European Organization for Research and Treatment of Cancer Lymphoma Cooperative Group and Groupe Pierre-et-Marie-Curie controlled clinical trial. J Clin Oncol. 1994;12(2):279–87.
32. Carde P, Hayat M, et al. Comparison of total nodal irradiation versus combined sequence of mantle irradiation with mechlorethamine, vincristine, procarbazine, and prednisone in clinical stages I and II Hodgkin's disease: experience of the European Organization for Research and Treatment of Cancer. NCI Monogr. 1988;(6):303–10.
33. Young RC, Chabner BA, et al. Maintenance chemotherapy for advanced Hodgkin's disease in remission. Lancet. 1973; 301(7816):1339–43.

34. Lowenbraun STAN, DeVita VT, et al. Combination chemotherapy with nitrogen mustard, vincristine, procarbazine and prednisone in previously treated patients with Hodgkin's disease. Blood. 1970;36(6):704–17.

35. Fisher RI, DeVita VT, et al. Prolonged disease-free survival in Hodgkin's disease with MOPP reinduction after first relapse. Ann Intern Med. 1979;90(5):761–3.

36. Arseneau JC, Sponzo RW, et al. Non lymphomatous malignant tumors complicating Hodgkin's disease: possible association with intensive therapy. N Engl J Med. 1972;287(22): 1119–22.

37. Weiden PL, Lerner KG, et al. Pancytopenia and leukemia in Hodgkin's disease: report of three cases. Blood. 1973;42(4): 571–7.

38. Sherins RJ, DeVita Jr VT. Effect of drug treatment for lymphoma on male reproductive capacity. Studies of men in remission after therapy. Ann Intern Med. 1973;79(2): 216–20.

39. Corder MP, Young RC, et al. Phytohemagglutinin-induced lymphocyte transformation: the relationship to prognosis of Hodgkin's disease. Blood. 1972;39(5):595–601.

40. Crowther D, Wagstaff J, et al. A randomized study comparing chemotherapy alone with chemotherapy followed by radiotherapy in patients with pathologically staged IIIA Hodgkin's disease. J Clin Oncol. 1984;2(8):892–7.

41. Nicholson WM, Beard ME, et al. Combination chemotherapy in generalized Hodgkin's disease. Br Med J. 1970;3(713): 7–10.

42. Ranson MR, Radford JA, et al. An analysis of prognostic factors in stage III and IV Hodgkin's disease treated at a single centre with MVPP. Ann Oncol. 1991;2(6):83–9.

43. Dady PJ, McElwain TJ, et al. Five years' experience with ChlVPP: effective low-toxicity combination chemotherapy for Hodgkin's disease CHLVPP advanced HL. Br J Cancer. 1982;45:851–9.

44. McElwain TJ, Toy J, et al. A combination of chlorambucil, vinblastine, procarbazine and prednisolone for treatment of Hodgkin's disease. Br J Cancer. 1977;36(276):280.

45. Luce JK, Gamble JF, et al. Combined cyclophosphamide vincristine, and prednisone therapy of malignant lymphoma. Cancer. 1971;28(2):306–17.

46. Bonadonna G, Monfardini S. Cardiac toxicity of daunorubicin. Lancet. 1969;1(7599):837.

47. Frei E, Luce JK, et al. 5-(3,3-Dimethyl-1-triazeno)imidazole-4-carboxamide (NSC-45388) in the treatment of lymphoma. Cancer Treat Rep. 1972;56(5):667–70.

48. O'Bryan RM, Luce JK, et al. Phase II evaluation of adriamycin in human neoplasia. Cancer. 1973;32(1):1–8.

49. Bonadonna G, Zucali R, et al. Combination chemotherapy of Hodgkin's disease with adriamycin, bleomycin, vinblastine, and imidazole carboxamide versus MOPP. Cancer. 1975;36(1):252–9.

50. Boleti E, Mead GM. ABVD for Hodgkin's lymphoma: full-dose chemotherapy without dose reductions or growth factors. Ann Oncol. 2007;18(2):376–80.

51. Bonadonna G, Santoro A, et al. Cyclic delivery of MOPP and ABVD combinations in Stage IV Hodgkin's disease: rationale, background studies, and recent results. Cancer Treat Rep. 1982;66(4):881–7.

52. Goldie JH, Coldman AJ. Analyzing the patterns of treatment failure. J Clin Oncol. 1986;4(6):825–6.

53. Santoro A, Bonadonna G, et al. Alternating drug combinations in the treatment of advanced Hodgkin's disease. N Engl J Med. 1982;306(13):770–5.

54. Canellos GP, Niedzwiecki D. Long-term follow-up of Hodgkin's disease trial. N Engl J Med. 2002;346(18):1417–8.

55. Aleman BM, Raemaekers JM, et al. Involved-field radiotherapy for advanced Hodgkin's lymphoma. N Engl J Med. 2003;348(24):2396–406.

56. Klimo P, Connors JM. MOPP/ABV hybrid program: combination chemotherapy based on early introduction of seven effective drugs for advanced Hodgkin's disease. J Clin Oncol. 1985;3(9):1174–82.

57. Radford JA, Crowther D, et al. Results of a randomized trial comparing MVPP chemotherapy with a hybrid regimen, ChlVPP/EVA, in the initial treatment of Hodgkin's disease. J Clin Oncol. 1995;13(9):2379–85.

58. Sieber M, Tesch H, et al. Treatment of advanced Hodgkin's disease with COPP/ABV/IMEP versus COPP/ABVD and consolidating radiotherapy: final results of the German Hodgkin's Lymphoma Study Group HD6 trial. Ann Oncol. 2004;15(2):276–82.

59. Duggan DB, Petroni GR, et al. Randomized comparison of ABVD and MOPP/ABV hybrid for the treatment of advanced Hodgkin's disease: report of an intergroup trial. J Clin Oncol. 2003;21(4):607–14.

60. Johnson PWM, Radford JA, et al. Comparison of ABVD and alternating or hybrid multidrug regimens for the treatment of advanced Hodgkin's lymphoma: results of the United Kingdom Lymphoma Group LY09 Trial (ISRCTN97144519). J Clin Oncol. 2005;23(36):9208–18.

61. Norton L, Simon R. Tumor size, sensitivity to therapy, and design of treatment schedules. Cancer Treat Rep. 1977;61: 1307–17.

62. Diehl V, Franklin J, et al. Standard and increased-dose BEACOPP chemotherapy compared with COPP-ABVD for advanced Hodgkin's disease. N Engl J Med. 2003;348(24): 2386–95.

63. Linch DC, Winfield D, et al. Dose intensification with autologous bone-marrow transplantation in relapsed and resistant Hodgkin's disease: results of a BNLI randomised trial. Lancet. 1993;341(8852):1051–4.

64. Schmitz N, Pfistner B, et al. Aggressive conventional chemotherapy compared with high-dose chemotherapy with autologous haemopoietic stem-cell transplantation for relapsed chemosensitive Hodgkin's disease: a randomised trial. Lancet. 2002;359(9323):2065–71.

65. Hasenclever D, Brosteanu O, et al. Modelling of chemotherapy: the effective dose approach. Ann Hematol. 2001;80 Suppl 3:B89–94.

66. Hasenclever D, Loeffler M, et al. German Hodgkin's Lymphoma Study Group. Rationale for dose escalation of first line conventional chemotherapy in advanced Hodgkin's disease. Ann Oncol. 1996;7(Suppl 4): 95–8.

67. Owadally WS, Sydes MR, et al. Initial dose intensity has limited impact on the outcome of ABVD chemotherapy for advanced Hodgkin lymphoma (HL): data from UKLG LY09 (ISRCTN97144519). Ann Oncol. 2010;21:568–73.

68. Brosteanu O, Hasenclever D, et al. Low acute hematological toxicity during chemotherapy predicts reduced disease control in advanced Hodgkin's disease. Ann Hematol. 2004; 83(3):176–82.

69. Ribrag V, Koscielny S, et al. Pharmacogenetic study in Hodgkin lymphomas reveals the impact of UGT1A1 polymorphisms on patient prognosis. Blood. 2009;113(14):3307–13.

70. Henry-Amar M, Hayat M, et al. EORTC Lymphoma Cooperative Group. Causes of death after therapy for early stage Hodgkin's disease entered on EORTC protocols. Int J Radiat Oncol Biol Phys. 1990;19(5):1155–7.

71. Van Leeuwen FE, Klokman WJ, et al. Second cancer risk following Hodgkin's-disease – a 20-year follow-up-study. J Clin Oncol. 1994;12(2):312–25.

72. Engert A, Diehl V, et al. Escalated-dose BEACOPP in the treatment of patients with advanced-stage Hodgkin's lymphoma: 10 years of follow-up of the GHSG HD9 study. J Clin Oncol. 2009;27(27):4548–54.

73. Engert A, Diehl V, et al. Two cycles of ABVD followed by involved field radiotherapy with 20 Gray (Gy) is the new standard of care in the treatment of patients with early-stage Hodgkin lymphoma: final analysis of the randomized German Hodgkin Study Group (GHSG) HD10. Study supported by the Deutsche Krebshilfe and in part by the Competence Network Malignant Lymphoma. ASH Annu Meet Abstr. 2009;114(22):716.

74. Bartlett NL, Rosenberg SA, et al. Brief chemotherapy, Stanford V, and adjuvant radiotherapy for bulky or advanced-stage Hodgkin's disease: a preliminary report. J Clin Oncol. 1995;13(5):1080–8.

75. Horning SJ, Williams J, et al. Assessment of the Stanford V regimen and consolidative radiotherapy for bulky and advanced Hodgkin's disease: Eastern Cooperative Oncology Group Pilot Study E1492. J Clin Oncol. 2000;18(5):972.

76. Horning SJ, Hoppe RT, et al. Stanford V and radiotherapy for locally extensive and advanced Hodgkin's disease: mature results of a prospective clinical trial. J Clin Oncol. 2002;20(3):630–7.

77. Gobbi PG, Levis A, et al. ABVD versus modified Stanford V versus MOPPEBVCAD with optional and limited radiotherapy in intermediate- and advanced-stage Hodgkin's lymphoma: final results of a Multicenter Randomized Trial by the Intergruppo Italiano Linfomi. J Clin Oncol. 2005;23(36):9198–207.

78. Hoskin PJ, Lowry L, et al. Randomized comparison of the Stanford V regimen and ABVD in the treatment of advanced Hodgkin's lymphoma: United Kingdom National Cancer Research Institute Lymphoma Group Study ISRCTN 64141244. J Clin Oncol. 2009;27(32):5390–6.

79. Radford JA, Rohatiner AZS, et al. ChlVPP/EVA hybrid versus the weekly VAPEC-B regimen for previously untreated Hodgkin's disease. J Clin Oncol. 2002;20(13):2988–94.

80. Green JA, Dawson AA, et al. Measurement of drug dosage intensity in MVPP therapy in Hodgkin's disease. Br J Clin Pharmacol. 1980;9:511–4.

81. Diehl V, Sieber M, et al.; The German Hodgkin's Lymphoma Study Group. BEACOPP: an intensified chemotherapy regimen in advanced Hodgkin's disease. Ann Oncol. 1997;8(2):143–8.

82. Diehl V, Haverkamp H, et al. Eight cycles of BEACOPP escalated compared with 4 cycles of BEACOPP escalated followed by 4 cycles of BEACOPP baseline with or without radiotherapy in patients in advanced stage Hodgkin lymphoma (HL): final analysis of the HD12 trial of the German Hodgkin Study Group (GHSG). ASCO Meet Abstr. 2009; 27(15S):8544.

83. Engert A, Franklin J, et al. HD12 randomised trial comparing 8 dose-escalated cycles of BEACOPP with 4 escalated and 4 baseline cycles in patients with advanced stage Hodgkin lymphoma (HL): an analysis of the German Hodgkin Lymphoma Study Group (GHSG), University of Cologne, D-50924 Cologne, Germany. ASH Annu Meet Abstr. 2006;108(11):99.

84. Kobe C, Dietlein M, et al. Positron emission tomography has a high negative predictive value for progression or early relapse for patients with residual disease after first-line chemotherapy in advanced-stage Hodgkin lymphoma. Blood. 2008;112(10):3989–94.

85. Federico M, Luminari S, et al. ABVD compared with BEACOPP compared with CEC for the initial treatment of patients with advanced Hodgkin's lymphoma: results from the HD2000 Gruppo Italiano per lo Studio dei Linfomi Trial. J Clin Oncol. 2009;27(5):805–11.

86. Gianni AM, Rambaldi A, et al. Comparable 3-year outcome following ABVD or BEACOPP first-line chemotherapy, plus pre-planned high-dose salvage, in advanced Hodgkin lymphoma (HL): a randomized trial of the Michelangelo, GITIL and IIL cooperative groups. ASCO Meet Abstr. 2008;26(15 Suppl):8506.

87. Proctor SJ, Mackie M, et al. A population-based study of intensive multi-agent chemotherapy with or without auto-transplant for the highest risk Hodgkin's disease patients identified by the Scotland and Newcastle Lymphoma Group (SNLG) prognostic index: a Scotland and Newcastle Lymphoma Group study (SNLG HD III). Eur J Cancer. 2002;38(6):795–806.

88. Federico M, Bellei M, et al. High-dose therapy and autologous stem-cell transplantation versus conventional therapy for patients with advanced Hodgkin's lymphoma responding to front-line therapy. J Clin Oncol. 2003;21(12):2320–5.

89. Arakelyan N, Berthou C, et al. Radiation therapy versus 4 cycles of combined doxorubicin, bleomycin, vinblastine, and dacarbazine plus myeloablative chemotherapy with autologous stem cell transplantation five-year results of a randomized trial on behalf of the GOELAMS group. Cancer. 2008;113(12):3323–30.

90. Young RC, Canellos GP, et al. Patterns of relapse in advanced Hodgkin's disease treated with combination chemotherapy. Cancer. 1978;42:1001–7.

91. Loeffler M, Brosteanu O, et al. Meta-analysis of chemotherapy versus combined modality treatment trials in Hodgkin's disease. International Database on Hodgkin's Disease Overview Study Group. J Clin Oncol. 1998;16(3):818–29.

92. Johnson PWM, Sydes MR, Hancock BW, Cullen MH, Radford JA, Stenning SP. Consolidation radiotherapy in patients with advanced Hodgkin lymphoma: survival data from the UKLG LY09 randomised controlled trial (ISRCTN97144519). Journal of Clinical Oncology. 2010;in press.

93. Diehl V, Loeffler M, et al. German Hodgkins' Study Group (GHSG). Further chemotherapy versus low-dose involved-field radiotherapy as consolidation of complete remission after six cycles of alternating chemotherapy in patients with advance Hodgkin's disease. Ann Oncol. 1995;6(9):901–10.

94. Ferme C, Sebban C, et al. Comparison of chemotherapy to radiotherapy as consolidation of complete or good partial response after six cycles of chemotherapy for patients with advanced Hodgkin's disease: results of the Groupe d'etudes

des Lymphomes de l'Adulte H89 trial. Blood. 2000;95(7): 2246–52.

95. Bonadonna G, Bonfante V, et al. ABVD plus subtotal nodal versus involved-field radiotherapy in early-stage Hodgkin's disease: long-term results. J Clin Oncol. 2004;22(14): 2835–41.

96. Engert A, Franklin J, et al. Two cycles of doxorubicin, bleomycin, vinblastine, and dacarbazine plus extended-field radiotherapy is superior to radiotherapy alone in early favorable Hodgkin's lymphoma: final results of the GHSG HD7 trial. J Clin Oncol. 2007;25(23):3495–502.

97. Ferme C, Eghbali H, et al. Chemotherapy plus involved-field radiation in early-stage Hodgkin's disease. N Engl J Med. 2007;357(19):1916–27.

98. Noordijk EM, Carde P, et al. Combined-modality therapy for clinical stage I or II Hodgkin's lymphoma: long-term results of the European Organisation for Research and Treatment of Cancer H7 randomized controlled trials. J Clin Oncol. 2006;24(19):3128–35.

99. Carde P, Hagenbeek A, et al. Clinical staging versus laparotomy and combined modality with MOPP versus ABVD in early-stage Hodgkin's disease: the H6 twin randomized trials from the European Organization for Research and Treatment of Cancer Lymphoma Cooperative Group. J Clin Oncol. 1993;11(11):2258–72.

100. Thomas J, Ferme C, et al. Results of the EORTC-GELA H9 Randomized Trials: The H9-F trial (comparing 3 radiation dose levels) and H9-U Trial (comparing 3 chemotherapy schemes) in patients with favorable or unfavorable early stage Hodgkin's lymphoma (HL). Haematologica. 2007; 92(s5):27.

101. Borchmann P, Diehl V, et al. Combined modality treatment with intensified chemotherapy and dose-reduced involved field radiotherapy in patients with early unfavourable Hodgkin lymphoma (HL): final analysis of the German Hodgkin Study Group (GHSG) HD11 Trial. ASH Annu Meet Abstr. 2009;114(22):717.

102. Advani R, Hoppe R, et al. Stage I/II Hodgkin's disease (HD) with bulky mediastinal disease or other risk factors (RF); the Stanford V experience. Haematologica. 2007; 92(s5):27.

103. Advani R, Maeda L, et al. Impact of positive positron emission tomography on prediction of freedom from progression after Stanford V chemotherapy in Hodgkin's disease. J Clin Oncol. 2007;25(25):3902–7.

104. Advani RH, Horning SJ. Treatment of early-stage Hodgkin's disease. Semin Hematol. 1999;36(3):270–81.

105. Horning S, Hoppe R, et al. Vinblastine, bleomycin and methotrexate: an effective adjuvant in favourable Hodgkin's disease. J Clin Oncol. 1988;6:1822–31.

106. Press OW, LeBlanc M, et al. Phase III randomized intergroup trial of subtotal lymphoid irradiation versus doxorubicin, vinblastine, and subtotal lymphoid irradiation for stage IA to IIA Hodgkin's disease. J Clin Oncol. 2001; 19(22):4238–44.

107. Nachman JB, Sposto R, et al. Randomized comparison of low-dose involved-field radiotherapy and no radiotherapy for children with Hodgkin's disease who achieve a complete response to chemotherapy. J Clin Oncol. 2002; 20(18):3765–71.

108. Meyer RM, Gospodarowicz MK, et al. Randomized comparison of ABVD chemotherapy with a strategy that includes radiation therapy in patients with limited-stage Hodgkin's lymphoma: National Cancer Institute of Canada Clinical Trials Group and the Eastern Cooperative Oncology Group. J Clin Oncol. 2005;23(21):4634–42.

109. Straus DJ, Portlock CS, et al. Results of a prospective randomized clinical trial of doxorubicin, bleomycin, vinblastine, and dacarbazine (ABVD) followed by radiation therapy (RT) versus ABVD alone for stages I, II, and IIIA nonbulky Hodgkin disease. Blood. 2004;104(12):3483–9.

110. Radford JA, O'Doherty M, et al. Results of the 2nd planned interim analysis of the RAPID trial (involved field radiotherapy versus no further treatment) in patients with clinical stages 1A and 2A Hodgkin lymphoma and a "negative" FDG-PET scan after 3 cycles ABVD. Blood. 2008; 112:369s.

111. Josting A, Rudolph C, et al. Time-intensified dexamethasone/cisplatin/cytarabine: an effective salvage therapy with low toxicity in patients with relapsed and refractory Hodgkin's disease. Ann Oncol. 2002;13(10):1628–35.

112. Aparicio J, Segura A, et al. ESHAP is an active regimen for relapsing Hodgkin's disease. Ann Oncol. 1999;10(5): 593–5.

113. Moskowitz CH, Nimer SD, et al. A 2-step comprehensive high-dose chemoradiotherapy second-line program for relapsed and refractory Hodgkin disease: analysis by intent to treat and development of a prognostic model. Blood. 2001;97(3):616–23.

114. Plunkett W, Huang P, et al. Gemcitabine: preclinical pharmacology and mechanisms of action. Semin Oncol. 1996; 23(5 Suppl 10):3–15.

115. Friedberg JW, Neuberg D, et al. Gemcitabine added to doxorubicin, bleomycin, and vinblastine for the treatment of de novo Hodgkin disease: unacceptable acute pulmonary toxicity. Cancer. 2003;98(5):978–82.

116. Sweetenham JW, Taghipour G, et al. High-dose therapy and autologous stem cell rescue for patients with Hodgkin's disease in first relapse after chemotherapy: results from the EBMT. Lymphoma Working Party of the European Group for Blood and Marrow Transplantation. Bone Marrow Transplant. 1997;20(9):745–52.

117. Moskowitz CH, Yahalom J, et al. High-dose chemo-radiotherapy for relapsed or refractory Hodgkin lymphoma and the significance of pre-transplant functional imaging. Br J Haematol. 148;890-897 2010.

118. Sweetenham JW, Carella AM, et al. High-dose therapy and autologous stem-cell transplantation for adult patients with Hodgkin's disease who do not enter remission after induction chemotherapy: results in 175 patients reported to the European Group for Blood and Marrow Transplantation. Lymphoma Working Party. J Clin Oncol. 1999;17(10):3101–9.

119. Bierman PJ, Bagin RG, et al. High dose chemotherapy followed by autologous hematopoietic rescue in Hodgkin's disease: long-term follow-up in 128 patients. Ann Oncol. 1993;4(9):767–73.

120. Ansell SM, Horwitz SM, et al. Phase I/II study of an anti-CD30 monoclonal antibody (MDX-060) in Hodgkin's lymphoma and anaplastic large-cell lymphoma. J Clin Oncol. 2007;25(19):2764–9.

121. Younes A, Romaguera J, et al. A pilot study of rituximab in patients with recurrent, classic Hodgkin disease. Cancer. 2003;98(2):310–4.

122. Ekstrand BC, Lucas JB, et al. Rituximab in lymphocyte-predominant Hodgkin disease: results of a phase 2 trial. Blood. 2003;101(11):4285–9.

123. Younes A, Forero-Torres A, et al. Multiple complete responses in a phase 1 dose escalation study of the antibody-drug conjugate SGN-35 in patients with relapsed or refractory CD30-positive lymphomas. Blood. 2008;112:s370.

124. Mendler JH, Kelly J, et al. Bortezomib and gemcitabine in relapsed or refractory Hodgkin's lymphoma. Ann Oncol. 2008;19(10):1759–64.

125. Younes A, Pro B, et al. Isotype-selective HDAC inhibitor MGCD0103 decreases serum TARC concentrations and produces clinical responses in heavily pretreated patients with relapsed classical Hodgkin lymphoma. Blood. 2007; 110(11):2566.

126. Sutcliffe S, Wrigley PFM, et al. MVPP chemotherapy regimen for advanced Hodgkin's disease. Br Med J. 1978; 6114:679–83.

127. Selby P, Patel P, et al. ChlVPP combination chemotherapy for Hodgkin's disease: long-term results. Br J Cancer. 1990; 62(2):279–85.

128. Viviani S, Bonadonna G, et al. Alternating versus hybrid MOPP and ABVD combinations in advanced Hodgkin's disease: ten-year results. J Clin Oncol. 1996;14(5): 1421–30.

129. Rodriguez J, Rodriguez MA, et al. ASHAP: a regimen for cytoreduction of refractory or recurrent Hodgkin's disease. Blood. 1999;93(11):3632–6.

130. Baetz T, Belch A, et al. Gemcitabine, dexamethasone and cisplatin is an active and non-toxic chemotherapy regimen in relapsed or refractory Hodgkin's disease: a phase II study by the National Cancer Institute of Canada Clinical Trials Group. Ann Oncol. 2003;14(12):1762–7.

131. Brice P, Marolleau JP, Pautier P, Makke J, Cazals D, Dombret H, et al. Hematologic recovery and survival of lymphoma patients after autologous stem-cell transplantation: comparison of bone marrow and peripheral blood progenitor cells. Leukemia & lymphoma. 1996;22(5-6): 449–56.

132. Andre M, Henry-Amar M, Pico JL, Brice P, Blaise D, Kuentz M, et al. Comparison of high-dose therapy and autologous stem-cell transplantation with conventional therapy for Hodgkin's disease induction failure: a case-control study. Societe Francaise de Greffe de Moelle. J Clin Oncol. 1999;17(1):222–9.

133. Ferme C, Mounier N, Divine M, Brice P, Stamatoullas A, Reman O, et al. Intensive salvage therapy with high-dose chemotherapy for patients with advanced Hodgkin's disease in relapse or failure after initial chemotherapy: results of the Groupe d'Etudes des Lymphomes de l'Adulte H89 Trial. J Clin Oncol. 2002;20(2):467–75.

134. Perz JB, Giles C, Szydlo R, O'Shea D, Sanz J, Chaidos A, et al. LACE-conditioned autologous stem cell transplantation for relapsed or refractory Hodgkin's lymphoma: treatment outcome and risk factor analysis in 67 patients from a single centre. Bone marrow transplantation. 2007; 39(1):41–7.

135. Johnson PWM, Sydes MR, Hancock BW, Cullen MH, Radford JA, Stenning SP. Consolidation radiotherapy in patients with advanced Hodgkin lymphoma: survival data from the UKLG LY09 randomised controlled trial (ISRCTN97144519). Journal of Clinical Oncology. 2010;in press.

# Treatment of Early Favorable Hodgkin Lymphoma

**10**

Elly Lugtenburg and Anton Hagenbeek

## Contents

E. Lugtenburg (✉)
Department of Haematology, Erasmus MC, University Medical Center, PO Box 2040, 3000 CA, Rotterdam, The Netherlands
e-mail: p.lugtenburg@erasmusmc.nl

A. Hagenbeek
Department of Haematology, Academic Medical Center, Meibergdreef 9, 1105 AZ, Amsterdam, The Netherlands
e-mail: a.hagenbeek@amc.uva.nl

## 10.1 Introduction

Historically, Hodgkin lymphoma (HL) was the first malignant disease that could be cured. In the past century, the first successful outcomes of radiotherapy employing large radiation fields were reported, in particular in patients with limited disease. Even bulky tumors melted away during intense irradiation. One might hypothesize that this can be explained by the radiosensitivity of the few malignant cells in HL (Hodgkin and Reed–Sternberg [H-RS] cells) amidst the majority of non-malignant surrounding cells in the microenvironment.

Further refinement of this initial treatment approach was achieved through carefully designed prospective randomized phase III clinical trials. In this context, the step-by-step development of uniformly accepted staging procedures and clear definitions of stages and response criteria was a major achievement. This allowed direct comparison of study results performed in different consortia worldwide.

Focusing on stage-adapted treatment of HL, these trials allowed the definition of clinical prognostic factors. These, in turn, lead to risk-adapted treatment, which became more refined with subsequent studies. In line with these advances, treatment strategies changed from radiotherapy only using extended field radiotherapy (EFRT) and later involved field radiation (IFRT) to combined modality treatment (CMT) and limited chemotherapy only.

Thanks to the long-term follow-up of thousands of patients treated within clinical trials over decades, significant late effects of treatment became apparent, in particular secondary malignancies and damage to the cardiovascular and respiratory systems. Based on these unexpected findings, which could only be retrieved for

A. Engert and S.J. Horning (eds.), *Hodgkin Lymphoma*,
DOI: 10.1007/978-3-642-12780-9_10, © Springer-Verlag Berlin Heidelberg 2011

the first time in oncology due to the high cure rate and accurately documented long-term follow-up of HL patients, the ingredients of curative regimens were further adjusted. As far as possible, non-carcinogenic cytostatic agents were introduced in newly developed chemotherapy regimens and radiation doses were further reduced. This has lead to the current major challenges in the treatment of early stage HL: maintaining the very high cure rates and at the same time reducing the incidence of devastating late effects. To define an optimal balance, it is thus strongly advocated to treat early stage HL patients within clinical trials and not ad hoc according to local guidelines.

This chapter deals with recent developments in the treatment of stage I and II HL with favorable prognostic factors comprising 40% of all early stage HL patients.

## 10.2 Defining Favorable Early Stage Disease

### 10.2.1 Staging

In HL patients, prognosis is distinctly worse with each progressive stage of disease and the selection of appropriate treatment depends on accurate staging of the extent of disease. The Ann Arbor staging classification was formulated in 1971 and is still the most commonly used staging system for HL [1]. During the Cotswold meeting in 1989, some modifications were introduced to account for new imaging techniques such as computerized tomography (CT) scanning. In addition, clinical involvement of liver and spleen were redefined, to formally introduce the concept of bulky disease and to draw the attention to the problem of equivocal complete remission [2]. Stage I indicates involvement of a single lymph node region or a single extranodal organ or site. In stage II disease, two or more lymph node regions on the same side of the diaphragm are involved, or there is localized involvement of an extranodal organ or site and of one or more lymph node regions on the same side of the diaphragm. The stage number is followed by the letter A or B indicating the absence (A) or presence (B) of one or more of the following constitutional symptoms: (a) unexplained fever with temperatures above 38°C during

the previous month, (b) drenching night sweats during the previous months, and (c) unexplained weight loss of more than 10% of body weight in the previous 6 months. Mediastinal bulk was defined by the ratio of the maximum transverse tumor diameter to the internal thoracic diameter at the level of the T5-6 vertebral interspace. A ratio exceeding one-third was considered bulky.

For the initial staging of HL, a detailed history, complete physical examination, bone marrow biopsy, and imaging studies are generally recommended. In patients with stage IA or IIA disease, a bone marrow biopsy has a very low yield and can be omitted [2, 3]. Laparotomy with lymph node dissection and splenectomy had been a routine staging procedure, but was replaced by CT scanning for the identification of nodal and extranodal involvement not detectable by clinical examination. Today, most centers perform chest radiographs and CT scans of the neck, thorax, abdomen, and pelvis. In case of specific symptoms or physical signs, special investigations and imaging studies may be performed to confirm clinical involvement at a given site. Only a limited number of studies have directly assessed the value of positron emission tomography using [18F]-fluoro-2-deoxy-D-glucose (FDG-PET, here referred to as PET) for the initial staging of HL [4, 5]. The sensitivity of PET scanning seems to be better than the sensitivity of CT scanning for detecting nodal and extranodal disease. This results in an upstaging of disease stage in approximately 15–20% of patients, with an impact on patient management in about 5–15% [4, 6]. However, the influence on treatment strategy varies markedly from study to study, so the actual impact on patient management and outcome remains to be shown. Moreover, care should be taken that patients with an excellent prognosis and at risk of over-treatment do not receive more intensive treatment solely based on the results of the PET scan. Also, CT detects some regions of disease with normal FDG uptake and, therefore, PET should always be combined with CT scans. Nevertheless, a pre-therapy PET can be useful for a more reliable interpretation of post-therapy PET [7]. See Chaps. 6 and 7 for a more comprehensive review of clinical evaluation and functional imaging.

About 7% of stage I–II HL patients present with infradiaphragmatic disease [8]. The specific features and treatment of stage I–II infradiaphragmatic HL patients are described in Chap. 12.

## 10.2.2 Prognostic Factors

The stage of the disease is not the only prognostic tool in HL. Several studies describing prognostic factors in early stage HL have been performed [9, 10]. They were derived from long-term follow-up of patient cohorts treated in a variety of phase III prospective randomized trials. These prognostic factors predict the likelihood of occult disease in the abdomen and the effectiveness of treatment. The prognostic significance of bulky disease particularly in the mediastinum has been well documented [9]. The presence of constitutional symptoms has always been considered one of the main prognostic indicators. There is also a strong correlation between erythrocyte sedimentation rate (ESR) and the number of involved lymph node regions (see Chap. 8 for prognostic factors). Different Lymphoma Collaborative Groups worldwide use varying combinations of prognostic factors to identify prognostic risk groups. These prognostic factors allow patients to be stratified into favorable or unfavorable prognostic groups. The current definitions of a favorable treatment group according to the different study groups in Europe and the United States are presented in Table 10.1. The Lymphoma Group of the European Organization for Research and Treatment of Cancer (EORTC) and the French–Belgian Groupe d'Etude des Lymphomes de l'Adulte (GELA) define clinical stage I–II patients as favorable if they present with the following characteristics: age <50 years and low ESR (<50 mm/h without and <30 mm/h with B-symptoms), no more than three involved lymph node regions, and no large mediastinal mass [11]. All these criteria need to be met to be "favorable." The German Hodgkin Study Group (GHSG) criteria differ slightly in that they substituted age <50 years with no extranodal

disease and specify no more than two involved nodal regions rather than ≤3 as in the EORTC [12]. In Canada and North America, it is common to define an early or limited stage risk group as stage I and IIA disease without bulky disease (see Table 10.1).

## 10.3 Radiotherapy Alone

The use of radiation therapy, pioneered at Stanford University in the 1960s by Henry Kaplan and Saul Rosenberg, offered patients with HL the first hope for cure. In the treatment of early stages, EFRT was considered the standard treatment modality for many years. With this technique, radiation was delivered not only to the clinically involved but also to the adjacent, clinically uninvolved sites. Because it was known that HL spreads to contiguous nodal sites, mantle field RT encompassed all nodal sites above the diaphragm. The combination of mantle field with inverted Y field and spleen irradiation was termed "subtotal nodal irradiation" (STNI). See Chap. 9 for definitions of field size.

Significant advances in the treatment of HL were then derived from clinical trials. Investigators at Stanford demonstrated that radiation therapy alone using total lymphoid irradiation or STNI is adequate treatment for nearly all patients with pathologic stage I–II. In a series of 109 patients, the freedom from relapse rate at 10 years was 77%. The likelihood of relapse after treatment with irradiation alone was much higher for patients with extensive mediastinal disease than minimal mediastinal involvement [13].

The Princess Margaret Hospital in Toronto, Canada, conducted a retrospective study of patients with clinical

**Table 10.1** Definition of early-stage favorable HL

| EORTC/GELA | GHSG | NCIC/ECOG |
|---|---|---|
| CS I–II without risk factors (supradiaphragmatic) | CS I–II without risk factors | CS I–IIA without risk factors (supradiaphragmatic) |
| No large mediastinal mass<br>Age <50 years<br>No elevated ESRᵃ<br>1–3 involved nodal regions | No large mediastinal mass<br>No extranodal disease<br>No elevated ESRᵃ<br>1–2 involved nodal regions | No large mediastinal mass<br>Age <40 years<br>ESR <50 mm/h<br>1–3 involved nodal regions<br>LPHL or NS histology |

*EORTC* European Organization for Research and Treatment of Cancer; *GELA* Groupe d'Etude des Lymphomes de l'Adulte; *GHSG* German Hodgkin Study Group; *NCIC* National Cancer Institute of Canada; *ECOG* Eastern Cooperative Oncology Group; *CS* clinical stage; *ESR* erythrocyte sedimentation rate; *LPHL* nodular lymphocyte predominant Hodgkin lymphoma; *NS* nodular sclerosis

ᵃESR <50 mm/h without B symptoms or ESR <30 mm/h with B symptoms stage I and II treated between 1978 and 1986 to determine the impact of patient selection and EFRT on outcome. The study involved 250 patients with supradiaphragmatic disease and no adverse prognostic factors selected for treatment with radiation alone. Patients with favorable prognostic features (age <50 years, ESR <40 mm/h, and lymphocyte-predominance or nodular sclerosis histology) treated with mantle and para-aortic-splenic irradiation had only 12.7% actuarial risk of relapse at 8 years [14].

Between 1964 and 1987, the EORTC performed four consecutive randomized clinical trials aiming to delineate the subsets of patients who could be safely treated with RT alone [15, 16] (Table 10.2). In the EORTC H1 trial, all 288 patients had clinical stage I or II disease [17]. No staging laparotomy was performed. Patients received mantle field RT in case of supradiaphragmatic disease and inverted-Y RT for subdiaphragmatic disease. Patients in complete remission were randomized between no further treatment and 2 years of a weekly vinblastine. The 15-year follow-up showed a significant advantage in disease-free survival for the combined treatment compared with RT alone (60 vs. 38%). The incidence of relapse in the para-aortic region was high in patients who received supradiaphragmatic RT only. However, the benefit of the combined treatment was more evident in patients with unfavorable characteristics. The overall survival did not differ significantly between both arms (65 vs. 58%).

The EORTC H2 trial compared staging laparotomy including splenectomy followed by mantle field and para-aortic RT with STNI without staging laparotomy in 300 patients with supradiaphragmatic clinical stage I–II disease [16, 18]. To assess the prognostic significance of the laparotomy findings, the results of the staging laparotomy did not change the treatment policy. It was found that positive laparotomy was associated with a higher relapse rates. However, the impact of positive laparotomy on disease-free survival was observed only in patients with favorable prognostic factors. At 12-year follow-up, the disease-free survival and overall survival did not differ significantly between the laparotomy and the no-laparotomy groups (76 vs. 68% and 79 vs. 77%, respectively). This trial showed that staging laparotomy could be omitted in certain subsets of patients, provided STNI was given instead of mantle field RT. Together with data from the H1 trial, a new set of clinical prognostic factors could be derived that identified groups of patients with a more favorable and unfavorable prognosis. This gave the opportunity to develop treatment regimens tailored to these prognostic factors, with the aim to minimize treatment intensity as much as possible in the favorable subgroups to spare them from unnecessary treatment toxicity.

In the next EORTC trial (H5F), patients with favorable characteristics (age ≤40 years; ESR ≤70 mm/h; clinical stage I or stage II without mediastinal involvement; and lymphocyte predominant or nodular sclerosing histology) underwent staging laparotomy [16, 19]. The laparotomy was used to select a group of patients with a good prognosis for whom RT alone might be sufficient. Patients (n = 198) with negative laparotomy remained in the favorable group and were randomized between mantle field RT and STNI. At 9-years follow-up there was no significant difference in disease-free survival and overall survival between the two treatment arms (69 vs. 70% and 94 vs. 91%, respectively). This trial showed that favorable patients with negative staging laparotomy could safely be treated with relatively limited RT alone.

The EORTC H6F trial investigated whether staging laparotomy was mandatory for the identification of the subset of patients that could be treated by STNI and splenic irradiation alone [20]. The favorable subgroup was characterized by clinical stages I or II with a maximum of two involved areas and no bulky mediastinum and ESR ≤50 mm/h if no B-symptoms present or ≤30 mm/h in case of B-symptoms. These patients (n = 262) were randomized between clinical staging plus STNI (mantle, spleen, and para-aortic RT) and staging laparotomy plus treatment adaptation. If the laparotomy was negative, patients with lymphocyte predominant or nodular sclerosing subtypes were treated with mantle field RT, and patients with mixed cellularity or lymphocyte depleted histology received mantle field and para-aortic RT (STNI). Again, no significant differences between the two treatment arms were found in this trial in disease-free survival and overall survival at 6-year follow-up (80 vs. 84% and 93 vs. 89%, respectively).

Taken together, these four randomized trials demonstrated that staging laparotomy could be safely omitted in patients with favorable clinical characteristics in early favorable HL and that these patients could be treated by STNI (40 Gy) with a similar outcome as obtained by staging laparotomy followed by mantle field RT (40 Gy). Another important finding was that the overall outcome had gradually improved over the years (Fig. 10.1).

**Table 10.2** Early-stage favorable HL: selection of randomized studies of radiotherapy alone

| Trial | Year | Study arms | Number of patients | Outcome | Overall survival | Reference |
|---|---|---|---|---|---|---|
| EORTC H1 | 1964–1971 | A. Mantle field or inverted Y RT B. The same RT followed by vinblastine | 288 | A. 38% DFS (15 years) B. 60% DFS (15 years) $p < 0.001$ | A. 58% OS (15 years) B. 65% OS (15 years) $p = 0.15$ (NS) | Tubiana et al. [17] |
| EORTC H2 | 1972–1976 | A. Laparotomy and mantle field+para-aortic lymph node RT B. STNI | 300 | A. 76% DFS (12 years) B. 68% DFS (12 years) $p = 0.18$ (NS) | A. 79% OS (12 years) B. 77% OS (12 years) $p = 0.38$ (NS) | Tubiana et al. [16, 18] |
| EORTC H5F | 1977–1982 | Laparotomy negative patients: A. Mantle field RT B. STNI | 198 | A. 69% DFS (9 years) B. 70% DFS (9 years) $p > 0.50$ (NS) | A. 94% OS (9 years) B. 91% OS (9 years) $p > 0.50$ (NS) | Carde et al. [19] |
| EORTC H6F | 1982–1987 | A. Laparotomy, if negative: Mantle field RT for LP or NSc histology STNI for MC or LD histology B. STNI | 262 | A. 84% RFS (6 years) B. 80% RFS (6 years) $p = 0.25$ (NS) | A. 89% OS (6 years) B. 93% OS (6 years) $p = 0.24$ (NS) | Carde et al. [20] |
| EORTC H7VF-H8VF | 1988–1993 | Mantle field RT | 40 | RFS 73% (6 years) | OS 95% (6 years) | Noordijk et al. [22], abstract |
| GHSG HD4 | 1988–1994 | A. STNI 40 Gy B. STNI 30 Gy+IFRT 10 Gy | 376 | A. 78% RFS (7 years) B. 83% RFS (7 years) $p = 0.093$ (NS) | A. 91% OS (7 years) B. 96% OS (7 years) $p = 0.16$ (NS) | Dühmke et al. [21] |

*EORTC* European Organization for Research and Treatment of Cancer; *GHSG* German Hodgkin Study Group; *DFS* disease-free survival; *OS* overall survival; *RFS* relapse-free survival; *STNI* subtotal nodal irradiation; *RT* radiotherapy; *IFRT* involved-field radiotherapy; *Gy* Gray; *NS* not significant; *LP* lymphocyte predominant; *NSc* nodular sclerosing; *MC* mixed cellularity; *LD* lymphocyte depleted

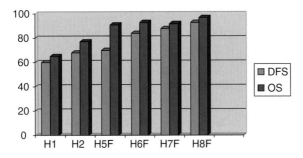

**Fig. 10.1** Disease-free survival and overall survival in consecutive EORTC Lymphoma Group trials on early-stage favorable Hodgkin lymphoma (HL). *DFS* disease-free survival; *OS* overall survival

The total radiation dose in these EORTC trials was always 40 Gy. The HD4 trial of the GHSG tested the hypothesis that dose reduction from 40 to 30 Gy in the extended field would be possible without a clinically relevant increase in the recurrence rate [21]. All patients ($n=376$) with pathologically staged stage I or II without adverse prognostic factors received 40 Gy radiation dose to the involved field, but were randomly assigned to receive either 40 or 30 Gy to the noninvolved extended field. The 7-year relapse-free and overall survival rates did not differ (78 vs. 83% and 91 vs. 96%, respectively). Hence, 30 Gy seems a sufficient dose for treating subclinical involvement of HL with RT alone.

Radiation in mantle field technique can potentially cause less long-term toxicity compared with STNI. However, in clinically staged patients, results with mantle irradiation alone have been disappointing. In the EORTC H7-VF and H8-VF trials, 40 female patients were treated with mantle field RT only. The respective prognostic factors were stage IA, aged <40 years, nodular sclerosing or lymphocyte predominant histology, and ESR <50 mm/h. These patients were expected to have a very low risk of occult abdominal involvement (5%). The relapse-free survival was however lower than expected: a total of 23% had relapsed at 6 years [22]. Because of this unacceptable rate, the very favorable subgroup has since been treated according to the EORTC strategy for the favorable subgroup.

Specht et al. reported on the influence of radiation field size on long-term outcome in early stage disease in a meta-analysis of eight randomized trials evaluating larger vs. smaller radiation fields [23]. These trials included almost 2,000 patients with both favorable and unfavorable prognosis stage I–II disease. A definite and substantial reduction in the risk of treatment failure was demonstrated if more extensive radiotherapy was

used. The 10-year risk of recurrence was 43% for patients treated with smaller-field irradiation compared to 31% for those treated with larger-field radiation therapy. The size of reduction in risk for failure in patients with different stages of disease, with and without B-symptoms, of different ages and staged with and without laparotomy was remarkably similar. Although the additional radiotherapy prevented a substantial proportion of recurrences, it did not significantly affect overall mortality. The lack of survival difference suggests that salvage chemotherapy for relapse after initial radiotherapy is effective enough to minimize the impact of any increase in relapse on survival.

To summarize, STNI was considered standard treatment for early favorable HL until the 1990s. However, 25–30% of patients eventually relapsed with subsequent 10-year survival rates of only 63% [24].

## 10.4 Late Treatment Effects and Mortality

As the number of patients surviving HL increased and there was longer follow-up, it became evident that their life expectancy did not revert completely to that of the age-matched general population. The higher mortality of HL patients is largely a result of the long-term effects of treatment. Important late effects comprise secondary malignancies, cardiovascular diseases, pulmonary problems, gonadal dysfunction, infectious complications, and fatigue. The incidence of the most life-threatening late side effects, i.e., secondary cancers and cardiovascular diseases, is significantly related to the radiation dose and field size, choice of cytostatic drugs, and total amount of drugs administered.

In patients with early favorable disease, mortality from causes other than HL has increased over time, exceeding HL-related mortality after 10–15 years [25, 26]. A large study with a median follow-up of more than 17 years examined case-specific mortality and absolute excess mortality, compared to population rates, in a cohort of 1,261 Dutch patients [25]. These patients were younger than 40 years when treated between 1965 and 1987. HL was the most frequent cause of death (55%), followed by secondary malignancies (22%) and cardiovascular diseases (9%). In the first 10 years following initial treatment, the excess mortality rate is largely due to the primary disease, while after 10 years causes other than HL contribute most to excess mortality. The actuarial risk

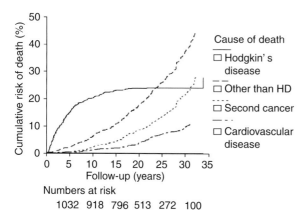

**Fig. 10.2** The actuarial risks of death from major disease categories in 1,261 Dutch HL patients. Data from Dutch database on Hodgkin lymphoma (Reprinted from [25] with permission)

**Table 10.3** Chemotherapy regimens used in early-stage favorable HL

| Regimen | Drug combinations |
|---|---|
| ABVD | Doxorubicin, vinblastine, bleomycin, dacarbazine |
| EBVP | Epirubicin, bleomycin, vinblastine, prednisone |
| MOPP | Mechlorethamine, vincristine, procarbazine, prednisone |
| MOPP/ABV | Mechlorethamine, vincristine, procarbazine, prednisone, doxorubicin, bleomycin, vinblastine |
| Stanford V | Vinblastine, doxorubicin, vincristine, bleomycin, mechlorethamine, etoposide, prednisone |
| VBM | Vinblastine, methotrexate, bleomycine |

of death is shown in Fig. 10.2. Even after 30 years of follow-up, there was no evidence of a decline in the relative risk of death from causes other than HL. In 30-year survivors, the annual excess mortality rate from all causes other than HL was nearly 3 per 100 patients. Solid tumors, especially in the digestive and respiratory tract, contributed most to this excess risk, followed by cardiovascular diseases [25]. Recently, the EORTC and the GELA published their results of a study analyzing the cause-specific excess mortality in adult patients with respect to treatment modality [27]. The study population consisted of 4,401 patients aged 15–69 in all stages, who were treated between 1964 and 2000. In patients with early stage disease, the overall excess mortality was associated with age $\geq$40 years ($p=0.007$), male gender ($p<0.001$), unfavorable prognostic features ($p<0.001$), treatment with EBVP (epirubicin, bleomycin, vinblastine, prednisone) plus IFRT ($p=0.002$), and mantle field irradiation alone ($p=0.003$). Therefore, excess mortality was linked to treatment modalities that were associated with poor failure-free survival resulting in a higher need for salvage treatment. Late treatment effects are covered in more detail in Chaps. 22, 23, 24, and 25.

## 10.5  Combined Modality Treatment

With the observation of high relapse rates and fatal long-term effects, most study groups abandoned STNI and EFRT from the treatment of early stage HL.

Studies were developed in an attempt to reduce long-term toxicity without increasing disease-specific mortality. Most randomized studies evaluated CMT in an attempt to define the optimal chemotherapy, number of cycles needed, as well as radiation field size and dose when combined with chemotherapy. Commonly used regimen and drug combinations are listed in Table 10.3.

### 10.5.1  Radiotherapy Alone vs. CMT

The high relapse rates after treatment with radiotherapy alone prompted several groups to study CMT as induction therapy. An earlier meta-analysis of individual patient data showed that CMT reduced the relapse risk compared with radiotherapy alone, but did not improve overall survival [23]. Most of the trials included in this analysis were conducted between 1967 and 1988 using MOPP or MOPP-like regimens, which produced unacceptable hematologic toxicity, frequently induced secondary malignancies, and rendered most recipients infertile. These studies were therefore only of historical interest and will not be discussed further. Later, based mainly on results of studies in advanced HL, the ABVD regimen became the standard of care in early favorable HL. When compared with MOPP, ABVD had a better efficacy and produced less toxicity [28]. In particular, secondary leukemias and infertility are less frequently observed than after alkylating-agent-containing regimens.

Two randomized studies, one in Europe and one in the United States, showed the benefit of adjuvant chemotherapy with a short course of ABVD or ABVD-like chemotherapy in early favorable patients: GHSG HD7 trial compared EFRT alone with CMT consisting of two cycles ABVD followed by EFRT in 650 early favorable patients [12]. A significant advantage in freedom from treatment failure (FFTF) was seen after CMT, mainly related to fewer relapses as compared with EFRT only (3 vs. 22%). There were no differences in overall survival between treatment arms. Importantly, with a median follow-up of 87 months, CMT was not associated with significantly more acute or long-term toxicity. The US trial included more than 300 patients and confirmed the benefit of adjuvant radiotherapy given after a short course of limited chemotherapy in clinically staged IA and IIA patients [29]. The study showed that three cycles of doxorubicin and vinblastine (AV) followed by STNI were well tolerated and gave a superior failure-free survival compared with STNI alone. The conclusion from these two studies is that the number of relapses can be reduced by the addition of ABVD or ABVD-like chemotherapy to large radiation fields. However, these extensive radiation fields can cause severe late side effects.

In a small randomized US trial, the VBM regimen was combined with mantle field radiotherapy and produced comparable results to STNI in clinically favorable stage I–II patients [30]. However, VBM was later abandoned due to concern of pulmonary toxicity. The Group Pierre-et-Marie-Curie showed that it was possible to replace the classic mantle field irradiation by a more limited radiotherapy to initially involved areas only. This novel approach termed IFRT involved the addition of chemotherapy to control occult disease in uninvolved areas [31]. IFRT reduced the irradiation of normal tissues, such as breast, heart, and lungs.

Therefore, several groups performed randomized trials comparing STNI with a combined modality approach in which patients received smaller radiation fields and combination chemotherapy. The results of a selection of some of the largest trials are listed in Table 10.4.

In the EORTC H7F trial in 333 patients with early favorable disease, six cycles of EBVP were followed by IFRT and randomly compared with STNI [32]. EBVP was assumed to be potentially less toxic but similarly effective compared to ABVD. There were significantly more treatment failures in the STNI arm, especially in non-irradiated lower abdominal and extranodal areas. EBVP combined with IFRT proved to be

effective in these favorable patients; the 10-year event-free survival rate after EBVP and IFRT was 10% better than after STNI alone, whereas overall survival was 92% in both arms. This trial demonstrated that EFRT could be replaced by CMT including IFRT. However, in early unfavorable patients, EBVP was significantly less efficient than MOPP/ABV [32]. Randomized comparisons of EBVP and ABVD have not been performed.

In the subsequent H8F trial by the EORTC-GELA, more than 500 favorable HL patients were randomized between STNI or CMT consisting of three cycles of MOPP/ABV hybrid followed by IFRT [11]. Patients in the CMT arm had a lower relapse rate, which resulted in a significantly higher event-free survival rate than for patients in the STNI arm (93 vs. 68% at 10 years). Importantly, patients in the combined modality arm also had a significantly higher overall survival than patients in the STNI arm (97 vs. 92% at 10 years) (see Fig. 10.3). The results of this study again demonstrated the superiority of CMT over EFRT alone and showed that IFRT is a sufficient treatment after chemotherapy for early favorable HL. However, due to its carcinogenic potential MOPP/ABV was abandoned in favor of ABVD. Therefore, this trial cannot be used to draw firm conclusions regarding the number of cycles of ABVD required as part of CMT.

## 10.5.2 Optimal Number of Cycles of Chemotherapy

The use of fewer cycles of ABVD could potentially reduce late side effects of combined-modality therapy. Between 1998 and 2003, the GHSG HD10 trial accrued more than 1,300 favorable prognosis stage I–II HL patients. Patients were randomized to four arms in a 2×2 factorial design: two cycles of ABVD followed by 30 Gy IFRT; two cycles of ABVD followed by 20 Gy IFRT; four cycles of ABVD followed by 30 Gy IFRT; and four cycles of ABVD followed by 20 Gy IFRT. This trial tested a possible reduction in the number of ABVD cycles as well as reduction of radiation dose when using IFRT. The final analysis of this trial was presented at the 2009 American Society of Hematology Congress: with a median follow-up of 79–91 months, there were no significant differences in FFTF and overall survival between four or two cycles

**Table 10.4** Early-stage favorable HL: selection of studies comparing STNI alone with combined modality treatment (CMT)

| Trial | Year | Study arms | Number of patients | Outcome | Overall survival | Reference |
|---|---|---|---|---|---|---|
| SWOG/CALGB | 1989–2000 | A. STNI (36–40 Gy) B. 3 AV + STNI (36–40 Gy) | 326 | A. 81% FFS (3 years) B. 94% FFS (3 years) $p<0.001$ | Follow-up too short | Press et al. [29] |
| Stanford-Kaiser Permanente | 1988–1995 | A. STNI (30–44 Gy) B. 6 VBM + mantle field RT | 78[*] | A. 92% PFS (5 years) B. 87% PFS (5 years) $p=0.73$ (NS) | A. 98% OS (5 years) B. 94% OS (5 years) $p=0.50$ (NS) | Horning et al. [30] |
| EORTC H7F | 1988–1993 | A. STNI (36 Gy) B. 6 EBVP + IFRT (36 Gy) | 333 | A. 78% EFS (10 years) B. 88% EFS (10 years) $p=0.0113$ | A. 92% OS (10 years) B. 92% OS (10 years) $p=0.79$ (NS) | Noordijk et al. [32] |
| EORTC/ GELA H8F | 1993–1999 | A. STNI (36 Gy) B. 3 MOPP/ABV + IFRT (36 Gy) | 542 | A. 68% EFS (10 years)B. 93% EFS (10 years) $p<0.001$ | A. 92% OS (10 years) B. 97% OS (10 years) $p=0.001$ | Fermé et al. [11] |
| GHSG HD7 | 1994–1998 | A. EFRT 30 Gy (IFRT 40 Gy) B. 2 ABVD + EFRT 30 Gy (IFRT 40 Gy) | 627 | A. 67% FFTF (7 years) B. 88% FFTF (7 years) $p<0.0001$ | A. 92% OS (7 years) B. 94% OS (7 years) $p=0.43$ (NS) | Engert et al. [12] |

*SWOG* Southwest Oncology Group; *CALGB* Cancer and Leukemia; *EORTC* European Organization for Research and Treatment of Cancer; *GELA* Groupe d'Etude des Lymphomes de l'Adulte; *GHSG* German Hodgkin Study Group; *STNI* subtotal nodal irradiation; *IFRT* involved-field radiotherapy; *EFRT* extended-field radiotherapy; *Gy* Gray; *FFS* failure-free survival; *PFS* progression-free survival; *EFS* event-free survival; *FFTF* freedom from treatment failure; *OS* overall survival; *NS* not significant

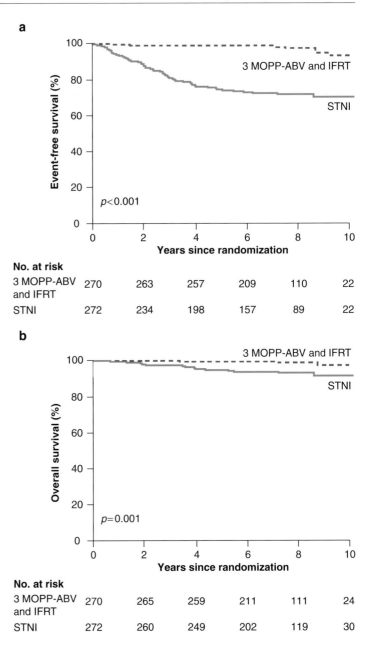

**Fig. 10.3** Kaplan–Meier estimates of event-free and overall survival among 542 patients with a favorable prognosis in the EORTC/GELA H8F trial. At 10 years, event-free survival was 93% in the group that received MOPP-ABV-IFRT and 68% in the STNI group ($p<0.001$) (**a**), and overall survival was 97 and 92%, respectively ($p=0.001$) (**b**). (Reprinted from [11] with permission)

of ABVD. In addition, there was also no difference between 30 and 20 Gy IFRT [33]. Importantly, there was also no significant difference in terms of overall survival, FFTF, and progression-free survival when all four arms were compared. The treatment arms with four cycles of ABVD and 30 Gy IFRT showed significantly more acute toxicity in comparison with two cycles of ABVD and 20 Gy IFRT. Two cycles of ABVD followed by 20 Gy IFRT is thus the new GHSG standard of care for HL patients in early favorable stages.

### 10.5.3 Optimal Chemotherapy Combination

Reduction of chemotherapy-induced toxicity is being pursued in the ongoing GHSG HD13 trial. This trial investigated whether drugs can be omitted from the ABVD regimen and randomized patients with early favorable HL to two cycles of either ABVD, AVD, ABV, or AV with all arms followed by 30 Gy IFRT. After the preliminary analysis in 2006, the ABV and AV arms were closed due to increased number of events (relapses and progressions). Therefore, it seems that dacarbazine is an important therapeutic agent in ABVD that cannot be deleted. Accrual for the ABVD and AVD arms were continued, exploring the role of bleomycin in the ABVD regimen (Engert 2009, personal communication).

The 12-week chemotherapy program, Stanford V, including radiotherapy to bulky lymphoma sites, is highly effective in locally extensive and advanced HL with 5-year freedom from progression of 89% and 5-year overall survival of 96% [34]. This regimen combines vinblastine, doxorubicin, vincristine, bleomycin, mechlorethamine, etoposide, and prednisone. A modified 8-week version, in which mechlorethamine was replaced by cyclophosphamide and the radiotherapy dose reduced to 20–30 Gy, is currently under study in phase II for stage I or IIA non-bulky HL in the United States.

## 10.5.4  Optimal Radiation Dose

Apart from the choice of cytostatic agents and the number of courses, the question of radiation field size and dose has also been evaluated (for a selection of randomized trials, see Table 10.5). A decline in late complications is expected with lower radiation doses as their incidence is correlated with the amount of radiation given.

Two randomized trials have investigated radiation doses in early favorable HL patients treated with CMT. In the EORTC/GELA H9F trial, 783 patients with stage I–II disease and favorable characteristics received six cycles of EBVP. Patients in complete remission after chemotherapy were randomized to receive standard dose IFRT (36 Gy), low-dose IFRT (20 Gy), or no RT at all. This trial thus evaluated the role of IFRT and potential differences in the radiation dose delivered. The experimental arm without RT was closed early due to an excess failure rate compared with the two RT arms: only 70% event-free survival at 4 years for the non-RT arm vs. 84 and 87% for the 20 and 36 Gy IFRT arms, respectively [35]. Therefore, it can be concluded that in favorable patients who achieve a complete remission after six cycles of EBVP, omission of IFRT leads to an unacceptable failure rate. Although no differences in outcome were reported between the two radiation dose levels, follow-up is too short to draw definite conclusions, including those on late effects.

As discussed in Sect. 10.5.2, the GHSG HD10 trial compared doses of 30 and 20 Gy IFRT after two or four cycles of ABVD. No significant differences were observed between patients receiving 30 Gy IFRT and 20 Gy IFRT in terms of overall survival (97.6 vs. 97.5%), FFTF (93.4 vs. 92.9%) and progression-free survival (93.7 vs. 93.2%), respectively [33]. Therefore, IFRT with a dose of 20 Gy seems to be sufficient after two cycles of ABVD.

## 10.5.5  Optimal Radiation Field Size

The rationale for reduced radiation therapy field size is to further improve the therapeutic ratio. Smaller radiation fields should also lead to a decrease in late complications such as cardiovascular and secondary cancers as the amount of irradiated normal tissue was reduced. Several randomized trials in early unfavorable HL have shown that after effective chemotherapy, IFRT is as effective as EFRT in terms of overall survival and FFTF [11, 36]. However, data from randomized trials in patients with early favorable HL are scarce.

Bonadonna et al. reported the long-term follow-up of 133 patients with early HL randomly assigned to IFRT or STNI after four cycles of ABVD and found no significant differences in overall survival (94 vs. 96%) or freedom from progression (94 vs. 93%) at 12 years [37] (see Table 10.5). The limited size of the patient sample, however, had no adequate statistical power to test for non-inferiority of IFRT vs. STNI.

Is it possible to further reduce the field size beyond IFRT? Based on the observation that in patients treated with chemotherapy alone, recurrences typically occur in sites of initial nodal involvement, the EORTC-GELA group introduced the concept of involved-node radiotherapy (INRT) [38, 39]. INRT only includes the initially involved lymph nodes with a small isotropic margin. Identifying and contouring involved lymph nodes is of outmost importance. Therefore, it is recommended that all patients have cervical and thoracic CT scans pre- and post-chemotherapy, preferably in the treatment position, and must be examined by the radiation oncologist before start of the chemotherapy [38, 40]. Better sparing of normal tissues such as salivary glands, heart, coronary arteries, and breast in female patients, is expected with the use of INRT compared to IFRT (Fig. 10.4). The new INRT concept is applied in the current EORTC-GELA

**Table 10.5** Early-stage favorable HL: selection of studies of RT field size and dose in CMT

| Trial | Year | Study arms | Number of patients | Outcome | Overall survival | Reference |
|---|---|---|---|---|---|---|
| Milan | 1990–1997 | A. 4 ABVD+STNI 36–40 Gy<br>B. 4 ABVD+IFRT 36–40 Gy | 133 | A. FFP 93% (12-years)<br>B. FFP 94% (12-years) | A. OS 96% (12-years)<br>B. OS 94% (12-years) | Bonadonna et al. [37] |
| EORTC/GELA H9F | 1998–2004 | A. 6 EBVP+IFRT 36 Gy<br>B. 6 EBVP+IFRT 20 Gy<br>C. 6 EBVP (no RT)<br>median follow-up 33 months | 783 | A. EFS 87% (4-years)<br>B. EFS 84% (4-years)<br>C. EFS 70% (4-years)<br>no RT arm closed because of excess failure rate ($p < 0.001$) | A. OS 98% (4-years)<br>B. OS 98% (4-years)<br>C. OS 98% (4-years) | Noordijk et al. [35], abstract |
| GHSG HD10 | 1998–2003 | A. 2 ABVD+IFRT 30 Gy<br>B. 2 ABVD+IFRT 20 Gy<br>C. 4 ABVD+IFRT 30 Gy<br>D. 4 ABVD+IFRT 20 Gy<br>median follow-up 91 months | 1,370 | No differences in FFTF between patients given two or four cycles of ABVD or 20 or 30 Gy IFRT (FFTF 91–93%) | No survival differences between patients given two or four cycles of ABVD or 20 or 30 Gy IFRT (OS 96–97%) | Engert et al. [33], abstract |

*EORTC* European Organization for Research and Treatment of Cancer; *GELA* Groupe d'Etude des Lymphomes de l'Adulte; *GHSG* German Hodgkin Study Group; *STNI* subtotal nodal irradiation; *IFRT* involved-field radiation; *RT* radiotherapy; *Gy* Gray; *FFP* freedom from progression; *OS* overall survival; *EFS* event-free survival; *FFTF* freedom from treatment failure

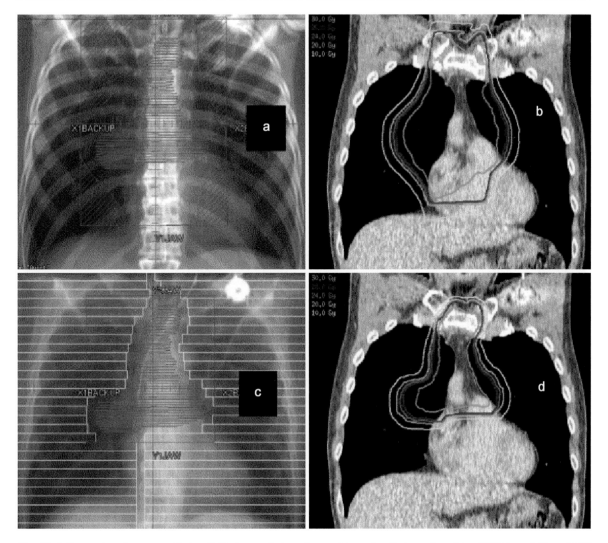

**Fig. 10.4** Comparison between radiation field sizes and the volume of heart irradiation using either IFRT (**a** and **b**) or INRT (**c** and **d**) for a mediastinal tumor mass (PTV in *red color*). (Reprinted from [38] with permission)

H10 randomized trial for patients with early stage HL (see Fig. 10.5 for the trial design).

Canadian researchers reported promising results with INRT in a retrospective study, although the definition of INRT was not exactly the same as that of the EORTC-GELA Group and a greater radiation margin was applied [41]. In British Columbia, patients with limited stage HL, defined as stage IA or IIA with tumor bulk less than 10 cm are treated according to province-wide guidelines consisting of combined chemotherapy and radiation therapy. The extent of the radiation therapy field size underwent serial changes during the last decades, from EFRT to IFRT and eventually since 2001 to INRT with margins from 1.5 to 5 cm. There

were no statistically significant differences among the three groups for progression-free survival and overall survival. There were also no marginal recurrences in the INRT patient group [41]. Clearly, the exact definition of INRT is still in evolution and requires further investigation prior to its incorporation into routine practice.

## 10.6  Chemotherapy Alone

The potentially life-threatening late side effects of radiotherapy for HL patients have raised the question

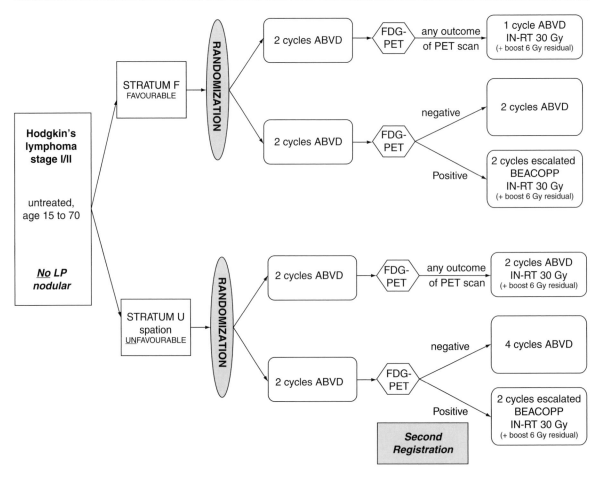

**Fig. 10.5** Design EORTC/GELA/ILL H10 trial for early-stage HL

whether those in early stage disease can be treated with chemotherapy alone. This question is particularly relevant for patients in whom the risk of RT-induced toxicity is deemed less acceptable. Chemotherapy-only protocols have been successfully used in children and adolescents (see Chap. 15 on pediatric HL). However, few data exist on their role in adults. Table 10.6 shows a selection of randomized trials performed in adult patients with early favorable HL dealing with the issue of chemotherapy alone. These trials encountered a number of problems with design, patient accrual, as well as variations in the type of chemotherapy and field size of radiation therapy utilized.

The use of chemotherapy alone is not a new concept. Two randomized trials published in the early 1990s compared MOPP as first-line therapy in early stage HL with radiotherapy: a preliminary analysis of a small randomized US trial in laparotomy-staged

patients suggested that MOPP alone was at least as effective as radiation in a subset of patients with more favorable prognostic features [42]. Another small trial from Italy performed in laparotomy-staged early favorable and unfavorable patients showed a very low overall survival at 8 years after MOPP (56%) compared with 93% in the EFRT arm, whereas freedom from progression- and relapse-free survival were similar in both groups. In contrast to the US study, the rescue rate of patients who relapsed after MOPP was significantly lower than that observed after radiotherapy [43]. However, the two studies are not comparable, because of the distinct criteria adopted for the selection of patients.

The National Cancer Institute of Canada (NCI-C) and the Eastern Cooperative Oncology Group (ECOG) conducted a randomized phase III trial addressing the role of chemotherapy alone (ABVD) for early favorable

**Table 10.6** Early-stage favorable HL: selection of randomized studies of chemotherapy alone in adult patients

| Trial | Year | Study arms | Number of patients | Outcome | Overall survival | Reference |
|---|---|---|---|---|---|---|
| NCI-US | 1978–1989 | A. 6–8 MOPP<br>B. Radiotherapy | 84 | A. DFS 82% (10-years)<br>B. DFS 67% (10-years)<br>$p$=NS | A. OS 90% (10-years)<br>B. OS 85% (10-years)<br>$p$=NS | Longo et al. [42] |
| Rome-Florence | 1979–1982 | A. Mantle field + para-aortic RT (36–44 Gy)<br>B. 6 MOPP | 89 | A. RFS 70% (8-years)<br>B. RFS 71% (8-years)<br>$p$=NS | A. OS 93% (8-years)<br>B. OS 56% (8-years)<br>$p$<0.001 | Biti et al. [43] |
| NCI-C/ECOG HD6 | 1994–2002 | A. 4–6 ABVD<br>B. STNI | 123 | A. EFS 87% (5-years)<br>B. EFS 88% (5-years)<br>$p$=0.6 (NS) | A. OS 97% (5-years)<br>B. OS 100% (5-years)<br>$p$=0.3 (NS) | Meyer et al. [44] |
| EORTC/GELA H9F | 1998–2004 | A. 6 EBVP+IFRT 36 Gy<br>B. 6 EBVP+IFRT 20 Gy<br>C. 6 EBVP (no RT)<br>median follow-up 33 months | 783 | A. EFS 87% (4-years)<br>B. EFS 84% (4-years)<br>C. EFS 70% (4-years)<br>no RT arm closed because of excess failure rate ($p$<0.001) | A. OS 98% (4-years)<br>B. OS 98% (4-years)<br>C. OS 98% (4-years) | Noordijk et al. [35], abstract |
| Memorial Sloan-Kettering Cancer Centre | 1990–2000 | A. 6 x ABVD<br>B. 6 x ABVD+RT | 152 | A. FFP 81% (5-years)<br>B. FFP 86% (5-years)<br>$p$=0.61 (NS) | A. OS 90% (5-years)<br>B. OS 97% (5-years)<br>$p$=0.08 (NS) | Strauss et al. [45] |

*NCI-US* National Cancer Institute United States; *EORTC* European Organization for Research and Treatment of Cancer; *NCI-C* National Cancer Institute of Canada; *ECOG* Eastern Cooperative Oncology Group; *GELA* Groupe d'Etude des Lymphomes de l'Adulte; *STNI* subtotal nodal irradiation; *IFRT* involved-field radiotherapy; *RT* radiotherapy; *Gy* Gray; *NS* not significant; *FFP* freedom from progression; *OS* overall survival; *DFS* disease-free survival; *RFS* relapse-free survival; *EFS* event-free survival and unfavorable HL. Favorable patients had following characteristics: age <40 years, ESR <50 mm/h, lymphocyte predominant or nodular sclerosing histology, no bulky disease, and less than four nodal sites involved. The experimental arm consisted of four cycles of ABVD alone if a complete remission was achieved after two cycles. Otherwise, patients received six cycles. The standard arm was STNI with 35 Gy. Among the favorable-risk patients, there was no difference between the two arms for event-free survival, freedom from disease progression, and overall survival after a median follow-up of 4.2 years [44]. However, longer follow-up is needed to determine late toxicities.

Only two randomized trials comparing CMT with chemotherapy alone in early favorable patients have been published. As discussed in Sect. 10.5.4, one was the EORTC-GELA H9F trial in which IFRT in 36 Gy was compared with 20 Gy or no radiotherapy in CR patients after six cycles of EBVP. The chemotherapy-only arm was prematurely closed due to an excessive number of relapses [35].

The Memorial Sloan-Kettering Cancer Centre randomized early non-bulky HL patients between six cycles of ABVD alone and six cycles of ABVD plus 36 Gy radiotherapy. Of the 76 patients randomized to radiotherapy, 11 received IFRT; the rest received modified EFRT. Due to the poor accrual rate, the trial was closed before completion and only 152 patients were randomized. No significant differences were observed between CMT and chemotherapy alone, but the sample size was insufficient [45].

From the abovementioned trials, it can be concluded that no published data are available on randomized trials testing the question of treatment with ABVD alone in comparison with the current standard treatment of ABVD plus IFRT in adult favorable early stage patients. Therefore, in these patients the use of chemotherapy alone outside of a clinical trial should be reserved for the few patients with contraindications to radiation therapy or those that refuse radiation therapy.

## 10.7 Treatment Adaptation Based on PET Scan Response

PET is becoming an important tool for staging and response assessment in HL (see Chap. 6). Functional imaging with FDG-PET enables evaluation of early metabolic changes rather than the morphologic changes occurring later during treatment. Several studies using PET after two or three cycles of ABVD have shown that early metabolic changes are predictive of the final treatment response and progression-free survival [5, 46–48]. Most studies with early interim PET were performed in patients with advanced stages. A negative interim PET has been associated with an event-free survival of 90% and higher, whereas a positive interim PET has been associated with event-free survival of only 0–13%. The negative predictive value of interim PET in HL is high with 94–100% rates reported on relatively short follow-up. However, the positive predictive value of interim PET has varied from 61 to 100% [49]. This understanding has led to the use of PET scanning for early treatment response assessment as surrogate test of chemosensitivity. Given that a substantial fraction of patients with early favorable HL might currently be overtreated, there is potential benefit in identifying patients who might be eligible for less intensive treatment. However, reduction of treatment based on negative interim PET has not been proven safe yet. Likewise, no data exist to support the hypothesis that intensification of therapy based on a positive interim PET improves the clinical outcome.

Several large randomized controlled trials have incorporated PET response-adapted therapy into their designs. Three ongoing trials currently investigate the effect of reducing treatment intensity by omitting radiotherapy for patients with negative interim PET. Moreover, in one of these trials the treatment is intensified in patients with a positive interim PET. The ongoing NCRI Lymphoma Group RAPID trial in the UK treats all patients with early HL with three ABVD cycles, followed by PET restaging. PET negative patients are randomized between 30 Gy IFRT or no radiotherapy, while PET positive patients receive a fourth ABVD cycle followed by IFRT. The GHSG HD16 trial in early favorable patients compares 20 Gy IFRT after two cycles of ABVD with no further treatment. All PET positive patients will receive 20 Gy IFRT. The ongoing EORTC/GELA/ILL (Intergruppo Italiano dei Linfomi) H10F trial is comparing a standard arm consisting of three cycles of ABVD followed by INRT with an experimental arm in which treatment is guided by early PET (see Fig. 10.5). Those with a negative PET after two cycles of ABVD receive another two cycles of ABVD and no radiotherapy. In contrast, patients with positive PET after two cycles of ABVD receive treatment intensification with two cycles of BEACOPP escalated followed by INRT.

Although the prognostic value of PET is established for HL patients, the results of these trials must be awaited before interim PET scan results can safely be used for treatment adaptation.

## 10.8  Recommendations and Future Directions

In most parts of the world, CMT strategies including two to three cycles of ABVD followed by 20–30 Gy IFRT is the current standard treatment for patients with early favorable HL. With this approach, FFTF rates of more than 90% and an overall survival of nearly 95% are reached. HL-related death is unusual and mortality is mainly due to late toxicity. Even strategies that provide very high freedom from recurrence may not be optimal, since, depending on the strategy used, treatment-related mortality at 10–20 years may exceed HL mortality in this low risk group. Therefore, choice of a given strategy must not only be judged by the tumor control, but also weighed against acute and chronic morbidities. In this respect, new criteria such as quality of life are also becoming more important [50].

Over the last decades, several strategies have attempted to reduce late complications in HL patients by giving less chemotherapy or radiotherapy. It should be realized that most long-term results are not known yet. Therefore, it remains to be seen which strategy provides the best balance between treatment efficacy and toxicity. At present, the goal in early favorable HL is to maintain the excellent efficacy with as little complications as possible. One of the key questions in early favorable HL is which patients might be safely treated with chemotherapy alone. Risk-adapted and response-adapted approaches based on results of interim PET are being evaluated. As this is a relatively new focus, the optimal strategy is probably not yet defined [51].

In summary, it is clear that HL is the ultimate type of malignancy in which the consecutive improvement in outcome was achieved by carefully planned subsequent prospective phase III randomized clinical trials performed by the various lymphoma groups throughout the world. The challenge for the next decade is to focus on targeted treatment, thereby preventing early and late toxicities due to damage of normal tissues by the cytostatic agents and radiation employed. In this respect, a variety of new developments in the treatment arena are currently recognized, among others targeting the microenvironment in HL, developing and testing new antibodies which specifically target Reed–Sternberg cells, and exploring a number of small molecules interfering with specific signal pathways that maintain the proliferation of Hodgkin cells, etc. These and future strategies are all based on better insight into the molecular pathology of HL. Further intensification of translational research is therefore of utmost importance, to provide our patients with patient-tailored treatment leading to the highest possible cure rates and at the same time preventing major toxic side effects.

## References

1. Carbone PP, Kaplan HS, Musshoff K, Smithers DW, Tubiana M. Report of the committee on Hodgkin's disease staging classification. Cancer Res. 1971;31:1860–1.
2. Lister TA, Crowther D, Sutcliffe SB, Glatstein E, Canellos GP, Young RC, et al. Report of a committee convened to discuss the evaluation and staging of patients with Hodgkin's disease: Cotswolds meeting. J Clin Oncol. 1989;7:1630–6.
3. Munker R, Hasenclever D, Brosteanu O, Hiller E, Diehl V; German Hodgkin's Lymphoma Study Group. Bone marrow involvement in Hodgkin's disease: an analysis of 135 consecutive cases. J Clin Oncol. 1995;13:403–9.
4. Hutchings M, Eigtved AI, Specht L. FDG-PET in the clinical management of HL. Crit Rev Oncol Hematol. 2004;52:19–32.
5. Hutchings M, Loft A, Hansen M, Pedersen LM, Berthelsen AK, Keiding S, et al. Position emission tomography with or without computed tomography in the primary staging of Hodgkin's lymphoma. Haematologica. 2006;91:482–9.
6. Juweid ME (2006) Utility of positron emission tomography (PET) scanning in managing patients with HL. Hematology Am Soc Hematol Educ Program. 259–65.
7. Juweid ME, Stroobants S, Hoekstra OS, Mottaghy FM, Dietlein M, Guermazi A, et al. Use of positron emission tomography for response assessment of lymphoma: consensus of the Imaging Subcommittee of International Harmonization Project in Lymphoma. J Clin Oncol. 2007;25:571–8.
8. Specht L, Nissen NI. Hodgkin's disease stages I and II with infradiaphragmatic presentation: a rare and prognostically unfavourable combination. Eur J Haematol. 1988;40:396–402.
9. Specht L. Prognostic factors in Hodgkin's disease. Semin Radiat Oncol. 1996;6:146–61.
10. Tubiana M, Henry-Amar M, van der Werf-Messing B, Henry J, Abbatucci J, Burgers M, et al. A multivariate analysis of prognostic factors in early stage Hodgkin's disease. Int J Radiat Oncol Biol Phys. 1985;11:23–30.

11. Fermé C, Eghbali H, Meerwaldt JH, Rieux C, Bosq J, Berger F, et al. Chemotherapy plus involved-field radiation in early stage Hodgkin's disease. N Engl J Med. 2007;357: 1916–27.

12. Engert A, Franklin J, Eich HT, Brillant C, Sehlen S, Cartoni C, et al. Two cycles of doxorubicin, bleomycin, vinblastine, and dacarbazine plus extended-field radiotherapy is superior to radiotherapy alone in early favorable Hodgkin's lymphoma: final results of the GHSG HD7 trial. J Clin Oncol. 2007;25:3495–502.

13. Hoppe RT, Coleman CN, Cox RS, Rosenberg SA, Kaplan HS. The management of stage I–II Hodgkin's disease with irradiation alone or combined modality therapy: the Stanford experience. Blood. 1982;59:455–65.

14. Gospodarowicz MK, Sutcliffe SB, Clark RM, Dembo AJ, Fitzpatrick PJ, Munro AJ, et al. Analysis of supradiaphragmatic clinical stage I and II Hodgkin's disease treated with radiation alone. Int J Radiat Oncol Biol Phys. 1992;22:859–65.

15. Raemaekers J, Kluin-Nelemans H, Teodorovic I, Meerwaldt C, Noordijk E, Thomas J, et al. The achievements of the EORTC Lymphoma Group. European Organisation for Research and Treatment of Cancer. Eur J Cancer. 2002;38 Suppl 4: S107–13.

16. Tubiana M, Henry-Amar M, Carde P, Burgers JM, Hayat M, Van der Schueren E, et al. Toward comprehensive management tailored to prognostic factors of patients with clinical stages I and II in Hodgkin's disease. The EORTC Lymphoma Group controlled clinical trials: 1964-1987. Blood. 1989;73: 47–56.

17. Tubiana M, Henry-Amar M, Hayat M, Breur K, van der Werf-Messing B, Burgers M. Long-term results of the E.O.R.T.C. randomized study of irradiation and vinblastine in clinical stages I and II of Hodgkin's disease. Eur J Cancer. 1979;15:645–57.

18. Tubiana M, Hayat M, Henry-Amar M, Breur K, van der Werf MB, Burgers M. Five-year results of the E.O.R.T.C. randomized study of splenectomy and spleen irradiation in clinical stages I and II of Hodgkin's disease. Eur J Cancer. 1981;17:355–63.

19. Carde P, Burgers JM, Henry-Amar M, Hayat M, Sizoo W, Van der Schueren E, et al. Clinical stages I and II Hodgkin's disease: a specifically tailored therapy according to prognostic factors. J Clin Oncol. 1988;6:239–52.

20. Carde P, Hagenbeek A, Hayat M, Monconduit M, Thomas J, Burgers MJ, et al. Clinical staging versus laparotomy and combined modality with MOPP versus ABVD in early stage Hodgkin's disease: the H6 twin randomized trials from the European Organization for Research and Treatment of Cancer Lymphoma Cooperative Group. J Clin Oncol. 1993; 11:2258–72.

21. Dühmke E, Franklin J, Pfreundschuh M, Sehlen S, Willich N, Ruhl U, et al. Low-dose radiation is sufficient for the noninvolved extended-field treatment in favorable early stage Hodgkin's disease: long-term results of a randomized trial of radiotherapy alone. J Clin Oncol. 2001;19:2905–14.

22. Noordijk EM, Carde P, Hagenbeek A, Mandard AM, Kluin-Nelemans JC, Thomas J, et al. Combination of radiotherapy and chemotherapy is advisable in all patients with clinical stage I-II Hodgkin's disease six-year results of the EORTC-GPMC controlled clinical trials H7-VF, H7-F and H7-U. Int J Radiat Oncol Biol Phys. 1997;39:173.

23. Specht L, Gray RG, Clarke MJ, Peto R; International Hodgkin's Disease Collaborative Group. Influence of more extensive radiotherapy and adjuvant chemotherapy on long-term outcome of early stage Hodgkin's disease: a meta-analysis of 23 randomized trials involving 3,888 patients. J Clin Oncol 1998;16:830–43.

24. Horwich A, Specht L, Ashley S. Survival analysis of patients with clinical stages I or II Hodgkin's disease who have relapsed after initial treatment with radiotherapy alone. Eur J Cancer. 1997;33:848–53.

25. Aleman BM, van den Belt-Dusebout AW, Klokman WJ, Van't Veer MB, Bartelink H, van Leeuwen FE. Long-term cause-specific mortality of patients treated for Hodgkin's disease. J Clin Oncol. 2003;21:3431–9.

26. Ng AK, Bernardo MP, Weller E, Backstrand KH, Silver B, Marcus KC, et al. Long-term survival and competing causes of death in patients with early stage Hodgkin's disease treated at age 50 or younger. J Clin Oncol. 2002;20:2101–8.

27. Favier O, Heutte N, Stamatoullas-Bastard A, Carde P, Van't Veer MB, Aleman BM, et al. Survival after HL: causes of death and excess mortality in patients treated in 8 consecutive trials. Cancer. 2009;115:1680–91.

28. Canellos GP, Anderson JR, Propert KJ, Nissen N, Cooper MR, Henderson ES, et al. Chemotherapy of advanced Hodgkin's disease with MOPP, ABVD, or MOPP alternating with ABVD. N Engl J Med. 1992;327:1478–84.

29. Press OW, LeBlanc M, Lichter AS, Grogan TM, Unger JM, Wasserman TH, et al. Phase III randomized intergroup trial of subtotal lymphoid irradiation versus doxorubicin, vinblastine, and subtotal lymphoid irradiation for stage IA to IIA Hodgkin's disease. J Clin Oncol. 2001;19:4238–44.

30. Horning SJ, Hoppe RT, Mason J, Brown BW, Hancock SL, Baer D, et al. Stanford-Kaiser Permanente G1 study for clinical stage I to IIA Hodgkin's disease: subtotal lymphoid irradiation versus vinblastine, methotrexate, and bleomycin chemotherapy and regional irradiation. J Clin Oncol. 1997; 15:1736–44.

31. Zittoun R, Audebert A, Hoerni B, Bernadou A, Krulik M, Rojouan J, et al. Extended versus involved fields irradiation combined with MOPP chemotherapy in early clinical stages of Hodgkin's disease. J Clin Oncol. 1985;3:207–14.

32. Noordijk EM, Carde P, Dupouy N, Hagenbeek A, Krol AD, Kluin-Nelemans JC, et al. Combined-modality therapy for clinical stage I or II Hodgkin's lymphoma: long-term results of the European Organisation for Research and Treatment of Cancer H7 randomized controlled trials. J Clin Oncol. 2006;24:3128–35.

33. Engert A, Diehl V, Pluetschow A, Eich H, Herrmann R, Doerken B, et al. Two cycles of ABVD followed by involved field radiotherapy with 20 Gray (Gy) is the new standard of care in the treatment of patients with early stage HL: Final analysis of the randomized German Hodgkin Study Group (GHSG) HD10. Blood. 2009;114:716.

34. Horning SJ, Hoppe RT, Breslin S, Bartlett NL, Brown BW, Rosenberg SA. Stanford V and radiotherapy for locally extensive and advanced Hodgkin's disease: mature results of a prospective clinical trial. J Clin Oncol. 2002;20:630–7.

35. Noordijk E, Thomas J, Ferme C, van't Veer M, Brice P, Divine M, et al. First results of the EORTC-GELA H9 randomized trials: the H9-F trial (comparing 3 radiation dose levels) and the H9-U trial (comparing 3 chemotherapy

schemes) in patients with favorable or unfavorable early stage Hodgkin's lymphoma (HL). J Clin Oncol. 2005; 23:6505.

36. Engert A, Schiller P, Josting A, Herrmann R, Koch P, Sieber M, et al. Involved-field radiotherapy is equally effective and less toxic compared with extended-field radiotherapy after four cycles of chemotherapy in patients with early stage unfavorable Hodgkin's lymphoma: results of the HD8 trial of the German Hodgkin's Lymphoma Study Group. J Clin Oncol. 2003;21:3601–8.

37. Bonadonna G, Bonfante V, Viviani S, Di Russo A, Villani F, Valagussa P. ABVD plus subtotal nodal versus involved-field radiotherapy in early stage Hodgkin's disease: long-term results. J Clin Oncol. 2004;22:2835–41.

38. Girinsky T, van der Maazen R, Specht L, Aleman B, Poortmans P, Lievens Y, et al. Involved-node radiotherapy (INRT) in patients with early HL: concepts and guidelines. Radiother Oncol. 2006;79:270–7.

39. Shahidi M, Kamangari N, Ashley S, Cunningham D, Horwich A. Site of relapse after chemotherapy alone for stage I and II Hodgkin's disease. Radiother Oncol. 2006; 78:1–5.

40. Girinsky T, Specht L, Ghalibafian M, Edeline V, Bonniaud G, Van Der Maazen R, et al. The conundrum of HL nodes: to be or not to be included in the involved node radiation fields. The EORTC-GELA lymphoma group guidelines. Radiother Oncol. 2008;88:202–10.

41. Campbell BA, Voss N, Pickles T, Morris J, Gascoyne RD, Savage KJ, et al. Involved-nodal radiation therapy as a component of combination therapy for limited-stage Hodgkin's lymphoma: a question of field size. J Clin Oncol. 2008; 26:5170–4.

42. Longo DL, Glatstein E, Duffey PL, Young RC, Hubbard SM, Urba WJ, et al. Radiation therapy versus combination chemotherapy in the treatment of early stage Hodgkin's disease: seven-year results of a prospective randomized trial. J Clin Oncol. 1991;9:906–17.

43. Biti GP, Cimino G, Cartoni C, Magrini SM, Anselmo AP, Enrici RM, et al. Extended-field radiotherapy is superior to MOPP chemotherapy for the treatment of pathologic stage I-IIA Hodgkin's disease: eight-year update of an Italian prospective randomized study. J Clin Oncol. 1992;10: 378–82.

44. Meyer RM, Gospodarowicz MK, Connors JM, Pearcey RG, Bezjak A, Wells WA, et al. Randomized comparison of ABVD chemotherapy with a strategy that includes radiation therapy in patients with limited-stage Hodgkin's lymphoma: National Cancer Institute of Canada Clinical Trials Group and the Eastern Cooperative Oncology Group. J Clin Oncol. 2005;23:4634–42.

45. Straus DJ, Portlock CS, Qin J, Myers J, Zelenetz AD, Moskowitz C, et al. Results of a prospective randomized clinical trial of doxorubicin, bleomycin, vinblastine, and dacarbazine (ABVD) followed by radiation therapy (RT) versus ABVD alone for stages I, II, and IIIA nonbulky Hodgkin disease. Blood. 2004;104:3483–9.

46. Gallamini A, Hutchings M, Rigacci L, Specht L, Merli F, Hansen M, et al. Early interim 2-[18F]fluoro-2-deoxy-D-glucose positron emission tomography is prognostically superior to international prognostic score in advanced-stage Hodgkin's lymphoma: a report from a joint Italian-Danish study. J Clin Oncol. 2007;25:3746–52.

47. Hutchings M, Mikhaeel NG, Fields PA, Nunan T, Timothy AR. Prognostic value of interim FDG-PET after two or three cycles of chemotherapy in HL. Ann Oncol. 2005;16: 1160–8.

48. Hutchings M, Loft A, Hansen M, Pedersen LM, Buhl T, Jurlander J, et al. FDG-PET after two cycles of chemotherapy predicts treatment failure and progression-free survival in HL. Blood. 2006;107:52–9.

49. Kasamon YL, Wahl RL. FDG PET and risk-adapted therapy in Hodgkin's and non-Hodgkin's lymphoma. Curr Opin Oncol. 2008;20:206–19.

50. Heutte N, Flechtner HH, Mounier N, Mellink WA, Meerwaldt JH, Eghbali H, et al. Quality of life after successful treatment of early stage Hodgkin's lymphoma: 10-year follow-up of the EORTC-GELA H8 randomised controlled trial. Lancet Oncol. 2009;10:1160–70.

51. Brepoels L, Stroobants S. PET scanning and prognosis in Hodgkin's lymphoma. Curr Opin Oncol. 2008;20:509–16.

# Treatment of Early Unfavorable HL

**11**

John M.M. Raemaekers and Andreas Engert

## Contents

J.M.M. Raemaekers (✉)
Department of Hematology, Radboud University Nijmegen
Medical Center, Geert Grooteplein Zuid 8, 6525GA Nijmegen,
The Netherlands
e-mail: J.Raemaekers@hemat.umcn.nl

A. Engert
Department I of Internal Medicine, University Hospital of
Cologne, Kerpener Strasse 62, 50937, Köln, Germany
e-mail: a.engert@uni-koeln.de

## 11.1 Why Early Unfavorable?

The Ann Arbor staging system with the Cotswolds modifications [1] is still being used worldwide in the staging of patients with HL. In the past, patients with limited stage I/II disease were treated with extended field radiotherapy (RT) whereas those with more advanced stages III or IV received multi-agent chemotherapy. Up to the nineties of the twentieth century, staging laparotomy was performed to more reliably identify patients with disease truly limited to one side of the diaphragm. The successful introduction of chemotherapy in advanced stages, its potential to eradicate occult disease, relapse rates of up to 30% after extended field RT alone, and the increasing awareness of serious long-term toxicity after extended field RT promoted the development of combined modality treatment approaches. Combined modality has the evident advantage of combining two efficacious treatment modalities. It is given as combination of a fixed number of chemotherapy cycles followed by a certain dose and extent of RT. As a result, the extent of both RT as well as chemotherapy could be reduced in the combined treatment design as compared to administering single treatment modalities. However, even in stages I/II, the extent of disease varies substantially requiring a risk-adapted treatment. In many early-stage patients, mediastinal bulky disease is present, which has been demonstrated as prognostically unfavorable. Other poor prognostic clinical factors include higher age, increased number of involved nodes, and elevated erythrocyte sedimentation rate (ESR), accompanied by B-symptoms. Though slight differences in definition exist between major cooperative groups, CS I/II HL patients in Europe are generally divided into an early favorable and an early unfavorable (intermediate) subgroup. In contrast, patients in North America presenting with adverse factors (mainly the presence of bulky disease) are treated like stage III–IV disease and are not included in clinical trials for CS I/II disease. At present, progression-free survival rates of 85–90% are common for patients with unfavorable CS I/II disease treated with a combined modality approach.

## 11.2 Prognostic Factors

The factors used by the European Organisation for Research and Treatment of Cancer (EORTC) Lymphoma Group, the German Hodgkin Study Group (GHSG), the National Cancer Institute of Canada (NCIC), and the Eastern Cooperative Oncology group (ECOG) are shown in Table 11.1 [1, 2]. We have to bear in mind that these risk factors and the resulting prognostic groups were originally defined in the context of treatment with extended field RT. In a combined modality setting the differences in prognosis between favorable and unfavorable disease are likely to be smaller. Moreover, in more recent series the treatment had already been tailored according to the prognostic groups. Thus, one would have anticipated that these prognostic factors today have less independent prognostic significance. However, there is one large recent randomized trial that included a joint experimental treatment arm for both favorable and unfavorable subgroups, thus possibly reflecting the current impact of predictive factors. In this trial, EORTC H7 [3], the unfavorable subset of patients was randomized between six cycles of EBVP (epirubicin, bleomycin,

vinblastine, prednisone), a combination presumed to be less toxic and equally effective to ABVD [4], and six cycles of MOPP/ABV (mechlorethamine, vincristine, procarbazine, prednisone, adriamycin, bleomycin, vinblastine, and dacarbazine), both followed by 30–36 Gy involved field RT (IF-RT). After a median follow-up of 9 years, patients treated with EBVP had a significantly higher rate of tumor progression and relapse than those treated with MOPP/ABV resulting in a significantly inferior 10-year event-free survival (EFS) of 68 vs. 88% ($p<0.001$). The favorable subset of patients was randomized between six cycles of EBVP followed by IF-RT and subtotal nodal irradiation (STNI), considered standard treatment at the time of initiation of the trial. Those treated with EBVP had a superior 10-year EFS compared to patients treated with STNI alone: 88 vs. 78% ($p=0.01$). While the less toxic EBVP regimen produced superior results in the favorable subset of patients, the poor results in the unfavorable patients reflect the necessity for a more potent and intense treatment for this subgroup. Thus, the clinical relevance of the prognostic factors appeared to be maintained. Indirect evidence for the impact of discriminating between favorable and unfavorable early stages can be found in two other trials including patients with adverse prognostic factors, though differently defined. In a trial performed by the Grupo Argentino de Tratamiento de la Leucemia Aguda (GATLA), the less intense AOPE (adriamycin, vincristine, prednisone, and etoposide) proved inferior to CVPP (cyclophosphamide, vincristine, procarbazine, prednisone) [5]. The Southwestern Oncology Group trial 9051 tested a less toxic combination of etoposide, vinblastine, and adriamycin (EVA) followed by STNI and found an

**Table 11.1** Definition of favorable and unfavorable (intermediate) early stage Hodgkin lymphoma

| | EORTC | GHSG | NCIC/ECOG |
|---|---|---|---|
| Risk factors | (a) Large mediastinal mass<br>(b) Age ≥50 years<br>(c) ESR ≥50 without B-symptoms or ≥30 with B-symptoms<br>(d) ≥4 nodal areas | (a) Large mediastinal mass<br>(b) Extranodal disease<br>(c) ESR ≥50 without B-symptoms or ≥30 with B-symptoms<br>(d) ≥3 nodal areas | (a) Histology other than LP/NS<br>(b) Age ≥40 years<br>(c) ESR ≥50<br>(d) ≥4 nodal areas |
| Favorable | CS I–II (supradiaphragmatic) without risk factors | CS I–II without risk factors | CS I–II without risk factors |
| Unfavorable | CS I–II (supradiaphragmatic) with ≥1 risk factors | CS I or CS IIA with ≥1 risk factors<br>CS IIB with (c) or (d) but without (a) and (b) | CS I–II with ≥ risk factors |

*EORTC* European Organisation for Research and Treatment of Cancer; *GHSG* German Hodgkin Study Group; *NCIC* National Cancer Institute of Canada; *ECOG* Eastern Cooperative Oncology group; *ESR* erythrocyte sedimentation rate; *LP* lymphocyte predominance; *NS* nodular sclerosis; *CS* clinical stage unacceptably high relapse rate mainly in non-irradiated areas indicating the inferiority of the chemotherapy [6].

## 11.3 Chemotherapy Regimens

After the initial Bonadonna report on ABVD [7] and the randomized trial on ABVD vs. MOPP vs. MOPP/ABVD in advanced disease [8], the NCIC/ECOG Intergroup trial on ABVD vs. MOPP/ABV hybrid set the stage for ABVD as standard chemotherapy due to equal efficacy but less toxicity as compared with MOPP/ABV [9]. In an attempt to reduce toxicity even further, the GOELAMS (Groupe Ouest-Est d'Étude des Leucémies et Autres Maladies du Sang) included both early favorable and unfavorable patients in their H90-NM study [10]. A total of 386 patients were randomized between ABVDm (ABVD plus methylprednisolone) and the potentially less toxic EBVMm, followed by extended field RT in responding patients. The ABVDm arm proved to be superior to the EBVMm treatment in terms of complete remission rates and FFS. Very similar to the conclusions of the EORTC H7 trial, these results highlight the need for sufficiently effective chemotherapy. Notwithstanding concerns on toxicity of chemotherapy and a reluctance to apply more intense treatment in CS I/II disease, one could argue that a 10–15% failure rate in the unfavorable subset of patients is too high and warrants improvement. In this respect, the trials summarized in Table 11.2 are

important. Both the EORTC H9U and the GHSG HD11 studies failed to show a significant PFS advantage for more intensive treatment comparing four cycles of BEACOPP baseline with four cycles of conventional ABVD [11, 12]. The GHSG follow-up trial for early unfavorable patients, HD14, compared four cycles of ABVD with two cycles of BEACOPP escalated followed by two cycles of ABVD ("2+2"). The decision for this combination was in part based on the higher effective dose (ED) model calculations [6, 13]. Here, four cycles of ABVD given over 16 weeks have an ED of 15 as compared with 15.2 for four cycles of BEACOPP baseline given over 12 weeks. In contrast, the "2+2" variant has an ED of 17.3. In both treatment arms of the HD14 study, additional IF-RT with 30 Gy was given. The third pre-planned interim analysis of this trial demonstrated a significantly better PFS for the more intensive "2+2" arm: PFS at 3 years was 97% with "2+2" treatment compared with 91% after ABVD ($p < 0.0017$) [14]. While an absolute improvement in PFS of only 6% appears rather modest at first glance and one can argue about clinical relevance, the results show that even an upfront intensification with only two cycles of BEACOPP escalated indeed improves outcome in this group of patients. It corroborates the claim for a start of treatment with the most effective regimen to prevent the development of early chemoresistance, but it remains to be seen whether this gain in PFS outbalances the putative increased toxicity, e.g., infertility and secondary malignancies. Similar considerations should also be applied in appreciating

**Table 11.2** Randomized clinical trials in unfavorable CS I/II disease on ABVD vs. alternative chemotherapy regimens

| Trial (ref) | Treatment | Number of patients included | PFS (years) | OS (years) | Remarks |
|---|---|---|---|---|---|
| EORTC/GELA H9U [12] | ABVDx6+IF-RT 30–36 Gy | 276 | 91% (4) | 95% (4) | Not final analysis |
| | ABVDx4+IF-RT 30–36 Gy | 277 | 87% (4) | 94% (4) | EFS instead of PFS |
| | BEACOPPx4+IF-RT 30–36 Gy | 255 | 90% (4) | 93% (4) | n.s. |
| GHSG HD11 [11] | ABVDx4+IF-RT 30 Gy | 356 | 87% (5) | 94% (5) | Final analysis |
| | ABVDx4+IF-RT 20 Gy | 347 | 82% (5) | 94% (5) | n.s. |
| | BEACOPPx4+IF-RT 30 Gy | 341 | 88% (5) | 95% (5) | |
| | BEACOPPx4+IF-RT 20 Gy | 351 | 87% (5) | 95% (5) | |
| GHSG HD14 [14] | ABVDx4+IF-RT 30 Gy | | 91% (3) | | $p < 0.01$ |
| | BEACOPPesc.x2+ABVD x2+IF-RT 30 Gy | | 96% (3) | | |
| Intergroup USA | ABVDx6+IF-RT 36 Gy | | | | Ongoing |
| | Stanford V+IF-RT 36 Gy | | | | |

*ref* reference; *PFS* progression-free survival; *OS* overall survival; *EORTC* European Organisation for Research and Treatment of Cancer; *GELA* Groupe d'Etude des Lymphomes de l'Adulte; *EFS* event-free survival; *IF-RT* involved field radiotherapy; *n.s.* statistically not significant; *GHSG* German Hodgkin Study Group whether the 12-week intense chemotherapy regimen Stanford V, with its mainly alkylating-agent-induced toxicity, can improve treatment outcome as compared with ABVD. This question is being addressed in the ongoing US Intergroup study. Based on current data, ABVD still appears to be the standard chemotherapy. However, the more intense BEACOPP escalated based "2×2" design reports superior PFS suggesting that is indeed possible to improve efficacy in this group of patients.

## 11.4 Number of Cycles of Chemotherapy

Only a few randomized trials have addressed the issue of number of cycles required. These studies show that four cycles of conventional chemotherapy are sufficient in a combined modality setting. In the EORTC/GELA H8U study, MOPP/ABV hybrid was used as standard chemotherapy regimen; four or six cycles followed by IF-RT were compared [15]. The EFS at 7 years did not differ significantly with rates of 86 and 84%, respectively. In the more recent EORTC/GELA H9U trial, 533 patients were randomized between four

and six cycles of ABVD followed by IF-RT [12]. The interim analysis showed an EFS of 87 and 91% at 4 years, which was not significantly different. While some cooperative groups consider early unfavorable CS I/II disease as advanced stage and treat accordingly with six cycles of chemotherapy, a number of four cycles in a combined modality setting is currently considered standard treatment.

## 11.5 Extent and Dose of RT

A number of randomized trials focused on the comparison of extended- and IF-RT in combined modality approaches (Table 11.3) [16, 17]. The important general conclusion from these trials was that extended field RT was not needed in combined modality treatment and was associated with more long-term adverse effects. Thus, IF-RT became standard of care in this setting.

In the era of extended field RT as single modality, the standard dose of RT was 36 Gy, often followed by a boost of 4–6 Gy to residual disease and/or initial bulky sites. When combined with chemotherapy, both, the field size and the RT dose could be reduced. In the GHSG HD11 trial, four cycles of ABVD or four cycles

**Table 11.3** Randomized trials on extent and dose of RT, combined with ABVD(-like) chemotherapy

| Trial (ref) | Treatment | Number of patients included | PFS (years) | OS (years) | Remarks |
|---|---|---|---|---|---|
| *Extent of RT* | | | | | |
| GHSG HD8 [16] | COPP/ABVDx2 + EF-RT 30–40 Gy | 532 | 85% (5) | 90% (5) | n.s. |
| | COPP/ABVDx2 + IF-RT 30–40 Gy | 532 | 84% (5) | 92% (5) | |
| Milan [27] | ABVDx4 + EF-RT | 65 | 96% | 100% | n.s. |
| | ABVDx4 + IF-RT | 68 | 93% | 96% | |
| EORTC/GELA H8U [15] | MOPP/ABVx6 + IF-RT 36–40 Gy | 336 | 84% (7) | 89% (7) | EFS instead of PFS |
| | MOPP/ABVx4 + IF-RT 36–40 Gy | 333 | 86% (7) | 90% (7) | n.s. |
| | MOPP/ABVx4 + STNI 36–40 Gy | 327 | 86% (7) | 90% (7) | |
| Anselmo et al. [17] | ABVDx4 + EF-RT | 102 | 94% (5) | 97% (5) | n.s. |
| | ABVDx4 + IF-RT | 107 | 91% (5) | 96% (5) | |
| *Dose of RT* | | | | | |
| GHSG HD11 [11] | ABVDx4 + IF-RT 30 Gy | 343 | 88% (5) | 95% (5) | Final analysis |
| | ABVDx4 + IF-RT 20 Gy | 339 | 83% (5) | 95% (5) | PFS *p* = 0.03, OS n.s. |
| | BEACOPPx4 + IF-RT 30 Gy | 332 | 89% (5) | 96% (5) | |
| | BEACOPPx4 + IF-RT 20 Gy | 337 | 89% (5) | 97% (5) | |

*ref* reference; *PFS* progression-free survival; *OS* overall survival; *GHSG* German Hodgkin Study Group; *EF-RT* extended field radiotherapy; *IF-RT* involved field radiotherapy; *n.s.* statistically not significant; *EORTC* European Organisation for Research and Treatment of Cancer; *GELA* Groupe d'Etudes des Lymphomes de l'Adulte; *STNI* subtotal nodal irradiation; *EFS* event-free survival of BEACOPP baseline were followed by IF-RT, either a 30 or 20 Gy dose. The final analysis showed no significant difference in PFS between the 30 and 20 Gy treatment arms for those patients receiving BEACOPP baseline. In contrast, those treated with four cycles of ABVD and 20 Gy IF-RT had a poorer tumor control as compared to those receiving 30 Gy IF-RT ($p = 0.048$) [11]. In the EORTC/GELA H9F trial randomizing between a dose of 36 and 20 Gy of IF-RT after EBVP chemotherapy, no differences in PFS were seen in the interim analysis, but this trial included only favorable stage I/II disease [12]. Thus the dose of IF-RT needed in the combined modality treatment of early unfavorable HL depends on the efficacy of the preceding chemotherapy.

## 11.6 Chemotherapy Alone

Several randomized trials performed in patients with advanced stages indicated that RT can be omitted without compromising outcome, providing a robust CR was achieved with six to eight cycles of chemotherapy such as MOP/BAP, MOPP/ABV hybrid, or BEACOPP

escalated [18, 19]. Positron emission tomography (PET) holds the promise of predicting more accurately which remission is robust and if residual masses will benefit from additional RT [20]. Conflicting data came out of a study from India [21]. Here, six cycles of ABVD were followed for patients in CR by IF-RT or no RT in a randomized fashion. Though patients who received RT had a significantly better PFS than those who did not, this study included many early stages, pediatric patients, and used suboptimal imaging methods. These data suggest that after an adequate number of cycles of effective chemotherapy and good response, additional RT will not further improve the outcome in patients with advanced stage disease. The question therefore arose whether RT can also be omitted in unfavorable early stages. Table 11.4 summarizes the results of the most relevant trials, all having their limitations. In the GATLA study [22], a nonstandard chemotherapy was used; other studies included pediatric patients or all stages of disease, used divergent definitions of unfavorable prognostic features, or had not enough statistical power to detect clinically significant differences in PFS between RT and non-RT arms. The NCIC/ECOG study on early stages is probably the most relevant at present though bulky disease as unfavorable prognostic factor

**Table 11.4** Randomized clinical trials in unfavorable CS I/II disease on combined modality treatment vs. chemotherapy alone

| Trial (ref) | Treatment | Number of patients included | PFS (years) | OS | Remarks |
|---|---|---|---|---|---|
| GATLA [22] | CVPPx3 + IF-RT 30 Gy + CVPPx3 CVPPx6 | 44 66 | 75% (7) 34% (7) | 84% 66% | PFS $p = 0.001$; OS n.s. |
| Aviles [28] | ABVDx6 + IF-RT 30 Gy ABVDx6 | | 76% (11) 48% (11) | 88% 59% | PFS and OS $p < 0.01$; only bulky IA and IIA |
| CCG children [29] | COPP/ABVx4-6 + IF-RT 21 Gy COPP/ABVx4-6 (only CR randomized for RT or no RT) | 501 | 93% (3) 85% (3) | n.s. | PFS $p = 0.02$; all stages (68% CS I/II); only children |
| Tata Memorial Hospital [21] | ABVDx6 + IF-RT 30Gy ABVDx6 (only CR randomized for RT or no RT) | 179 | 88% (8) 76% (8) | 100% 89% | PFS $p = 0.01$; OS $p = 0.002$; all stages (55% CS I/II) and children (50%) included |
| MSKCC [30] | ABVDx6 + IF-RT or EF-RT ABVDx6 | 76 76 | 86% (5) 81% (5) | 97% 90% | n.s.; non-bulky CS IB, IIB, IIIA; only powered for differences in PFS >20% |
| NCIC/ECOG [23] | ABVDx2 + STNI 35 Gy ABVDx4-6 no RT | 139 137 | 95% (5) 88% (5) | 92% (5) 95% (5) | PFS $p = 0.004$ OS n.s.; B-symptoms and bulky disease excluded |

*ref* reference; *PFS* progression-free survival; *OS* overall survival; *GATLA* Grupo Argentino Tratamiento de la Leucemia Aguda; *IF-RT* involved field radiotherapy; *n.s.* statistically not significant; *CCG* Children's Cancer study Group; *MSKCC* Memorial Sloan Kettering Cancer Center; *EF-RT* extended field radiotherapy; *NCIC* National Cancer Institute of Canada; *ECOG* Eastern Cooperative Oncology Group; *STNI* subtotal nodal irradiation was an exclusion criterion for entry into the study: this study failed to show a survival benefit for adding RT to ABVD in the early unfavorable cohort of patients, notwithstanding a significant advantage in PFS for those who received the outdated large-field RT [23]. Thus, the question on the role of RT in early unfavorable stages disease cannot yet be answered unequivocally. Until there is generally accepted evidence that RT can really be omitted in unfavorable stages I/II without jeopardizing the long-term outcome, combined modality treatment remains the preferred treatment approach for patients with unfavorable CS I/II disease.

## 11.7 Special Situations

### 11.7.1 Bulky Mediastinal Tumor

The presence of a bulky mediastinal tumor, defined as a mediastinum/thorax ratio of $\geq 0.35$, is one of the most prominent negative prognostic factors in HL patients with CS I/II disease. Some groups treat these patients according to protocols for advanced disease. Upon treatment, the nodular sclerosing histology is associated with inherent slow regression particularly of bulky mediastinal tumors. When evaluated by conventional CT scans, a reliable and reproducible interpretation of response after chemotherapy is often difficult. In case of post-chemotherapy residual masses with uncertain dignity, investigators may easily conclude a partial remission and advocate additional RT. That would possibly not be wrong from a tumor control point of view; however, mediastinal radiation fields are typically associated with severe adverse long-term effects such as secondary malignancies (e.g., breast and bronchus carcinoma) and early cardiovascular events (see Chaps. 22 and 23 for more details). There are no randomized data specifically addressing the need for RT in patients with bulky mediastinal disease based on modern imaging techniques. Although being a single-arm study on a fixed combined modality approach, the experience with Stanford V chemotherapy followed by IF-RT provides the most appropriate data in this respect, including response evaluation with FDG-PET [24]. Patients with a persistent positive FDG-PET scan after Stanford V had a significantly higher relapse rate even after additional IF-RT when compared to those patients with

a negative FDG-PET scan post-chemotherapy who also received RT as planned.

In future studies, patients who really need additional RT and those who will not benefit might be better identified by FDG-PET-based response evaluation. This would hopefully secure optimal tumor control and spare subgroups of patients already cured by chemotherapy alone from long-term RT-induced toxicity. For the time being, however, combined modality treatment remains the standard treatment for patients with CS I/II disease with bulky mediastinal disease.

### 11.7.2 Concomitant Disease

For patients who cannot tolerate chemotherapy or for whom chemotherapy is contraindicated due to concomitant disease, large-field RT at doses of 36–40 Gy is still an alternative treatment option. However, patients with unfavorable CS I/II disease have a relapse rate of more than 40% after RT alone and will probably also experience considerable toxicity from large-field RT. Thus a balance on an individual basis between tumor control and avoidance of serious toxicity has to be found.

## 11.8 Future

The most important challenge is the identification of patients who are adequately treated with ABVD alone, those who need combined modality treatment, and those who need intensified chemotherapy such as BEACOPP escalated. The recent data from the GHSG HD14 study show that more intense chemotherapy significantly improves tumor control. On the other hand, in these patients with localized disease, we also aim at minimizing early and late toxicity of treatment. New clinical prognostic factors are unlikely to allow for selecting patients needing more or less intensive treatment. Biomarkers could become useful but at present no individual marker or set of markers has been sufficiently reliable. New functional imaging techniques will very likely become valid tools to identify subsets of patients requiring different treatment approaches early in the course of treatment (see Chap. 7). The currently ongoing EORTC/GELA/IIL (Intergruppo

Italiano di Linfomi) H10 trial is pivotal in this respect. In this trial, the standard combined modality approach with four cycles of ABVD followed by involved node RT is randomly being compared to an early FDG-PET scan directed approach: if the FDG-PET scan is negative after two cycles of ABVD, treatment continues with chemotherapy alone up to a total of six cycles, whereas in case of persistent FDG-PET positivity after two cycles of ABVD, treatment continues with two cycles of BEACOPP escalated followed by involved node RT [25].

In the meantime, new RT techniques will further evolve and especially the reduction of the involved field to the involved node principle in the combined modality treatment setting could reduce toxicity while maintaining the high efficacy [26] (see Chap. 9). The involved node principle has already been incorporated in the abovementioned EORTC/GELA/IIL H10 trial and will be randomly compared with IF-RT in the ongoing GHSG HD17 trial for unfavorable CS I/II disease.

# References

1. Lister TA, Crowther D, Sutcliffe SB, et al. Report of a committee convened to discuss the evaluation and staging of patients with Hodgkin's disease: Cotswolds meeting. J Clin Oncol. 1989;7:1630–6.
2. Specht L, Raemaekers J. Do we need an early unfavorable (intermediate) stage of Hodgkin's lymphoma? Hematol Oncol Clin North Am. 2007;21:881–96.
3. Noordijk EM, Carde P, Dupouy N, et al. Combined-modality therapy for clinical stage I or II Hodgkin's lymphoma: long-term results of the European Organisation for Research and Treatment of Cancer H7 randomized controlled trials. J Clin Oncol. 2006;24:3128–35.
4. Hoerni B, Orgerie MB, Eghbali H, et al. New combination of epirubicine, bleomycin, vinblastine and prednisone (EBVP II) before radiotherapy in localized stages of Hodgkin's disease. Phase II trial in 50 patients. Bull Cancer. 1988;75:789–94.
5. Pavlovsky S, Schvartzman E, Lastiri F, et al. Randomized trial of CVPP for three versus six cycles in favorable-prognosis and CVPP versus AOPE plus radiotherapy in intermediate-prognosis untreated Hodgkin's disease. J Clin Oncol. 1997;15:2652–8.
6. Wasserman TH, Petroni GR, Millard F, et al. Sequential chemotherapy (etoposide, vinblastine, and doxorubicin) and subtotal lymph node radiation for patients with localized stages of Hodgkin's disease and unfavorable prognostic features: a phase II Cancer and Leukemia Group B Study (9051). Cancer. 1999;86:1590–5.
7. Bonadonna G, Zucali R, Monfardini S, De LM, Uslenghi C. Combination chemotherapy of Hodgkin's disease with adriamycin, bleomycin, vinblastine, and imidazole carboxamide versus MOPP. Cancer. 1975;36:252–9.
8. Canellos GP, Niedzwiecki D. Long-term follow-up of Hodgkin's disease trial. N Engl J Med. 2002;346:1417–8.
9. Duggan DB, Petroni GR, Johnson JL, et al. Randomized comparison of ABVD and MOPP/ABV hybrid for the treatment of advanced Hodgkin's disease: report of an intergroup trial. J Clin Oncol. 2003;21:607–14.
10. Le Maignan C, Desablens B, Delwail V, et al. Three cycles of adriamycin, bleomycin, vinblastine, and dacarbazine (ABVD) or epirubicin, bleomycin, vinblastine, and methotrexate (EBVM) plus extended field radiation therapy in early and intermediate Hodgkin disease: 10-year results of a randomized trial. Blood. 2004;103:58–66.
11. Borchmann P, Dieh V, Goergen H, et al. Combined modality treatment with intensified chemotherapy and dose-reduced involved field radiotherapy in patients with early unfavourable Hodgkin lymphoma (HL): final analysis of the German Hodgkin Study Group (GHSG) HD11 trial [abstract]. Blood. 2009;114:299–300.
12. Thomas J, Ferme C, Noordijk E, et al. Results of the EORTC-GELA H9 randomized trials: the H9-F trial (comparing 3 radiation dose levels) and H9-U trial comparing 3 chemotherapy schemes) in patients with favorable or unfavorable early stage Hodgkin's lymphoma [abstract]. Haematologica. 2007;92:27.
13. Hasenclever D, Loeffler M, Dieh V; German Hodgkin's Lymphoma Study Group. Rationale for dose escalation of first line conventional chemotherapy in advanced Hodgkin's disease. Ann Oncol. 1996;7:95–8.
14. Engert A, Borchmann P, Pluetschow A, et al. Dose-intensified combined modality treatment with 2 cycles of BEACOPP escalated followed by 2 cycles of ABVD and involved field radiotherapy (IF-RT) is superior to 4 cycles of ABVD and IF-RT in patients with early unfavourable Hodgkin lymphoma (HL): an analysis of the German Hodgkin Study Group (GHSG) HD 14 trial [abstract]. Haematologica. 2009;94:553.
15. Ferme C, Eghbali H, Meerwaldt JH, et al. Chemotherapy plus involved-field radiation in early-stage Hodgkin's disease. N Engl J Med. 2007;357:1916–27.
16. Engert A, Schiller P, Josting A, et al. Involved-field radiotherapy is equally effective and less toxic compared with extended-field radiotherapy after four cycles of chemotherapy in patients with early-stage unfavorable Hodgkin's lymphoma: results of the HD8 trial of the German Hodgkin's Lymphoma Study Group. J Clin Oncol. 2003;21:3601–8.
17. Anselmo AP, Cavalieri E, Osti FM, et al. Intermediate stage Hodgkin's disease: preliminary results on 210 patients treated with four ABVD chemotherapy cycles plus extended versus involved field radiotherapy. Anticancer Res. 2004;24:4045–50.
18. Aleman BM, Raemaekers JM, Tirelli U, et al. Involved-field radiotherapy for advanced Hodgkin's lymphoma. N Engl J Med. 2003;348:2396–406.
19. Diehl V, Franklin J, Pfreundschuh M, et al. Standard and increased-dose BEACOPP chemotherapy compared with COPP-ABVD for advanced Hodgkin's disease. N Engl J Med. 2003;348:2386–95.

20. Kobe C, Dietlein M, Franklin J, et al. Positron emission tomography has a high negative predictive value for progression or early relapse for patients with residual disease after first-line chemotherapy in advanced-stage Hodgkin lymphoma. Blood. 2008;112:3989–94.
21. Laskar S, Gupta T, Vimal S, et al. Consolidation radiation after complete remission in Hodgkin's disease following six cycles of doxorubicin, bleomycin, vinblastine, and dacarbazine chemotherapy: is there a need? J Clin Oncol. 2004;22:62–8.
22. Pavlovsky S, Maschio M, Santarelli MT, et al. Randomized trial of chemotherapy versus chemotherapy plus radiotherapy for stage I-II Hodgkin's disease. J Natl Cancer Inst. 1988;80:1466–73.
23. Meyer RM, Gospodarowicz MK, Connors JM, et al. Randomized comparison of ABVD chemotherapy with a strategy that includes radiation therapy in patients with limited-stage Hodgkin's lymphoma: National Cancer Institute of Canada Clinical Trials Group and the Eastern Cooperative Oncology Group. J Clin Oncol. 2005;23:4634–42.
24. Horning SJ, Hoppe RT, Breslin S, et al. Stanford V and radiotherapy for locally extensive and advanced Hodgkin's disease: mature results of a prospective clinical trial. J Clin Oncol. 2002;20:630–7.
25. Andre M, Reman O, Federico M, et al. First report on the H10 EORTC/GELA/IIL randomized Intergroup trial on early FDG-PET scan guided treatment adaptation versus standard combined modality treatment in patients with supradiaphragmatic stahe I/II Hodgkin's lymphoma, for the Groupe d'Etude des Lymphomes de l'Adulte (GELA), European Organisation for the Research and Treatment of Cancer (EORTC) Lymphoma Group and the Intergruppo Italiano Linfomi (IIL). Blood. 2009;114:44–5.
26. Girinsky T, van der Maazen R, Specht L, et al. Involved-node radiotherapy (INRT) in patients with early Hodgkin lymphoma: concepts and guidelines. Radiother Oncol. 2006;79:270–7.
27. Bonadonna G, Bonfante V, Viviani S, et al. ABVD plus sub-total nodal versus involved-field radiotherapy in early-stage Hodgkin's disease: long-term results. J Clin Oncol. 2004;22:2835–41.
28. Aviles A, Delgado S. A prospective clinical trial comparing chemotherapy, radiotherapy and combined therapy in the treatment of early stage Hodgkin's disease with bulky disease. Clin Lab Haematol. 1998;20:95–9.
29. Nachman JB, Sposto R, Herzog P, et al. Randomized comparison of low-dose involved field radiotherapy and no radiotherapy for children with Hodgkin's disease who achieve a complete response to chemotherapy. J Clin Oncol. 2002;20:3765–71.
30. Straus DJ, Portlock CS, Qin J, et al. Results of a prospective randomized clinical trial of doxorubicin, bleomycin, vinblastine, and dacarbazine (ABVD) followed by radiation therapy (RT) versus ABVD alone for stages I, II, and IIIA nonbulky Hodgkin disease. Blood. 2004;104:3483–9.

# Treatment of Advanced Stage Hodgkin Lymphoma

**12**

Peter Borchmann and Volker Diehl

## Contents

P. Borchmann
German Hodgkin Study Group (GHSG), Köln, Germany

V. Diehl (✉)
Klinik I für Innere Medizin, Universitätsklinikum Köln,
Kerpener Str. 62, 50937, Köln, Germany
e-mail: v.diehl@uni-koeln.de

## 12.1 From MOPP to MOPP/ABVD to ABVD

Before the introduction of combination chemotherapy, more than 95% of patients with advanced HL succumbed to their disease within 5 years. Thus, remission rates in excess of 50% achieved with MOPP (mechlorethamine, vincristine, procarbazine, and prednisone) were a major breakthrough in oncology [1, 2]. MOPP was successfully introduced almost 40 years ago and used for many years for advanced stage disease, resulting in long-term remission of nearly 50% [1, 3]. It was then replaced by ABVD (adriamycin, bleomycin, vinblastine, and dacarbazine), after a series of large multicenter trials had investigated ABVD vs. alternating MOPP/ABVD or MOPP alone [3–5].

Bonadonna et al. were the first to report on the relevance of ABVD and anthracyclines for the treatment of advanced stage HL [3]. Patients were randomly assigned to receive either MOPP or MOPP alternated monthly with ABVD. All 88 evaluable patients had not received chemotherapy and 25 had had a relapse after primary irradiation. The complete remission (CR) rate with MOPP/ABVD was 88.9%, and with MOPP alone 74.4%. The 8-year results reported that MOPP/ABVD was superior to MOPP in terms of freedom from progression (FFP) (64.6 vs. 35.9%; $p<0.005$), relapse-free survival (RFS) (72.6 vs. 45.1%; $p<0.01$), and overall survival (OS) (83.9 vs. 63.9%; $p<0.06$). This study impressively showed the benefit of ABVD in terms of efficacy when added to MOPP (Table 12.1).

Also ABVD alone when compared to MOPP gave superior results, favoring ABVD. Santoro et al investigated 3xMOPP+RT+3xMOPP vs. 3xABVD+RT+3x ABVD. In this trial, the 7-year results indicated that ABVD was superior to MOPP in terms of FFP (80.8

A. Engert and S.J. Horning (eds.), *Hodgkin Lymphoma*,
DOI: 10.1007/978-3-642-12780-9_12, © Springer-Verlag Berlin Heidelberg 2011

**Table 12.1** MOPP/ABVD in randomized trials

| Trial and references | Publication year | Therapy regimen | Number of patients | Outcome | FU and comments |
|---|---|---|---|---|---|
| Bonadonna [3] | 1986 | A. MOPP/ABVD alternating | 43 | 64.6% (FFP); 83.9% (OS) | FU 8 years |
| | | B. MOPP | 45 | 35.9% (FFP); 63.9% (OS) | |
| Santoro [5] | 1987 | A. 3xMOPP-RT-3xMOPP | 114 | 62.8% (FFP); 77.4% (OS) | FU 7 years (Sub)-total nodal irradiation in all patients |
| | | B. 3xABVD-RT-3xABVD | 118 | 80.8% (FFP); 67.9% (OS) | |
| US Intergroup [4] | 2003 | A. ABVD (six cycles) | 433 | 63% (FFS); 82% (OS) | FU 5 years; MDS and sAML only in MOPP treated patients |
| | | B. MOPP/ABV hybrid (six cycles) | 419 | 66% (EFS); 81% (OS) | |
| Viviani [7] | 1996 | A. MOPP/ABVD alternating | 211 | 67% (FFP); 74% (OS) | FU 10 years |
| | | B. MOPP/ABVD hybrid | 204 | 69% (FFP); 72% (OS) | |
| Connors [8] | 1997 | A. MOPP/ABVD hybrid (eight cycles) | 252 | 71% (FFS); 81% (OS) | FU 5 years |
| | | B. MOPP/ABVD alternating (eight cycles) Radiotherapy after cycle six for PR | 248 | 67% (FFS); 83% (OS) | |
| GHSG HD6 [9] | 2003 | A. COPP/ABV/IMEP (hybrid 4x) | 223 | 54% (FFTF); 73% (OS) | FU 7 years |
| | | B. COPP/ABVD (alternating 4x) | 245 | 56% (FFTF); 73% (OS) | |

*GHSG* German Hodgkin Study Group; *RT* radiotherapy; *FFS* failure-free survival; *FFP* freedom from progression; *EFS* event-free survival; *OS* overall survival; *FU* follow-up; *FFTF* freedom from treatment failure

vs. 62.8%; $p < 0.002$), RFS (87.7 vs. 77.2%; $p = 0.06$), and most importantly OS (77.4 vs. 67.9%; $p = 0.03$) [5]. Another US trial also tested six to eight cycles of ABVD against six to eight cycles of MOPP or MOPP alternating with ABVD for 12 cycles [6]. Of 361 eligible patients, 123 received MOPP, 123 received MOPP alternating with ABVD, and 115 received ABVD alone. The overall response rate was 93%, with a CR rate of 77%: MOPP 67%, ABVD 82%, and MOPP-ABVD 83% ($p = 0.006$ for the comparison of MOPP with the other two doxorubicin-containing regimens). The rates of failure-free survival at 5 years were 50% for MOPP, 61% for ABVD, and 65% for MOPP-ABVD. OS at 5 years was 66% for MOPP, 73% for ABVD, and 75% for MOPP-ABVD ($p = 0.28$ for the comparison of MOPP with the doxorubicin regimens). MOPP was associated with more severe hematologic toxicity. Since ABVD was equally effective and less toxic than MOPP-ABVD, this trial supported the use of ABVD alone as first-line therapy for advanced stage HL.

Finally, a large American intergroup trial ($n = 856$) tested ABVD vs. MOPP/ABV hybrid. The rates of CR (76 vs. 80%, $p = 0.16$), failure-free survival at 5 years (63 vs. 66%, $p = 0.42$), and OS at 5 years (82 vs. 81%, $p = 0.82$) were similar for ABVD and MOPP/ABV, respectively [4]. However, clinically significant acute pulmonary and hematologic toxicity were more common with MOPP/ABV ($p = 0.06$ and 0.001, respectively). More therapy-associated fatal outcomes were reported for the hybrid regimen (ABVD = 9, MOPP/ABV = 15, $p = 0.057$). Also, secondary malignancies occurred more often with MOPP/ABV, without reaching statistical significance. Out of 13 patients developing MDS or acute leukemia, 11 were initially treated with MOPP/ABV, and only two with ABVD. Both subsequently received MOPP-containing regimens and radiotherapy before developing leukemia ($p = 0.011$) [4]. Therefore, it was concluded from this study that ABVD and MOPP/ABV hybrid are equally effective therapies for HL, but due to significant less toxicity,

ABVD should be considered the standard regimen for treatment of advanced stage HL.

This conclusion is supported by the fact that the alkylating agents within the MOPP regimen led to more severe toxicity in most studies. The comparative iatrogenic morbidity showed that irreversible gonadal dysfunction as well as acute leukemia occurred only in patients subjected to MOPP [5].

Also, the evaluation of rapidly alternating and non-cross-resistant regimens was not successful. Alternating MOPP/ABVD was tested against the MOPP/ABV hybrid regimen, alternating COPP/ABV/IMEP against the COPP/ABVD hybrid, and alternating MOPP/ABVD against the MOPP/ABVD hybrid, all without improving patient outcome [7–9].

Taken together, ABVD has become widely accepted as the standard regimen for advanced stage HL. A major advantage of this regimen is its tolerability. ABVD is a safe outpatient treatment without the need for close white blood cell monitoring and can be administered also in developing countries [10]. One has to keep in mind, though, that a long-term follow-up report of 123 patients treated with ABVD for advanced HL revealed a failure-free survival of only 47% and an OS of 59% after 14.1 years [11]. Since 40% mortality among young patients suffering from a curable malignancy is unacceptably high, many alternative approaches have been developed to improve these results.

## 12.2 Fourth-Generation Regimens

### 12.2.1 Hybrid and Alternating Regimens

Up-front ABVD has been further tested vs. the Stanford V regimen (see below) and the MOPP/EBV/CAD schedule in an Italian cooperative study, and vs. alternating or hybrid multidrug regimens such as ChlVPP/PABlOE and ChlVPP/EVA in a UK study [12, 13].

The Italian cooperative study was a multicenter, prospective, randomized clinical trial investigating two chemotherapy regimens (i.e., Stanford V: doxorubicin, vinblastine, mechlorethamine, vincristine, bleomycin, etoposide, and prednisone; and MOPPEBVCAD: mechlorethamine, vincristine, procarbazine, prednisone, epidoxorubicin, bleomycin, vinblastine, lomustine,

doxorubicin, and vindesine), which were compared to ABVD [12]. Radiotherapy was limited to less than and equal to two sites of either previous bulky or partially remitting disease. The CR rates for ABVD, Stanford V, and MOPPEBVCAD were 89, 76, and 94%, respectively; 5-year failure-free survival and progression-free survival (PFS) rates were 78, 54, 81%, and 85, 73, and 94%, respectively ($p < 0.01$ for comparison of Stanford V with the other two regimens). Corresponding 5-year OS rates were 90, 82, and 89% for ABVD, Stanford V, and MOPPEBVCAD, respectively. Stanford V was more myelotoxic than ABVD but less myelotoxic compared with MOPPEBVCAD. The authors concluded that ABVD still is the standard treatment when combined with optional, limited irradiation. The reported failure-free survival for ABVD is high compared to other studies. This might be in part explained by the fact that stage IIB patients without additional risk factors were enrolled into this study, resulting in a relatively high percentage of good prognosis patients according to the international prognostic score (IPS) (35%).

The UK study compared ABVD with two multidrug regimens, that is, alternating chlorambucil, vinblastine, procarbazine, and prednisolone (ChlVPP) with prednisolone, doxorubicin, bleomycin, vincristine, and etoposide (PABlOE), or hybrid ChlVPP/etoposide, vincristine, and doxorubicin (EVA) [13]. Radiotherapy was planned for incomplete response or initial bulky disease. At 52 months median follow-up, the primary objective EFS at 3 years was 75% (95% CI, 71–79%) for ABVD and 75% (95% CI, 70–79%) for multidrug regimens (hazard ratio (HR) = 1.05; 95% CI, 0.8–1.37). The 3-year OS rates were 90% (95% CI, 87–93%) in patients allocated to ABVD and 88% (95% CI, 84–91%) in patients allocated to multidrug regimens (HR = 1.22; 95% CI, 0.84–1.77). Patients receiving multidrug regimens experienced more grade 3/4 side effects including infection, mucositis, and neuropathy. To conclude, in the absence of a significant difference in EFS or OS between ABVD and multidrug regimens, ABVD remained the standard treatment of advanced HL. It should be mentioned that this study reported a better EFS and OS for ABVD than other trials. This is explained by the fact that this trial included patients with stage I/II disease that had systemic symptoms, multiple sites of involvement, or bulky disease. Looking at stage III and IV patients only, the 5-year EFS and OS was 65 and 82%, respectively, and thus clearly lower.

Taken together, in both trials hybrid regimens did not show any superiority over ABVD.

The Manchester group followed a different approach. They developed the hybrid ChlVPP/EVA to enhance the outcome of MOPP [14]. Patients in the hybrid arm of this trial had a higher CR rate (68.1 vs. 55.3%) and a lower failure rate (2.4 vs. 12.5%). With a median follow-up period for survivors of 4.5 years (range 0–9), actuarial 5-year PFS for all cases was 80% in the hybrid arm and 66% in the MOPP arm ($p = 0.005$) with a trend towards better OS. ChlVPP/EVA had, therefore, been adopted as standard first-line therapy in this group. This regimen was then tested against VAPEC-B, an abbreviated 11-week chemotherapy program. After 5 years, event-free survival and OS were significantly better with ChlVPP/EVA than with VAPEC-B (EFS: 78 vs. 58%; OS: 89 vs. 79%) [15]. Later on, ChlVPP/EVA was tested against ABVD and did not show superiority, so ABVD remained the gold standard [13].

## 12.2.2 Stanford V

Stanford V was developed as a short-duration, reduced-toxicity program, and was applied weekly over 12 weeks. Consolidating radiotherapy to sites of initial disease was employed [16]. Unfortunately, data were generated in a single-center setting with a very limited number of patients. 142 patients with stage III or IV or locally extensive mediastinal stage I or II HL received Stanford V chemotherapy for 12 weeks followed by 36-Gy RT to initial sites of bulky (≥5 cm) or macroscopic splenic disease. With a median follow-up of 5.4 years, the 5-year FFP was 89% and the OS was 96%. However, FFP was significantly inferior among patients with an IPS 3 and higher (94 vs. 75%, $p = 0.0001$). One hundred and twenty nine of 142 patients (91%) received additional radiotherapy. A prospectively randomized multicenter comparison of Stanford V with MOPPEBVCAD and ABVD showed that this regimen was inferior in terms of response rate (76 vs. 89 and 94%) and PFS (73 vs. 85 and 94%) in a multicenter setting [12]. These conflicting results might be partially explained by the use of less radiotherapy in the randomized setting and the better treatment quality in single-center studies. Furthermore, in a large intergroup trial including all US cooperative study groups,

Stanford V was compared to ABVD±RT [17]. In this multicenter, prospective, randomized controlled trial, weekly alternating Stanford V was compared to the standard twice-weekly ABVD regimen. Patients had stage IIB, III, or IV disease, or stage I to IIA disease with bulky disease or other adverse features. Radiotherapy was administered in both arms to sites of previous bulk (>5 cm) and to splenic deposits, although this was omitted in the latter part of the trial for patients achieving CR in the ABVD arm. Five hundred patients received protocol treatment, and radiotherapy was administered to 73% in the Stanford V arm and to 53% in the ABVD arm. The overall response rates after completion of all treatment were 91% for Stanford V and 92% for ABVD. During a median follow-up of 4.3 years, there was no difference in the projected 5-year PFS and OS rates (76 and 90%, respectively, for ABVD; 74 and 92%, respectively, for Stanford V). Thus, in this large, randomized trial, Stanford V was not superior to standard ABVD when given in combination with radiotherapy. However, 20% more patients had to be irradiated in the Stanford V arm and the 5-year PFS was about 15% lower than reported in the single-center setting. This inferiority in terms of PFS is in the magnitude seen in the Intergruppo Italiano Linfomi [12]. Finally, a large US intergroup (E2496) study comparing Stanford V to ABVD has been fully recruited and results will be available soon. To summarize, the compelling single-center phase II data could not be confirmed in multicenter randomized trials so far.

## 12.2.3 BEACOPP Escalated

The BEACOPP regimen (bleomycin, etoposide, adriamycin, cyclophosphamide, vincristine, procarbazine, and prednisone) has been introduced by the German Hodgkin Study Group (GHSG) in its baseline and dose-escalated variants, with a substantial increase of dose density and dose intensity compared to ABVD and hybrid regimens. Although some indications for a role of dose intensity were available in the early 1990s, no prospective randomized trial had been undertaken. In order to obtain an impression of the shape of the essential dose–response characteristic, Hasenclever et al. developed a novel statistical model to analyze a set of data in which dose variations had been used. The model took tumor growth and chemotherapy effects into account and was applied to correlate tumor control in relation to treatment intensity. It was fitted to the data of 706 patients who had received COPP/ABVD-like regimens and revealed considerable heterogeneity in chemosensitivity, but showed a positive slope for dose–response relationship. The model was used to simulate the effect of dose escalation and changes of schedule and architecture of the COPP/ABVD regimen. On the basis of such simulations the model predicted that shortening cycle intervals from 4 to 3 weeks should lead to small benefits (about 3% in 5-year tumor control rates), but a moderate average dose escalation by 30% of a standard chemotherapy would lead to a potential benefit in the range of 10–15% in tumor control at 5 years. On the basis of this theoretical model, the BEACOPP scheme was designed. G-CSF was introduced to compensate for the myelotoxic effects. In a phase II study, the optimal dosage of the BEACOPP baseline and BEACOPP escalated regimen were determined [18]. The subsequent HD9 trial of the GHSG found the predicted dose–response curve to be correct. In this trial, COPP/ABVD, BEACOPP baseline, and BEACOPP escalated were compared. Results from 1,195 randomized patients showed a clear superiority of BEACOPP escalated over BEACOPP baseline and COPP/ABVD at 5 years [19]. The follow-up data at 10 years confirmed these results: with a median follow-up of 112 months, the FFTF and OS rates were 64 and 75% in the COPP/ABVD group, 70 and 80% in the BEACOPP baseline group, and 82 and 86% in the BEACOPP escalated group, respectively [20]. The 10-year update of the HD9 study did not only confirm a significant improvement in long-term FFTF and OS for BEACOPP escalated, but also showed that this advantage is particularly evident in the subset of intermediate prognosis patients, as defined by the IPS (2–3). Importantly, this is the largest subset of patients (IPS 0–1: 28%, IPS 2–3: 38%, IPS 4–7: 13%) [20].

However, toxicity of this more aggressive approach remained a concern. The subsequent GHSG HD12 trial thus aimed at de-escalating chemo- and radiotherapy by comparing four courses of BEACOPP escalated with four courses of escalated and four courses of baseline BEACOPP ("4+4") [21]. Furthermore, in the HD12 trial, the role of radiotherapy was tested by a second randomization between consolidating radiation to initial bulky and residual disease and no

radiotherapy. At 5 years, OS was 91%, FFTF 85.5%, and PFS 86.2%. However, there was no statistical difference between 8xBEACOPP escalated and the 4+4 arm in all outcome parameters. There was also no significant difference between the RT or no-RT arms in this study, with the caveat that a high number of high-risk patients (~10%) received RT based on the blinded panel decision. Since some subgroup analyses in the HD12 trial are pending, the GHSG still considers eight cycles of BEACOPP escalated as standard of care for advanced stage HL patients (Table 12.2).

## 12.3  What Is the Standard Treatment Today?

ABVD is widely accepted as gold standard for the treatment of advanced stage HL. As pointed out above, the only long-term follow-up report of 123 patients treated with ABVD for advanced HL revealed a failure-free survival of 47% and an OS of 59% after 14.1 years [11]. Since supportive care and salvage therapy have been improved over the last decades, the outcome might be slightly better today; however, in the trials reported so far, 5-year progression-free survival is between 60 (in most studies) and 75% (in few studies) with only about half of the relapsed patients surviving [4–6, 12, 13, 17]. Therefore, ABVD is certainly a good regimen – but not good enough.

Two different strategies are commonly being used today:

1. Starting with the less toxic ABVD regimen and accepting a RFS of 60–70% at 5 years trying to salvage relapsing patients with high-dose chemotherapy (HDCT) and autologous stem cell transplantation (ASCT) (including substantial toxicities for patients undergoing this procedure) [4, 6].

2. Starting with the aggressive BEACOPP escalated regimen (FFTF at 5 years 87%) in order to cure as many patients as possible with the first-line therapy accepting an excess of toxicity for those patients who could have been cured with a less intensive therapy [20]. These opposing treatment strategies have been discussed very intensively in the past, leading to a series of large international ongoing trials. These will, hopefully, provide evidence in the near future regarding which strategy is more benefi-

**Table 12.2** Fourth-generation trials

| Trial and references | Publication year | Therapy regimen | Number of patients | Outcome | FU and comments |
|---|---|---|---|---|---|
| Intergroup Italy [12] | 2005 | A. ABVD (six cycles)<br>B. Stanford V (12 weeks)<br>C. MEC hybrid (six cycles)<br>(+ RT initial bulk/residual mass) | 98<br>89<br>88 | 83% (FFS); 91% (OS)<br>67% (FFS); 89% (OS)<br>85% (FFS); 87% (OS) | FU 5 years<br>Patients in stage IIB without additional risk factors included |
| UK Lymphoma Group [13] | 2005 | A. ABVD (six cycles)<br>B. ChlVPP/EVA (six cycles)<br>C. ChlVPP/PABIOE (3x alternating) | 391<br>109<br>275 | 77% (EFS); 86% (FFP); 90% (OS)<br>77% (EFS); 76% (FFP); 83% (OS)<br>74% (EFS); 93% (FFP); 90% (OS) | FU 3 years<br>Stage I and II included; stage III and IV at FU 5 years: 65% (EFS); 81% (OS) |
| Intergroup GB and Italy [15] | 2002 | A. ChlVPP/EVA hybrid (six cycles)<br>B. VAPEC-B (11 weeks)<br>(±RT initial bulk/residual mass) | 144<br>138 | 82% (FFP); 78% (EFS); 89% (OS)<br>62% (FFP); 58% (EFS); 79% (OS) | FU 5 years |
| Stanford V [16] | 2002 | Single arm phase II Stanford V 36-Gy RT to initial sites of bulky (≥5 cm) or macroscopic splenic disease | 142 | 89% (FFP); 96% (OS)<br>In patients IPS ≥3: 75% (FFP) | FU 5 years; patients with stage I or II with risk factor LMM included; 129 of 152 patients (91%) received additional radiotherapy |
| UKNCRI [17] | 2009 | A. ABVD (six to eight cycles)<br>B. Stanford V 36-Gy RT to initial sites of bulky (≥5 cm) or splenic deposits | 252<br>248 | 76% (PFS); 90% (OS)<br>74% (PFS); 92% (OS) | FU 5 years<br>Patients in stage I and II with bulky disease included<br>20% more patients irradiated after S V (73%) |
| GHSG HD9 [19] | 2003 | A. COPP/ABVD (four cycles)<br>B. BEACOPP baseline (eight cycles)<br>C. BEACOPP escalated (eight cycles) | 260<br>469<br>466 | 69% (FFTF); 83% (OS)<br>76% (FFTF); 88% (OS)<br>87% (FFTF); 91% (OS) | FU 5 years |
| GHSG HD9 [20] | 2009 | A. COPP/ABVD (four cycles)<br>B. BEACOPP baseline (eight cycles)<br>C. BEACOPP escalated (eight cycles) | 260<br>469<br>466 | 64% (FFTF); 75% (OS)<br>70% (FFTF); 80% (OS)<br>82% (FFTF); 86% (OS) | FU 10 years |
| GHSG HD12 [21] | | A. 8 BEA escalated<br>B. 8 BEA escalated<br>C. 4 BEA esc. +4 BEA baseline<br>D. 4 BEA esc. +4 BEA baseline<br>(A.+C.: +RT bulk/residual mass) | 887<br>887 | A+B: 88% (PFS); 92% (OS)<br>C+D: 85% (PFS); 90% (OS) | FU 5 years |

*GHSG* German Hodgkin Study Group; *RT* radiotherapy; *FFS* failure-free survival; *FFP* freedom from progression; *EFS* event-free survival; *PFS* progression-free survival; *OS* overall survival; *FFTF* freedom from treatment failure; *FU* follow-up; *UKNCRI* United Kingdom National Cancer Research Institute cial for the cohort of HL patients in question, short- and long-term.

Since so far no mature results of these trials are available, only an indirect comparison is possible. Taking the 5-year relapse rate of about 30–40% for ABVD into account, the pivotal question is, obviously, how many of these relapsing patients can be rescued. With regard to this issue, the results from two randomized studies comparing conventional chemotherapy and HDCT followed by ASCT are not too encouraging. In the BNLI trial, patients were treated with conventional-dose mini-Beam (carmustine, etoposide, cytarabine, and melphalan) or high-dose BEAM with ASCT; the actuarial 3-year event-free survival was significantly better in patients who received high-dose therapy (53 vs. 10%), but still rather low [22]. In the HDR1 study conducted by the GHSG in cooperation with the EBMT, patients were randomly assigned to four courses of mini-Beam plus dexamethasone (dexa-mini-Beam) or two courses of dexa-mini-Beam followed by BEAM and ASCT: the final analysis showed that FFP was significantly higher in the BEAM + ASCT group (55 vs. 34%) [23]. The HDR2 follow-up study tried to improve these results by introducing a new induction regimen (dexamethasone, high-dose cytarabine, and cisplatinum) [24]. With a median follow-up of 30 months (range 3–61 months), freedom from second failure (FF2F) and OS were 59 and 78% for all patients, respectively. FF2F and OS for patients with early relapse were 62 and 81%, for late relapse 65 and 81%; for progressive disease 41 and 48%, respectively.

To summarize these data, about a half of all relapsing HL patients might be salvaged by ASCT. With a 5-year relapse rate of 30–40%, one would expect to have an OS of around 80–85% for ABVD. This is exactly the number that was found in most prospectively randomized trials [4–6, 13]. Those trials reporting a better OS had included early-stage patients [12, 17]. The corresponding number for BEACOPP escalated is 91%, as confirmed in two large randomized studies [19, 21]. Thus, there is strong indirect evidence that the number needed to treat (NNT) with BEACOPP escalated to safe one life in patients with advanced stage HL compared to ABVD is 10–15. Of course, a direct comparison delivers a better level of evidence. Fortunately, and trials investigating this important question are underway.

## 12.3.1  ABVD vs. BEACOPP

Three studies have been initiated comparing these two approaches in a prospective randomized setting. So far, only one trial has undergone final analysis. Immature data have been reported for the second, and no data are available for the third. The final results of the HD2000 trial showed a significant superiority of BEACOPP over ABVD in terms of FFP but not for OS [25]. At 5 years, the FFP rate was 68% for ABVD and 81% for BEACOPP (4 escalated + 2 baseline, "4+2"); the OS was 84% for ABVD and 92% for BEACOPP, respectively. However, the lack of significance is likely due to the low power of this study that enrolled 307 patients in three different treatment arms. In the IIL-GITIL-Michelangelo study, ABVD (six to eight courses) or BEACOPP given in 4+4 fashion plus pre-planned high-dose salvage produced a comparable 3-year outcome [26]. BEACOPP up-front showed a superior 3-year FFP (87 vs. 71%, $p < 0.04$). Finally, a large intergroup trial organized by the EORTC is currently ongoing (#20012). In this trial, ABVD is compared to BEACOPP 4+4; results are pending (Table 12.3).

To summarize, the difference in FFTF at 3–5 years is around 15% resulting in an OS difference of once a sufficient median observation time (5 years) is reached. Thus, the described indirect evidence of 8% a clinically meaningful superiority of BEACOPP escalated over ABVD in terms of OS is strongly supported by the existing data set.

## 12.4  Outcome Prediction

## 12.4.1  The International Prognostic Score

Overall, it would be preferable to treat each advanced stage patient according to his/her individual risk profile in order to better balance efficacy and toxicity. Accordingly, some current concepts also include prognostic factors into the treatment plan by using the IPS for risk stratification [27].

The score was derived from 5,141 patients who had been treated with a COPP/ABVD-like regimen with or without radiotherapy. The end point was FFP of disease. Seven factors had similar independent

**Table 12.3** ABVD vs. BEACOPP

| Trial and references | Publication year | Therapy regimen | Numbers of patients | Outcome | FU and comments |
|---|---|---|---|---|---|
| Gruppo Italiano per lo Studio dei Linfomi [25] | 2009 | A. ABVD (six cycles)<br>B. BEACOPP (4 esc + 4 base)<br>C. COPPEBVCAD (six cycles) | 103<br>102<br>102 | 61% (PFS); 84% (OS)<br>81% (PFS); 92% (OS)<br>78% (PFS); 91% (OS) | FU 5 years<br>Significant reduction of progressive disease in the BEACOPP arm |
| Michelangelo, GITIL and IIL cooperative groups [26] | 2008 | A. ABVD (six cycles)<br>B. BEACOPP<br>(4 esc + 4 base)<br>30 Gy of radiotherapy to sites of initial bulky disease or of residual mass | 166<br>155 | 71% (FFP); 91% (OS)<br>87% (FFP); 90% (OS) | FU 3 years |
| EORTC 20012 | | A. ABVD<br>(eight cycles)<br>B. BEACOPP<br>(4 esc + 4 base) | 550 | | |

*EORTC* European Organisation for Research and Treatment of Cancer; *FFP* freedom from progression; *PFS* progression-free survival; *OS* overall survival; *FU* follow-up

prognostic effects: serum albumin of less than 4 g/dL, hemoglobin level of less than 10.5 g/dL, male sex, age of 45 years or older, stage IV disease (according to the Ann Arbor classification), leukocytosis (white-cell count of at least 15,000/mm³), and lymphocytopenia (lymphocyte count of less than 600/mm³, or less than 8% of the white-cell count, or both). The IPS is currently being used for a risk-adapted therapy in an Israelian phase II study (NCT00392314). Patients in good prognostic advanced stages (IPS 0–2) are treated with ABVD, and patients with an IPS ≥3 receive BEACOPP escalated induction therapy. This strategy is supported by the excellent outcome of IPS 0–2 patients after ABVD or BEACOPP. However, a distinct group of patients at very high risk cannot be identified on the basis of routinely documented demographics and clinical characteristics as used in the IPS.

### 12.4.2 Positron Emission Tomography

The IPS is more and more being challenged by response-adapted risk evaluation. It has been demonstrated for HL patients that response to chemotherapy has an impact on the final treatment outcome [28, 29]. However,

response as measured by computed tomography (CT) scan might occur with some delay in advanced HL. This is likely due to the fibrotic tissue infiltrating lymph nodes in this disease, which often results in residual masses remaining several months after therapy, especially in cases of bulky disease. For example, in the GHSG HD15 trial, 311 of 817 patients (38%) showed residual disease >2.5 cm as determined by CT after the completion of chemotherapy [30]. However, 79% (n=245) of these patients at the same time had a negative FDG-PET scan. These patients did not receive any additional radiotherapy and, with a rather short median observation time of 18 months, their outcome was not inferior compared to patients reaching a CR after chemotherapy. These data indicate, at least, that the biologic response determined by FDG-PET is superior to the morphologic response in terms of its negative predictive value. PET is discussed in detail elsewhere in this book (see Chap. 6); nevertheless, the work by Gallamini et al. must be mentioned in this context. They were able to show that the early PET response (after two cycles of ABVD) overshadows the prognostic value of the IPS and thus is an important tool for planning risk-adapted treatment in advanced HL [31, 32].

Therefore, current concepts include early response evaluation, guided by FDG-PET, into treatment strategies and will hopefully define a new standard of care in which each patient receives as much therapy as needed.

## 12.5 Current Concepts: Response-Adapted Therapy

### 12.5.1 De-escalating BEACOPP

The HD15 trial of the GHSG was the first large trial to investigate the negative predictive value of PET in advanced HL, which was used to guide therapy after completion of chemotherapy. Patients were randomized between eight courses of BEACOPP escalated, six courses of BEACOPP escalated, or eight courses of BEACOPP-14 (a time-intensified variant of BEACOPP baseline) [33]. As described above, additional radiotherapy was applied only to residual lesions >2.5 cm positive by PET, and a high negative predictive value for progression or early relapse was found (NPV = 94%). Encouraged by these results and by reports from other studies, the GHSG decided to test a PET-guided strategy in the current HD18 trial [32, 34]. In this study, PET is used to assess the early response after two cycles of BEACOPP escalated and, in case of negativity, therapy is reduced to a total of four cycles (and compared to the standard of eight cycles). This is a de-escalating approach based on the excellent negative predictive value of PET in HL. First results from the Israeli group have recently been published and support this approach [35]. Patients with advanced stage HL and an IPS ≥3 received two initial cycles of BEACOPP escalated and were then evaluated by PET/CT scan. In case of PET negativity, they were treated by four cycles of ABVD. After a median follow-up of 48 months, PFS and OS at 4 years were 78 and 95%, respectively. Though the PFS of 78% in this trial published by Avigdor et al. looks disappointing at the first glance, this is within the expected range. In the HD9 trial, FFTF for patients in the unfavorable risk group (IPS 4–7) was 82% at 5 years. However, looking at the PET results, the 4-year PFS for early PET-negative patients (n = 31) and early PET-positive patients (n = 13) was 87 and 53%, respectively (p = 0.01). Though the absolute patient number is small, these data suggest that a de-escalating approach in early PET-negative patients after two cycles of BEACOPP escalated might be feasible.

### 12.5.2 Escalating ABVD

Several groups follow the alternative approach of escalating treatment in patients not responding to two cycles of ABVD as defined by PET positivity. These patients have a very poor outcome with ABVD or ABVD-like therapy. The 2-year PFS is reported as low as 6% [36]. So far, only very preliminary data are available from ongoing trials. However, first results of the GITIL (Gruppo Italiano Terapie Innovative nei Linfomi) trial were published in 2009 [37]. In this trial, PET-positive patients receive two cycles of ABVD followed by eight cycles of BEACOPP (4 + 4). Out of 164 enrolled patients, 24 (15%) were PET-2-positive and 136 PET-2-negative, respectively. The two cohorts of patients were well matched in terms of prognostic factors and the IPS ≥3 was equally frequent in both arms (29 and 28%, p = 0.95). Of the 24 PET-positive patients, 15 (62%) were in continuous CR (CCR) after BEACOPP and 9 progressed; the mean duration of CR for the responding patients was 18 months (11–37). 127/136 PET-negative patients (93.5%) were in CCR after standard ABVD and nine progressed or relapsed. The 2-year PFS of PET-positive patients was 56% only and 93% for the PET-negative patients, respectively.

These data can be compared with those published by Dann et al. who used two cycles of BEACOPP baseline as induction and increased the dose to BEACOPP escalated in PET-positive cases. In this study, the 5-year PFS was 85% for these high-risk patients, accounting for a difference of almost 30% as compared to the induction with ABVD. A possible explanation for this observation is the longer duration (8 vs. 6 weeks for 2x ABVD vs. 2x BEACOPP) and a lower dose intensity in the first 2 months, which are possibly most relevant for long-term outcome, allowing the Hodgkin and Reed–Sternberg cells to develop chemoresistance. This hypothesis was developed many years ago and was termed the "Kairos principle," referring to the god of the right moment in the ancient Greek mythology. Another observation supports this hypothesis: the most relevant improvement when using BEACOPP escalated occurs in the early treatment phase with the reduction of the number of patients suffering from progressive disease compared to ABVD (difference around 8%) [25]. However, also other cooperative groups are studying the ABVD escalation approach and mature results have to be awaited.

The SWOG is currently conducting a study (NCT00822120) in which treatment intensification in PET-positive patients after two cycles of ABVD using six cycles of BEACOPP escalated is being evaluated. The design of a cooperative trial including UK-NCRI, Italian, and Nordic centers is very similar. In this study,

PET-positive patients receive two cycles of ABVD followed by four to six cycles of dose dense BACOPP-14 or four to six cycles of BEACOPP escalated. The IIL (Italian Lymphoma Intergroup) increases the chemotherapy intensity in case of a positive PET scan after two cycles of ABVD using the IGEV regimen (ifosfamide, gemcitabine, vinorelbine) followed by HDCT and ASCT (NCT00784537). A similar approach in the "pre-PET era" randomized patients with unfavorable HL (defined as the presence of two poor risk factors consisting of high serum LDH, large mediastinal mass, greater than one extranodal site, low hematocrit, or inguinal involvement) who achieved a CR or PR after four courses of ABVD chemotherapy to either ASCT or four cycles of conventional chemotherapy [38]. ASCT was not superior to conventional dose therapy in terms of PFS or OS. However, early PET-positive patients represent a very poor-prognosis group and might have a greater benefit from this very aggressive strategy than a patient population selected by two baseline risk factors.

To summarize, the early PET-guided escalation approach after ABVD induction is currently being investigated in several studies, one of which has been presented as interim analysis so far. In this analysis, the PFS at 2 years was poor with only 56%. Though this is better than in a historical control with patients treated with ABVD only, it is much worse than the PFS for PET-positive patients after two cycles BEACOPP baseline induction, as discussed earlier [34, 37]. So far, these data support the Kairos hypothesis, which favors an early escalation and thus an aggressive induction therapy. However, more mature results of the ongoing trials must consolidate this hypothesis before final conclusions can be drawn.

## 12.6 The Role of Radiotherapy

The role of consolidating radiotherapy for advanced HL depends on the efficacy of the prior chemotherapy. After MOPP or MOPP-like regimen, there might be a potential advantage of IFRT as detected by a meta-analysis of 16 randomized studies, whereas this advantage is not evident after ABVD or ABVD-like regimens [39, 40]. A randomized EORTC study demonstrated that consolidation with IFRT did not improve the outcome in CR patients after six to eight courses of alternating MOPP and ABV, but potentially improved the

outcome of PR patients [41]. A randomized GELA trial showed that consolidation with IFRT after doxorubicin-induced CR was not superior to two additional cycles of chemotherapy [42]. The GHSG HD12 study randomized consolidating radiotherapy to residual disease vs. observation only and showed a noninferiority of the observation arm [21]. Unfortunately, the study was biased by the central review. Experts in this panel were blinded to the randomization result and recommend radiotherapy independent of randomization in patients deemed at high risk of relapse without additional radiotherapy. On the basis of the expert panel recommendation almost 10% of patients were irradiated who had originally been randomized to the observation arm. These patients obviously represent a high-risk group which might need consolidative therapy, e.g., IFRT or possibly HDCT + SCT, as has been shown also in the HD15 trial, where around 15–20% were PET-positive after induction chemotherapy and received IFRT. In addition, so far unpublished data from the HD12 trial indicate a benefit of radiotherapy to residual disease >1.5 cm in terms of PFS.

To conclude, in patients achieving a CR with chemotherapy, consolidating radiotherapy does not seem to improve the overall results. However, FDG-PET scan might be helpful to identify patients with residual disease and the need for consolidating therapy [30]. Whether or not radiotherapy will suffice to rescue these 15–20% high-risk patients still needs to be determined.

## 12.7 Summary

Advanced stage HL has become a curable disease for the majority of patients. First-line treatment with six to eight cycles of ABVD is the widely accepted standard. However, the more aggressive BEACOPP escalated regimen induces a clinically relevant superior PFS, which translates into an improved OS in indirect comparisons. Ongoing well-designed prospectively randomized studies are currently evaluating these two approaches and valid results will be available in the near future. It might well be, though, that in the meantime the early PET response-adapted design of the latest study generation will render this question obsolete. Scientific interest is currently focused on the questions whether (1) two cycles of the less toxic regimen ABVD should be escalated to the more aggressive BEACOPP schedule in case of PET-2 positivity, or (2) if after an aggressive induction therapy with two cycles of BEACOPP further treatment can be de-escalated. Both approaches promise to find the best balance between toxicity and efficacy for the benefit of each individual patient. Unfortunately, these different approaches are not tested against each other within a single randomized trial and, therefore, the current debate on the standard treatment of advanced stage HL will continue to keep us excited.

# References

1. Longo DL, Young RC, Wesley M, Hubbard SM, Duffey PL, Jaffe ES, et al. Twenty years of MOPP therapy for Hodgkin's disease. J Clin Oncol. 1986;4:1295–306.
2. DeVita Jr VT, Simon RM, Hubbard SM, Young RC, Berard CW, Moxley JH, et al. Curability of advanced Hodgkin's disease with chemotherapy. Long-term follow-up of MOPP-treated patients at the National Cancer Institute. Ann Intern Med. 1980;92:587–95.
3. Bonadonna G, Valagussa P, Santoro A. Alternating non-cross-resistant combination chemotherapy or MOPP in stage IV Hodgkin's disease. A report of 8-year results. Ann Intern Med. 1986;104:739–46.
4. Duggan DB, Petroni GR, Johnson JL, Glick JH, Fisher RI, Connors JM, et al. Randomized comparison of ABVD and MOPP/ABV hybrid for the treatment of advanced Hodgkin's disease: report of an intergroup trial. J Clin Oncol. 2003; 21:607–14.
5. Santoro A, Bonadonna G, Valagussa P, Zucali R, Viviani S, Villani F, et al. Long-term results of combined chemotherapy-radiotherapy approach in Hodgkin's disease: superiority of ABVD plus radiotherapy versus MOPP plus radiotherapy. J Clin Oncol. 1987;5:27–37.
6. Canellos GP, Anderson JR, Propert KJ, Nissen N, Cooper MR, Henderson ES, et al. Chemotherapy of advanced Hodgkin's disease with MOPP, ABVD, or MOPP alternating with ABVD. N Engl J Med. 1992;327:1478–84.
7. Viviani S, Bonadonna G, Santoro A, Bonfante V, Zanini M, Devizzi L, et al. Alternating versus hybrid MOPP and ABVD combinations in advanced Hodgkin's disease: ten-year results. J Clin Oncol. 1996;14:1421–30.
8. Connors JM, Klimo P, Adams G, Burns BF, Cooper I, Meyer RM, et al. Treatment of advanced Hodgkin's disease with chemotherapy--comparison of MOPP/ABV hybrid regimen with alternating courses of MOPP and ABVD: a report from the National Cancer Institute of Canada clinical trials group. J Clin Oncol. 1997;15:1638–45.
9. Sieber M, Tesch H, Pfistner B, Rueffer U, Paulus U, Munker R, et al. Treatment of advanced Hodgkin's disease with COPP/ABV/IMEP versus COPP/ABVD and consolidating radiotherapy: final results of the German Hodgkin's Lymphoma Study Group HD6 trial. Ann Oncol. 2004;15:276–82.
10. Stefan DC, Stones D: How much does it cost to treat children with Hodgkin lymphoma in Africa? Leuk Lymphoma. 2009;50:196–9.
11. Canellos GP, Niedzwiecki D: Long-term follow-up of Hodgkin's disease trial. N Engl J Med. 2002;346:1417–8.
12. Gobbi PG, Levis A, Chisesi T, Broglia C, Vitolo U, Stelitano C, et al. ABVD versus modified stanford V versus MOPPEBVCAD with optional and limited radiotherapy in intermediate- and advanced-stage Hodgkin's lymphoma: final results of a multi-center randomized trial by the Intergruppo Italiano Linfomi. J Clin Oncol. 2005;23:9198–207.
13. Johnson PW, Radford JA, Cullen MH, Sydes MR, Walewski J, Jack AS, et al. Comparison of ABVD and alternating or hybrid multidrug regimens for the treatment of advanced Hodgkin's lymphoma: results of the United Kingdom Lymphoma Group LY09 Trial (ISRCTN97144519). J Clin Oncol. 2005;23:9208–18.
14. Radford JA, Crowther D, Rohatiner AZ, Ryder WD, Gupta RK, Oza A, et al. Results of a randomized trial comparing MVPP chemotherapy with a hybrid regimen, ChlVPP/EVA, in the initial treatment of Hodgkin's disease. J Clin Oncol. 1995;13:2379–85.
15. Radford JA, Rohatiner AZ, Ryder WD, Deakin DP, Barbui T, Lucie NP, et al. ChlVPP/EVA hybrid versus the weekly VAPEC-B regimen for previously untreated Hodgkin's disease. J Clin Oncol. 2002;20:2988–94.
16. Horning SJ, Hoppe RT, Breslin S, Bartlett NL, Brown BW, Rosenberg SA. Stanford V and radiotherapy for locally extensive and advanced Hodgkin's disease: mature results of a prospective clinical trial. J Clin Oncol. 2002;20:630–7.
17. Hoskin PJ, Lowry L, Horwich A, Jack A, Mead B, Hancock BW, et al. Randomized comparison of the stanford V regimen and ABVD in the treatment of advanced Hodgkin's Lymphoma: United Kingdom National Cancer Research Institute Lymphoma Group Study ISRCTN 64141244. J Clin Oncol. 2009;27:5390–6.
18. Diehl V. Dose-escalation study for the treatment of Hodgkin's disease. The German Hodgkin Study Group (GHSG). Ann Hematol. 1993;66:139–40.
19. Diehl V, Franklin J, Pfreundschuh M, Lathan B, Paulus U, Hasenclever D, et al. Standard and increased-dose BEACOPP chemotherapy compared with COPP-ABVD for advanced Hodgkin's disease. N Engl J Med. 2003;348:2386–95.
20. Engert A, Diehl V, Franklin J, Lohri A, Dorken B, Ludwig WD, et al. Escalated-dose BEACOPP in the treatment of patients with advanced-stage Hodgkin's lymphoma: 10 years of follow-up of the GHSG HD9 study. J Clin Oncol. 2009;27:4548–54.
21. Diehl V, H. H, Mueller RP, Eich HT, Mueller-Hermelink H, Cerny T, et al. Eight Cycles of BEACOPP Escalated Compared with 4 Cycles of BEACOPP Escalated Followed by 4 Cycles of BEACOPP Baseline with Or without Radiotherapy in Patients in Advanced Stage Hodgkin Lymphoma (HL): Final Analysis of the Randomised HD12 Trial of the German Hodgkin Study Group (GHSG). Blood (ASH Annual Meeting Abstracts). 2008; Abstract 1558.
22. Linch DC, Winfield D, Goldstone AH, Moir D, Hancock B, McMillan A, et al. Dose intensification with autologous bone-marrow transplantation in relapsed and resistant Hodgkin's disease: results of a BNLI randomised trial. Lancet. 1993; 341:1051–4.

23. Schmitz N, Pfistner B, Sextro M, Sieber M, Carella AM, Haenel M, et al. Aggressive conventional chemotherapy compared with high-dose chemotherapy with autologous haemopoietic stem-cell transplantation for relapsed chemosensitive Hodgkin's disease: a randomised trial. Lancet. 2002;359:2065–71.

24. Josting A, Rudolph C, Mapara M, Glossmann JP, Sieniawski M, Sieber M, et al. Cologne high-dose sequential chemotherapy in relapsed and refractory Hodgkin lymphoma: results of a large multicenter study of the German Hodgkin Lymphoma Study Group (GHSG). Ann Oncol. 2005;16:116–23.

25. Federico M, Luminari S, Iannitto E, Polimeno G, Marcheselli L, Montanini A, et al. ABVD compared with BEACOPP compared with CEC for the initial treatment of patients with advanced Hodgkin's lymphoma: results from the HD2000 Gruppo Italiano per lo Studio dei Linfomi Trial. J Clin Oncol. 2009;27:805–11.

26. Gianni AM, Rambaldi A, Zinzani PL, Levis A, Brusamolino E, Pulsoni A: Comparable 3-year outcome following ABVD or BEACOPP first-line chemotherapy, plus pre-planned high-dose salvage, in advanced Hodgkin lymphoma: a randomized trial of the Michelangelo, GITIL and IIL cooperative groups. J Clin Oncol. 2008;26:Abstract 8506.

27. Hasenclever D, Diehl V: A prognostic score for advanced Hodgkin's disease. International Prognostic Factors Project on Advanced Hodgkin's Disease. N Engl J Med. 1998; 339:1506–14.

28. Carde P, Koscielny S, Franklin J, Axdorph U, Raemaekers J, Diehl V, et al. Early response to chemotherapy: a surrogate for final outcome of Hodgkin's disease patients that should influence initial treatment length and intensity? Ann Oncol. 2002;13 Suppl 1:86–91.

29. Colonna P, Jais JP, Desablens B, Harousseau JL, Briere J, Boasson M, et al. Mediastinal tumor size and response to chemotherapy are the only prognostic factors in supradiaphragmatic Hodgkin's disease treated by ABVD plus radiotherapy: ten-year results of the Paris-Ouest-France 81/12 trial, including 262 patients. J Clin Oncol. 1996; 14: 1928–35.

30. Kobe C, Dietlein M, Franklin J, Markova J, Lohri A, Amthauer H, et al. Positron emission tomography has a high negative predictive value for progression or early relapse for patients with residual disease after first-line chemotherapy in advanced-stage Hodgkin lymphoma. Blood. 2008; 112:3989–94.

31. Gallamini A, Hutchings M, Rigacci L, Specht L, Merli F, Hansen M, et al. Early interim 2-[18F]fluoro-2-deoxy-D-glucose positron emission tomography is prognostically superior to international prognostic score in advanced-stage Hodgkin's lymphoma: a report from a joint Italian-Danish study. J Clin Oncol. 2007;25:3746–52.

32. Hutchings M, Loft A, Hansen M, Pedersen LM, Buhl T, Jurlander J, et al. FDG-PET after two cycles of chemotherapy predicts treatment failure and progression-free survival in Hodgkin lymphoma. Blood. 2006;107:52–9.

33. Sieber M, Bredenfeld H, Josting A, Reineke T, Rueffer U, Koch T, et al. 14-day variant of the bleomycin, etoposide, doxorubicin, cyclophosphamide, vincristine, procarbazine, and prednisone regimen in advanced-stage Hodgkin's lymphoma: results of a pilot study of the German Hodgkin's Lymphoma Study Group. J Clin Oncol. 2003;21:1734–9.

34. Dann EJ, Bar-Shalom R, Tamir A, Haim N, Ben-Shachar M, Avivi I, et al. Risk-adapted BEACOPP regimen can reduce the cumulative dose of chemotherapy for standard and high-risk Hodgkin lymphoma with no impairment of outcome. Blood. 2007;109:905–9.

35. Avigdor A, Bulvik S, Levi I, Dann EJ, Shemtov N, Perez-Avraham G, et al. Two cycles of escalated BEACOPP followed by four cycles of ABVD utilizing early-interim PET/CT scan is an effective regimen for advanced high-risk Hodgkin's lymphoma. Ann Oncol. 2010;21:126–32.

36. Gallamini A, Rigacci L, Merli F, Nassi L, Bosi A, Capodanno I, et al. The predictive value of positron emission tomography scanning performed after two courses of standard therapy on treatment outcome in advanced stage Hodgkin's disease. Haematologica. 91:475–81.

37. Gallamini A, Fiore F, Sorasio R, Rambaldi A, Patti C, Stelitano C, et al. Early chemotherapy intensification with BEACOPP in high-risk, interim-pet positive advanced stage Hodgkin lymphoma, improves the overall treatment outcome of ABVD: a GITIL multicenter clinical study. Annuanl EHA Meeting. 2009; Abstract Number 0502.

38. Federico M, Bellei M, Brice P, Brugiatelli M, Nagler A, Gisselbrecht C, et al. High-dose therapy and autologous stem-cell transplantation versus conventional therapy for patients with advanced Hodgkin's lymphoma responding to front-line therapy. J Clin Oncol. 2003;21:2320–5.

39. Andrieu JM, Yilmaz U, Colonna P. MOPP versus ABVD and low-dose versus high-dose irradiation in Hodgkin's disease at intermediate and advanced stages: analysis of a meta-analysis by clinicians. J Clin Oncol. 1999;17:730–4.

40. Loeffler M, Brosteanu O, Hasenclever D, Sextro M, Assouline D, Bartolucci AA, et al. Meta-analysis of chemotherapy versus combined modality treatment trials in Hodgkin's disease. International Database on Hodgkin's Disease Overview Study Group. J Clin Oncol. 1998;16: 818–29.

41. Aleman BM, Raemaekers JM, Tirelli U, Bortolus R, van 't Veer MB, Lybeert ML, et al. Involved-field radiotherapy for advanced Hodgkin's lymphoma. N Engl J Med. 2003; 348:2396–406.

42. Ferme C, Mounier N, Casasnovas O, Brice P, Divine M, Sonet A, et al. Long-term results and competing risk analysis of the H89 trial in patients with advanced-stage Hodgkin lymphoma: a study by the Groupe d'Etude des Lymphomes de l'Adulte (GELA). Blood. 2006;107: 4636–42.

# Relapsed and Refractory Hodgkin Lymphoma

## 13

Andreas Josting and Philip J. Biermann

## Contents

A. Josting (✉)
German Hodgkin Lymphoma Study Group (GHSG),
Gleueler Str. 269–271, 50935 Köln, Germany
e-mail: andreas.josting@uni-koeln.de

P.J. Biermann
984455 Nebraska Medical Ctr.,
Omaha, NE 68198–4455, USA
e-mail: pjbierma@unmc.edu

## 13.1 Introduction

Depending on stage and risk factor profile, up to 95% of patients diagnosed with Hodgkin lymphoma (HL) at first presentation reach complete remission (CR) after the initial standard treatment including radiotherapy, combination chemotherapy, or combined modality treatment. Patients who relapse after first CR can achieve a second CR with salvage treatment including radiotherapy for localised relapse in previously non-irradiated areas, conventional salvage chemotherapy, or high-dose chemotherapy (HDCT) followed by stem cell transplantation (SCT) [1].

## 13.2 Prognostic Factors in Relapsed and Refractory Hodgkin Lymphoma

The length of remission to first-line chemotherapy has a marked effect on the ability of patients to respond to subsequent salvage treatment [2]. In 1992, the National Cancer Institute (NCI) updated these findings with the long-term follow-up of patients who had relapsed after polychemotherapy [3]. Derived primarily from investigations involving failures after treatment with mechlorethamine, vincristine, procarbazine, and prednisone (MOPP) and its variants, these conclusions were also relevant for other chemotherapy regimens. On this basis, chemotherapy failures can be divided into three subgroups:

A. Engert and S.J. Horning (eds.), *Hodgkin Lymphoma*,
DOI: 10.1007/978-3-642-12780-9_13, © Springer-Verlag Berlin Heidelberg 2011

- Primary progressive HL – these are patients who never achieved a CR
- Early relapse – relapse within 12 months of CR
- Late relapse – relapse after CR lasting more than 12 months

Virtually no patient with primary progressive disease survives more than 8 years when treated with conventional chemotherapy. In contrast, the projected 20-year survival for patients with early relapse or late relapse in earlier studies was 11 and 22%, respectively [3].

## 13.3 Primary Progressive Hodgkin Lymphoma

Patients with primary progressive disease, defined as progression during induction treatment or within 90 days after the end of treatment, have a particularly poor prognosis. Conventional salvage regimens have given disappointing results in the vast majority of patients: response to salvage treatment is low and the duration of response is usually short. The 8-year overall survival (OS) ranges between 0 and 8% [3, 4].

The German Hodgkin Study Group (GHSG) retrospectively analysed 206 patients with primary progressive HL to determine outcomes after salvage therapy and to identify prognostic factors [5]. The 5-year freedom from second failure (FF2F) and OS for all patients was 17 and 26%. As reported from transplant centres, the 5-year FF2F and OS for patients treated with HDCT was 42 and 48%, respectively, but only 33% of all patients were treated with HDCT. The low percentage of patients actually receiving HDCT was due to rapidly progressing fatal disease or life-threatening severe toxicity after salvage therapy. Other reasons not to proceed to HDCT were insufficient stem cell harvest, poor performance status, and advanced age. In multivariate analysis, Karnofsky performance score at progress ($p<0.0001$), age ($p=0.019$), and attaining at least a temporary remission to first-line chemotherapy ($p=0.0003$) were significant prognostic factors for survival. Patients with none of these risk factors had a 5-year OS of 55% compared with 0% for patients with all three of these unfavourable prognostic factors.

## 13.4 Prognostic Factors in Relapsed Hodgkin Lymphoma

The overall prognosis is bad for patients relapsing after first-line chemotherapy when treated with conventional chemotherapy. At present, HDCT followed by autologous stem cell transplant (ASCT) is the treatment of choice for patients with relapsed HL after first-line polychemotherapy. The results reported with HDCT in patients with late relapse were better than those reported in most series of conventional chemotherapy. However, the use of HDCT in late relapses has been an area of controversy because patients with late relapse have satisfactory second CR rates when treated with conventional chemotherapy and OS ranges from 40 to 55%. As far as randomised clinical trials are concerned, HDR-1 performed by the GHSG showed improved FFTF after HDCT compared with conventional chemotherapy in patients with late relapse [6].

Many prognostic factors have been described for patients relapsing after first-line chemotherapy. These include age, sex, histology, site of relapse, stage at relapse, bulky disease, B-symptoms, performance status, and extranodal relapse. The impact of these factors is difficult to assess due to confounding factors such as small numbers of patients and inclusion of primary progressive HL. In addition, multivariate analyses were often not performed [7–9].

Brice et al. reported one of the largest studies evaluating prognostic factors in relapsed HL. One-hundred and eighty-seven patients who relapsed after a first CR were included. At first relapse, treatment was conventional (chemo- and/or radiotherapy) in 44% and HDCT followed by ASCT in 56%. By multivariate analysis, two prognostic factors were identified to correlate with both FF2F and OS. These factors were the initial duration of first remission (i.e. <12 months or >12 months; $p<0.0001$) and stage at relapse (I–II vs. III–IV; $p=0.0013$). FF2F was 62 and 32%; OS 44 and 87%, respectively, according to the presence of zero or two parameters. Laboratory data were not available for this retrospective analysis [10].

The GHSG also performed a retrospective analysis including 422 relapsed patients. The analysis of prognostic factors suggests that the prognosis of a patient with relapsed HL can be estimated according to several risk factors. The most relevant factors were combined into a prognostic score (Table 13.1). This score included duration of first remission, stage at relapse, and the presence or absence of anaemia at relapse. Early recurrence within

**Table 13.1** Prognostic score in relapsed Hodgkin disease evaluated in 422 patients Josting et al. [11]

| Factor | | Groups with 4-year OS (%) |
|---|---|---|
| Duration of first remission | Early relapse vs. Late relapse | 47 73 |
| Stage at relapse | Stage III/IV vs. Stage I/II | 46 77 |
| Hemoglobin | F < 10.5 g/dL; M < 12.0 g/dL vs. | 40 |
| | F > 10.5 g/dL; M > 12.0 g/dL | 72 |

3–12 months after the end of primary treatment, relapse stage III or IV, and haemoglobin <10.5 g/dL in female or <12 g/dL in male patients contributed to a score with values 0–3 in order of worsening prognosis [11]. This prognostic score allowed to distinguish between different prognostic groups. The actuarial 4-year FF2F and OS for patients relapsing after chemotherapy with three unfavourable factors was 17 and 27%, respectively. In contrast, patients with none of the unfavourable factors had FF2F and OS at 4 years of 48 and 83%, respectively. In addition, the prognostic score was also predictive for other patient groups such as those relapsing after radiotherapy, for patients relapsing after chemotherapy who were treated with conventional treatment or HDCT followed by ASCT, and for patients under 60 years having a Karnofsky performance status ≥90%. These were the major candidate groups for dose intensification. This prognostic score used clinical characteristics that can be easily collected at the time of relapse separating groups of patients with clearly different outcomes.

The prognostic factors identified may be useful in tailoring treatment for subgroups of patients, defining homogenous cohorts for prospective randomised trials, and identifying more precisely patients with poor-risk relapse who should be treated with innovative approaches.

## 13.5 Treatment Strategies

Patients who relapse following radiation therapy only for localised HL achieve satisfactory results with combination chemotherapy and are not considered candidates for HDCT and ASCT. The survival of patients relapsing after radiotherapy-treated early-stage disease is at least equal to that of advanced-stage patients initially treated with chemotherapy. OS and disease-free survival (DFS) range from 57 to 71% [12, 13].

Salvage radiotherapy has been used in patients with relapsed HL and has resulted in long-term PFS ranging between 25 and 35% especially in localised relapse without B-symptoms [43, 44]. Conventional salvage chemotherapy is now being used to reduce tumour burden prior to HDCT and ASCT. Several regimens have been published (Table 13.2). However, so far no randomised trial compared different conventional salvage chemotherapy regimens.

HDCT followed by ASCT has been shown to produce 30–65% long-term DFS in selected patients with refractory or relapsed HL [14–17]. In addition, the reduction of early transplant-related mortality ranging from 10 to 25% in earlier studies to less than 5% in more recent studies led to the widespread acceptance

**Table 13.2** Response rates (RR) and treatment related mortality (TRM) of selected conventional salvage chemotherapy regimens in patients with relapsed/refractory HL

| Regimen | n | RR (%) Overall | Relapse | Progress | TRM (%) | Author |
|---|---|---|---|---|---|---|
| DHAP | 102 | 88 | 92 | 65 | 0 | Josting et al, Ann Oncol 2002 |
| IGEV | 91 | 81 | 93 | 61 | 0 | Santorro, Ann Oncol 2007 |
| ICE | 65 | 88 | n.e. | n.e. | 2 | Moschkowitz, Blood 2001 |
| ASHAP | 57 | 70 | 85 | 51 | 0 | Rodriguez, Blood 1999 |
| Dexa-BEAM | 55 | 60 | 70 | 52 | 4 | Pfreundschuh, JCO, 1994 |
| Mini-BEAM | 44 | 74 | 85 | 52 | 0 | Linch, Lancet 1993 |
| GDP | 23 | 70 | n.e. | n.e. | 0 | Baetz, Ann Oncol 1993 |
| ESHAP | 22 | 73 | 73 | 0 | 5 | Aparicio, Ann Oncol 1999 |

of HDCT and ASCT. Although results of HDCT have generally been better than those observed after conventional dose salvage therapy, the validity of these results has been questioned due to the lack of randomised trials. The most compelling evidence for the superiority of HDCT and ASCT in relapsed HL comes from two reports: one was conducted by the British National Lymphoma Investigation (BNLI) and the other by the GHSG together with the EBMT (European Group for Blood and Marrow Transplantation). In the BNLI trial, patients with relapsed or refractory HL were treated with a combination of carmustine (BCNU), etoposide, cytarabine, and melphalan at a conventional-dose level (mini-BEAM) or a high-dose level (BEAM) that was supported by autologous bone-marrow transplantation [18]. The actuarial 3-year event-free survival (EFS) was significantly better in patients who received HDCT (53 vs. 10%). The second randomised multi-center trial in this setting was performed by the GHSG/EBMT to determine the benefit of HDCT in relapsed HL. Patients who relapsed after polychemotherapy were randomly assigned to four cycles of Dexa-BEAM (dexamethasone, BCNU, etoposide, Ara-C, and melphalan) or two cycles of Dexa-BEAM followed by HDCT (BEAM) and ABMT/PBSCT. The final analysis of 144 evaluable patients revealed that for 117 patients in PR or CR after two cycles of chemotherapy, FFTF in the HDCT group was 55% compared with 34% for patients receiving additional two cycles of conventional dose chemotherapy. OS was not significantly different [6].

A potential alternative to the commonly used multi-agent HDCT regimens was sequential HDCT. This approach had increasingly been employed in the treatment of solid tumours as well as in haematologic and lymphoproliferative malignancies. Initial results from phase I/II studies indicated that this approach was safe and effective [19–24]. In accordance with the Norton–Simon hypothesis [25], few non-cross-resistant agents were given after initial cytoreduction at short time intervals. In general, the transplantation of PBSC and the use of growth factors allowed the application of the putatively most effective drugs at highest possible doses and intervals of 1–3 weeks. Sequential HDCT thereby enabled the highest possible dosing over a minimum period of time (dose intensification).

In 1997, a multicenter phase II trial with a high-dose sequential chemotherapy program and a final myeloablative course evaluated feasibility and efficacy

of this novel regimen in patients with relapsed HL [26]. Eligibility criteria included patients aged 18–60 years, histologically proven relapsed or primary progressive HL, second relapse with no prior HDCT, and ECOG performance status 0–1. The treatment program consisted of two cycles of DHAP (dexamethasone, ara-C, cisplatin) in the first phase in order to reduce tumour burden before HDCT. Patients with PR or CR after two cycles of DHAP received sequential HDCT consisting of cyclophosphamide 4 $g/m^2$ i.v.; methotrexate 8 $g/m^2$ i.v. plus vincristine 1.4 $mg/m^2$ i.v.; and etoposide 2 $g/m^2$ i.v. The final myeloablative course was BEAM followed by PBSCT with at least $2 \times 10^6$ CD34+ cells/kg. At the final evaluation, 102 patients were available for analysis. Of these patients, 10 had multiple relapses, 16 progressive disease, 20 early relapse, and 44 late relapse. At 18 months of median follow-up (range 3–31 months) results were as follows: response rate (RR) after DHAP 87% (23% CR, 64% PR) and RR at final evaluation 77% (68% CR, 9% PR). Toxicity was tolerable with no treatment-related deaths. FFTF and OS for patients with early relapse were 64 and 87% for early relapse; 68 and 81% for late relapse; 30 and 58% for patients with progressive disease as well as 55 and 88% for patients with multiple relapse [26].

Based on these challenging results, the GHSG, EORTC, GEL/TAMO, and EBMT started a prospective randomised study in 2001 to compare the effectiveness of a standard HDCT regimen (BEAM) with a sequential HDCT after initial cytoreduction using two cycles of DHAP. Patients with histologically confirmed early or late relapsed HL, and patients in second relapse with no prior HDCT fulfilling the entry criteria received two cycles of dexamethasone and high-dose cytarabine and cisplatin (DHAP) followed by G-CSF. Patients achieving NC, PR, or CR after DHAP were centrally randomised to receive either BEAM followed by PBSCT (arm A of the study) or high-dose cyclophosphamide, followed by high-dose MTX plus vincristine, followed by high-dose etoposide and a final myeloablative course with BEAM (arm B of the study).

A total of 284 patients with relapsed HL were included in this largest randomised trial performed in this setting so far; 241 patients were randomised after DHAP. The median follow-up was 42 months. There were no major differences in patient characteristics between the arms with most of the patients in late first relapse (CR >12 months). The intensified

**Table 13.3** Results of randomized trials in patients with relapsed/refractory Hodgkin lymphoma

| Design | $n$ | Results | $p$ | TRM | Author |
|---|---|---|---|---|---|
| 2 x DHAP + BEAM vs.<br>2 x DHAP + HDSCT + BEAM | 284 | 72% vs.<br>67% (3y-PFS) | n.s. | 2% vs.<br>2% | Josting et al, in press |
| 4 x Dexa-BEAM vs.<br>2 x Dexa Beam + Beam | 161 | 34% vs.<br>55% (3y-FFTF) | 0.019 | 14% vs.<br>10% | Schmitz et al, Lancet, 2002 |
| Mini-Beam vs.<br>BEAM | 40 | 10% vs.<br>53% (3y-EFS) | 0.025 | 5 vs.<br>9 | Linch et al, Lancet, 1993 |

experimental arm showed significantly longer mean treatment duration, more frequent WHO Grade IV toxicity before BEAM and more frequent protocol violations ($p < 0.05$). Mortality was nearly identical in both arms (20 and 18%) and there were no differences in terms of FFTF, PFS, and OS. The respective 3-year-rates for the standard arm and the intensified arm were FFTF 71 vs. 65%, PFS 72 vs. 67%, and OS 87 vs. 80%. Patients with Ann Arbor stage IV, early or multiple relapse, and anaemia had a significantly higher risk of recurrence (all single bivariate $p < 0.05$, combined $p < 0.001$). In conclusion, both regimens tested showed equally favourable results in outcome and survival. Since further intensification did not improve results, two cycles of conventional chemotherapy (DHAP) followed by HDCT (BEAM) and autologous stem cell transplantation are the current standard of care for patients with relapsed HL.

Table 13.3 summarizes the results of the three randomized trials performed so far in patients with relapsed HL.

## 13.6 Allogeneic Transplantation After Reduced Conditioning in Hodgkin Lymphoma

Allogeneic transplantation (alloSCT) has clear advantages when compared with autologous transplantation: donor marrow cells unaffected by malignancy are used thus avoiding the risk of infusing occult tumour cells which may contribute to relapse in treated patients. In addition, donor lymphoid cells can potentially mediate a graft-versus-lymphoma effect. Generally, donor availability and age constraints have limited a broader application of alloBMT in HL. Moreover, alloBMT is associated with a high treatment-related mortality of up

to 75% in patients with induction failure, which casts doubt on the feasibility of this approach in HL [27–30]. In most cases, allogeneic transplantation from HLA-identical siblings or matched unrelated donors is not recommended for patients with HL. The reduced relapse rate associated with a potential graft-versus-tumour effect is offset by lethal graft-versus-host toxicity.

Nevertheless, patients with induction failure or relapsed patients with additional risk factors face a poor prognosis after HDCT and ASCT. Therefore, the role of alloBMT should be further evaluated within clinical trials in these patients. To reduce treatment-related mortality associated with allografting, allogeneic stem cell transplant combined with nonmyeloablative therapy have been assessed. As described in detail in Chap. 19, several groups recently updated their findings with nonmyeloablative conditioning regimens [31–33].

## 13.7 Future Directions

Alternative strategies have been developed to improve the outcome of relapsed or resistant HL. These approaches include new cytostatic drugs and biological agents with proven efficacy in preclinical models as well as the use of new imaging techniques to better predict the outcome (Chap. 6).

One of the promising new cytostatic drugs is the vinca alkaloid vinorelbine, which has demonstrated activity in HL patients pretreated with vincristine or vinblastine [34]. The use of vinorelbine in first- and second-line treatment is under investigation. The pyrimidine analogue gemcitabine represents a new mechanism of action – a "self-potentiating" effect leads to an enhanced accumulation and prolonged retention of gemcitabine in the malignant cell. The results of gemcitabine in advanced relapsed HL are promising, with an overall RR of up to 53% in relapsed patients [35].

Although some clinical efficacy has been demonstrated in clinical trials with immunotoxins (IT), none of the currently available IT seems to be suited for a clinical phase III study [36, 37]. Bispecific monoclonal antibodies (BiMoab) such as CD30×CD64 or CD16×CD30 constructs and the monoclonal anti-CD20 antibody rituximab were clinically evaluated and are undergoing further clinical development [38–40]. The use of recombinant DNA technology for site-directed modifications and the development of humanised ITs might optimise their efficacy [41, 42]. To this end, the auristatin-linked anti-CD30 monoclonal antibody construct SGN35 has given promising data in phase I and phase II trials [43, 44]. An array of other biological response modifiers such as lenalidomide, bevacizumab, different histone deacetylase inhibitors, and other small molecules are currently being investigated in preclinical models and early clinical studies [45]. In the future, combining standard chemo-/radiotherapy with biological agents might result in the elimination of residual tumour cells and subsequently more relapse-free long-term survivors.

Several groups have evaluated the use of early 2-[fluorine-18]fluoro-2-deoxy-D-glucose positron emission tomography (FDG-PET) prior to HDCT and ASCT to predict outcome. Preliminary results suggest that a positive PET prior to HDCT might indicate a poorer outcome PET. Whether patients with positive PET should be considered candidates for more intensive or investigational approaches warrants further controlled studies [46].

# References

1. Josting A, Wolf J, Diehl V. Hodgkin's disease. Prognostic factors and treatment strategies. Curr Opin Oncol. 2000;12: 403–11.
2. Fisher R, De VV, Hubbard S, et al. Prolonged disease-free survival in Hodgkin disease with MOPP reinduction after first relapse. Ann Intern Med. 1979;90:761–5.
3. Longo D, Duffey P, Young R, et al. Conventional-dose salvage combination chemotherapy in patients relapsing with Hodgkin disease after combination chemotherapy: the low probability for cure. J Clin Oncol. 1992;10:210–8.
4. Bonfante V, Santoro A, Viviani S, et al. Outcome of patients with Hodgkin disease failing after primary MOPP/ABVD. J Clin Oncol. 1997;15:528–34.
5. Josting A, Rueffer U, Franklin J, et al. Prognostic factors and treatment outcome in primary progressive Hodgkin's lymphoma – a report from the German Hodgkin's Lymphoma Study Group (GHSG). Blood. 2000;96(4):1280–6.
6. Schmitz N, Pfistner B, Sextro M, et al. Aggressive conventional chemotherapy compared with high-dose chemotherapy with autologous haemopoietic stem-cell transplantation for relapsed chemosensitive Hodgkin disease: a randomised trial. Lancet. 2002;359(9323):2065–71.
7. Lohri A, Barnett M, Fairey RN, et al. Outcome of treatment of first relapse of Hodgkin disease after primary chemotherapy: identification of risk factors from the British Columbia experience 1970 to 1988. Blood. 1991;77(10): 2292–8.
8. Fermè C, Bastion Y, Lepage E, et al. The MINE regimen as intensive salvage chemotherapy for relapsed and refractory Hodgkin disease. Ann Oncol. 1995;6(6):543–9.
9. Reece D, Barnett M, Shepherd J, et al. High-dose cyclophosphamide, carmustine (BCNU), and etoposide (VP16-213) with or without cisplatin (CBV +/– P) and autologous transplantation for patients with Hodgkin disease who fail to enter a complete remission after combination chemotherapy. Blood. 1995;86:451–8.
10. Brice P, Bastion Y, Divine M, et al. Analysis of prognostic factors after the first relapse of Hodgkin disease in 187 patients. Cancer. 1996;78(6):1293–9.
11. Josting A, Franklin J, May M, et al. A new prognostic score based on treatment outcome of patients with relapsed Hodgkin lymphoma registered in the database of the German Hodgkin Lymphoma Study Group (GHSG). J Clin Oncol. 2002;20(1):221–30.
12. Cannellos G, Young RC, De Vita VD. Combination chemotherapy for advanced Hodgkin's disease in relapse following extensive radiotherapy. Clin Pharm Ther. 1972;13:750–8.
13. Santoro A, Viviani S, Villarreal C, et al. Salvage chemotherapy in Hodgkin disease irradiation failures: superiority of doxorubicin-containing regimens over MOPP. Cancer Treat Rep. 1986;70:343–51.
14. Josting A, Katay I, Rueffer U, et al. Favorable outcome of patients with relapsed or refractory Hodgkin disease treated with high-dose chemotherapy and stem cell rescue at the time of maximal response to conventional salvage therapy (Dexa-BEAM). Ann Oncol. 1998;9:289–96.
15. Biermann PJ, Bagin RG, Jagannath S, et al. High dose chemotherapy followed by autologous hematopoietic rescue in Hodgkin's disease: long term follow-up in 128 patients. Ann Oncol. 1993;4:767–73.
16. Reece DE, Connors JM, Spinelli JJ, et al. Intensive therapy with cyclophosphamide, carmustine, etoposide +/– cisplatin, and autologous bone marrow transplantation for Hodgkin's disease in first relapse after combination chemotherapy. Blood. 1994;83(5):1193–9.
17. Armitage JO, Biermann PJ, Vose JM, et al. Autologous bone marrow transplantation for patients with relapsed Hodgkin's disease. Am J Med. 1991;91:605–10.
18. Linch D, Winfield D, Goldstone A, et al. Dose intensification with autologous bone marrow transplantation in relapsed and resistant Hodgkin disease: results of a BNLI randomised trial. Lancet. 1993;341:1051–4.
19. Gianni AM, Siena S, Bregni M, Lombardi F, et al. High-dose sequential chemo-radiotherapy with peripheral blood progenitor cell support for relapsed or refractory Hodgkin's disease – a 6-year update. Ann Oncol. 1993;4:889–91.
20. Gianni AM, Bregni M, Siena S. 5-year update of the Milan Cancer Institute randomized trial of high-dose sequential

(HDS) *vs* MACOP-B therapy for diffuse large-cell lymphomas. Proc ASCO. 1994;13:373 (A1263).

21. Patrone F, Ballestrero A, Ferrando F, Brema F, Moraglio L, Valbonesi M, et al. Four-step high-dose sequential chemotherapy with double hematopoetic progenitor-cell rescue for metastatic breast cancer. J Clin Oncol. 1995;13:840–6.

22. Shea T, Mason JR, Storniolo AM, et al. Sequential cycles of high-dose carboplatin administered with recombinat human granulocyte-makrophage colony-stimulating factor and repeated infusions of autologous peripheral-blood progenitor cells: a novel and effective method for delivering multiple courses of dose-intensive therapy. J Clin Oncol. 1992;10:464–73.

23. Gianni AM, Taella C, Bregni M, et al. High-dose sequential chemo-radiotherapy, a widely applicable regimen, confers survival benefit to patients with high-risk multiple myeloma. J Clin Oncol. 1994;12:503–9.

24. Caracciolo D, Gavarotti P, Aglietta M, et al. High-dose sequential chemotherapy with blood and marrow cell autograft as salvage treatment in very poor prognosis, relapsed non-Hodgkin's lymphoma. Bone Marrow Transplant. 1993;12:621–5.

25. Norton L, Simon R. The Norton-Simon hypothesis revisited. Canc Treat Rep. 1986;70:163–9.

26. Josting A, Rudolph C, Mapara M, et al. Cologne high-dose sequential chemotherapy in relapsed and refractory Hodgkin lymphoma – results of a large multicenter study of the German Hodgkin Lymphoma Study Group (GHSG). Blood. 2003;102(11 Suppl 1):1461.

27. Anderson JE, Litzow MR, Appelbaum FR, et al. Allogeneic, syngeneic, and autologous marrow transplantation for Hodgkin's disease: the 21-year Seattle experience. J Clin Oncol. 1993;11:2342–50.

28. Phillips GL, Reece DE, Barnett MJ, et al. Allogeneic marrow transplantation for refractory Hodgkin's disease. J Clin Oncol. 1989;7:1039–45.

29. Jones RJ, Piantadosi S, Mann RB, et al. High-dose cytotoxic therapy and bone marrow transplantation for relapsed Hodgkin's disease. J Clin Oncol. 1990;8:527–37.

30. Milpied N, Fielding AK, Pearce RM, et al. Allogeneic bone marrow transplantation is not better than autologous transplant for patients with relapsed Hodgkin's disease. J Clin Oncol. 1996;14:1291–6.

31. Carella AM, Cavaliere M, Beltrami G, et al. Immunosuppressive nonmyeloablative allografting as salvage therapy in advanced Hodgkin disease. Haematologica. 2001;86(11):1121–3.

32. Sureda A, Robinson S, Canals C, et al. Reduced-intensity conditioning compared with conventional allogeneic stem-cell transplantation in relapsed or refractory Hodgkin lymphoma: an analysis from the Lymphoma Working Party of the European Group for Blood and Marrow Transplantation. J Clin Oncol. 2008;26(3):455–62.

33. Schmitz N, Sureda A, Robinson S. Allogeneic transplantation of hematopoietic stem cells after nonmyeloablative conditioning for Hodgkin disease: indications and results. Semin Oncol. 2004;31(1):27–32.

34. Devizzi L, Santaro A, Bonfante V, et al. Vinorelbine: an active drug for the management of patients with heavily pretreated Hodgkin's disease. Ann Oncol. 1994;5:817–20.

35. Santoro A, Bredenfeld H, Devizzi L, et al. Gemcitabine in the treatment of refractory Hodgkin disease: results of a multicenter phase II study. J Clin Oncol. 2000;18:2615–9.

36. Engert A, Diehl V, Schnell R, et al. A phase I study of an anti-CD25 ricin A chain immunotoxin (RFT5-SMPT-dgA) in patients with refractory Hodgkin's lymphoma. Blood. 1997;15:403–10.

37. Schnell R, Stark O, Borchmann P, et al. A phase I study with an anti-CD30 ricin A-chain Immunotoxin (Ki-4.dgA) in patients with refractory CD30 positive Hodgkins and non-Hodgkin's lymphoma. Clin Canc Res. 2002;8(6):1779–86.

38. Hartmann F, Renner C, Jung W, et al. Treatment of refractory Hodgkin's disease with an anti-CD16/CD30 bispecific antibody. Blood. 1997;15:2042–7.

39. Borchmann P, Schnell R, Fuss I, et al. Phase 1 trial of the novel bispecific molecule H22xKi-4 in patients with refractory Hodgkin lymphoma. Blood. 2002;100:3101–7.

40. Younes A, Romaguera J, Hagemeister F, et al. A pilot study of rituximab in patients with recurrent, classic Hodgkin disease. Cancer. 2003;98(2):310–4.

41. Borchmann P, Morschhauser F, Parry A, et al. The human anti-CD30 antibody 5F11 shows in vitro and in vivo activity against malignant lymphoma. Blood. 2003;102(10):3737–3742.

42. Reiners KS, Gossmann A, von Strandmann EP, et al. Effects of the anti-VEGF monoclonal antibody bevacizumab in a preclinical model and in patients with refractory and multiple relapsed Hodgkin lymphoma. J Immunother. 2009;32(5):508–12.

43. Evens A, et al. Phase I analysis of the safety and pharmacodynamics of the Novel Broad Spectrum Histone Deacetylase Inhibitor PCI-24781 in relapsed and refractory lymphoma. Blood. 2009;114(22):2726A.

44. Younes A, et al Personal communication (August 2010).

45. Younes A, et al. Novel targeted therapy for relapsed Hodgkin lymphoma. Hematology Am Soc Hematol Educ Program. 2009;1:507–19.

46. Crocchiolo R, Canevari C, Assanelli A, et al. Pre-transplant 18FDG-PET predicts outcome in lymphoma patients treated with high-dose sequential chemotherapy followed by autologous stem cell transplantation. Leuk Lymphoma. 2008;49(4):727–33.

# Pediatric Hodgkin Lymphoma

Georgina Hall, Cindy Schwartz, Stephen Daw,
and Louis S. Constine

**14**

## Contents

G. Hall (✉)
Pediatric Haematology/Oncology Unit, John Radcliffe
Hospital, Headley Way, Headington, Oxford OX3 9DU, UK
e-mail: georgina.hall@paediatrics.ox.ac.uk

C. Schwartz
Division of Pediatric Hematology/Oncology, Hasbro Children's
Hospital, 593 Eddy Street, Providence, RI 02903, USA

S. Daw
Children & Young People's Cancer Services, Divison of
Paediatrics, University College Hospital, 250 Euston Road,
London NW1 1PQ University College Hospital London,
London, UK
e-mail: stephen.daw@uclh.nhs.uk

L.S. Constine
Department of Radiation Oncology, University of Rochester
Medical Center, Rochester, NY, USA

## 14.1 Introduction

### 14.1.1 Comparison of Pediatric/ Adolescent vs. Adult HL

A comparison of the demographics of clinical presentations of PHL compared with adult HL is presented in Table 14.1. The first of the bimodal incidence peaks in Hodgkin lymphoma (HL) occurs in teenagers and young adults (15–25 year age group). HL represents less than 5% of malignancies in children under the age of 15 years. In contrast, it represents 16–20% of malignancies in adolescents making it the most common malignancy of this age group.

Childhood HL is biologically indistinguishable from HL of young and middle aged adults other than the relative incidence of specific disease histologies. Mixed cellularity (MC) and nodular lymphocyte predominant (nLP) HL are the common forms of HL in the preadolescent child; adolescents and young adults are most frequently (85%) afflicted with nodular sclerosing (NS) HL [1]. Only a third of children will have advanced disease; approximately 25% will have B symptoms. The incidence of HL with adverse features increases with age. Although there were no discernable differences in clinical presentation, response to therapy, or long-term outcome noted for adolescents (16–21 years) vs. young adults (22–45 years) treated similarly for HL [2], the treatment of children/adolescents and adults has diverged over the years.

A. Engert and S.J. Horning (eds.), *Hodgkin Lymphoma*,
DOI: 10.1007/978-3-642-12780-9_14, © Springer-Verlag Berlin Heidelberg 2011

**Table 14.1** Demographic and clinical characteristics at presentation of pediatric HL (modfied from [71, 72])

| | Childhood HL | AYA HL | Adult HL |
|---|---|---|---|
| Age range (years) | ≤14 | 15–35 | ≥35 |
| Prevalence of HL cases (%) | 10–12 | 50.00 | |
| Gender | | | |
| Male:female | 2–3:1 | 1:1–1.3:1 | |
| Histology | | | |
| Nodular sclerosis (%) | 40–45 | 65–80 | |
| Mixed cellularity (%) | 30–45 | 10–25 | |
| Lymphocyte depleted (%) | 0–3 | 1–5 | |
| LPHL (%) | 8–20 | 2–8 | |
| EBV associated | 27–54% Risk factors: male, younger age, mixed cellularity histology, economically disadvantaged countries | 20–25% | 34.00–40% |
| Other risk factors | Lower SES Increasing family size | Higher SES Smaller family size Early birth order | |
| Stage at presentation | 30–35% with Stage III or IV disease 25% with B symptoms | 40% with Stage III or IV disease 30–40% with B symptoms | |
| Relative survival rates at 5 years | 94% (<20 years) | 90% (<50 years) | |

*AYA*, adolescents and young adults; *IPS*, International Prognostic Score; *SES*, socioeconomic status

## 14.1.2 Classical Pediatric Hodgkin Lymphoma (PHL)

### 14.1.2.1 Overall Strategies

The adverse consequences of therapy have driven the pediatric treatment paradigm of care. Clinical trials for pediatric and adolescent HL have been designed to both reduce long-term organ injury and to increase efficacy. Pediatric oncologists responded first to developmental issues in the young child, and later to the long-term treatment consequences in all young survivors in the design of treatment approaches. Recognition of musculoskeletal hypoplasia in young children with HL treated with high-dose radiation (shortened sitting height, thin necks, narrow shoulders and chest [3–6] precipitated the development of pediatric-specific regimens for HL. Combined-modality treatments, even for low stage disease, allowed for the reduction of radiation dose [7] and field size, thus sparing normal structures (Fig. 14.1). This strategy for care was extended to older children and adolescents when hypothyroidism [8, 9], secondary cancers, and valvular and atherosclerotic heart disease [10, 11] were also found to be attributable to high-dose radiation.

Low dose radiation of 15–25 Gy has been the standard in childhood and adolescent HL for decades. This reduced the potential for long term risk without adversely impacting event free survival. A convergence of treatment approaches may be emerging as recent adult trials have begun to address these issues and reduce radiation doses. With overall survival over 90%, the quality of survival becomes paramount.

Early response to therapy was recognized [12, 13] as highly predictive of outcome. In Europe and the US, response-based, risk-adapted approach to treating HL [14] allows therapy to be tailored to each individual, within the context of clinical trials. Dose-dense regimens used are similar to those used by adult groups [15, 16], but the pediatric algorithms use the enhanced efficacy to support reduction of therapy.

### 14.1.2.2 Low-Risk (Early Favorable) Disease

Although there have been differing definitions of low-risk disease (Table 14.2), risk adapted approaches aim to define a cohort of patients that is curable with minimal

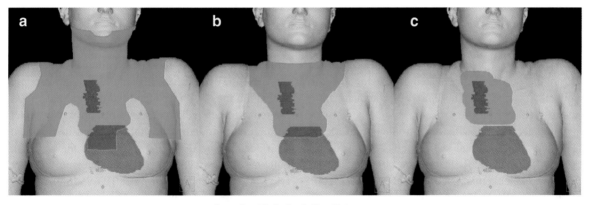

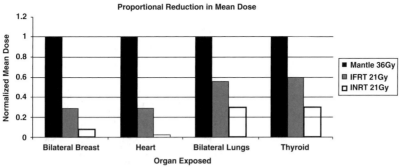

**Fig. 14.1** CT-based planning images depicting a historic mantle RT, compared to standard involved-field radiation treatment (IFRT), and involved node RT (INRT) for a patient with stage I disease involving the mediastinum. The postchemotherapy volume of initially involved paratracheal nodes is depicted in *dark red* and the cardiac silhouette is also evident. (**c**) Demonstration of the reduction in dose to breast, lung, heart, and thyroid for the female patient shown in (**a**). (From Hodgson et al. [70])

**Table 14.2** Risk groups employed by selected pediatric study groups (modified from [71, 72])

| Study group | Risk features (RF) | Low risk | Intermediate/early unfavorable risk | High risk |
|---|---|---|---|---|
| *Pediatric* | | | | |
| Children's Oncology Group [14, 73] | | IA/IIA no bulk or extranodal extension | IA bulk or "E" extension<br>IB<br>IIA bulk or "E" extension<br>IIB<br>IIIA<br>IVA | IIIB, IVB |
| German Multicenter Studies (Pediatric) [32, 74] | | IA/B<br>IIA | IIB<br>IIIEA<br>IIIB | IIEB<br>IIIEA/B<br>IIIB<br>IVA/B |
| St. Jude/Stanford/ Dana-Farber [28, 38, 68, 75] | Categorized as favorable or unfavorable risk by IPS | IA/IIA no bulk | IA bulk<br>IB<br>IIA bulk<br>IIB<br>III<br>IV | |
| Children's Cancer Group [32, 63] | Hilar lymphadenopathy<br>>4 sites nodal disease<br>Bulky disease | IA/B without RFs<br>IIA without RFs | IA/B with RFs<br>IIA with RFs<br>IIB<br>IIIA/B | V |

*RF*, refractory fever

therapy. Treatment group allocation, risk stratification, and response assessment varies according to each study group (Table 14.2) but all treatment groups define low-risk based on stage and bulky disease. Patients with nLP HL are increasingly being treated on specific low-dose regimens separate from those used for the treatment of classical HL.

In the decade following the introduction of MOPP, secondary leukemia and sterility emerged as significant concerns [17–20]. During the 1980s, alkylator exposure and leukemia risk was reduced by alternating MOPP and ABVD [21, 22]. The goal was to avoid reaching thresholds of toxicity for any specific agent. The Pediatric Oncology Group (POG) compared four cycles of MOPP/ABVD plus 25.5 Gy to six cycles of chemotherapy alone without detecting differences in efficacy [12]. However, the profound sensitivity of testes to procarbazine continued to cause sterility in boys, even with only two cycles of procarbazine-containing chemotherapy [23]. Although early attempts to avoid procarbazine were unsuccessful [24], more recent regimens have achieved this goal.

ABVD is used routinely in adults [25], but is not standard of care in children with early favorable HL. Successful regimens have been devised by the German Paediatric Oncology Hodgkin's Group (GPOH) [26] using OEPA (vincristine, etoposide, prednisone, and doxorubicin) in males (see Table 14.3), by the French Society of Pediatric Oncology [27] using EBVP (etoposide, bleomycin, vincristine, prednisone), by Donaldson et al. [28] using VAMP (vincristine, doxorubicin, methotrexate, and prednisone) and by the Pediatric Oncology Group (POG) using ABVE (doxorubicin, bleomycin, vincristine, etoposide)[29]. With these approaches, EFS of 88–92% can be achieved without significant radiation or alkylator toxicity. Patients treated on these newer regimens receive less than 200 mg/m$^2$ of doxorubicin plus or minus 20–25 Gy of involved field radiation.

The traditional approach of most pediatric HL treatment groups has been to use combined-modality therapy. Currently, these study groups are involved in evaluating methods to define low-risk patients who may be cured without radiotherapy, i.e., with chemotherapy alone. However, patients with early-stage HL treated with chemotherapy alone most frequently relapse in the initially involved lymph node(s) [30]. Therefore, an effort has also been made to reduce further the size of the radiation field size by including only the initially involved lymph node(s) – so called involved node radiation (INRT) [31].

Nachman et. al. showed an increased relapse rate in patients who did not receive radiation despite achieving CR at the end of chemotherapy [32]. Late-response evaluation may not have identified the optimal cohort for reduction of radiation. Early response may better define the profoundly chemotherapy-sensitive patient who does not need radiation. Based on the excellent outcomes of low-risk HL patients achieving CR after two cycles of chemotherapy [12], HD-95 trial [26, 33], three groups (COG, the St. Jude/DFCI/Stanford consortium, and the EuroNet PHL group) are examining early response criteria to determine who does or does not require radiation postchemotherapy.

The prognostic importance of early chemotherapy response rather than end-of-chemotherapy response has led to the use of early response assessment (after 6–9 weeks) to titrate individual therapy and dense regimens to maximize the early response rates. The most recent COG study (AHOD0431) evaluated whether early assessment by PET after one cycle is a predictor of recurrence [Keller et al. 2009, Personal Communication]. The current EuroNet PHL-C1 classical HL trial is evaluating PET activity after two intensive cycles of OEPA (cumulative dose of anthracycline is 160 mg/m$^2$) to predict who does not require radiotherapy [34]. All such reductions in treatment may increase the risk of relapse; hence adverse outcomes such as the need for high-dose salvage therapy (e.g., stem cell transplant or high-dose radiation) must be closely monitored.

### 14.1.2.3 High-Risk (Advanced, Unfavorable) Disease

For children with advanced-stage disease, improving efficacy while limiting long-term toxicity is even more challenging. The approach in pediatric HL has been to increase the number of agents so as to limit cumulative doses of individual agents. Regimens used in the 1980–1990s alternated MOPP/ABVD [22, 35] or used the hybrid COPP/ABV [32] to avoid the cumulative doses of doxorubicin (300–400 mg/m$^2$) and bleomycin (120–160 mg/m$^2$) associated with six to eight cycles of the four-drug ABVD regimen [21, 25].

Minimalistic dose regimens in combined-modality protocols, such as VEPA (Table 14.4) that eliminated traditional alkylating agents, were not successful and

**Table 14.3** Treatment results for early, favorable pediatric HL

| Group or institution | Patients (n) | Stage | Chemotherapy | Radiation (Gy), field | Survival (%) Overall | DFS, EFS, or RFS | Follow-up interval (years) | References |
|---|---|---|---|---|---|---|---|---|
| *Combined-modality trials* | | | | | | | | |
| POG 8625 (2006) | 81 | CS I–IIIA | 4 MOPP/ABVD | 25.5 IF | 97 | 91 | 8 | [12, 75] |
| U.S. CCG (2002) | 294 | CS IA/B, IIA | 4 COPP/ABV | 21, IF | 100 | 97 | 3 | [32, 63] |
| SFOP MDH-90 (2000) | 171 | I–II | 4 VBVP, good responders | 20, IF | 97.5 | 91 | 5 | [27, 66] |
|  | 27 | I–II | 4 VBVP 1–2 OPPA, poor responders | 20, IF | | 78 | 5 | |
| Germany–Austria HD-95 (2001) | 326 | I, IIA | 2 OEPA/OPPA | 20–35, IF for PR; | 97 | 91 | 3 | [32, 74] |
|  | 224 | IIB, IIIA | 2 OEPA/OPPA + 2 COPP | No RT if CR | 97 | 94 | 3 | |
| Germany–Austria HD-90 (1996) | 275 | IA/IB–IIA | 2 OEPA/OPPA | 25, IF | 99 | 94/95 | 5 | [76–79] |
|  | 124 | IIB–IIIA | 2 OEPA/OPPA 2 COPP | 25, IF | 97 | 90/96 | 5 | |
| Royal Marsden (1997) | 125 | II | 6–10 ChlVPP | 35, IF | 92 | 85 | 10 | [79, 80] |
| *Chemotherapy alone* | | | | | | | | |
| USA-CCG (2002) | 106 | CS IA/B, IIA | 4 COPP/ABV | None | 100 | 91 | 3 | [32, 63] |
| POG 8625 (2006) | 78 | CS I–IIIA | 6 MOPP/ABVD | None | 94 | 83 | 8 | [12, 75] |

*ABVD*, adriamycin, bleomycin, vinblastine, and dacarbazine; *AEIOP*, Italian Association of Hematology and Pediatric Oncology; *CCG*, Children's Cancer Group; *ChlVPP*, chlorambucil, vinblastine, procarbazine, and prednisolone; *COPP*, cyclophosphamide, vincristine (Oncovin), prednisone, and procarbazine; *COPP/ABV*, cyclophosphamide, vincristine (Oncovin), procarbazine, prednisone, adriamycin, bleomycin, and vinblastine; *CR*, complete response; *CS*, clinical stage; *EF*, extended field; *EFS*, event-free survival; *HD*, Hodgkin's disease; *IF*, involved field; *MDH*, multicenter trial; *MH*, multicenter Hodgkin's trial; *MOPP*, nitrogen mustard, vincristine (Oncovin), procarbazine, and prednisone; *MT*, mediastinal/thoracic ratio; *OEPA*, vincristine (Oncovin), etoposide, prednisone, and adriamycin; *OPA*, vincristine (Oncovin), prednisone, and adriamycin; *OPPA*, vincristine (Oncovin), procarbazine, prednisolone, and adriamycin; *PR*, partial response; *PS*, pathologic stage; *R*, regional; *RFS*, relapse-free survival; *RT*, radiotherapy; *SFOP*, French Society of Pediatric Oncology; *VAMP*, vinblastine, adriamycin, methotrexate, and prednisone; *VBVP*, vinblastine, bleomycin, etoposide (VP-16), and prednisone
Mediastinal thoracic ratio <0.33, lymph node <6 cm
Some patients were clinically staged

**Table 14.4** Treatment Results for Advanced, Unfavorable Pediatric Hodgkin's Lymphoma

| Group or institution | Patients (n) | Stage | Chemotherapy | Radiation (Gy), field | Survival, % Overall | DFS, EFS, or RFS | Follow-up interval (yr) | Reference |
|---|---|---|---|---|---|---|---|---|
| *Combined-modality trials* | | | | | | | | |
| Germany Austria HD-90 (1996) | 179 | $II_E B$, $III_E A/B$, IIIB, IVA/B | 2 OEPA/OPPA + 4 COPP | 20, IF | 98/89 | 83/91 | 5 | [76–79] |
| Germany Austria HD-95 (2001) | 280 | $II_E B$, $III_E A/B$, IIIB, IVA/B | 2 OEPA/OPPA + 4 COPP | PR:20–35, IF CR: no RT | 97 | 84 | 3 | [32, 74] |
| Gustave-Roussy (1985) | 60 | I–IV | 3–6 MOPP | 40, IF | 93 | 86 | 5 | [4, 76] |
| SFOP MDH-82 (1992) | 40 | CS III | 3 MOPP/3 ABVD | 20–40, EF | | 82 | 6 | [44, 77] |
| | 21 | CS IV | 3 MOPP/3 ABVD | 20–40, EF | | 62 | 6 | |
| AEIOP MH-83 (1993) | 49 | Group 3 IIIB–IV | Group 3 5 MOPP/5 ABVD | 20–40, EF | 60 | | 7 | [[9, 81] |
| | 24 | I–IV | CCOPP/CAPTe | 30–40, IF | | 83 | 5 | |
| Royal Marsden (1997) | 80 | III | 6–10 ChlVPP | 35, IF | 84 | 73 | 10 | [79, 80] |
| | 27 | IV | 6–10 ChlVPP | 35, IF | 71 | 38 | 10 | |
| U.S. POG (1997) | 80 | CS/PS IIB, $IIIA_2$, IIIB, IV | 4 MOPP/4 ABVD | 21, EF | 87 | 80 | 5 | [13, 29] |
| Stanford, St. Jude, Dana Farber (2002) | 56 | CS I/II bulky (n=26) CS III/IV(n=30) | 6 VEPA | 15–25.5, IF | 81.9 | 67.8 | 5 | [7, 36] |
| U.S. CCG (2002) | 394 | CS I/II[a], CS IIB, CS III | 6 COPP/ABV | 21, IF | 95 | 87 | 3 | [32, 63] |
| | 141 | CS IV | COPP/ABV + CHOP + AraC/VP-16 | 21, IF | 100 | 90 | 3 | |
| St. Jude's, Stanford, DFCI (2004) | | CS IB/IIB or bulky>6cm | 6 VAMP/COP | 15 IF if CR | 93 | 76 | 5 | [68, 75] |
| 159 | | CS III/IV | | 25.5 IF if PR | | | | |
| COG – P9425 (2009) | 216 | CS IB,IIB, $IIIA_2$,IIIB,IV $IIA/IIIA_1$, "bulk" | RER:3 ABVE-PC SER:5 ABVE-PC | 21 IF 21 IF | 95 | 86 84 | 5 | [14, 73] |

*Chemotherapy alone*

| | | | | | | | | |
|---|---|---|---|---|---|---|---|---|
| UKCCSG (2002) | 67 | CS IV | 6–8 ChlVPP | None[b] | 80.8 | 55.2 | 5 | [55, 82] |
| U.S. CCG (2002) | 394 | CS I/II[a], CS IIB, CS III | 6 COPP/ABV | None | 100 | 83 | 3 | [32, 63] |
| | 141 | CS IV | COPP/ABV, CHOP, AraC/VP-16 | None | 94 | 81 | 3 | |
| U.S. POG (1997) | 81 | CS IIB, III₂A, IIIB, IV | 4 MOPP/4 ABVD | None | 96 | 79 | 5 | [13, 29] |

*ABVD*, adriamycin, bleomycin, vinblastine, and dacarbazine; *ABVE-PC*, adriamycin, bleomycin, vincristine, etoposide, prednisone, and cyclophosphamide; *AEIOP*, Italian Association of Hematology and Pediatric Oncology; *AraC*, cytosine arabinoside; *CAPTe*, cyclophosphamide, adriamycin, prednisone, and teniposide; *CCG*, Children's Cancer Group; *CCOPP*, vincristine (Oncovin), procarbazine, and prednisone; *ChlVPP*, chlorambucil, vinblastine, procarbazine, and prednisolone; *CHOP*, cyclophosphamide, hydroxy-davnamycin, vincristine (Oncovin), and prednisone; *COMP*, cyclophosphamide, vincristine (Oncovin), methotrexate, and prednisolone; *COPP*, cyclophosphamide, vincristine (Oncovin), prednisone, and procarbazine; *COPP/ABV*, cyclophosphamide, vincristine (Oncovin), procarbazine, prednisone, adriamycin, bleomycin, and vinblastine; *CR*, complete response; *CS*, clinical stage; *CVPP*, cyclophosphamide, vinblastine, procarbazine, and prednisone; *DFS*, disease-free survival; *EF*, extended field; *EFS*, event-free survival; *HD*, Hodgkin's disease; *IF*, involved field; *MDH*, multicenter trial; *MH*, multicenter Hodgkin's trial; *MOPP*, nitrogen mustard, vincristine (Oncovin), procarbazine, and prednisone; *NR*, no response; *OEPA*, vincristine (Oncovin), etoposide, prednisone, and adriamycin; *OPA*, vincristine (Oncovin), prednisone, and adriamycin; *OPPA*, vincristine (Oncovin), procarbazine, prednisolone, and adriamycin; *POG*, Pediatric Oncology Group; *PR*, partial response; *PS*, pathologic stage; *R*, regional; *RFS*, relapse-free survival; *RT*, radiotherapy; *SFOP*, French Society of Pediatric Oncology; *TLI*, total lymphoid irradiation; *UKCCSG*, United Kingdom Children's Cancer Study Group; *VAMP*, vinblastine, doxorubicin, methotrexate, and prednisone; *VEEP*, vincristine, etoposide, epirubicin, and prednisolone; *VEPA*, vinblastine, etoposide, prednisone, and adriamycin.

† Presence of adverse features = (t)hila, >4 nodal sites, bulk

[a] 12 patients received 20–35 Gy, IF; 2 received whole lung irradiation

resulted in a 70 and 49% 5-year EFS for Stage III and IV HD, respectively [36].

It has been known for decades that outcome in HL is optimized by dose intensity. Only recently has this knowledge been considered a clue to improving outcome [37–39]. ABVE-PC was developed by the COG (by adding prednisolone and cyclophosphamide to ABVE) for the treatment of advanced HL and dose density was increased by the use of 3-week cycles [14]. This regimen is similar to dose-dense regimens such as Stanford V and BEACOPP, developed simultaneously in the adult groups [15, 16]. BEACOPP and escalated BEACOPP are dose-intensive regimens with improved efficacy compared to COPP/ABVD. Instead of further cumulative dose escalation, the COG and EuroNet PHL take advantage of dose-dense delivery to limit cumulative cytotoxic therapy. Such dose-intensive regimens also limit the cumulative dose of agents delivered to the early responders.

ABVE-PC is the backbone for all new COG trials. This dose-dense approach allows for the elimination of procarbazine and the limitation of the doxorubicin and etoposide dose. The first such study (POG 9425) resulted in 5-year EFS of 84% and 5-year overall survival (OS) of 95% for advanced HL. Early responders (after three cycles of ABVE-PC) on this study proceeded directly to receive 21 Gy regional RT. Others received two more cycles (total five ABVE-PC in 15 weeks) prior to 21 Gy RT.

Low-dose, involved field radiation remains a significant modality of therapy in high-risk disease. The multicenter trial GPOH-HD 95 used OPPA/COPP for girls and OEPA/COPP for boys with radiation dose determined by end of chemotherapy response. For the intermediate- and higher-risk groups (TG2 and TG4), outcome was significantly better for those receiving radiation therapy (TG2:0.78 vs. 0.92; TG 2 +3:0.79 vs. 0.91) [26]. The Children's Cancer Group also noted improved outcome for patients treated with radiation, despite CR at the end of chemotherapy [32]. Kelly et al. [40] reported excellent results using a modified approach to BEACOPP that reduced doses of chemotherapy for girls and for boys with a rapid response. Nonetheless, this regimen is not being used currently because cumulative doses of chemotherapy remain high. Current trials in both the COG and in Europe are addressing early response directed approaches to limit need for radiation.

### 14.1.2.4 Future Considerations in Classical Pediatric and Adolescent HL

Progress has been made in the treatment of children with HL with all stages of disease and risk factors, but several issues remain to be resolved. Response to chemotherapy may define both the total amount of chemotherapy required, and the need for radiotherapy (RT). For early stage patients, the balance between chemotherapy dose and radiation exposure continues to be explored. Restriction of RT to initially involved lymph nodes (involved node irradiation) rather than chains (or regions) of nodes may affect the balance of risk. For high-risk disease, dose-dense chemotherapy improves efficacy and supports tailoring of therapy to the patient's response. RT is clearly effective in enhancing the local control of PHL, but has a dose-dependent toxicity profile favoring a limited volume/dose approach. Ongoing studies are needed to assess the role of RT for initial bulk disease, to residual postchemotherapy disease (particularly if it is PET negative), and to involved organs. Carefully designed and sequential evidence-based studies are needed to continue to improve efficacy while limiting toxicity.

### 14.1.3 Lymphocyte-Predominant HL (LPHL)

An indolent, more NHL-like disease, LPHL was recognized in the early 1990s as a clinico-pathologically distinct form of HL [41]. Unlike classical HL, LPHL is a CD20-positive lymphoma that is not associated with EBV genomic integration. The most common form of LPHL is the nodular variant (hence LPHL); the diffuse form represents approximately 20% of cases. In children, LPHL can represent 10–20% of HL [1] vs. 3–8% in adults [42]; it is rarely reported in adolescents. There is a distinct male predominance (ratio 2–3:1) with nearly 90% of pediatric patients having early stage disease (IA/ IIA). Peripheral lymphadenopathy is the most common presentation, occasionally having been present for months or years. The natural history of LPHL can be quite indolent.

Adults with early stage LPHL are usually treated with involved field radiotherapy. Children have received standard pediatric HL therapy, often with combined-modality chemoradiotherapy [43]. Children with fully resected early stage nLPHD have been cured without the need for any chemoradiotherapy [44–46], but the specific situations in which this strategy is appropriate have not been well defined. On-going studies in Europe and the United States intend to determine this. Salvage therapy is effective for late or even multiple relapses if they are of early stage [47]. Unfortunately, there appears to be a predilection (in about 5% of cases) for transformation to NHL [48], including diffuse large B cell lymphoma (DLBCL). The clonal origin of the NHL is the same as the original LP [49], suggesting that this event represents transformation rather than a therapy-induced second malignancy. Risk factors for transformation are unknown and incidence rates in children appear very low.

European and US cooperative groups have ongoing trials that are evaluating minimal therapy for LPHL. The EuroNet PHL-L1 trial is investigating surgery alone for resectable IA disease and low-dose chemotherapy for unresectable or IIA early stage disease (using conventional and FDG-PET imaging). The COG AHOD03P1 LP trial is studying a surgical approach only for those with a single resected node. Both groups use limited chemotherapy for others with IA/IIA disease (EuroNetPHL-LI: CVP (cyclophosphamide, vinblastine, and prednisolone) vs. COG's: doxorubicin, vincristine, prednisone, cyclophosphamide).

Low-dose RT is used for those with PR in the COG trial. Final results are needed to determine the acceptability of surgical approaches and the efficacy of the different regimens.

Rituximab has been studied in adults for use in this CD20-positive tumor [50]. Although responses are documented, no evidence is available that confirms benefit in a curative regimen. The pediatric community would need to carefully consider the safety of using Rituximab, particularly the impact on immune status/memory in young children, before integrating this agent into regimens for children with a highly curable disease.

### 14.1.4 Recurrence, Relapse, and Salvage in PHL

#### 14.1.4.1 Introduction

Relapsed and refractory classical Hodgkin Lymphoma (HL) remains a clinical and therapeutic challenge.

Approximately 10% of patients with early stage, and up to 30% with advanced stage disease, relapse after first-line chemotherapy. Cure can still be achieved in patients with recurrent disease but there is no uniform approach to salvage therapy. No pediatric trials have compared standard dose chemotherapy regimens to high-dose chemotherapy followed by autologous stem cell transplantation HDCT/ASCT. Radiotherapy has an important role in salvage, but must be individualized based on previous radiation exposure, in or out field recurrence, stage at recurrence, and the toxicities of total treatment burden.

#### 14.1.4.2 Standard Dose Salvage Chemotherapy Regimens

After recurrence is noted, the first step is reinduction with a salvage regimen. There is no "best" chemotherapy regimen at salvage, and there are no randomized studies comparing standard dose chemotherapy regimens. The choice of regimen should take account of primary therapy, use of non-cross-resistant drugs, and cumulative drug toxicities. The aim of salvage therapy is to obtain cytoreduction and to demonstrate chemosensitivity. It also facilitates collection of peripheral stem cells for ASCT. Salvage regimes can be divided into intensive conventional regimens[1] (mini-BEAM), cisplatin based regimens[2] (ESHAP, DHAP (ESHAP, DHAP, APPE, DECAL)), ifosfamide based regimens[3] (EPIC, IEP, ICE, IV), or others[4] (GV, IGEV). The COG uses IV as its standard regimen because of efficacy and with the intent of avoiding etoposide-induced secondary malignancy after stem cell transplantation [51]. The decision to continue salvage therapy with RT for consolidation vs. use of high-dose chemotherapy and stem cell transplantation is based on assessment of predictive factors.

---

[1]Mini-BEAM; BCNU, etoposide, cytarabine, melphalan
[2]*ESHAP*, etoposide, methylprednisolone, cytarabine, cisplatin; *DHAP*, dexamethasone, cytarabine, cisplatin; *APPE*, cytarabine, cisplatin, prednisone, etoposide; *DECAL*, cytarabine, cisplatin, prednisone, etoposide, asparaginase
[3]*EPIC*, etoposide, vincristine epirubicin, prednisolone; *IEP*, ifosfamide, etoposide, prednisolone; *ICE*, ifosfamide, carboplatin, etoposide; *IV*, ifosfamide, vinorelbine
[4]*GV*, gemcitabine, vinorelbine; *IGEV*, ifosfamide, gemcitabine, vinorelbine, prednisolone

### 14.1.4.3 Prognostic Factors at Relapse in Pediatric HL: Standard Dose Chemoradiotherapy vs. High-Dose Chemotherapy/Stem Cell Transplantation

Prognostic factors at relapse may be used to allocate patients to a risk stratified salvage approach. Response to retrieval chemotherapy is particularly relevant in determining likelihood of curative intent. FDG PET CT is increasingly used for response assessment.

Early relapse and primary progressive disease is associated with lower OS and EFS in pediatric studies [52–54]. Chemosensitivity to standard dose chemotherapy and disease status at transplantation is also predictive of outcome. In one study, 5-year FFS was 35% for patients with chemosensitive disease vs. 9% with chemoresistant disease [52]. Another group found 68% OS and 59% FFS at 5 years in chemosensitive patients vs. 18 and 0% in chemoresistant patients [53]. Several particularly adverse factors have been noted. Chemoresistant patients had 5-year FFS of 0% with HDCT/ASCT [53]. Adolescents with B symptoms at recurrence had poor OS even after HDCT/ASCT (11 year OS 27% with B disease vs. 60% without) [55]. No difference in OS or FFS between age subgroups or in comparison with adult cohorts is reported by several studies [52, 53, 56].

The largest pediatric review of outcome after recurrent/refractory HL defined prognostic factors [57] in 176 pediatric patients diagnosed with HL and treated on the DAL/GPOH studies over a 17-year period. HDCT/ASCT was used only in a subgroup (30%) with an unfavorable prognosis. The 10-year DFS and OS were 62 and 75%, respectively. Length of time between primary therapy and disease recurrence was the strongest prognostic factor with DFS of 41, 55, and 86% for those with refractory disease, early relapse, and late relapse, respectively. Stage IV, extranodal disease, and female gender were associated with lower OS. This study showed that salvage can be risk adapted.

### 14.1.4.4 High-Dose Chemotherapy and Autologous Stem Cell Transplant

Patients with limited stage, late relapse, and chemotherapy-responsive disease are usually salvaged with standard dose chemotherapy plus RT. The COG protocols have studied HDCT/ASCT and immunomodulatory therapy in all patients except the lowest risk group (late relapse without bulky disease or B symptom in those initially treated for IA/IIA disease with minimal systemic therapy) [58]. In Europe, HDCT/ASCT has a recognized role in salvage for those with higher risk features, primary progressive HL and poor response to reinduction. Intermediate-risk patients who achieve a complete FDG-PET defined response after two cycles of SDCT receive more chemotherapy plus RT.

There are no studies that define the most effective HDCT; BEAM and CVB (cyclophosphamide, etoposide, carmustine) are commonly used. TBI-containing regimens confer no benefit and are associated with increased toxicity and late effects. Transplant-related mortality is down to 0–2% in some series. A higher TRM rate has been associated with history of atopy, thoracic irradiation, multiple chemotherapy regimens, and multiple relapses.

Series with HDCT/ASCT in pediatric and adolescent patients are small and report EFS rates of 31–67% [52, 53, 56, 59]; outcome for children is similar to adults with HDCT/ASCT [52, 56]. Studies that evaluate survival benefit rather than event-free survival after disease recurrence often rely on transplant after second or later recurrence to achieve good OS [53, 60]. Patients with primary progressive disease and those resistant to salvage regimens remain a huge challenge. SDCT with radiotherapy will not afford a chance of cure, but even HDCT/ASCT is inadequate therapy for most such patients. New approaches to such patients such as use of allogeneic SCT or immunomodulatory therapy may prove beneficial [58].

Long-term follow-up is required post-HDCT for detection of late relapse and development of second cancers, which have been reported at a rate of 5–10% at 5 years and substantially higher at 20 years or more in some series. Thirty-eight percent of deaths occurred 4–12 years after ASCT; 85% of relapses occur within 2 years of ASCT [54].

### 14.1.4.5 High-Dose Chemotherapy and Allogeneic Stem Cell Transplantation

Allogeneic transplantation is not recommended as the initial transplant approach [61] due to high nonrelapse mortality (NRM) rate, mainly caused by graft vs. host disease and infection. Reduced intensity conditioning

(RIC) ameliorates the NRM while maintaining theoretical graft vs. lymphoma effect. Allogeneic-SCT may be an option for relapse post-HDCT/ASCT and for patients with refractory advanced stage HL and chemoresistant disease at salvage.

Children and adolescents allografted for HL had an OS of 45% and PFS of 30% at 5 years [62]. All were heavily pretreated, almost half with HDCT/ASCT. Those with chemosensitive disease and good performance status achieved 3-year OS of 83% and PFS of 60%. NRM was $21 \pm 4\%$ in both the RIC and myeloablative conditioning groups. RIC was associated with a significantly higher relapse risk compared to myeloablative conditioning. Graft vs. host disease did not affect relapse rate.

Although studies based on "registry" data are useful, prospective trials are required to gain a better understanding of the role of allogeneic transplantation. The indications, optimal time point, conditioning regimen, and GVHD prophylaxis all still need to be better defined.

## 14.1.5 Late Effects

Long-term adverse sequelae of greatest concern in children treated for HL (particularly with regimens including high-dose radiation) include impairment of muscle and bone development [3] and injury to the lungs [63], heart [10, 64], thyroid gland [8, 9], and reproductive organs [65]. Cardiovascular dysfunction, pulmonary fibrosis, and secondary malignancies significantly compromise the quality and length of life in survivors [66].

### 14.1.5.1 Cardiac Toxicities

High-dose (>3 Gy) radiation to the mediastinum has been associated with significant long-term effects in patients with HL. Stanford investigators reported that the actuarial risk of developing cardiac disease necessitating pericardectomy was 4% at 17 years in a series of long-term survivors of childhood HL who had received high-dose radiation [11]. Screening echocardiogram, exercise stress test, and resting and 24-h ECG identified numerous clinically significant cardiac abnormalities in HL patients who had mediastinal irradiation at a median age of 16.5 years (range, 6.4–25 years). Significant valvular defects were detected in 42%, autonomic dysfunction in 57%, persistent tachycardia in 31%, and reduced hemodynamic response to exercise in 27% of patients [67]. With the introduction of techniques that reduce the radiation dosage to the heart, the rates of radiation-associated cardiac injury have declined dramatically.

Mediastinal irradiation given for HL may further predispose patients with PHL to anthracycline-related myocardiopathy [11, 68]. Cardiac dysfunction after anthracycline therapy itself can be noted, with the highest risk in those receiving high cumulative doses or in [11, 68] young children who may be affected by an adverse effect on cardiac myocyte growth. Fortunately, most pHL patients are adolescents and current pHL regimens doses are significantly lower than those used in adult ABVD regimens.

### 14.1.5.2 Pulmonary Toxicities

Chronic pneumonitis and pulmonary fibrosis should be rare in the current era of treatment for primary HL (Fig. 14.1). Predisposing therapies include thoracic radiation and bleomycin chemotherapy [63, 64]. The bleomycin in ABVD can cause both acute pulmonary compromise and late pulmonary fibrosis and can be augmented by the fibrosis that can be associated with pulmonary radiation. Asymptomatic pulmonary dysfunction that improves over time has been observed after contemporary combined-modality treatment.

### 14.1.5.3 Thyroid Toxicities

Thyroid sequelae are common after RT for PHL. Hypothyroidism, hyperthyroidism, thyroid nodules, and thyroid cancer have been observed in long-term survivors [8, 9]. Of these, hypothyroidism, particularly compensated hypothyroidism, defined as thyroid-stimulating hormone (TSH) elevation in the presence of a normal thyroxine (T4) level, is the most common thyroid abnormality. Risk factors for hypothyroidism include younger age at trea tment and higher cumulative radiation dosage. As many as 78% of patients treated with radiation dosages greater than 26 Gy demonstrate thyroid dysfunction, as indicated by elevated TSH levels [8].

**Table 14.5** Secondary cancers after childhood HL

| Reference | Cohort size | Time period studied | Number of secondary cancers | Cumulative incidence (%) (years) | Standardized incidence ratio |
|---|---|---|---|---|---|
| Stanford [83] | 694 | 1960–1995 | 59 | Males: 9.7% (20 years) Females: 16.8% (20 years) | Males: 10.6 Females: 15.4 |
| LESG [73] | 1,641 | 1940s to 1991 | 62 | 18% (30 year) | 7.7 |
| Roswell [84] | 182 | 1960–1989 | 28 | 26.7% (30 year) | 9.4 |
| LESG [85] | 1,380 | 1955–1986 | 135 | 31.2% (30 year) | 17.9 |
| US/European [86] | 5,925 | 1935–1994 | 195 | Solid tumors: 11.7% (25 year) | 7.7 |
| University of Rochester/Johns Hopkins/University of Florida/St. Jude/ Dana-Farber [69] | 930 | 1960–1990 | 102 | 19% (25 year) | Males: 8.41 Females: 19.93 |

#### 14.1.5.4 Secondary Malignancies

The overall cumulative risk of developing a subsequent malignancy after treatment for PHL has been reported to range from 7 to 10% at 15 years from diagnosis and rises to 16–28% by 20 years (Table 14.5) [69]; these data are based on patients treated in earlier decades. The most common secondary malignacies historically included both secondary acute myeloid leukemia (MDS/secondary AML) and solid tumors. However, leukemias are now infrequent due to changes in chemotherapy. Female breast cancer is a particular concern but is likely to be less common with current radiation doses and techniques, since it is associated with RT fields that include breast tissue (especially mantle fields), and higher radiation doses (Fig. 14.1)

### 14.1.6 Summary/Future Directions

Tremendous strides have been made in treating children with HL, both in terms of cure and reduction of toxicity. Devising new strategies to treat children with HL is problematic because of the overall success of current treatment regimens. However, grouping patients into different risk categories, using response-based therapy and newer imaging techniques, allows investigators to construct protocols intended to diminish therapy-induced toxicity for patients with favorable prognoses. These protocols also aim to improve efficacy of treatment for patients with intermediate and unfavorable prognoses. Unfortunately, the ability to conduct clinical trials, where the difference in survival between treatment arms is likely to be small, is compromised by the large patient numbers required to detect such differences. If a reduction in treatment toxicity is the intended goal of a new regimen, then many years of follow-up are necessary to prove efficacy. For patients with refractory, or multiply relapsed, disease, phase II studies, investigating the use of monoclonal anti-CD30 antibodies, HDAC, and mTOR inhibitors in children are being planned internationally. The importance of investigators working together throughout the world to share data, and new treatment approaches, in order to cure children with HL safely, is clear.

**Acknowledgments** With thanks to Ann Muhs, Rochester, for her help with the manuscript, particularly the references.

### References

1. Hochberg J, Waxman IM, Kelly KM, et al. Adolescent non-Hodgkin lymphoma and Hodgkin lymphoma: state of the science. Br J Haematol. 2009;144:24–40.
2. Foltz LM, Song KW, Connors JM. Hodgkin's lymphoma in adolescents. J Clin Oncol. 2006;24:2520–6.
3. Donaldson SS, Kaplan HS. Complications of treatment of Hodgkin's disease in children. Cancer Treat Rep. 1982;66:977–89.

4. Mauch PM, Weinstein H, Botnick L, et al. An evaluation of long-term survival and treatment complications in children with Hodgkin's disease. Cancer. 1983;51:925–32.

5. Merchant TE, Nguyen L, Nguyen D, et al. Differential attenuation of clavicle growth after asymmetric mantle radiotherapy. Int J Radiat Oncol Biol Phys. 2004;59:556–61.

6. Probert JC, Parker BR, Kaplan HS. Growth retardation in children after megavoltage irradiation of the spine. Cancer. 1973;32:634–9.

7. Donaldson SS, Glatstein E, Rosenberg SA, Kaplan HS. Pediatric Hodgkin's disease. II. Results of therapy. Cancer. 1976;37:2436–47.

8. Constine LS, Donaldson SS, McDougall IR, et al. Thyroid dysfunction after radiotherapy in children with Hodgkin's disease. Cancer. 1984;53:878–83.

9. Sklar C, Whitton J, Mertens A, et al. Abnormalities of the thyroid in survivors of Hodgkin's disease: Date from the Childhood Cancer Survivor Study. J Clin Endocrinol Metab. 2000;85:3227–32.

10. Adams MJ, Hardenbergh PH, Constine LS, et al. Radiation-associated cardiovascular disease. Crit Rev Oncol Hematol. 2003;45:55–75.

11. Hancock SL, Donaldson SS, Hoppe RT. Cardiac disease following treatment of Hodgkin's disease in children and adolescents. J Clin Oncol. 1993;11:1208–15.

12. Kung FH, Schwartz CL, Ferree CR, et al. POG 8625: a randomized trial comparing chemotherapy with chemoradiotherapy for children and adolescents with Stages I, IIA, IIIA1 Hodgkin Disease: a report from the Children's Oncology Group. J Pediatr Hematol Oncol. 2006;28:362–8.

13. Weiner M, Leventhal B, Brecher M, et al. Randomized study of intensive MOPP-ABVD with or without low-dose total nodal radiation therapy in the treatment of stages IIB, IIIA2, IIIB, and IV Hodgkin's disease in pediatric patients: a Pediatric Oncology Group study. J Clin Oncol. 1997;15:2769–79.

14. Schwartz CL, Constine LS, Villaluna D, et al. A risk-adapted, response-based approach using ABVE-PC for children and adolescents with intermediate- and high-risk Hodgkin lymphoma: the results of P9425. Blood. 2009;114:2051–9.

15. Diehl V, Franlin J, Pfreundschuh M, et al. Standard and increased-dose BEACOPP chemotherapy compared with COPP-ABVD for advanced Hodgkin's disease. N Engl J Med. 2003;348:2386–99.

16. Horning SJ, Hoppe RT, Breslin S, et al. Stanford V and radiotherapy for locally extensive and advanced Hodgkin's disease: Mature results of a prospective clinical trial. J Clin Oncol. 2002;20:630–7.

17. Kaldor JM, Day NE, Clarke EA, et al. Leukemia following Hodgkin's disease. N Engl J Med. 1990;322:7–13.

18. Mackie E, Radford M, Shalet S. Gonadal function following chemotherapy for childhood Hodgkin's disease. Med Pediatr Oncol. 1996;27:74–8.

19. Ortin TT, Shostak CA, Donaldson SS. Gonadal status and reproductive function following treatment for Hodgkin's disease in childhood: the Stanford experience. Int J Rad Oncol Biol Phys. 1990;19:873–80.

20. van den Berg H, Furstner F, van den Bos C, Behrendt H. Decreasing the number of MOPP courses reduces gonadal damage in survivors of childhood Hodgkin disease. Pediatr Blood Cancer. 2004;42:210–5.

21. Canellos GP, Anderson JR, Propert KJ, et al. Chemotherapy of advanced Hodgkin's disease with MOPP, ABVD, or MOPP alternating with ABVD. N Engl J Med. 1992;327:1478–84.

22. Hunger S, Link M, Donaldson S. ABVD/MOPP and low-dose involved-field radiotherapy in pediatric Hodgkin's disease: the Stanford experience. J Clin Oncol. 1994;12:2160–6.

23. Bramswig J, Heimes U, Heiermann E, et al. The effects of different cumulative doses of chemotherapy on testicular function. Results in 75 patients treated for Hodgkin's disease during childhood or adolescence. Cancer. 1990;65:1298–302.

24. Schellong G, Hornig I, Bramswig J, et al. Significance of procarbazine in the chemotherapy of Hodgkin's disease–a report of the Cooperative Therapy Study DAL-HD-85. Klin Pädiatr. 1988;200:205–13.

25. Bonadonna G, Santoro A. ABVD chemotherapy in the treatment of Hodgkin's disease. Cancer Treat Rev. 1982;9:21–35.

26. Doerffel W, Luders H, Ruhl U, et al. Preliminary results of the multicenter trial GPOH-HD 95 for the treatment of Hodgkin's disease in children and adolescents: analysis and outlook. Klin Padiatr. 2003;215:139–45.

27. Landman-Parker J, Pacquement H, Leblanc T, et al. Localized childhood Hodgkin's disease: response-adapted chemotherapy with etoposide, bleomycin, vinblastine, and prednisone before low-dose radiation therapy-results of the French Society of Pediatric Oncology Study MDH90. J Clin Oncol. 2000;18:1500–7.

28. Donaldson S, Hudson M, Lamborn K, et al. VAMP and low-dose, involved-field radiation for children and adolescents with favorable, early-stage Hodgkin's disease: results of a prospective clinical trial. J Clin Oncol. 2002;20:3081–7.

29. Tebbi CKMN, Schwartz C, Williams J, et al. Response dependent treatment of stages IA, IIA, and IIIA1 micro Hodgkin's disease with ABVE and low dose involved field irradiation with or without dexrazoxane. Leuk Lymphoma. 2001;42:100.

30. Shahidi M, Kamangari N, Ashley S, et al. Site of relapse after chemotherapy alone for stage I and II Hodgkin's disease. Radiother Oncol. 2006;78:1–5.

31. Girinsky T, van der Maazen R, Specht L, et al. Involved-node radiotherapy (INRT) in patients with early Hodgkin lymphoma: concepts and guidelines. Radiother Oncol. 2006;79:270–7.

32. Nachman JB, Sposto R, Herzog P, et al. Randomized comparison of low-dose involved-field radiotherapy and no radiotherapy for children with Hodgkin's disease who achieve a complete response to chemotherapy. J Clin Oncol. 2002;20:3765–71.

33. Korholz D, Claviez A, Hasenclever D, et al. The concept of the GPOH-HD 2003 therapy study for pediatric Hodgkin's disease: evolution in the tradition of the DAL/GPOH studies. Klin Pädiatr. 2004;216:150–6.

34. Korholz D, Kluge R, Wickmann L, et al. Importance of F18-fluorodeoxy-D-2-glucose positron emission tomography (FDG-PET) for staging and therapy control of Hodgkin's lymphoma in childhood and adolescence – consequences for the GPOH-HD 2003 protocol. Onkologie. 2003;26:489–93.

35. Weiner MA, Leventhal BG, Marcus R, et al. Intensive chemotherapy and low-dose radiotherapy for the treatment of advanced-stage Hodgkin's disease in pediatric patients: a Pediatric Oncology Group study. J Clin Oncol. 1991;9:1591–8.

36. Friedmann AM, Hudson MM, Weinstein HJ, et al. Treatment of unfavorable childhood Hodgkin's disease with VEPA and low-dose, involved-field radiation. J Clin Oncol. 2002;20:3088–94.

37. Carde P, MacKintosh FR, Rosenberg SA. A dose and time response analysis of the treatment of Hodgkin's disease with MOPP chemotherapy. J Clin Oncol. 1983;1:146–53.

38. DeVita VT, Hubbard SM, Longo DL. Treatment of Hodgkin's disease. J Natl Cancer Inst Monogr. 1990;10:19–28.

39. van Rijswijk RE, Haanen C, Dekker AW, et al. Dose intensity of MOPP chemotherapy and survival in Hodgkin's disease. J Clin Oncol. 1989;7:1776–82.

40. Kelly KM, Hutchinson RJ, Sposto R, et al. Feasibility of upfront dose-intensive chemotherapy in children with advanced-stage Hodgkin's lymphoma: preliminary results from the Children's Cancer Group Study CCG-59704. Ann Oncol. 2002;13 Suppl 1:107–11.

41. Mason DY, Banks PM, Chan J, et al. Nodular lymphocyte predominance Hodgkin's disease: a distinct clinico-pathological entity. Am J Surg Pathol. 1994;18:526–30.

42. Diehl V, Sextro M, Franklin J, et al. Clinical presentation, course, and prognostic factors in lymphocyte-predominant Hodgkin's disease and lymphocyte-rich classical Hodgkin's disease: report from the European Task Force on Lymphoma Project on Lymphocyte-Predominant Hodgkin's Disease. J Clin Oncol. 1999;17:776–83.

43. Sandoval C, Venkateswaran L, Billups C, et al. Lymphocyte-predominant Hodgkin disease in children. J Pediatr Hematol Oncol. 2002;24:269–73.

44. Mauz-Korholz C, Gorde-Grosjean S, Hasenclever D, et al. Resection alone in 58 children with limited stage, lymphocyte-predominant Hodgkin lymphoma-experience from the European network group on pediatric Hodgkin lymphoma. Cancer. 2007;110:179–85.

45. Murphy SB, Morgan ER, Katzenstein HM, et al. Results of little or no treatment for lymphocyte-predominant Hodgkin disease in children and adolescents. J Pediatr Hematol Oncol. 2003;25:684–7.

46. Pellogrino B, Terrier-Lacobe MJ, Oberlin O, et al. Lymphocyte-predominant Hodgkin's lymphoma in children: therapeutic abstenstion after initial lymph node resection – A study of the French Society of Pediatric oncology. J Clin Oncol. 2003;21:2984–92.

47. Hall GW, Katzilakis N, Pinkerton CR, et al. Outcome of children with nodular lymphocyte predominant Hodgkin lymphoma - a Children's Cancer and Leukaemia Group report. Br J Haematol. 2007;138:761–8.

48. Miettinen M, Franssila KO, Saxen E. Hodgkin's disease, lymphocyte predominance nodular: Increased risk of subsequent non-Hodgkin's lymphoma. Cancer. 1983;51:2293–300.

49. Wickert RS, Weisenburger DD, Tierens A, et al. Clonal relationship between lymphocytic predominance Hodgkin's disease and concurrent or subsequent large-cell lymphoma of B lineage. Blood. 1995;86:2312–20.

50. Nogova L, Reineke T, Brillant C, et al. Lymphocyte-predominant and classical Hodgkin's lymphoma: a compre-hensive analysis from the German Hodgkin Study Group. J Clin Oncol. 2008;26:434–9.

51. Bhatia S, Robison LL, Francisco L, et al. Late mortality in survivors of autologous hematopoietic-cell transplantation: report from the Bone Marrow Transplant Survivor Study. Blood. 2005;105:4215–22.

52. Baker KS, Gordon BG, Grass TG, et al. Autologous hematopoetic stem-cell transplantation for relapsed or refractory Hodgkin's disease in children and adolescents. J Clin Oncol. 1999;17:825–31.

53. Claviez A, Sureda A, Schmitz N. Haematopoietic SCT for children and adolescents with relapsed and refractory Hodgkin's lymphoma. Bone Marrow Transplant. 2008;42 Suppl 2:S16–24.

54. Lieskovsky YE, Donaldson SS, Torres MA, et al. High-dose therapy and autologous hematopoietic stem-cell transplantation for recurrent or refractory pediatric Hodgkin's disease: results and prognostic indices. J Clin Oncol. 2004;22:4532–40.

55. Akhtar S, El Weshi A, Rahal M et al. (2009) High-dose chemotherapy and autologous stem cell transplant in adolescent patients with relapsed or refractory Hodgkin's lymphoma. Bone Marrow Transplant. 2010 Mar;45(3):476-82. Epub 2009 Sep 7

56. Williams CD, Goldstone AH, Pearce R, et al. Autologous bone marrow transplantation for pediatric Hodgkin's disease: a case-matched comparison with adult patients by the European Bone Marrow Transplant Group Lymphoma Registry. J Clin Oncol. 1993;11:2243–9.

57. Schellong G, Dorffel W, Claviez A, et al. Salvage therapy of progressive and recurrent Hodgkin's disease: results from a multicenter study of the pediatric DAL/GPOH-HD study group. J Clin Oncol. 2005;23:6181–9.

58. Chen AR, Hutchison R, Hess A, et al. Clinical outcomes of patients with recurrent/refractory Hodgkin disease receiving cyclosporine, interferon-V and interleukin-2 immunotherapy to induce autoreactivity after autologous stem cell transplantation with BEAM: A COG study. Blood 2007;110:Abstract 1896.

59. Frankovich J, Donaldson SS, Lee Y, et al. High-dose therapy and autologous hematopoietic cell transplantation in children with primary refractory and relapsed Hodgkin's disease: atopy predicts idiopathic diffuse lung injury syndromes. Biol Blood Marrow Transplant. 2001;7:49–57.

60. Stoneham S, Ashley S, Pinkerton CR, et al. Outcome after autologous hemopoietic stem cell transplantation in relapsed or refractory childhood Hodgkin disease. J Pediatr Hematol Oncol. 2004;26:740–5.

61. Bradley MB, Cairo MS. Stem cell transplantation for paediatric lymphoma: past, present and future. Bone Marrow Transplant. 2008;41:149–58.

62. Claviez A, Canals C, Dierickx D, et al. Allogeneic hematopoietic stem cell transplantation in children and adolescents with recurrent and refractory Hodgkin lymphoma: an analysis of the European Group for Blood and Marrow Transplantation. Blood. 2009;114:2060–7.

63. Marina NM, Greenwald CA, Fairclough DL, et al. Serial pulmonary function studies in children treated for newly diagnosed Hodgkin's disease with mantle radiotherapy plus cycles of cyclophosphamide, vincristine, and procarbazine alternating with cycles of doxorubicin, bleomycin, vinblastine, and dacarbazine. Cancer. 1995;75:1706–11.

64. Mefferd JM, Donaldson SS, Link MP. Pediatric Hodgkin's disease: pulmonary, cardiac, and thyroid function following combined modality therapy. Int J Radiat Oncol Biol Phys. 1989;16:679–85.

65. Green DM, Hall B. Pregnancy outcome following treatment during childhood or adolescence for Hodgkin's disease. Pediatr Hematol Oncol. 1988;5:269–77.

66. Hudson MM, Poquette CA, Lee J, et al. Increased mortality after successful treatment for Hodgkin's disease. J Clin Oncol. 1998;16:3592–600.

67. Adams MJ, Lipsitz SR, Colan SD, et al. Cardiovascular status in long-term survivors of Hodgkin's disease treated with chest radiotherapy. J Clin Oncol. 2004;22:3139–48.

68. Green DM, Hyland A, Chung CS, et al. Cancer and cardiac mortality among 15-year survivors of cancer diagnosed during childhood or adolescence. J Clin Oncol. 1999;17: 3207–15.

69. Constine LS, Tarbell N, Hudson MM, et al. Subsequent malignancies in children treated for Hodgkin's disease: associations with gender and radiation dose. Int J Radiat Oncol Biol Phys. 2008;72:24–33.

70. Hodgson DC, Hudson MM, Constine LS. Pediatric hodgkin lymphoma: maximizing efficacy and minimizing toxicity. Semin Radiat Oncol. 2007;17:230–42.

71. Rubin P, Williams JP, Deveson SS, Travis LB, Constine LS. Semin Radiat Oncol. 2010 Jan 20(1):3-11..

72. Punnett A, Tsang R, Hodgson DC. Hodgkin lymphoma across the age spectrum: epidemiology, therapy, and late effects. Semin Radiat Oncol. 2010;20(1):30–44.

73. Sankila R, Garwicz S, Olsen JH, et al. Risk of subsequent malignant neoplasms among 1, 641 Hodgkin's disease patients diagnosed in childhood and adolescence: a population-based cohort study in the five Nordic countries. Association of the Nordic Cancer Registries and the Nordic Society of Pediatric Hematology and Oncology. J Clin Oncol. 1996;14:1442–6.

74. Rühl U, Albrecht M, Dieckmann K, et al. Response-adapted radiotherapy in the treatment of pediatric Hodgkin's disease: an interim report at 5 years of the German GPOH-HD 95 trial. Int J Radiat Oncol Biol Phys. 2001;51:1209–18.

75. Hudson MM, Krasin M, Link MP, et al. Risk-adapted, combined-modality therapy with VAMP/COP and response-based, involved-field radiation for unfavorable pediatric Hodgkin's disease. J Clin Oncol. 2004;22:4541–50.

76. Oberlin O, Boilletot A, Leverger G, et al. Clinical staging, primary chemotherapy and involved-field radiotherapy in childhood Hodgkin's disease. Eur Paediatr Oncol. 1985; 2:65–70.

77. Oberlin O, Leverger G, Pacquement M, et al. Low-dose radiation therapy and reduced chemotherapy in childhood Hodgkin's disease: the experience of the French Society of Pediatric Oncology. J Clin Oncol. 1992;10:1602–8.

78. Schellong G. The balance between cure and late effects in childhood Hodgkin's lymphoma: the experience of the German-Austrian Study-Group since 1978. Ann Oncol. 1996;7 Suppl 4:67–72.

79. Schellong G. Treatment of children and adolescents with Hodgkin's disease: the experience of the German-Austrian Paediatric Study Group. Bailliere's Clin Haematol. 1996;9: 619–34.

80. Shankar A, Ashley S, Radford M, et al. Does histology influence outcome in childhood Hodgkin's disease? Results from the United Kingdom Children's Cancer Study Group. J Clin Oncol. 1997;15:2622–30.

81. Vecchi V, Pileri S, Burnelli R, et al. Treatment of pediatric Hodgkin disease tailored to stage, mediastinal mass, and age. Cancer. 1993;72:2049–57.

82. Atra A, Higgs E, Capra M, et al. ChlVPP chemotherapy in children with stage IV Hodgkin's disease: results of the UKCCSG HD 8201 and HD 9201 studies. Br J Haematol. 2002;119:647–51.

83. Wolden SL, Lamborn KR, Cleary SF, et al. Second cancers following pediatric Hodgkin's disease. J Clin Oncol. 1998;16:536–44.

84. Green DM, Hyland A, Barcos MP, et al. Second malignant neoplasms after treatment for Hodgkin's disease in childhood or adolescence. J Clin Oncol. 2000;18:1492–9.

85. Bhatia S, Robison LL, Oberlin O, et al. Breast cancer and other second neoplasms after childhood Hodgkin's disease. N Engl J Med. 1996;334:745–51.

86. Metayer C, Lynch CF, Clarke EA, et al. Second cancers among long-term survivors of Hodgkin's disease diagnosed in childhood and adolescence. J Clin Oncol. 2000;18: 2435–43.

# Lymphocyte-Predominant Hodgkin Lymphoma

# 15

## Andreas Engert and Anas Younes

## Contents

A. Engert (✉)
Department of Hematology and Oncology, University Hospital
of Cologne, Kerpener Strasse 62, 50924, Köln, Germany
e-mail: a. engert@uni-koeln. de

A. Younes
Department of Lymphoma and Myeloma, M.D. Anderson
Cancer Center, 1515 Holcombe Boulevard, Houston,
TX 77030, USA

## 15.1  Introduction

Lymphocyte-predominant Hodgkin lymphoma (LPHL) was first described in 1944 by Jackson and Parker as nodular paragranuloma [1]. Other synonyms used were lymphocytic predominant Hodgkin disease, lymphocytic and histiocytic (L&H) predominant Hodgkin disease, nodular lymphocyte-predominant Hodgkin disease, and nodular LPHL [2–5]. This term has become the one that is currently being used. LPHL represents 5% of all HL cases and is a rare disease with an estimated incidence of 1.5 per million [6]. LPHL differs from classical Hodgkin lymphoma in pathological and clinical characteristics.

This chapter describes pathological and clinical characteristics, differential diagnosis, risk factors, and treatment of LPHL.

## 15.2  Pathology of LPHL

LPHL has a number of distinctive pathologic characteristics. The main feature is a malignant cell population that was originally termed L&H. These cells were reclassified in the WHO 2008 classification as LP cells [5]. LP cells carry one large single folded or polylobated vesiculated nucleus (Table 15.1). In contrast to H–RS cells, the number of nucleoli in LPHL is increased. These features have resulted in the more descriptive term "popcorn cells" [7]. In rare cases, however, LP cells can resemble classical or laguna-type Hodgkin and Reed–Sternberg (H–RS) cells.

H–RS tumor cells of classical Hodgkin lymphoma appeared to be derived from germinal center (GC) B- cells that normally would have undergone apoptosis.

**Table 15.1** Characteristics of classical Hodgkin lymphoma and LPHL (histology and immunophenotype)

|  | Classical Hodgkin lymphoma | LPHL |
|---|---|---|
| Pattern | Diffuse, interfollicular, nodular | Nodular, at least in part |
| Tumor cells | Diagnostic RS cells; mononuclear or lacunar cells | LP or "popcorn" cells |
| Background | Lymphocytes, histiocytes, eosinophils, plasma cells | Lymphocytes, histiocytes |
| Fibrosis | Common | Rare |
| CD15 | + | − |
| CD30 | + | − |
| CD20 | ± | + |
| CD79 | − | + |
| EBV | + (~50%) | − |

*EBV* Epstein–Barr virus; *LPHL* lymphocyte-predominant Hodgkin lymphoma

In contrast, LP cells originate from GC B-cells that were positively selected. Single-cell polymerase chain reaction assays demonstrated that LP cells typically contain rearranged immunoglobulin (Ig) genes and variably express immunoglobulin mRNA [8–11]. The Ig heavy chain can show evidence of somatic hypermutation in line with the germinal center origin of LP cells, which express G-chain in most cases. Different chromosomal abnormalities in up to two-third of LPHL cases have been described [12]. Although some genetic lesions were identified, little is known on the pathogenesis of LP cells in LPHL (Chap. 3). Constitutive activity of NF-κB, the JAK/STAT pathway, and the BCL-6 transcription factors appear to be involved. Mutations in the genes coding for the NF-κB regulating factors IκBα and A20 are uncommon [13].

LP cells are embedded in a nodular or follicular background that is dominated by small B-lymphocytes. More diffuse growth pattern can also be observed. A follicular infiltrate by follicular dendritic cells is usually present forming meshworks in the nodules. There was some controversy as to the existence of both a more nodular and a diffuse subtype. However, since the diffuse subtype was reported in less than 1% of all diagnoses and at least a partial nodular pattern is required for the diagnosis of LPHL, it remains controversial whether purely diffuse cases really exist. For simplicity, we refer to LPHL.

Immunophenotyping is usually needed to establish the correct diagnosis of LPHL. LP cells present a B-cell phenotype expressing CD20, CD75, and frequently CD79a. In contrast to H–RS cells, LP cells are negative for CD15, CD30, and EBV. Occasionally a weak positivity for CD30 can be observed in LPHL but these cells are typically non-neoplastic extrafollicular immunoblasts. B-cell transcription factors such as BOB.1 and OCT-2 are usually positive; BCL-6 and the activation-induced cystidine deaminase (AID) are expressed. In smaller lesions, B-cells dominate the background where histiocytes and T-cells are more prominent during the evolution of LPHL. This can result in LPHL cases becoming very difficult to distinguish from T-cell-rich B-cell lymphoma (TCRBCL). Figure 15.1 shows typical LPHL and classical Hodgkin lymphoma histology, and Fig. 15.2 immunostaining of CD20. The main characteristics of LPHL and classical Hodgkin lymphoma are shown in Table 15.1.

## 15.3 Differential Diagnosis

The discrimination of LPHL from classical Hodgkin lymphoma or other related lymphoma is difficult. A consortium of European and American expert pathologists evaluating 426 cases that had initially been classified as LPHL highlighted this problem [6]. Using classical morphology and immunohistochemistry, 51% of cases were confirmed as LPHL, 27% were reclassified as lymphocyte-rich classical Hodgkin lymphoma (LRcHL), and 5% as classical Hodgkin lymphoma. The remaining 17% of cases were identified as non-Hodgkin lymphoma (3%); reactive lesions (3%) or were not assessable (11%). These findings underscore the need for immunohistochemistry and expert pathology review particularly for the diagnosis of LPHL.

**Fig. 15.1** HE-stained tumor sections showing LPHL (**a**) and lymphocyte-rich classical Hodgkin lymphoma (**b**)

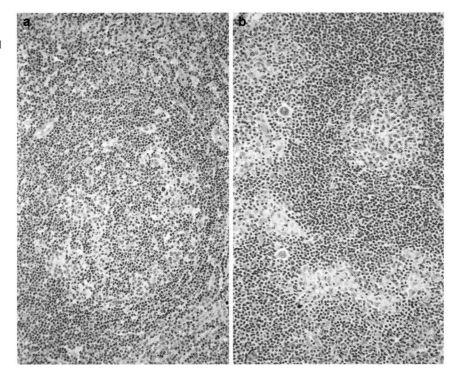

**Fig. 15.2** CD20 immunostaining of LPHL (**a**) and classical Hodgkin lymphoma (**b**)

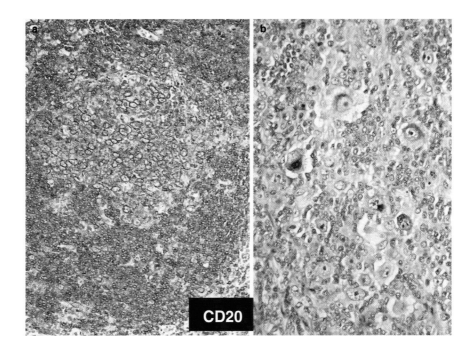

## 15.4 LPHL and T-Cell-Rich B-Cell Lymphoma

TCRBCL is a variant of diffuse large B-cell lymphoma in which malignant B-cells are surrounded by non-malignant T-cells [14]. TCRBCL comprises less than 5% of all diffuse large B-cell lymphoma. Earlier studies had described striking similarities between LPHL and TCRBCL in terms of histology. In the latest WHO classification, TCRBCL was characterized by a "limited number of scattered, large, atypical B-cells embedded in a background of abundant T-cells and frequently histiocytes" [5]. Median age at presentation is in the 40s with a male predominance. The majority of TCRBCL patients presents with advanced disease and often shows involvement of spleen, liver, and bone marrow. Although they are distinct tumors, there are morphological and biological similarities between LPHL and TCRBCL, which can make the differential diagnosis difficult. The most reliable morphological differences are seen between the tumor cells. In LPHL, most malignanT-cells are LP cells with their characteristic popcorn appearance. H–RS cells are extremely rare. The neoplastic cells in TCRBCL resemble centroblasts or immunoblasts and rarely appear as LP cells. A follicular environment is retained in LPHL as documented by the presence of meshworks of follicular dendritic cells, which are absent in TCRBCL [14]. Small B-cells are abundant in LPHL but rare in TCRBCL. T-cells in LPHL are mainly CD4+, CD7+ rosette-forming follicular cells [15], whereas CD8+ cytotoxic T-cells and histiocytes dominate in TCRBCL, and T-cell rosettes are rarely seen [16]. CD79A and Bcl-2 are more frequently expressed in TCRBCL than in LPHL [17]. The transcription factor PU.1, which is associated during early B-cell differentiation, is expressed in LPHL but absent in TCRBCL [18].

Recent reports show that LPHL will eventually transform into large B-cell lymphoma even 15–20 years after the initial diagnosis [19]. TCRBCL is the most common histology of transformed LPHL cases [20]. Similarly, there are many examples showing that LPHL is clonally related to TCRBCL [21, 22]. Comparative genetic studies revealed numerous genomic imbalances with only a few overlapping genetic abnormalities in both entities. Thus, the genetic link between LPHL and TCRBCL might be among these recurrent chromosomal abnormalities.

## 15.5 Lymphocyte-Rich Classical Hodgkin Lymphoma

LRcHL was introduced as a new subtype of classical Hodgkin lymphoma in the REAL classification [3] and later confirmed by the WHO [4, 5]. This is also a rare entity representing less than 5% of all Hodgkin lymphoma cases. In tissues involved, few H–RS cells on a background of small mature lymphocytes characterize LRcHL. There are both nodular and diffuse growth patterns. LRcHL can be difficult to differentiate from LPHL with conventional staining (Fig. 15.1). Exact diagnosis often requires immunohistochemistry. Here, the malignanT-cells in LRcHL display the typical immunophenotype of classical Hodgkin lymphoma (CD30+CD15+CD20−). In contrast, LP cells are CD30−CD15−CD20+.

Analyses conducted by the GHSG comprising 2,750 patients with biopsy-proven HL reported an average age of 38 years for LRcHL patients and 40 years for LPHL patients, which contrasts with 33 years average for other classical Hodgkin lymphoma patients. Similar to LPHL, LRcHL patients usually present with early stages of disease and treatment outcome is excellent. For a group of 100 LRcHL patients identified in a recent retrospective analysis, there was 100% overall response to treatment. The event-free survival and the overall survival rates were 97% at 32 months [23]. Only three patients died; all deaths were due to treatment-related toxicities. Similar differences in clinical parameters between LRcHL and classical Hodgkin lymphoma were observed by the European Task Force [6]. Thus, very similar to LPHL, special emphasis should be taken to reduce toxicity in this entity.

## 15.6 Transformation to Non-Hodgkin Lymphoma

In a comprehensive individual patient data analysis by the "International Database on Hodgkin's Disease" (IDHD), a significantly higher risk for secondary NHL in LPHL patients was described [24]. The risk was increased by a factor of 1.8 for LPHL patients as compared with classical Hodgkin lymphoma. Higher incidence of secondary non-Hodgkin lymphoma after primary diagnosis of LPHL was also reported from other studies [6]. In the ETFL database, there were 6 of 219 patients with secondary NHL at a median follow-up of 6.8 years. This compares with 0.9% of secondary NHL in the IDHD database comprising 12,411 HL patients. Based on these studies, LPHL patients seem to have a two- to threefold higher risk of secondary NHL as compared to other Hodgkin patients. However, these findings were not confirmed in the GHSG database [25]. Given the natural history of LPHL eventually transforming to TCRBCL and the lack of reference pathology review in some of these studies, this issue requires longer follow-up for a final answer.

## 15.7 Clinical Characteristics

The most comprehensive clinical data derive from the European Task Force on Lymphoma (ETFL) analysis [6]. In this study, patient data from 17 European and American centers were included and a total of 219 patients with histology-confirmed LPHL were evaluated. Here, a median age of 35 years for both LPHL and classical Hodgkin lymphoma patients was described. A comprehensive analysis performed by the GHSG compared 394 reference pathology-confirmed LPHL cases with 7,904 classical HL patients from their database describing an average age of 37 years for LPHL patients and 33 years for classical Hodgkin lymphoma [26]. Seventy percent in the EFTL and 73% in the GHSG analysis were male patients (Table 15.2).

In the EFTL analysis, 53% of all LPHL patients were in stage I, 28% in stage II, 14% in stage III, and 6% in stage IV. In addition, 24% of patients had purely infradiaphragmatic disease, 7% presented with mediastinal mass, 13% bulky disease, and 8% spleen involvement. B symptoms were present in 10% of patients. In the GHSG analysis, 63% of LPHL patients were in early favorable stages, 16% in early unfavorable and 21% in advanced stages, in contrast to 22, 39, and 39% of classical Hodgkin lymphoma patients, respectively. Compared with classical Hodgkin lymphoma patients, fewer LPHL patients had B symptoms (9 vs. 40%) three or more nodal areas involved (28 vs. 55%), elevated ESR (4 vs. 45%), mediastinal bulky disease (31 vs. 55%), extranodal involvement (6 vs. 14%), or elevated lactate dehydrogenase (16 vs. 32%) (Table 15.2).

**Table 15.2** Characteristics of LPHL and classical Hodgkin lymphoma patients, Nogova et al. [25]

| Patient characteristics | LPHL (n=394) | cHL (n=7,904) |
|---|---|---|
| Median age (years) | 37 | 33 |
| Female (%) | 25 | 44 |
| Male (%) | 75 | 56 |
| Early favorable (%) | 63 | 22 |
| Early unfavorable (%) | 16 | 39 |
| Advanced (%) | 21 | 39 |
| B symptoms (%) | 9 | 40 |
| Three nodal areas (%) | 28 | 55 |
| Mediastinal bulk (%)[a] | 31 | 55 |
| Elevated ESR (%) | 4 | 45 |
| Extranodal involvement (%) | 6 | 14 |
| Serum LDH >ULN (%) | 16 | 32 |

*LPHL* lymphocyte-predominant Hodgkin lymphoma; *cHL* classical Hodgkin lymphoma; *ESR* erythrocyte sedimentation rate; *LDH* lactate dehydrogenase; *ULN* upper limit of normal
[a]Bulk one third of maximum thoracic diameter; information provided in 3,335 of 8,298 patients
ESR 50 mm/h without B symptoms and 30 mm/h with B symptoms

The relevant prognostic risk factors of classical Hodgkin lymphoma such as large mediastinal mass or bulky disease are rare in LPHL. Also infrequent is extranodal disease with 6% of patients having spleen involvement, 3% liver, 1% lung and bone marrow, respectively. Involvement of peripheral lymph nodes however is common and includes inguinal and cervical areas. In the GHSG analysis, negative prognostic factors for tumor control (FFTF) were advanced stage ($p=0.0092$), hemoglobin less than 10.5 g/dL ($p=0.0171$), and lymphopenia (<8% of white cell count; $p=0.01$). Hemoglobin <10.5 g/dL ($p=0.0014$), age older than 45 years ($p=0.0125$) and advanced stage ($p=0.0153$) were negative prognostic factors for overall survival (Table 15.3).

## 15.8 Treatment of Early Favorable LPHL

In early favorable stages, LPHL patients have an excellent prognosis with an overall survival of close to 100% in IA staged patients. There are different approaches in

**Table 15.3** Multivariate analysis for OS including international prognostic score and follicular lymphoma international prognostic index modified according to the GHSG risk factors

| Risk factor | LPHL | cHL |
|---|---|---|
| Male sex | 0.7556 | <0.0001 |
| Age 45 years | 0.0125 | <0.0001 |
| Advanced stage | 0.0153 | 0.6858 |
| Albumin <4 g/dL | 0.6730 | 0.6759 |
| Hemoglobin <10.5 g/dL | 0.0014 | 0.0112 |
| Leukocytes >15,000/L | 0.1244 | 0.0209 |
| Lymphopenia | 0.9946 | 0.1608 |
| Serum LDH >ULN | 0.2353 | 0.0471 |
| Three nodal areas | 0.1205 | <0.0001 |
| Elevated ESR[a] | 0.0894 | 0.0010 |
| Extranodal involvement | 0.5794 | <0.0001 |

Note, lymphopenia <8% of white blood count
OS overall survival; GHSG German Hodgkin Study Group; LPHL lymphocyte-predominant Hodgkin lymphoma; cHL classical Hodgkin lymphoma; LDH lactate dehydrogenase; ULN upper limit of normal; ESR erythrocyte sedimentation rate
[a]ESR 50 mm/h without B symptoms and 30 mm/h with B-symptoms

these patients including a watch and wait strategy, radiotherapy in small (IFRT) or large field technique (EFRT), multiagent chemotherapy, combined modality treatment and, more recently, monoclonal anti-CD20 antibodies.

The treatment of LPHL patients in early stages is clearly aimed at inducing as little acute and late toxicity as possible. Particularly in children with LPHL, treatment strategies focus on avoiding long-term side effects including secondary malignancies, infertility, growth retardation, hypothyroidism, and damage of heart and lung. In an attempt to postpone treatment, a watch and wait strategy after diagnostic lymphadenectomy was compared in smaller series of patients [27, 28]. In one study of 27 pediatric patients, 13 underwent lymphadenectomy only, 10 were treated with combined modality, one patient had IFRT and three patients chemotherapy only. At a median follow-up of 70 months, the overall survival for all 27 patients was 100% with an event-free survival of 69%. The event-free survival in the watch and wait group was 42% compared with 90% of those having additional treatment. Patients

with residual lymphoma after the diagnostic operation clearly had inferior EFS when receiving no further treatment. Thus, watch and wait has to be regarded experimental and should not be routinely recommended in clinical practice. More studies are needed such as the one currently conducted by the EORTC. Here, stage IA LPHL patients with infradiaphragmatic stage IA are followed by watch and wait after complete tumor resection.

An American group of pediatric oncologists reported 15 children and adolescents at a median age of 11 years with localized LPHL [28]. Patients received a selected therapy: those with stage I disease that were disease-free after the diagnostic biopsy were carefully followed without further treatment. Patients with stage I or II who had incomplete resection were treated with brief chemotherapy consisting of vincristine, doxorubicin, cyclophosphamide, and prednisone. All these patients reached complete remission; one patient in stage II relapsed six years after the initial diagnosis.

For most LPHL patients in early favorable stages, radiotherapy is the mainstay of treatment. There are two retrospective analyses including a smaller series of 36 stage I/IIA patients that were either treated with IFRT or a modified localized radiation with an event-free survival of 95% and overall survival of 100% after 5 years [29]. A larger Australian series analyzed 208 stage I/II patients treated with radiotherapy in mantle field technique or reverted Y. In this group of patients, the progression-free survival was 82% with an overall survival of 83% at a median follow-up of 8.8 years. The authors conclude that a reduction of field size in this group of patients is feasible and safe and suggested radiotherapy alone as treatment of choice for early-stage LPHL [30]. In their studies, the GHSG treated a total of 131 stage IA LHPL patients with different treatment modalities including EFRT (45 patients), IFRT (45 patients) and combined modality treatment (41 patients) [31]. Median follow-up was 78 months for the EF-treated group, 40 months for those with IFRT and 17 months for combined modality treatment. Overall 99% patients reached a complete remission. As shown in Fig. 15.3, there was no difference in terms of FFTF between these different treatments. Although longer follow-up is required for a more comprehensive picture, the efficacy and tolerability of IFRT has resulted in this treatment modality being recommended by the GHSG for patients with stage IA LPHL. The EORTC has also adopted IFRT as standard of care of

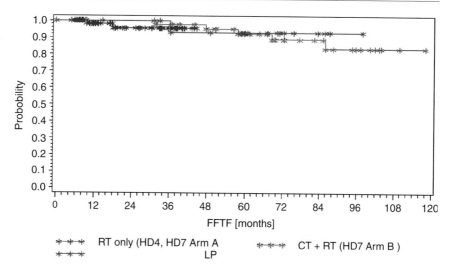

**Fig. 15.3** Stage IA LPHL in GHSG clinical trials, FFTF according to different treatments, Nogova et al. (2005)

stage IA LPHL [32]. Similarly, the guidelines panel of the US National Cancer Center Network (NCCN) recommends small field radiotherapy as treatment of choice for stage IA LPHL [33]. A French group analyzed 500 patients with Hodgkin lymphoma including 42 LPHL, 144 classical Hodgkin Lymphoma without mediastinal involvement and 314 patients with mediastinal involvement. The mortality rates after 15 years were similarly low in those LPHL and classical Hodgkin lymphoma patients without mediastinal involvement. They reported an excellent prognosis after brief antracylin-based chemotherapy followed by EFRT [34]. More recently, long-term follow-up of 113 patients with stage I/II LPHL treated between 1970 and 2005 was reported [35]. The overall survival and progression-free survival were similar among patients who received limited-field, regional-field, or extended-field radiation therapy. The 10-year progression-free survival was 85% for patients with stage I, and 61% for patients with stage II disease, with an overall survival of 94 and 97%, respectively.

## 15.9 Treatment of Early Unfavorable and Advanced Stages

The treatment of LPHL patients with early unfavorable (intermediate) and advanced stage LPHL is usually identical to the treatment of classical Hodgkin lymphoma. This is based on larger analyses performed by several groups. The GHSG analysis including 394 LPHL patients and 7,904 classical Hodgkin lymphoma patients reported that 91% of patients in early favorable, 86% in early unfavorable and 79% in advanced stages reached CR [26]. This compares with rates of 86, 83 and 75% in classical Hodgkin lymphoma patients. There were only 0.3% of LPHL patients with progressive disease as compared with 3.7% of classical Hodgkin lymphoma patients. Although the overall relapse rate was very similar (LPHL 8.1 vs. 7.9% classical Hodgkin lymphoma) early relapses were more frequent in patients with classical Hodgkin lymphoma (3.2 vs. 0.8%). The tumor control at a median follow-up of 41 months for patients with early unfavorable and advanced stage LPHL was 88% with an overall survival of 96% as compared with 82 and 92% for classical Hodgkin lymphoma. Similar data were reported by the EFTL [6]. Here, 96% of patients with advanced stage LPHL reached CR. The FFTF for LPHL patients was 95% at a median follow-up of 8 years as compared with 74% for classical Hodgkin lymphoma patients. Overall survival was 89% in both groups. Figure 15.4 shows FFTF and overall survival of LPHL and classical Hodgkin lymphoma patients; FFTF of LPHL patients according to clinical stage is shown in Fig. 15.5.

Because LPHL shares clinical and immunophenotypic featured with indolent B-cell NHL, the M.D. Anderson Cancer Center group is currently piloting the use of R-CHOP, a regimen commonly used for the treatment of patients with NHL, in patients with

**Fig. 15.4** (**a**) LPHL and classical HL, FFTF, Nogova et al. [26]. (**b**) LPHL and classical HL, overall survival, Nogova et al. [26]

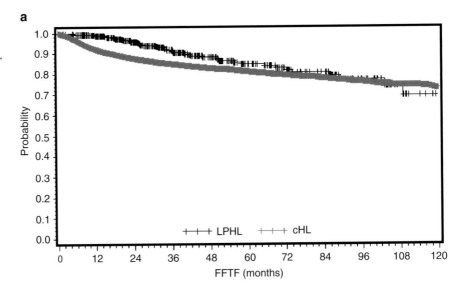

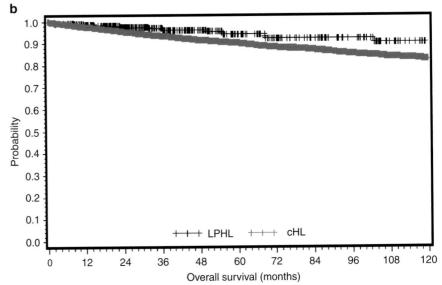

advanced stage LPHL [36]. Whether this approach will be more effective than regimens that are traditionally used for the treatment of patients with classical HL will require a randomized study through international cooperation.

## 15.10 Treatment of Relapsed LPHL

If possible, LPHL patients with suspected relapse should undergo a renewed biopsy since the transformation into a more aggressive non-Hodgkin lymphoma

should be excluded. In the ETFL study, 14% of LPHL relapses were identified as classical Hodgkin lymphoma and 10% as non-Hodgkin lymphoma. Patients with LPHL showed a tendency to more favorable survival after relapse as compared with classical Hodgkin Lymphoma patients ($p=0.05$). This however has to be handled with care since more LPHL patients had been in early stages at primary diagnosis and were treated with less intensive first-line treatment [6, 26, 35, 36]. Surprisingly, there were no differences in the prognosis of relapses between LPHL and classical Hodgkin lymphoma patients treated in three GHSG study generations. The relapse rate was very similar for LPHL

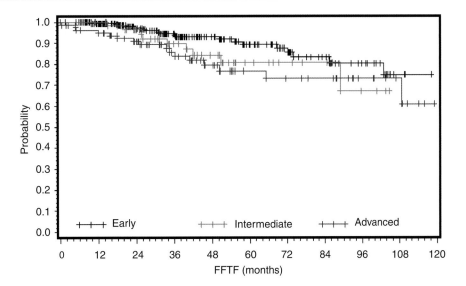

**Fig. 15.5** LPHL, FFTF according to clinical risk groups ($n = 394$), Nogova et al. (2008)

patients (8.1%) and classical Hodgkin lymphoma patients (7.9%).

Due to the restricted number of LPHL patients, prospectively randomized trials are not available and will be difficult to conduct. Although patients with early unfavorable and advanced stage LPHL have a slightly better prognosis as compared with classical Hodgkin lymphoma patients, the current standard treatment recommendation is identical to those for classical Hodgkin lymphoma.

With the advent of the anti-CD20 monoclonal antibody rituximab and the efficacy combined with excellent tolerability observed in clinical trials with other lymphoma entities, this antibody was subsequently evaluated in phase II studies in patients with relapsed or refractory LPHL. This was based on the fact that in LPHL not only the reactive background usually stains strongly for CD20 but, importantly, also the malignant LP cells are CD20 positive (Fig. 15.2a). In a study conducted by the GHSG, 14 patients were treated with weekly rituximab at doses of 375 mg/m² for 4 weeks [37]. The overall response rate was 86%; eight patients achieved CR and 4 patients PR. At a short median follow-up of 12 months, 9 patients were in remission. An up-date on this study with 21 patients included, of whom 15 had reconfirmed LPHL, reported an overall response rate of 94% [25]. With a median follow-up of 63 months, the median time to progression was 33 months, with the median overall survival not reached (Fig. 15.6). Similar results were reported in 22 less intensively or previously untreated patients from

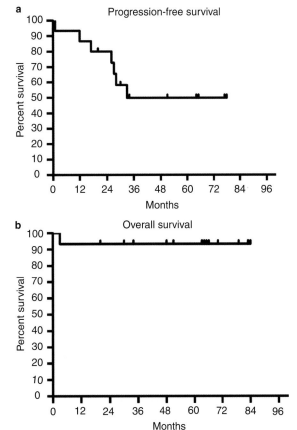

**Fig. 15.6** Time to progression and overall survival of LPHL patients on rituximab, Schulz et al. 2008 [35]. (**a**) Kaplan–Meier analysis of time to progression for 8 of 15 LPHL patients, progression-free survival. (**b**) Kaplan–Meier analysis of overall survival for 14 of 15 LPHL patients

Stanford [38]. In their study, the response rate was 100% with 9/22 complete remissions (41%). However, 9/22 patients had relapsed at a median follow-up of 13 months with two of five patients transformed to large cell Hodgkin lymphoma. On the basis of high efficacy and excellent tolerability, rituximab was evaluated in 30 previously untreated stage IA patients that did not have additional risk factors. The results of this study will be available shortly. Another treatment option for LPHL is the more recently described fully human anti-CD20 monoclonal antibody Ofatumumab that is currently undergoing clinical trials in this disease [39].

Due to the rare LPHL cases, the role of autologous stem cell transplant in the treatment of patients with relapsed LPHL remains undefined. In a recent retrospective study, 28 patients with relapsed LPHL who underwent ASCT were reported. The 5-year event-free survival was 69%, and the overall survival was 76% [40]. Thus, ASCT may be considered for selected patients with relapsed LPHL, especially at the time of histologic transformation.

# References

1. Jackson H, Parker F. Hodgkin's disease II. Pathology. N Engl J Med. 1944;231.
2. Lukes R, Butler J, Hicks E. Natural history of Hodgkin's disease as related to its pathological picture. Cancer. 1966; 19:317.
3. Harris NL, Jaffe JS, Stein H. A revised European-American classification of lymphoid neoplasms: a proposal from the International Lymphoma Study Group. Blood. 1994;84: 1361.
4. Jaffe E, Harris NL, Stein H, et al. Pathology and genetics of tumours of haematopoietic and lymphoid tissues. Lyon: IARC; 2001. p. 240–3.
5. Swerdlow SH, Campo E, Harris ES, Jaffe NL, Pileri SA, Stein H, et al., editors. WHO classification of tumours of haematopoietic and lymphoid tissues. Geneva: WHO Press; 2008.
6. Diehl V, Sextro M, Franklin J, et al. Clinical presentation, course, and prognostic factors in lymphocyte predominant Hodgkin's disease: report from the European Task Force on Lymphoma (ETFL) Project on lymphocyte-predominant hodgkin's disease. J Clin Oncol. 1999;17:776–83.
7. Mason DY, Banks PM, Chan J, et al. Nodular lymphocyte-predominance Hodgkin's disease. A distinct clinicopathological entity. Am J Surg Pathol. 1994;18:526–30.
8. Boudova L, Torlakovic E, Delabie J, et al. Nodular lymphocyte-predominant Hodgkin lymphoma with nodules resembling T-cell/histiocyte-rich B-cell lymphoma: differential diagnosis between nodular lymphocyte-predominant Hodgkin lymphoma and T-cell/histiocyte-rich B-cell lymphoma. Blood. 2003;102:3753–8.
9. Küppers R, Rajewsky K, Zhao M, et al. Hodgkin disease: Hodgkin and Reed–Sternberg cells picked from histological sections show clonal immunoglobulin gene rearrangements and appear to be derived from B-cells at various stages of development. Proc Natl Acad Sci USA. 1994;91:10962–6.
10. Delabie J, Tierens A, Wu G, et al. Lymphocyte predominance Hodgkin's disease: lineage and clonality determination using a single-cell assay. Blood. 1994;84:3291–8.
11. Marafioti T, Hummel M, Anagnostopoulos I, et al. Origin of nodular lymphocyte-predominant Hodgkin's disease from a clonal expansion of highly mutated germinal center B-cells. N Engl J Med. 1997;337:453–8.
12. Ohno T, Stribley JA, Wu G, et al. Clonality in nodular lymphocyte-predominant Hodgkin's disease. N Engl J Med. 1997;337:459–65.
13. Schumacher AM, Schmitz R, Brune V, et al. Mutations in the genes coding for den NJ-κB regulation factors IκBα and A20 are uncommon in nodular lymphocyte-predominant Hodgkin lymphoma. Haematologica. 2010;95:153–7.
14. Rüdiger TO, Ott MM, Müller-Deubert SM, et al. Differential diagnosis between classical Hodgkin's lymphoma, T-cell-rich B-cell lymphoma and paragranuloma by paraffin immunochemistry. Am J Surg Pathol. 1998;22:1184–91.
15. Poppema S. The nature of the lymphocytes surrounding Reed–Sternberg cells in nodular lymphocyte predominance and in other types of Hodgkin's disease. Am J Pathol. 1989;135:351–7.
16. Felgar RE, Steward KR, Cousar JB, et al. T-cell-rich large B-cell lymphomas contain non-activated CD8+ cytolytic T-cells, show increased tumor cell apoptosis, and have lower Bcl-2 expression than diffuse large-B-cell lymphomas. Am J Pathol. 1998;153:1707–15.
17. Alkan S, Ross CW, Hanson CA, et al. Epstein–Barr virus and BCL-2 protein overexpression are not detected in the neoplastic cells of nodular lymphocyte predominance Hodgkin's disease. Mod Pathol. 1995;8:544–7.
18. Torlakovic E, Tierens A, Dang HD, et al. The transcription factor PU.1, necessary for B-cell development is expressed in lymphocyte predominance, but not classical Hodgkin's disease. Am J Pathol. 2001;159:1807–14.
19. Sundeen JT, Gossman J, Jaffe ES. Lymphocyte predominant Hodgkin's disease nodular subtype with coexistent "large cell lymphoma". Histological progression or composite malignancy? Am J Surg Pathol. 1988;12:599–606.
20. Huang JZ, Weisenburger DD, Vose JM, et al. Diffuse large B-cell lymphoma arising in nodular lymphocyte predominant Hodgkin lymphoma: a report of 21 cases from the Nebraska Lymphoma Study Group. Leuk Lymphoma. 2004; 45:1551–7.
21. Rüdiger T, Gascoyne RE, Jaffe ES, et al. Workshop on the relationship between nodular lymphocyte predominant Hodgkin's lymphoma and T-cell/histiocyte-rich B-cell lymphoma. Ann Oncol. 2002;13 suppl 1:44–51.
22. Greiner TC, Gascoyne RD, Anderson ME, et al. Nodular lymphocyte-predominant Hodgkin's disease associated with large-cell lymphoma: analysis of Ig gene rearrangements by V-J polymerase chain reaction. Blood. 1996;88:657–66.
23. Shimabukuro-Vornhagen A, Haverkamp H, Engert A, et al. Lymphocyte-rich classical Hodgkin's lymphoma: clinical presentation and treatment outcome in 100 patients treated within German Hodgkin's Study Group trials. J Clin Oncol. 2005;23:5739–45.

24. Henry-Amar M. Second cancer after treatment for Hodgkin's disease: a report from the International Database on Hodgkin's disease. Ann Oncol. 1992;3 suppl 4:117.
25. Schulz H, Rehwald U, Morschhauser F, et al. Rituximab in relapsed lymphocyte predominant Hodgkin lymphoma: long-term results of a phase 2 trial of the German Hodgkin Lymphoma Study Group (GHSG). Blood. 2008;111:109–11.
26. Nogova L, Reineke T, Brillant C, et al. Lymphocyte-predominant and classical Hodgkin's lymphoma: a comprehensive analysis from the German Hodgkin Study Group. J Clin Oncol. 2008;26:434–9.
27. Pellegrino B, Terrier-Lacombe MJ, Oberlin O, et al. Lymphocyte-predominant Hodgkin's lymphoma in children: therapeutic abstention after initial lymph node resection – a study of the French Society of Pediatric Oncology. J Clin Oncol. 2003;21:2948–52.
28. Murphy SB, Morgan ER, Katzenstein HM, et al. Results of little for not treatment for lymphocyte-predominant Hodgkin disease in children and adolescents. J Pediatr Hematol Oncol. 2003;25:684–7.
29. Schlembach PJ, Wilder RB, Jones D, et al. Radiotherapy alone for lymphocyte-predominant Hodgkin's disease. Cancer J. 2002;8:377–83.
30. Wirth A, Yuen K, Barton M, et al. Long-term outcome after radiotherapy alone for lymphocyte-predominant Hodgkin lymphoma: a retrospective multicenter study of the Australasian Radiation Oncology Lymphoma Group. Cancer. 2005;104:1221–9.
31. Nogova L, Reineke T, Eich HT, et al. Extended field radiotherapy combined modality treatment or involved field radiotherapy for patients with stage IA lymphocyte-predominant Hodgkin's lymphoma: a retrospective analysis from the German Hodgkin Study Group (GHSG). Ann Oncol. 2005;16:1683–7.
32. Raemaekers J, Kluin-Nelemans H, Teodorovic I, et al. The achievements of the EORTC Lymphoma Group. European Organisation for Research and Treatment of Cancer. Eur J Cancer. 2002;38 suppl 4:107–13.
33. JNCCN – The Journal of the National Comprehensive Cancer Network. 2008;6(6) http://www.nccn.org/JNCCN/toc/2008jul.asp#hodgkins
34. Feugier P, Labouyrie E, Djeridane M, et al. Comparison of initial characteristics and long-term outcome of patients with lymphocyte-predominant Hodgkin lymphoma and classical Hodgkin lymphoma at clinical stages IA and IIA prospectively treated by brief anthracycline-based chemotherapies plus extended high-dose irradiation. Blood. 2004;104:2675–81.
35. Chen RC, Chin MS, Ng AK, et al. Early-stage, lymphocyte-predominant Hodgkin's lymphoma: patient outcomes from a large, single-institution series with long follow-up. J Clin Oncol. 2010;28:136–41.
36. Fanale MA, Younes A. Nodular lymphocyte predominant Hodgkin's lymphoma. Cancer Treat Res. 2008;142:367–81.
37. Rehwald U, Schulz H, Reiser M, et al. Treatment of relapsed CD20+ Hodgkin lymphoma with the monoclonal antibody rituximab is effective and well tolerated: results of a phase 2 trial of the German Hodgkin Study Group. Blood. 2003;101:420–4.
38. Ekstrand BC, Lucas JB, Horwitz SM, et al. Rituximab in lymphocyte-predominant Hodgkin disease: results of a phase 2 trial. Blood. 2003;101:4285–9.
39. Hagenbeek A, Gadeberg O, Johnson P, et al. First clinical use of Ofatumumab, a novel fully human anti-CD20 monoclonal antibody in relapsed or refractory follicular lymphoma: results of a phase I/II trial. Blood. 2008;111:5486–95.
40. Popat U, Hosing C, Fanale M, et al. Autologous transplantation for nodular lymphocyte-predominant Hodgkin lymphoma (LPHL). Blood (ASH Annual Meeting Abstracts) 2009;114:2310.

# The Management of Hodgkin Lymphoma During Pregnancy

**16**

Veronika Bachanova and Joseph M. Connors

## Contents

## 16.1 Introduction

Hodgkin lymphoma (HL) is the fourth most frequent cancer diagnosis among pregnant females and the most common hematologic malignancy complicating pregnancy [1]. The estimated incidence of HL ranges from 1:1,000 to 1:3,000 deliveries. Between 0.5 and 1.0% of cases of HL present coincident with pregnancy, which leads to the problem of optimally managing the lymphoma while giving the developing fetus the best chance of reaching term fully intact. Essentially, two patients need to be managed: one with lymphoma and the other without but affected by the toxicity of any treatments. The potentially life-threatening nature of HL diagnosis induces fear and anxiety in the pregnant patient and therapeutic decisions must be made in a complex milieu mixing the religious, ethical, psychological, social and cultural beliefs, and attitudes of the patient, her family, and her physicians. When HL is diagnosed during pregnancy, much of the discussion requires that the advising clinician balance provision of expertise and knowledge about treatment options and prognosis with respect for ethical principles, compassion, and acceptance of patient autonomy.

Fortunately, when HL is discovered during pregnancy, it is almost always possible to control the lymphoma and allow the pregnancy to go to full term. A multidisciplinary team composed of a hemato-oncologist knowledgeable in the treatment of HL, an obstetrician experienced in the management of high-risk pregnancy, a pediatrician/neonatologist familiar with hematologic problems in the neonate, and a nurse coordinator must work together closely to plan the overall management (Table 16.1 and 16.2). High-quality clinical evidence identifying the best approach to management of coincident HL and pregnancy is

V. Bachanova (✉)
Division of Hematology, Oncology and Transplantation, University of Minnesota, 420 Delaware Street, Minneapolis, MN 55455, USA
e-mail: bach0173@umn.edu

J.M. Connors
Lymphoma Tumor Group, BC Cancer Agency, 600 West 10th Avenue, Vancouver, BC, Canada V5Z 4E6

A. Engert and S.J. Horning (eds.), *Hodgkin Lymphoma*,
DOI: 10.1007/978-3-642-12780-9_16, © Springer-Verlag Berlin Heidelberg 2011

**Table 16.1** Characteristics of the multidisciplinary team for treatment of a pregnant patient with concomitant HL

| Obstetrician | Often makes the diagnosis, referral to heme/onc |
|---|---|
| | Provides experience in high-risk pregnancies (prenatal care in patients with active malignancy) |
| | Makes primary decisions regarding pregnancy |
| | Counsels the patient if pregnancy termination is recommended by the team |
| | Establishes the timing and method of delivery |
| | Administers antenatal steroids if appropriate |
| | Counsels about effective postpartum contraception methods for a minimum of 2 years after conclusion of HL treatment (greatest risk of relapse) |
| Hematologist/medical oncologist | Plans the diagnostic work-up and staging methods to minimize the adverse effects on fetus |
| | Coordinates with other team members to establish plan of care |
| | Administers the chemotherapy if deemed necessary |
| | Provides supportive care for patients treated with chemotherapy to keep Hgb≥10 g/dL and platelet count ≥30×109/L |
| | Reviews safety of medications used for supportive care during pregnancy |
| | Coordinates delivery planning and chemotherapy administration to ensure that platelet count is ≥50×109/L at the time of delivery |
| | Provides oncology follow-up after delivery to complete appropriate staging and treatments |
| | Provides oncologic follow-up to monitor for relapse |
| Neonatologist | Relies on prior experience in high-risk pregnancies |
| | Provides expertise in management of childhood hematologic disorders |
| | Examines placenta and arranges histopathologic evaluation for presence of metastasis |
| | Coordinates postnatal care of the newborn |
| | Registers the newborn in central registry of children born to pregnant mothers with HL |
| | Counsels about breastfeeding |
| | Schedules long-term follow-up of newborn |
| Nurse coordinator | Coordinates communication among the specialists |
| | Encourages close communication with the patient |
| | Provides emotional support to the patient and family |

**Table 16.2** Counseling the pregnant patient with coincident HL – points of discussion

| |
|---|
| Diagnosis, natural history of HL, curability, and prognosis |
| Staging and prognostic significance |
| Lack of evidence that HL by itself has an adverse effect on pregnancy or fetus |
| Option of terminating pregnancy for patients with early gestation |
| Treatment choices |
| Chemotherapy agents and associated side-effects and risks (vinblastine, ABVD) for mother and fetus |
| Expected outcomes |
| Need for multidisciplinary team to manage the patient |
| Discussions regarding patients preference, values, and ethical considerations |

limited. Decision making must therefore be guided by a judicious mix of careful clinical judgment, the experience of involved team members, knowledge of the usual natural history of HL, and consideration of the patient's personal beliefs and desires [2–4].

## 16.2 Diagnostic Algorithm for HL Staging During Pregnancy

When planning the diagnostic evaluation of HL in a pregnant patient, one has to balance the need for accurate disease assessment with the need to minimize the use of invasive procedures. The histopathologic diagnosis of HL should be based on tissue examination obtained by excisional or incisional tissue biopsy. Fine

**Table 16.3** Tests required for staging of HL discovered during pregnancy

| Complete history searching for B symptoms or other symptomatic problems suggesting more advanced disease | |
|---|---|
| Physical examination for lymphadenopathy or organomegaly | |
| Complete blood cell counts | |
| Serum creatinine, alkaline phosphatase, lactate dehydrogenase, bilirubin, and protein electrophoresis ( including albumin level) | |
| Chest radiograph, PA view only, with appropriate shielding | |
| Abdominal ultrasound for retroperitoneal lymphadenopathy | |
| Certain tests are only required for specific HL presentations | |
| *Test* | *Presentation/condition* |
| Bone marrow biopsy | B symptoms or WBC $<4.0 \times 10^9$/L or Hgb $<12$ g/dL or platelets $<125 \times 10^9$/L |
| ENT examination | Stage IA or IIA disease with upper cervical lymph node involvement (supra-hyoid) |

needle aspiration is inadequate in most cases. The initial evaluation should include a complete history and physical examination with careful documentation of B-symptoms (Table 16.3). Thorough palpation of all node-bearing areas should be performed. Standard laboratory tests should include hemoglobin, complete differential white blood cell count, platelet count, erythrocyte sedimentation rate, liver and renal function assessment, and lactate dehydrogenase. It is important to recall that pregnancy can affect the results of some of these tests (e.g., ESR, alkaline phosphatase) complicating interpretation.

In contrast to the imaging assessment of the usual patient with HL, which is designed to comprehensively characterize all sites of disease, the guiding principle in the pregnant patient is to restrict radiologic staging to the minimum necessary to identify disease that seriously threatens the immediate well-being of mother or child. Limiting radiation exposure to the fetus is critical, especially during early stages of gestation. Computed tomography (CT) and positron emission tomography (PET) scans should be avoided. A single postero-anterior radiograph of the chest, with proper shielding, should be obtained to characterize the extent of mediastinal and pulmonary disease. Abdominal ultrasonography can identify the extent and size of retroperitoneal nodal disease with sufficient detail for proper management [3]. Magnetic resonance imaging (MRI) without use of gadolinium can also be used and is, at least theoretically, free of potential toxicity to the fetus [5]; however, the amount of detail provided in excess of what can be found with ultrasonography is

unnecessary and the safety of the intensive magnetic fields required is not fully established.

Additional specific assessments can be helpful. Bone marrow biopsy is recommended for patients with B symptoms or abnormalities found in peripheral blood such as anemia, thrombocytopenia, or leucopenia (Table 16.3). Patients with upper cervical lymphadenopathy should undergo focused otolaryngologic examination. Echocardiography may be used to assess left ventricular function if chemotherapy is planned. Other tests should only be performed if decisions regarding immediate management would be influenced. The goal of clinical and radiologic staging is to provide guidance about disease aggressiveness, to explain specific symptoms such as cough or pain, and to identify organ compromise, all clues that may indicate the need to initiate treatment without delay.

## 16.3 Treatment

### 16.3.1 General Principles

The complexity of issues involved in caring for a pregnant patient with HL requires a multidisciplinary team of experts working together to develop an individualized management plan. What little we know about managing pregnant HL patients comes from several small series of cases and anecdotal descriptions. However, this limited evidence can provide useful guidance when complemented by careful clinical judgment and knowledge of the natural history of HL. The clinical dilemma lies in determining the effect of treatment delay on maternal survival vs. the risk of abortion, fetal malformation, and adverse perinatal outcomes associated with the use of chemotherapy and radiotherapy. Continuous communication with the patient and her family is crucial to ensure understanding and alleviate anxiety and fear.

Available recent evidence suggests that pregnancy itself does not affect the course of disease, response to therapy, or the overall survival rate when compared with age- and stage-equivalent nonpregnant controls [6, 7]. In addition, some reports found no difference in survival among women who had therapeutic abortion in comparison to those who did not [8, 9]. It has also been suggested by several authors that HL by itself does not appear to have an adverse effect on the course of pregnancy, the product of conception, labor, or

puerperium [10, 11]. Therefore, therapeutic abortion is not necessary to assure the best prognosis.

The majority of patients with HL during pregnancy require no immediate intervention. As a general rule, any treatment, such as radiation or chemotherapy, should be avoided during the first trimester unless severe, life-threatening symptoms are present (Fig. 16.1). Almost all chemotherapy agents have been documented to be teratogenic in animals or humans, although for some drugs only experimental data exist. Chemotherapy during the first trimester may increase the risk of spontaneous abortion, fetal death, and major malformation; the fetus is extremely vulnerable from the second to the eighth week of gestation during which time organogenesis occurs. Even after primary organogenesis several organs including the eyes, genitalia, hematopoietic system, and central nervous system remain vulnerable to chemotherapy and radiation therapy. Although

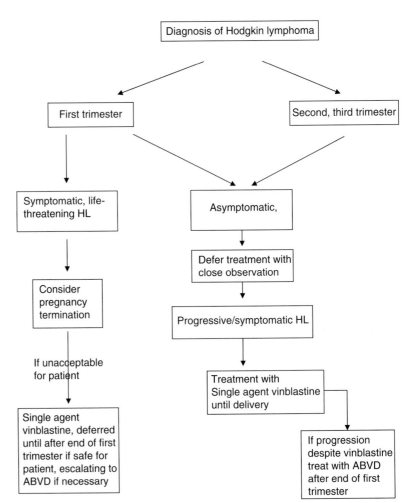

Fig. 16.1 Suggested algorithm for the treatment for pregnancy-associated Hodgkin lymphoma (HL)

generally unnecessary, the option of pregnancy termination needs to be considered for the rare patient whose first trimester is complicated by severely symptomatic or life-threatening disease, where the need for immediate chemotherapy may affect fetal development. Much more often, if intervention is required, especially after the first trimester, selected patients can be treated with single-agent or modified multiagent chemotherapy regimens, which have been used frequently in the second and third trimester with favorable outcomes for both mother and newborn [3, 4].

## 16.3.2 Early Stage HL in the Pregnant Patient

Over 70% of HL patients diagnosed during pregnancy have stage IA or IIA disease and are asymptomatic or minimally symptomatic. These patients require close monitoring and can often be followed through the entire pregnancy without treatment, which can be reserved for the development of severe symptoms or organ compromise. More than 50% of such patients can continue the pregnancy to term without any treatment for the lymphoma. This approach has been demonstrated to be safe in small case series such as those from Stanford (17 patients) and Royal Mardsen Hospital (19 patients) [12, 13]. Patients with stage IA–IIA HL with localized or stable disease can have chemotherapy safely deferred until normal full-term delivery after which they can complete appropriate staging and initiate treatment. In the more recent studies performed to date, with some of the HL patients opting to delay treatment until after delivery, there does not seem to be significant difference in birth weight, mean gestational age, or method or delivery compared to products of normal pregnancies [6, 11].

For symptomatic patients with upper body stage IB or IIB HL or patients with respiratory symptoms due to enlarging mediastinal masses, some authorities have recommended irradiation with special shielding [6, 8, 14, 15]. If the total dose of scatter irradiation to the fetus is less than 10 cGy, the risk to fetal development appears to be minimized [16]. The inverted Y field is not an option at any time during pregnancy. Anecdotally, mantle and upper para-aortic abdominal radiotherapy have been used successfully with meticulous shielding until the third trimester of pregnancy when the uterus starts to impinge on

the field. Estimates of radiation exposure to the fetus using this modality are typically less than 15 cGy [17]. However, use of any therapeutic radiation during pregnancy may have deleterious effects on the fetus due to direct or scatter irradiation, which may not be evident until many years later. For example, a known risk for the fetus from radiation in the second half of gestation is acquisition of blood dyscrasias or leukemia later in life [18].

Because radiation unnecessarily endangers the fetus, a better choice is systemic chemotherapy. What little is known about the effects of chemotherapy is drawn from several small clinical series and anecdotal descriptions [6–8, 11, 13, 15, 19, 20]. Single-agent vinblastine used in monotherapy appears to be a preferred agent if an early stage HL patient requires treatment because it does not cross the placenta and has been safely used in patients in all trimesters [8, 21–23].

## 16.3.3 Use of Chemotherapy for Symptomatic or Advanced Stage HL in the Pregnant Patient

Management of HL with bulky disease, visceral involvement, B symptoms, sub-diaphragmatic disease, or rapid disease progression remains controversial. Limited data have been reported on the use of standard multidrug regimens for the treatment of advanced stage HL in pregnant patients. MOPP or MOP (mechlorethamine, vincristine, prednisone with or without procarbazine) and cyclophosphamide as single agent or in combination appear to increase the risk of spontaneous abortion and fetal malformations, especially if administered during the first or second trimester of pregnancy [6, 7, 12, 13, 19, 20]. Based on these observations and the known carcinogenicity and teratogenicity of alkylating agents such as mechlorethamine, cyclophosphamide, procarbazine, and chlorambucil, this class of agents should be avoided. On the other hand, ABVD (doxorubicin, bleomycin, vinblastine, and dacarbazine) has been used during pregnancy, and the limited experience that has been reported has not identified obvious negative effects on the fetus, although the number of patients is still quite small and whether the trimester of exposure is important is unclear [15, 19, 24]. Recent reports suggest that ABVD used even in first trimester for patients with HIV-associated HL may be associated with favorable outcomes for the patient and fetus [25, 26].

Rather than expose the fetus to the potential adverse effects of multiple agents, an alternative approach using single-agent chemotherapy should be considered for symptomatic disease. Vinblastine was first described for this use more than 40 years ago [21, 27] and is a particularly attractive agent because of its high level of effectiveness against HL in treatment-naïve patients (>75% response rate) and modest acute toxicity. Although teratogenic effects have been reported in mice, neither teratogenic nor carcinogenic effects are apparent in humans at doses therapeutic for lymphoma. The combination of a high level of effectiveness, minimal acute toxicity, and low likelihood of a negative effect on the fetus make vinblastine an attractive agent to suppress HL during pregnancy. Infrequent doses at intervals of several weeks or longer can be given to control HL until delivery at term, minimizing risks to mother and child. Progression despite vinblastine, which occurs quite infrequently, should be treated with full-dose ABVD because evidence of chemotherapy resistance signifies aggressive disease requiring multiagent chemotherapy. Standard dosing of 6 mg/m$^2$ is quite unlikely to cause significant myelosuppression, but careful timing to avoid a blood cell count nadir near delivery is prudent.

We have managed 17 pregnant patients with coincident HL at the British Columbia Cancer Agency over the past 21 years using the approach described above. Eleven patients remained off treatment through term delivery and 6 required vinblastine to control disease. Thirteen of the 17 patients are still alive and well and 4 have died, 2 from HL and 1 each from acute myeloid leukemia and a retroperitoneal sarcoma. All 17 delivered normal children who now range in age from 2 to 21 years (median 15). Although these children have not been systematically assessed, no overt abnormality has become apparent [3]. Management built around conservative use of single-agent vinblastine has allowed normal term delivery of the children and effective management of the mother's HL with a minimum of psychological stress and appears to be a reasonable approach to this rare problem of coincident pregnancy and HL.

### 16.3.4 Supportive Care

Attention to symptom control is important for the well-being of a pregnant patient who requires chemotherapy. Vinblastine, as a single agent, is usually well tolerated and is not emetogenic. For multiagent programs, such as ABVD, the standard anti-nausea drugs – such as ondansteron or its derivatives, metoclopramide and lorazepam – are pregnancy category B agents with no known associated risks to fetal development. Dexamethasone has been linked to increased risk of fetal encepalo-leucomalacia and should not be routinely used. Given the potential for neutropenia with systemic chemotherapy, pregnant women with HL may require a course of antibiotics. Three groups of antibiotics that should be avoided are quinolones, sulfonamides, and tetracyclines. Quinolone use has been connected to the development of arthropathy in growing cartilage and is contraindicated for children. Sulfonamides, like other folate antagonists, have been associated with neural tube defects and cardiac malformations and should be avoided when possible. Tetracycline and its derivatives may affect bone and teeth development. Experience with treatment of neutropenia with growth factors such as filgrastim is limited, but no teratogenic effects have been reported. The common principle for pharmacological management during pregnancy is to use minimal effective doses to ameliorate the side-effect or symptoms and incorporate behavioral and nonpharmacological techniques to improve quality of life.

## 16.4 Delivery Care Planning and Postpartum Chemotherapy

One of the important considerations in the overall management of the pregnant patient with HL is to establish the timing and the mode of delivery. If HL therapy was deferred, then gestation should be allowed to progress to full term. If necessary, delivery may be induced after fetal pulmonary maturation is ensured, at least beyond 34–36 weeks of gestation. Short-course antenatal corticosteroids are frequently administered to expedite fetal lung maturity, and amniocentesis can be performed to assess the response [28].

Patients who have been able to complete the pregnancy without treatment for the lymphoma can be fully staged and treated appropriately after delivery. Most authorities strongly recommend against nursing due to variable excretion of cytotoxic drugs into the breast milk. For patients with HL who received chemotherapy during the third trimester, consideration should be given to planning the delivery 3–4 weeks following the last treatment cycle to allow bone marrow recovery. Furthermore, neonates have limited capacity to metabolize and excrete drugs due to liver and renal immaturity, and postponing the delivery will allow fetal elimination via the placenta. Patients who required vinblastine or other chemotherapy can no longer be accurately staged and therefore should be treated with a full course of 6–8 cycles of multiagent chemotherapy. Pathologic examination of the placenta should be performed after birth because this has been a site of documented, albeit exceedingly rare, metastases [29].

## 16.5  Outcomes of Children Born to Patients with HL

Although there are limited data on the effects of in vivo exposure to multiagent drugs using ABVD, it appears that this regimen has no adverse effects on the status of newborn babies at the time of birth. Few studies, however, have evaluated subsequent growth and development. Aviles reported 84 such children, 36 of which were exposed to chemotherapy in the first trimester and 27 of which were born to a mother with HL [30]. Children were examined for physical health; growth; development; and hematological, cytogenetic, neurological, psychological, and learning disorders and occurrence of cancer or acute leukemia. In all of the children studied, including the 12 second-generation children and median follow-up of 18.7 years, the birth weight was normal; learning and educational performance were normal; and no congenital, neurological, or psychological abnormalities were observed, and no cancer or acute leukemia has been observed. These results suggest that chemotherapy to treat HL at full doses can be considered, even during the first trimester, if the clinical situation requires immediate intervention.

## 16.6  Survival of HL Patients with Concurrent Pregnancy

The reciprocal influence of pregnancy on the natural history and prognosis of HL has long been debated. Two case-control comparative studies have systematically analyzed this question. In an Italian study, 21 pregnant patients were treated with radiation therapy (stage IA–IIA), MOPP chemotherapy, or their combination. Treatment was often delayed, interrupted, or discontinued and then completed after delivery.

Patients presented with similar clinical characteristics and stage distribution and similar survival at 5 and 12 years compared to 155 contemporaneous age- and stage-matched nonpregnant controls [7]. Lishner et al. reported similar 20-year survival rates for 48 pregnant females with HL in comparison to nonpregnant matched women with similar stage of disease, age, and year of treatment [6]. In both studies, pregnancy did not seem to induce a higher HL relapse rate.

## 16.7  Conclusions

Diagnosis of HL during pregnancy represents a unique clinical situation, where the expectant mother's life is endangered by malignant disease, albeit highly curable under standard circumstances. Treatment of HL, generally safe and highly effective, may seriously distress the development and vitality of the fetus. Multidisciplinary care should always involve the mother, the fetus, and the family during the pregnancy and long term follow-up is advisable. If possible, chemotherapy should be avoided in the first trimester and pregnancy should be carried to term. When the clinical course requires intervention, we recommend chemotherapy with single-agent vinblastine with intent to stabilize the disease. For symptomatic HL resistant to control with single-agent vinblastine, ABVD is the multiagent regimen of choice; its use appears to be safe for fetal development when used in any trimester; however even in aggregate, the reported cases are few and moderate levels of delayed toxicity in the child may well have been missed suggesting particular caution during the first trimester. Continued efforts to collect data on all HL patients who elect to continue coincidental pregnancy and establishment of a central registry of children born to HL patients would be of great value to capture long-term effects on both mother and child and inform broader recommendations.

## References

1. Smith LH, Danielsen B, Allen ME, Cress R. Cancer associated with obstetric delivery: results of linkage with the California cancer registry. Am J Obstet Gynecol. 2003;189(4):1128–35.
2. Connors JM. Clinical manifestations and natural history of Hodgkin's lymphoma. Cancer J. 2009;15(2):124–8.

3. Connors JM. Challenging problems: coincident pregnancy, HIV infection, and older age. Hematology Am Soc Hematol Educ Program. 2008:334–9.

4. Bachanova V, Connors JM. How is Hodgkin lymphoma in pregnancy best treated? ASH evidence-based review 2008. Hematology Am Soc Hematol Educ Program. 2008:33–4.

5. Nicklas AH, Baker ME. Imaging strategies in the pregnant cancer patient. Semin Oncol. 2000;27(6):623–32.

6. Lishner M, Zemlickis D, Degendorfer P, Panzarella T, Sutcliffe SB, Koren G. Maternal and foetal outcome following Hodgkin's disease in pregnancy. Br J Cancer. 1992;65(1):114–7.

7. Gobbi PG, Attardo-Parrinello A, Danesino M, Motta C, Di Prisco AU, Rizzo SC, et al. Hodgkin's disease and pregnancy. Haematologica. 1984;69(3):336–41.

8. Nisce LZ, Tome MA, He S, Lee III BJ, Kutcher GJ. Management of coexisting Hodgkin's disease and pregnancy. Am J Clin Oncol. 1986;9(2):146–51.

9. Jacobs C, Donaldson SS, Rosenberg SA, Kaplan HS. Management of the pregnant patient with Hodgkin's disease. Ann Intern Med. 1981;95(6):669–75.

10. Barry RM, Diamond HD, Craver LF. Influence of pregnancy on the course of Hodgkin's disease. Am J Obstet Gynecol. 1962;84:445–54.

11. Aviles A, Diaz-Maqueo JC, Talavera A, Guzman R, Garcia EL. Growth and development of children of mothers treated with chemotherapy during pregnancy: current status of 43 children. Am J Hematol. 1991;36(4):243–8.

12. Gelb AB, van de Rijn M, Warnke RA, Kamel OW. Pregnancy-associated lymphomas. A clinicopathologic study. Cancer. 1996;78(2):304–10.

13. Thomas PR, Biochem D, Peckham MJ. The investigation and management of Hodgkin's disease in the pregnant patient. Cancer. 1976;38(3):1443–51.

14. Byram D, Foulstone P. Radiotherapy for Hodgkin's disease in pregnancy. Australas Radiol. 1997;41(4):407–8.

15. Anselmo AP, Cavalieri E, Enrici RM, Pescarmona E, Guerrisi V, Paesano R, et al. Hodgkin's disease during pregnancy: diagnostic and therapeutic management. Fetal Diagn Ther. 1999;14(2):102–5.

16. Sutcliffe SB. Treatment of neoplastic disease during pregnancy: maternal and fetal effects. Clin Invest Med. 1985;8(4):333–8.

17. Friedman E, Jones GW. Fetal outcome after maternal radiation treatment of supradiaphragmatic Hodgkin's disease. CMAJ. 1993;149(9):1281–3.

18. Latourette HB. Induction of lymphoma and leukemia by diagnostic and therapeutic irradiation. Radiol Clin N Am. 1968;6(1):57–61.

19. Ebert U, Loffler H, Kirch W. Cytotoxic therapy and pregnancy. Pharmacol Ther. 1997;74(2):207–20.

20. Tawil E, Mercier JP, Dandavino A. Hodgkin's disease complicating pregnancy. J Can Assoc Radiol. 1985;36(2):133–7.

21. Rozenzweig AI, Crews Jr QE, Hopwood HG. Vinblastine sulfate in Hodgkin's disease in pregnancy. Ann Intern Med. 1964;61:108–12.

22. Lacher MJ, Geller W. Cyclophosphamide and vinblastine sulfate in Hodgkin's disease during pregnancy. JAMA. 1966;195(6):486–8.

23. Dilek I, Topcu N, Demir C, Bay A, Uzun K, Gul A, et al. Hematological malignancy and pregnancy: a single-institution experience of 21 cases. Clin Lab Haematol. 2006;28(3):170–6.

24. Cardonick E, Iacobucci A. Use of chemotherapy during human pregnancy [see comment]. Lancet Oncol. 2004;5(5):283–91.

25. Klepfish A, Schattner A, Shtalrid M, Shvidel L, Berrebi A, Bentwich Z. Advanced Hodgkin's disease in a pregnant HIV seropositive woman: favorable mother and baby outcome following combined anticancer and antiretroviral therapy. Am J Hematol. 2000;63(1):57–8.

26. Okechukwu CN, Ross J. Hodgkin's lymphoma in a pregnant patient with acquired immunodeficiency syndrome. Clin Oncol (R Coll Radiol). 1998;10(6):410–1.

27. Armstrong JG, Dyke RW, Fouts PJ. Vinblastine sulfate treatment of Hodgkin's disease during a pregnancy. Science. 1964;143:703.

28. Peleg D, Ben-Ami M. Lymphoma and leukemia complicating pregnancy. Obstet Gynecol Clin N Am. 1998;25(2):365–83.

29. Dildy III GA, Moise Jr KJ, Carpenter Jr RJ, Klima T. Maternal malignancy metastatic to the products of conception: a review. Obstet Gynecol Surv. 1989;44(7):535–40.

30. Aviles A, Neri N. Hematological malignancies and pregnancy: a final report of 84 children who received chemotherapy in utero. Clin Lymphoma. 2001;2(3):173–7.

# The Management of HIV-Hodgkin Lymphoma

# 17

Michele Spina and Umberto Tirelli

## Contents

M. Spina (✉) and U. Tirelli
Division of Medical Oncology A, National Cancer Institute,
Via Franco Gallini 2, 33081, Aviano (PN), Italy
e-mail: mspina@cro.it

## 17.1 Introduction

Since 1996, the availability of highly active antiretroviral therapy (HAART) has led to improvements in immune status among HIV-infected persons, reducing AIDS-related morbidity, and prolonging survival. However, despite the impact of HAART on HIV-related mortality, malignancies remain an important cause of death in the current era [1, 2]. The use of HAART was also associated with reduced incidence of the two major AIDS-associated malignancies – Kaposi's sarcoma (KS) and high-grade non-Hodgkin lymphoma (NHL) [3]. However, among non-AIDS-defining cancers, an increased risk of Hodgkin lymphoma (HL), anal cancer, lung cancer and hepatocarcinoma has been observed recently [4].

HIV-associated HL (HIV-HL) displays several peculiarities when compared with HL of the general population. First, HIV-HL exhibits an unusually aggressive clinical behavior, which mandates the use of specific therapeutic strategies and is associated with a poor prognosis. Second, the pathologic spectrum of HIV-HL differs markedly from that of HL in the general population [5, 6]. In particular, the aggressive histological subtypes of classic HL (cHL), namely mixed cellularity (MC) and lymphocyte depletion (LD), predominate among HIV-HL and the tumor tissue is characterized by an unusually large proportion of neoplastic cells, termed Reed–Sternberg (RS) cells [5]. Finally, despite the great improvement in chemotherapy and supportive care, optimal staging and treatment is still a matter of controversy.

A. Engert and S.J. Horning (eds.), *Hodgkin Lymphoma*,
DOI: 10.1007/978-3-642-12780-9_17, © Springer-Verlag Berlin Heidelberg 2011

## 17.2 Epidemiology

In the HIV-negative population of Western countries, HL is one of the most common malignancies diagnosed in young adults with 6 cases per 100,000 inhabitants under 45 years of age occurring each year [7], even if an increase in incidence rate in the last decade has been observed [8]. The epidemiology of HL is characterized by a peculiar age distribution pattern – a bimodal incidence curve with a first peak around the age of 30 and the second peak around the age of 50 years – that has been taken as suggestive of an infectious etiology.

In immune-suppressed patients, HL occurs more frequently than in the general population of the same age and gender. Given the relative high frequency of HL in the population groups at high risk for HIV infection, epidemiological studies conducted during the first years of the HIV epidemic in North America and in Europe had difficulties in including HL in the spectrum of HIV-associated cancers. However, with the spread of the epidemic and longer survival of infected people, the impact of HL could be better recognized. A summary of epidemiological studies that assess the HL risk of HIV-positive people is reported in Table 17.1. All studies [4, 9–20] strongly support the evidence that HIV-infected persons have, overall, a tenfold higher risk of developing HL than HIV-negative persons. Such an excess risk is more pronounced in HIV-infected individuals with moderate immune suppression, where the MC type is more frequent, and, noteworthy, is in sharp contrast with the pattern observed for KS or NHL [4]. Thus, the epidemiological pattern of HL in the HAART era substantially differs from those observed for KS or NHL – two neoplasms which drastically decreased after the introduction of HAART – and pose several new questions with regard to the relationship between degree of immunodeficiency, persistent viral infections, and cancer. Of some interest is the recent observation of Powles et al. who investigated the occurrence of cancers in a prospective cohort of 11,112 HIV-positive individuals, with 71,687 patient-years of follow-up [21].

Standardized incidence ratios (SIRs) were calculated using general population incidence data. The incidence of HL in the HIV cohort was higher than in the general population (SIR 13.85; 95% CI, 9.64–19.26). There was a significant increase in the SIRs across the three study periods (1983–1995: 4.5; 1996–2001: 11.1

and 2002–2007: 32.4). Multivariate analysis demonstrated that HAART was associated with an increased risk of disease (SIR 2.67; 95% CI, 1.19–6.02). Further multivariate modeling by class of antiretroviral agent showed that of the three classes of antiretroviral therapy, only the non-nucleoside reverse transcriptase inhibitors were associated with a significant increase in the incidence of HIV-HL (HR 2.20; 95% CI, 1.03–4.69). This might be explained because the risk of HL peaks when CD4 counts range from 150 to 199 CD4 cells/$\mu$L [4]. As the overall effect of HAART is to increase the CD4 count level, it paradoxically increases HL incidence, leading to speculate that, with severe immune suppression, the cellular background surrounding the RS cells may be altered. A potential mechanism emphasizes the role of the RS cells producing several growth factors that increased the influx of CD4 cell and inflammatory cells, which, in turn, provide proliferation signals for the RS neoplastic cells. One can imagine that in the case of severe immune suppression, leading to an unfavorable milieu, the progression of the RS neoplastic cells can be compromised [22–24]. In addition, HIV-HL is EBV-associated in almost all cases, in contrast to what is observed in the general population, in which this association is only observed in 20–50% according to histological type and age at diagnosis [25]. Usurpation of physiologically relevant pathways by EBV-encoded latent membrane protein 1 (LMP1) may lead to the simultaneous or sequential activation of signaling pathways involved in the promotion of cell activation, growth, and survival, contributing thus to most of the features of HIV-HL. Whether this change affects its categorization as HL or whether it delays HL development is unknown.

In summary, HAART use has improved immunity of HIV-infected persons, diminishing the risks of developing other cancers or other opportunistic infections, and paradoxically increasing the risk of HL.

## 17.3 Pathological Features

HIV-HL displays different pathological features in comparison with those of HL in HIV-negative patients [5]. In fact, HIV-HL is characterized by the high incidence of unfavorable histological subtypes (i.e., MC and LD) [5, 6]. In the pre-HAART era, among HIV-infected persons, MC was the most

**Table 17.1** Main results reported from epidemiological studies on HL risk among HIV-infected individuals

| First author/ publication year | Study period | Country | Main results |
|---|---|---|---|
| Biggar 1987 [9] | 1973–1984 | United States | Analysis of changes in the risk of malignancies from 1973 to 1978 through 1984 in never married men (a surrogate group of homosexual men) in high- or low-risk areas for AIDS. A non-significant ($p=0.13$) excess risk for HL was noted |
| Hessol 1992 [10] | 1978–1989 | United States | Cohort study of 6,704 HIV-positive homosexual men. This was the first study to demonstrate a statistically significant excess risk for HL in HIV-positive persons (RR = 5.0, 95% CI: 2.0–10.3) |
| Serraino 1993 [11] | 1985–1992 | Italy | Use of a clinical case series to compare the distributions of HL types between HIV-positive and HIV-negative persons. The findings put in evidence a fourfold increase of the mixed cellularity (MC) type and a 12-fold increase of the lymphocyte depletion (LD) type in HIV-positives |
| Serraino 1997 [12] | 1985–1995 | Italy | Cohort study on 1,255 HIV-positive persons with known date of seroconversion. First observation, based on only three observed cases, of an excess HL risk of nearly tenfold (95% CI: 8–111) in Europe |
| Franceschi 1998 [13] | 1985–1993 | Italy | Record linkage of the National AIDS registry with population-based cancer registries. The increased HL risk was confirmed (RR = 8.9, 95% CI: 4.4–16.0) by means of a higher number of observed HL cases |
| International Collaboration on HIV and Cancer 2000 [14] | 1985–1999 | Australia, Europe, and United States | Cancer incidence data collected from 23 studies that followed-up 47,936 persons with HIV infection. One of the first and largest evaluations of the impact of highly active antiretroviral therapy (HAART) on the spectrum of HIV-associated cancers. With regard to HL, this meta-analysis found no difference in incidence rates before (1992–1996) or after (1997–1999) the use of HAART (RR = 0.8, 95% CI: 0.3–1.9) |
| Gruilich 2002 [15] | 1985–1999 | Australia | This record linkage study of HIV, AIDS, and cancer registries confirmed, in Australia, the excess risk for HL (RR = 7.8, 95% CI: 4.4–13.0) previously noted in the United States and Europe |
| Dal Maso 2003 [16] | 1985–1998 | Italy | Update of the record linkage study between the national AIDS registry and population-based cancer registries. After 5 years, the relative risk nearly doubled (RR = 16.2, 95% CI: 11.8–21.7) |
| Herida 2003 [17] | 1992–1999 | France | Evaluation of HL risk of 77,025 HIV-positive persons during pre- and post-HAART periods, as compared to the general population of France of the same age and sex. HL risk seemed higher in the post-HAART (RR = 31.7) period than in the pre-HAART (RR = 22.8) one |
| Clifford 2005 [18] | 1985–2003 | Switzerland | Record linkage between the Swiss HIV Cohort and cancer registries. As seen in France, the findings of the study pointed to a higher risk for HL in HIV-positive persons treated with HAART (RR = 36.2), as compared to those who were never treated (RR = 11.4) |
| Biggar 2006 [4] | 1991–2002 | United States | The study focused on the relationship between degree of immune suppression and risk of HL. The findings indicated that incidence rates increased with increasing number of CD4+ cells in HIV-positive persons treated with HAART |
| Serraino 2007 [19] | 1985–2005 | France and Italy | Cohort study of 8,074 HIV-positive persons: the risk of HL did not significantly vary between those treated (RR = 9.4) or not treated (RR = 11.1) with HAART before HL occurrence |
| Engels 2008 [20] | 1991–2002 | United States | Record linkage study of 57,350 HIV-infected persons recruited from 1991 to 2002 with cancer registries. Whereas the incidence of KS and of NHL declined over time, that of HL increased (RR = 2.7, 95% CI: 1.0–7.1, 1996–2002 vs. 1991–1995). The study findings pointed to a shift in the spectrum of cancers associated with HIV infection determined by HAART treatment |

frequent HL subtype and nodular sclerosis (NS) was less frequent than in HIV-uninfected persons. For each HL subtype, incidence decreased with declining CD4 counts, but NS subtype decreased more precipitously than MC subtype, thereby increasing the proportion of MC subtype of HL seen in persons with HIV/AIDS. Thus, the greater proportion of MC and LD subtypes appears specifically related to severe immune compromise in HIV, while in the HAART era HIV-infected patients with modest immune compromise are more at risk for development of the NS subtype [4].

HIV-HL exhibits special features related to the cellular background (presence of fibrohistiocytoid stromal cell proliferation) and the high number of the neoplastic cell, and both these features may pose relevant difficulties in diagnosing and classifying the disease (Fig. 17.1). This finding contrasts with the rather low population of neoplastic cells usually found in HIV-unrelated HL [5, 26]. Moreover, a high frequency of EBV association has been shown in HL (80–100%) tissues from HIV-HL [27, 28]. The EBV genomes in such cases have been reported to be episomal and clonal, even when detected in multiple independent lesions. The elevated frequency of EBV association with HIV-HL indicates that EBV probably does represent a relevant factor involved in the pathogenesis of HIV-HL. An etiologic role of EBV in the pathogenesis of HIV-HL is further supported by data showing that LMP-1 is expressed in virtually all HIV-HL cases [5, 26–29]. On these bases, HL in HIV-infected persons appears to be an EBV-related lymphoma expressing LMP1 (Fig. 17.2).

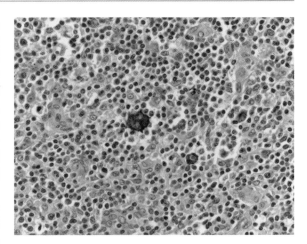

**Fig. 17.2** An RS positive for LMP-1. Immunostain with H counter stain (original magnification 25×)

Finally, RS cells of classical HL of HIV-negative patients represent transformed B-cells that originate from pre-apoptotic germinal center (GC) B-cells [30]. Most HIV-related HL cases express LMP1 and display the BCL6–/CD138+/MUM1 IRF4+ (for *Mu*ltiple *M*yeloma-1 *I*nterferon *R*egulatory *F*actor-4) phenotype, thus reflecting post-GC B cells [27, 30]. The possible contribution of LMP1 to the loss of BCL6 expression seems plausible given that LMP1 can downregulate many B-cell specific genes [31]. Loss of B-cell identity occurs during the normal differentiation of a GC B-cell into plasma cell or memory B-cell.

## 17.4 Clinical Aspects and Treatment

Similarly to that observed in HIV-NHL, one of the most peculiar features of HIV-HL is the widespread extent of the disease at presentation and the frequency of systemic "B" symptoms, including fever, night sweats, and/or weight loss >10% of the normal body weight. At the time of diagnosis 70–96% of the patients have "B" symptoms and 74–92% have advanced stages of disease with frequent involvement of extranodal sites, the most common being bone marrow (40–50%), liver (15–40%), and spleen (around 20%) [6, 32–34]. HIV-HL tends to develop as an earlier manifestation of HIV infection with higher median CD4+ cell count, ranging from 275 to 306/μL

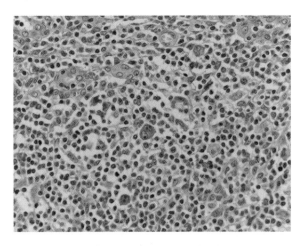

**Fig. 17.1** Reed–Sternberg (RS) cells of HIV-HL with polylobate nuclei and prominent nucleoli (H&E original magnification 25×)

[6, 32–34]. The widespread use of HAART has resulted in substantial improvement in the survival of patients with HIV infection and lymphomas, due to the reduction of the incidence of opportunistic infections, to the opportunity to allow more aggressive chemotherapy, and to the less aggressive presentation of lymphoma in patients in HAART in comparison with those lymphomas that arise in patients who never received HAART [6, 32–35].

Within the Italian Cooperative Group on AIDS and Tumors (GICAT), we have collected data on 290 patients with HIV-HL. Two hundred and eighty-one patients (87%) were males and the median age was 34 years (range 19–72 years) and 69% of patients were intravenous drug users. The median CD4 cell count was 240/μL (range 4–1,100/μL) and 57% of patients had a detectable HIV viral load.

MC was diagnosed in 53% of cases, followed by NS in 24% and LD in 14%. Advanced stages of disease were observed in 79% of patients and 76% had B symptoms. The overall extranodal involvement was 59% with bone marrow, spleen, and liver involved in 38%, 30%, and 17% respectively. With the aim to evaluate the impact of HAART on clinical presentation and outcome of our patients, we split the series into two subgroups: in the first group we included those patients who received HAART since 6 months before the onset of HL (84 patients); in the second group we included those patients who never received HAART before the diagnosis of HL or less than 6 months (206 patients). Briefly, in comparison to never experienced HAART, patients in HAART before the onset of HL are older, have less B symptoms, a higher leukocyte, neutrophil count, and hemoglobin level. The following parameters were associated with a better overall survival (OS): MC subtype, the absence of extranodal involvement, the absence of B symptoms, and prior use of HAART. Interestingly, three parameters were associated with a better time to treatment failure: a normal value of alkaline phosphatase, prior exposure to HAART, and an international prognostic score (IPS) less than 3 [36]. Table 17.2 summarizes these data. A similar study was carried out within the Spanish group GESIDA where the authors compared the clinical characteristics and outcome of 104 patients with HIV-HL, and treated (83 patients) or not (21 patients) with HAART. No differences were found between groups at baseline, but the complete remission (CR) rate was significantly higher in HAART

**Table 17.2** Clinical differences in 290 patients with HIV-HL according to prior HAART exposure

| Characteristics | Prior-HAART 84 patients (%) | HAART-naïve 206 patients (%) | p value |
|---|---|---|---|
| *Risk group* | | | |
| Intravenous drug users | 45 | 72 | |
| Heterosexual contacts | 30 | 13 | |
| Homosexual contacts | 25 | 14 | 0.0002 |
| *Age, years* | | | |
| <30 | 5 | 47 | |
| 31–40 | 46 | 40 | |
| >41 | 49 | 13 | <0.0001 |
| B symptoms | 68 | 80 | 0.03 |
| *White blood cells* | | | |
| <4,000 | 30 | 51 | |
| >4,000 | 70 | 49 | 0.002 |
| *Neutrophil count* | | | |
| <2,500 | 33 | 54 | |
| >2,500 | 67 | 46 | 0.002 |
| *Hemoglobin level* | | | |
| <10.5 | 35 | 49 | |
| ≥10.5 | 65 | 51 | 0.03 |

group (91 vs. 70%, p=0.023). The median OS was not reached in the HAART group and was 39 months in the no-HAART group (p=0.0089); the median disease free survival (DFS) was not reached in the HAART group and was 85 months in the no-HAART group (p=0.129). Factors independently associated with CR were a CD4 cell count >100 cells/μL and the use of HAART; CR was the only factor independently associated with OS [37].

Optimal therapy for HIV-HL has not been defined. Because most patients have advanced stages of disease, they have been treated with combination chemotherapy regimens but the CR rate remains lower than that of HL of the general population with the OS being approximately 1.5 years [6, 32–34]. Due to the low incidence of the disease, no randomized controlled trials have been conducted in this setting. However, several phase II studies have evaluated the feasibility and activity of different regimens. In a prospective trial, conducted within the GICAT between March 1989 and March 1992, 17 previously untreated patients with

**Table 17.4** Proposed criteria for PET interpretation after two cycles of chemotherapy

| | |
|---|---|
| *Negative* | |
| 0 | No uptake |
| 1 | Uptake ≤ mediastinum |
| 2 | Uptake > mediastinum but ≤ liver |
| *Positive* | |
| 3 | Uptake > liver in some sites even if uptake ≤ liver or mediastinum at other sites |
| 4 | Uptake > liver in over 90% of sites or development of new uptake consistent with progressive disease |

with a favorable outcome. Significance of residual uptake at sites of disease, however, needs further evaluation (e.g., biopsy). However, the use of FDG in the follow-up of HIV-HL patients who achieved CR cannot routinely recommend and further studies are warranted prior to any definite conclusion.

## 17.6 Conclusions

The outcome of patients with HIV-HL has improved with better combined antineoplastic and antiretroviral approaches. The main important challenges for the next years are (a) to demonstrate in a randomized trial that ABVD is the standard regimen in an HIV setting; (b) to validate the role of PET scan both in the staging and in the evaluation of response; (c) to better understand the interactions between chemotherapy and antiretroviral therapy in order to reduce the toxicity of both approaches; (d) to evaluate the use of new drugs (i.e., bortezomib) in this setting; (e) to evaluate the long-term toxicity of the treatment in cured patients.

## References

1. Bonnet F, Burty C, Lewden C, et al. Changes in cancer mortality among HIV-infected patients: the Mortalité 2005 Survey. Clin Infect Dis. 2009;48(5):633–9.
2. Serraino D, Dal Maso L, De Paoli A, et al. On changes in cancer mortality among HIV-infected patients: is there an excess risk of death from pancreatic cancer? Clin Infect Dis. 2009;49(3):481–2.
3. Engels EA, Pfeiffer RM, Goedert JJ, et al. Trends in cancer risk among people with AIDS in the United States 1980-2002. AIDS. 2006;20:1645–54.
4. Biggar RJ, Jaffe ES, Goedert JJ, et al. Hodgkin lymphoma and immunodeficiency in persons with HIV/AIDS. Blood. 2006;108:3786–91.
5. Grogg KL, Miller RF, Dogan A. HIV infection and lymphoma. J Clin Pathol. 2007;60:1365–72.
6. Tirelli U, Errante D, Dolcetti R, et al. Hodgkin's disease and human immmunodeficiency virus infection: clinicopathologic and virologic features of 114 patients from the Italian Cooperative Group on AIDS and Tumors. J Clin Oncol. 1995;13:1758–67.
7. Curado M P, Edwards B, Shin HR, et al., editors. Cancer incidence in five continents, Vol. IX IARC Scientific Publications No. 160. Lyon: IARC; 2007.
8. Hjalgrim H, Askling J, Pukkala E, et al. Incidence of Hodgkin's disease in Nordic countries. Lancet. 2001;358:297–8.
9. Biggar RJ, Horm J, Goedert JJ, et al. Cancer in a group at risk of acquired immunodeficiency syndrome (AIDS) through 1984. Am J Epidemiol. 1987;126:578–86.
10. Hessol NA, Katz MH, Liu JY, et al. Increased incidence of Hodgkin disease in homosexual men with HIV infection. Ann Intern Med. 1992;117:309–11.
11. Serraino D, Carbone A, Franceschi S, et al. Increased frequency of lymphocyte depletion and mixed cellularity subtypes of Hodgkin disease in HIV-infected patients. Italian Cooperative Group on AIDS and Tumours. Eur J Cancer. 1993;29A:1948–50.
12. Serraino D, Pezzotti P, Dorrucci M, et al. Cancer incidence in a cohort of human immunodeficiency virus seroconveters. HIV Italian Seroconverters Study Group. Cancer. 1997;79:1004–8.
13. Franceschi S, Dal Maso L, Arniani D, et al. Risk of cancer other than Kaposi sarcoma and non-Hodgkin's lymphoma in persons with AIDS in Italy. Cancer and AIDS Registry Linkage Study. Br J Cancer. 1998;78:966–70.
14. International Collaboration on HIV and Cancer. Highly active antiretroviral therapy and incidence of cancer in human immunodeficiency virus-infected adults. J Natl Cancer Inst. 2000;92:1823–30.
15. Grulich AE, Li Y, McDonald A, et al. Rates of non-AIDS-defining cancers in people with HIV infection before and after AIDS diagnosis. AIDS. 2002;16:1155–61.
16. Dal Maso L, Franceschi S, Polesel J, et al. Risk of cancer in persons with AIDS in Italy, 1985–1998. Br J Cancer. 2003;89:94–100.
17. Herida M, Mary-Krause M, Kaphan R, et al. Incidence of non AIDS-defining cancers before and during the highly active antiretroviral therapy era in a cohort of human immunodeficiency virus-infected patients. J Clin Oncol. 2003;21:3447–53.
18. Clifford GM, Polesel J, Rickenbach M, et al. Cancer risk in the Swiss HIV cohort study: associations with immunodeficiency, smoking, and highly active antiretroviral therapy. J Natl Cancer Inst. 2005;97:425–32.
19. Serraino D, Piselli P, Busnach G, et al. Risk of cancer following immunosuppression in organ transplant recipients and in HIV-positive individuals in southern Europe. Eur J Cancer. 2007;43:2117–23.
20. Engels EA, Biggar RJ, Hall HI, et al. Cancer risk in people infected with human immunodeficiency virus in the United States. Int J Cancer. 2008;123:187–94.

21. Powles T, Robinson D, Stebbing J, et al. Highly active anti-retroviral therapy and the incidence of non-AIDS-defining cancers in people with HIV infection. J Clin Oncol. 2009; 27(6):884–90.

22. Levine AM. Hodgkin lymphoma: to the HAART of the matter. Blood. 2006;108:3630.

23. Gloghini A, Carbone A. Why would the incidence of HIV-associated Hodgkin lymphoma increase in the setting of improved immunity? Int J Cancer. 2007;120:2753–4.

24. Carbone A, Cabras A, Gloghini A. HIV-associated Hodgkin's lymphoma. Antiapoptotic pathways and mechanisms for immune escape by tumor cells in the setting of improved immunity. Int J Biol Markers. 2007;22:161–3.

25. Dolcetti R, Boiocchi M, Gloghini A, Carbone A. Pathogenetic and histogenetic features of HIV-associated Hodgkin's disease. Eur J Cancer. 2001;37(10):1276–87.

26. Said JW. Immunodeficiency-related Hodgkin lymphoma and its mimics. Adv Anat Pathol. 2007;14:189–94.

27. Carbone A, Gloghini A, Larocca LM, et al. Human immuno-deficiency virus associated Hodgkin's disease derives from post-germinal center B cells. Blood. 1999;93:2319–26.

28. Rezk SA, Weiss LM. Epstein-Barr virus-associated lymphoproliferative disorders. Hum Pathol. 2007;38:1293–304.

29. Carbone A, Gloghini A, Dotti G. EBV-associated lymphoproliferative disorders: classification and treatment. Oncologist. 2008;13:577–85.

30. Klein U, Dalla-Favera R. Germinal centres: role in B-cell physiology and malignancy. Nat Rev Immunol. 2008;8: 22–33.

31. Vockerodt M, Morgan S, Kuo M, et al. The Epstein-Barr virus oncoprotein, latent membrane protein-1, reprograms germinal centre B cells towards a Hodgkin's Reed-Sternberg-like phenotype. J Pathol. 2008;216(1):83–92.

32. Tirelli U, Vaccher E, Serraino D, et al. Comparison of presenting clinical and laboratory findings of patients with persistent generalized lymphadenopathy (PGL) syndrome and malignant lymphoma (ML). Haematologica. 1987;72: 563–5.

33. Andrieu JM, Roithmann S, Tourani JM, et al. Hodgkin's disease during HIV-1 infection: the French registry experience. Ann Oncol. 1993;4:635–41.

34. Rubio R. disease associated with human immunodeficiency virus infection. A clinical study of 46 cases. Cancer. 1994;73: 2400–7.

35. Vaccher E, Spina M, Talamini R, et al. Improvement of systemic human immunodeficiency virus-related NHL in the era of HAART. Clin Infect Dis. 2003;37:1556–64.

36. Chimienti E, Spina M, Gastaldi R, et al. Clinical characteristics and outcome of 290 patients (pts) with Hodgkin's disease and HIV infection (HD-HIV) in pre and HAART (highly active antiretroviral therapy) era. Ann Oncol 2008;19:iv136, abstract 168.

37. Berenguer J, Miralles P, Ribera JM, et al. Characteristics and outcome of AIDS related Hodgkin Lymphoma before and after the introduction of highly active antiretroviral therapy. J Acquir Immune Defic Syndr. 2008;47:422–8.

38. Errante D, Tirelli U, Gastaldi R, et al. Combined antineoplastic and antiretroviral therapy for patients with Hodgkin's disease and human immunodeficiency virus infection. A prospective study of 17 patients. Cancer. 1994; 73:437–44.

39. Errante D, Gabarre J, Ridolfo AL, et al. Hodgkin's disease in 35 patients with HIV infection: an experience with epirubicin, bleomycin, vinblastine and prednisone chemotherapy in combination with antiretroviral therapy and primary use of G-CSF. Ann Oncol. 1999;10:189–95.

40. Levine AM, Li P, Cheung T, et al. Chemotherapy consisting of doxorubicin, bleomycin, vinblastine and dacarbazine with granulocyte-colony-stimulating factor CSF in HIV infected patients with newly diagnosed Hodgkin's disease: a prospective, multi-institutional AIDS Clinical Trials Group study (ACTG 149). J Acquir Immune Defic Syndr. 2000;24: 444–50.

41. Gastaldi R, Martino P, Gentile G, et al. Hodgkin's disease in HIV-infected patients: report of eight cases usefully treated with doxorubicin, bleomycin, vinblastine and dacarbazine (ABVD) plus granulocyte colony-stimulating factor. Ann Oncol. 2002;13(7):1158–60.

42. Spina M, Gabarre J, Rossi G, et al. Stanford V and concomitant HAART in 59 patients with Hodgkin's disease and HIV infection. Blood. 2002;100:1984–8.

43. Hartmann P, Rehwald U, Salzberger B, et al. BEACOPP therapeutic regimen for patients with Hodgkin's disease and HIV infection. Ann Oncol. 2003;14:1562–9.

44. Xicoy B, Ribera JM, Miralles P, et al. Results of treatment with doxorubicin, bleomycin, vinblastine and dacarbazine and highly active antiretroviral therapy in advanced stage human immunodefiency virus-related Hodgkin's lymphoma. Haematologica. 2007;92:191–8.

45. Xicoy B, Ribera JM, Romeu J, et al. Response to highly active antiretroviral therapy as the only therapy in an HIV-infected patient with interfollicular Hodgkin's lymphoma. Haematologica. 2007;92:191–8.

46. Spina M, Rossi G, Antinori A, et al. VEBEP regimen and highly active antiretroviral therapy (HAART) in patients (pts) with HD and HIV infection (HD-HIV). Ann Oncol 2008;19:iv152, abstract 227.

47. Gabarre J, Marcelin AG, Azar N, et al. High-dose therapy plus autologous hematopoietic stem cell transplantation for human immunodeficiency (HIV)-related lymphoma: results and impact on HIV disease. Haematologica. 2004;89: 1100–8.

48. Re A, Cattaneo C, Michieli M, et al. High-dose therapy and autologous peripheral blood stem cell transplantation as salvage treatment for HIV-associated lymphoma in patients receiving highly active antiretroviral therapy. J Clin Oncol. 2003;21:4423–7.

49. Krishnan A, Molina A, Zaia J, et al. Durable remission with autologous stem cell transplantation for high-risk HIV-associated lymphomas. Blood. 2005;105:874–8.

50. Serrano D, Carrion R, Balsalobre P, et al. HIV-associated lymphoma successfully treated with peripheral blood stem cell transplantation. Exp Hematol. 2005;33:487–94.

51. Re A, Michieli M, Casari S, et al. High-dose therapy and autologous peripheral blood stem cell transplantation as salvage treatment for AIDS-related lymphoma: long-term results of the Italian Cooperative Group on AIDS and Tumors (GICAT) study with analysis of prognostic factors. Blood. 2009;114(7):1306–13.

52. Spitzer TR, Ambinder RF, Lee JY, et al. Dose-reduced Busulfan, Cyclophosphamide, and autologous stem cell transplantation for human immunodeficiency virus-associated

lymphoma: AIDS Malignancy Consortium Study 020. Biol Blood Marrow Transpl. 2008;14:59–66.

53. Cheson BD, Pfistner B, Juweid ME, et al. Revised response criteria for malignant lymphoma. J Clin Oncol. 2007;25(5): 579–86.

54. Juweid ME, Stroobants S, Hoekstra OS, et al. Use of positron emission tomography for response assessment of lymphoma: consensus of the Imaging Subcommittee of International Harmonization Project in Lymphoma. J Clin Oncol. 2007;25(5):571–8.

55. Gallamini A, Rigacci L, Merli F, et al. The predictive value of positron emission tomography scanning performed after two courses of standard therapy on treatment outcome in advanced stage Hodgkin's disease. Haematologica. 2006;91(4):475–81.

56. Hutchings M, Loft A, Hansen M, et al. FDG-PET after two cycles of chemotherapy predicts treatment failure and progression-free survival in Hodgkin lymphoma. Blood. 2006;107(1):52–9.

57. Weihrauch MR, Manzke O, Beyer M, et al. Elevated serum levels of CC thymus and activation-related chemokine (TARC) in primary Hodgkin's disease: potential for a prognostic factor. Cancer Res. 2005;65(13):5516–9.

58. Just PA, Fieschi C, Baillet G, et al. 18F-fluorodeoxyglucose positron emission tomography/computed tomography in AIDS-related Burkitt lymphoma. AIDS Patient Care STDs. 2008;22(9):695–700.

59. Goshen E, Davidson T, Avigdor A, et al. PET/CT in the evaluation of lymphoma in patients with HIV-1 with suppressed viral loads. Clin Nucl Med. 2008;33(9):610–4.

# The Management of Elderly Patients with Hodgkin Lymphoma

# 18

Peter Borchmann, Teresa Halbsguth, and Stephen J. Proctor

## Contents

P. Borchmann (✉) and T. Halbsguth
German Hodgkin Study Group (GHSG)
e-mail: peter.borchmann@uni-koeln.de

Klinik I für Innere Medizin, Universitätsklinikum Köln,
Kerpener Straße 62, 50937, Köln, Germany

S.J. Proctor
Northern Institute for Cancer Research, Newcastle University,
Newcastle, NE 4HH, UK

## 18.1 Introduction

The treatment of Hodgkin lymphoma (HL) has been substantially improved during the past decades. Using stage-adapted poly-chemotherapy regimens and innovative radiation techniques, the 5-year progression-free survival (PFS) has reached almost 90% in young patients [1–3]. Since the median age at first diagnosis is around 32 years, these excellent results account for the majority of patients. Unfortunately, this progress did not translate into a major benefit for older patients, especially for advanced stage disease [4–8]. "Older age" is currently defined as age over 60 years, mainly due to the poor tolerability of aggressive chemotherapy regimens above the age of 60 years. Accordingly, these patients are often excluded from randomized controlled trials (RCTs). Thus, the percentage of older patients is underestimated using data from RCTs [9]. On the other hand, population studies estimate that patients over 60 years account for a substantial proportion of patients in clinical practice, i.e., about 20% of the total HL population [10]. Because only a few of them are being treated within clinical trials at all, a "standard of care" for this patient cohort has not been defined [11]. The lack of improvement in outcome for these patients will become an increasing problem, as the number of older people (over 65 years) will double during the next 50 years [12]. Malignant disorders in the elderly will become one of most important topics in oncology, and also the absolute number of older HL patients will increase. Obviously, there is an important and so far unmet medical need to improve outcome for older HL patients, especially in advanced stages and for patients with comorbidity. In this chapter, we summarize the currently available data on the management of older patients with HL and address the particular issues that

A. Engert and S.J. Horning (eds.), *Hodgkin Lymphoma*,
DOI: 10.1007/978-3-642-12780-9_18, © Springer-Verlag Berlin Heidelberg 2011

should be incorporated into prospective studies in order to improve the outcome in the future [13].

## 18.2 Epidemiology

In contrast to non-Hodgkin lymphomas (NHLs), the incidence of HL seems to be constant at 2–3 cases per 100,000 people in recent decades [14, 15]. The previously described bimodal age distribution with a first incidence peak around 30 years and a second around 50 years cannot be detected any longer in more recent analyses. This might be due to an improved hematopathologic workup including immunohistochemistry and the close cooperation with reference pathologists in most study groups. As a result, many HL cases were reclassified as NHL (e.g., T-cell anaplastic large cell lymphoma, Ki-1 anaplastic lymphoma, or T-cell rich B-cell lymphoma) [16].

Since the majority of studies and RCTs have excluded older patients on the basis of age or fitness rating, only 5–10% of all patients included into RCTs are older than 60 years [5, 17, 18]. The most accurate assessments appear to come from population-based studies. Two Swedish studies covering the years from 1979 to 1988 and from 1973 to 1994 showed a proportion of 31 and 26% of HL patients older than 60 years, respectively [7, 19]. The Scotland and Newcastle Lymphoma Group (SNLG) data demonstrated that

from 1979 to 2003, 624 (20%) of 3,373 patients registered on the population registry were over 60 years (see Fig. 18.1) [20]. For the registry period 1994–2003, 399 of 1,701 patients were >60 years (23%) (see Fig. 18.1). This is a percentage confirmed in the Northern UK regional survey of elderly HL, where the age-specific incidence was 1.97/100,000 for patients aged 60–69 and 2.18/100,000 for patients aged 70 or older [10, 11]. The incidence is somewhat higher than that reported by trial study groups since the SNLG data is population-based and, therefore, likely to have fewer exclusions. An analysis of the British National Lymphoma Investigation Group (BNLI) found about 15% of all HL patients older than 65 years, but only 5% had been included in BNLI studies [18]. In addition, another recent study confirms the proportion of about 20% of older HL patients [10].

## 18.3 Histopathology

With regard to the different patterns of histology subtypes, the German Hodgkin Study Group (GHSG) has published a comprehensive retrospective review of elderly patients [5]. Mixed cellularity was more evident in elderly patients (35%) as compared with younger (19%) ($p < 0.001$). By contrast, nodular sclerosis was less frequent among elderly patients with 41 vs. 66% in younger patients ($p < 0.001$). However, this

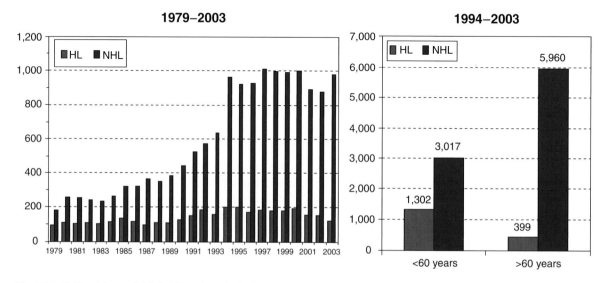

**Fig. 18.1** Epidemiology of elderly HL patients in the Scotland and Newcastle Lymphoma Group (SNLG)

subtype still remains the most common in both groups. The remaining rare subtypes, lymphocyte predominant/lymphocyte rich, and lymphocyte depleted, were represented with the same frequency in elderly and younger patients.

Comparable results have been obtained in some smaller studies. A higher frequency of the mixed cellularity subtype has also been reported by the Nebraska Study Group and the CALGB (The Cancer and Leukemia Group B) [6, 8, 17]. This difference in the incidence of mixed cellularity and nodular sclerotic subtypes, however, does not result in a different clinical outcome in these elderly patients [10, 21].

Jarrett et al. have drawn attention to the issue of Epstein–Barr virus (EBV) positivity in the Hodgkin and Reed–Sternberg (H-RS) cells at diagnosis [22]. EBV-associated disease was more often present in patients aged 50 years and older as compared to patients aged 15–34 years and 35–49 years. Importantly, EBV positivity was recognized as a poor prognostic factor for clinical outcome in patients over 50 years but not in the other groups [22]. The EBV-associated disease was also recognized as a negative prognostic factor by Stark et al. [10]. The EBV-positive status was also associated with advanced stage disease. It is speculated that such patients have failure of immune response to EBV and present with an enhanced state of immunodeficiency and hence more advanced stage disease [12]. The situation is reflected by the revised WHO (World Health Organization) classification of lymphomas that included a new entity for age-related Epstein–Barr virus–associated B-cell lymphoproliferative disorders (aEBVLPD). This disease group is characterized by EBV associated large B-cell lymphoma in the elderly without predisposing immunodeficiency. In about one-third of cases, aEBVLPD occurs as a polymorphous subtype with reactive cell-rich components, bearing a morphologic similarity to classic Hodgkin lymphoma (cHL), but shows an even poorer clinical course than cHL [23].

## 18.4  Clinical Presentation

There are two registry-based publications on the clinical presentation of older HL patients, both of them with a rather limited number of patients [7, 8]. In a study of Erdkamp et al. there were significantly more patients in stage II among younger patients ($p < 0.001$) [8]. Enblad et al. reported in their study more patients with advanced stages among elderly patients ($p = 0.02$) [7]. However, Stark et al. describe more patients in early stages in patients aged >70 years as compared to those aged 60–69 years [10]. Taken together, these publications draw a very heterogeneous picture. However, the comprehensive analysis of elderly HL patients treated within clinical trials of the GHSG among 372 patients aged ≥60 years also found a significant difference in clinical stage with more pronounced incidence of the very early and very advanced stages in the elderly population [5]. This finding is accordance with the above cited studies.

With regard to the clinical symptoms, Erdkamp et al. report a trend for a higher number of patients over 50 years presenting with B-symptoms [8]. In accordance with this report, a trend toward more patients suffering from B-symptoms was also detected by Enblad [7]. The GHSG analysis showed statistically significant more female patients, and more patients presenting with B-symptoms, elevated erythrocyte sedimentation rate, and a higher ECOG. Furthermore, there were less patients with large mediastinal mass and bulky disease as compared with 3,879 patients aged <60 years. Additionally, the Nebraska Study Group described statistically significant more patients with poor performance status, with B-symptoms at diagnosis and less with bulky disease [6].

To summarize, compared to younger patients older patients with HL seem to present more often with B-symptoms, in a poorer performance status, but with less bulky disease. The stage distribution also is different with more patients in very early or advanced stage disease and less patients in intermediate clinical stages.

## 18.5  Age Issues Affecting Treatment and Outcome

### 18.5.1  Comorbidity

It remains highly unlikely that only biologic and disease-associated factors are responsible for the unsatisfactory outcome in older HL patients. Van Sprosen et al. analyzed 194 HL patients and 904 NHL patients registered between 1993 and 1996 with regard to their age-specific comorbidities and the potential impact on the outcome. The most frequent comorbidity in the HL patient cohort was cardiovascular disease (18%), followed by chronic obstructive lung disease (13%), diabetes mellitus (10%), and hypertension (3%). Taken together, 56% of HL patients aged over 60 years suffered from severe comorbidity. This finding was true for early and advanced stages. Accordingly, patients with severe comorbidity received less frequently systemic chemotherapy and had a poorer overall survival (OS) especially within the first 4 months after first diagnosis of the HL. This clearly indicates that the comorbidities do have an impact on the survival [24]. This analysis is in line with the report from Levis at al. who found comorbidities in 35% of 105 older HL patients treated with VEPEMB. A multivariate analysis of this cohort identified comorbidity as an independent prognostic factor for poorer survival [25]. Guinee et al. compared the outcome of patients aged 60–70 years and 40–59 years, respectively. They investigated the time period between 1977 and 1983. As compared to the younger patients, the older patients had a twofold increased risk of dying due to HL, but even a fourfold increased risk of dying due to other reasons. Surprisingly, the response rates (RR) were not different between the two cohorts with an overall RR of 84% for the older patients and 88% for the younger patients [21]. To summarize the available data, comorbidity obviously is a major prognostic factor for the outcome of older patients with HL.

There are existing objective tools to assess comorbidity, one of which is described by the National Institute of Ageing/National Cancer Institute, designated ACE-27 [26]. Such a system used by Janssen-Heijnen et al. in a population of NHL patients showed double the mortality rate with high comorbidity, a finding that was confirmed by another report [27, 28]. There are several validated comorbidity scores for older patients available as reviewed elsewhere [29, 30]. Nonetheless, only the CIRS (Cumulative Illness Rating Scale) is currently being used for decision making in a cooperative study group (the German CLL Study Group) and no data are available for HL patients. This clearly indicates the urgent need to incorporate the assessment of comorbidity into clinical trials and daily practice. So far, there is only one study, i.e., the SHIELD study, in which a modified ACE-27 comorbidity score is being utilized and excludes patients from aggressive chemotherapy (VEPEMB), if the patient fails the assessment [31]. Results from this study will be available during 2010.

### 18.5.2 Comprehensive Geriatric Assessments and Frailty Measures

There are now recommendations from the International Society of Geriatric Oncology on the use of comprehensive geriatric assessment (CGA) tools in oncology studies in the elderly [46]. Such tools include functional assessments: activities of daily living (ADL), instruments of daily living (IDL), medical comorbidity, nutritional status, cognitive function, social/psychological status, and medication requirement. Currently, a specific CGA tool is not available and validated for routine use [32]. A self-administered frailty assessment approach is undergoing evaluation by the Cancer and Leukaemia B Cooperative Group [13]. Certainly, the use of ECOG status and Karnofsky status are helpful in younger patients but less so in the elderly [33]. There is a clear need for the development of an age-specific prognostic tool in elderly HL, to incorporate comorbidity, frailty, and functional and biological parameters, which is a defined aim of the SHIELD study. However, this will require a substantial patient population with appropriate parameters for analysis [20].

### 18.5.3 Quality of Life

The importance in clinical research of determining the health status of patients both before medical treatment and their well-being at endpoints resulting from medical treatment is well documented [34]. Health-related quality of life (HRQOL) assessments in HL have historically been conducted on long-term survivors [35–39]. There have been few HRQOL assessment of HL patients at diagnosis, during treatment, and end of treatment phase, and none in the elderly [40]. In the case of elderly HL patients, therapeutic intervention may only have a small impact on clinical endpoints and any gains in survival must be weighed against negative impact on HRQOL. It is important to recognize that HRQOL in clinical medicine represents the functional effect of an illness and its consequent therapy upon a patient as perceived by the patient. The above-mentioned SHIELD study measures the patient's perceived HRQOL at pre-treatment, end of treatment, and years 2 and 5 for those patients undertaking the VEPEMB regimen.

### 18.5.4 Therapy-Associated Toxicity

It is also clear that therapy-associated toxicities have a major impact on the treatment of older HL patients. The reduced tolerability of conventional chemotherapy results in more severe toxicities including fatal outcomes, the inability to maintain the scheduled dose density, and a shorter survival for relapsing or progressing patients [6–8, 19, 41–43]. This was also shown in the GHSG analysis, in which the reduced dose density and the increased mortality during therapy were identified as the major determinants for an inferior outcome of older patients [5]. Unfortunately, dose-dense aggressive chemotherapy is the most important positive prognostic factor for advanced stage HL. But even in patients younger than 60 years, who are being treated with BEACOPP escalated, the incidence of fatal events show a steep increase with age, mostly due to neutropenic infections. Accordingly, the full administration of the planned therapy is very unlikely in the cohort of older patients, especially in patients with advanced stage disease. As in younger patients, the most prominent toxicities were leucopenia, infections, and cardiopulmonary events [5, 41, 44, 45]. The early termination of the scheduled therapy in older patients had a negative impact on the survival [5, 19]. The incidence of severe therapy-associated toxicities varies in the literature for commonly used polychemotherapy regimens between 8 and 20% [6–8, 21, 44, 45]. Using COPP/ABVD, 19% acute toxic deaths have been reported [46]. This high number was confirmed for MOPP/ABVD with 18%. Today, ABVD is regarded as standard of care for most HL patients including the older patients. Unfortunately, no prospectively randomized studies have been published in older patients using this schedule and a reliable statement on its toxicity in these patients cannot be given. There is only one study currently ongoing using ABVD as the standard arm and comparing it with VEPEMB (vinblastine, cyclophosphamide, procarbazine, prednisolone, etoposide, mitoxantrone, and bleomycin). The most recent interim analysis did not show any therapy-associated deaths, but the final analysis must be awaited [47]. Additionally in the SHIELD program, ABVD is the curative therapy most commonly used in patients less than 70 years who are not in the VEPEMB study; it is anticipated that more information on ABVD tolerability and efficacy will emerge.

Other new regimens, specifically designed for older HL patients, had a low toxicity, but also a low efficacy [46, 48, 49]. To overcome the most apparent problem, i.e., neutropenic infections, the use of granulocyte colony-stimulating factors (G-CSF) was thought to be beneficial [41, 50, 51]. However, in randomized studies in older NHL patients, no impact on the incidence of severe infections and mortality could be documented [52]. This result is strongly supported by a recent meta-analysis of Cochrane Hematological Malignancies Group (CHMG) [53]. Thus, the role of G-CSF for the prevention of severe infections in older HL patients still has to be assessed. There seems to be a general problem with the use of dose-dense aggressive conventional polychemotherapy in older HL patients indicating that a substantial improvement of their outcome might only be reachable by using different therapeutic modalities. Among them are immunomodulatory drugs (e.g., lenalidomide), histone deacetylase inhibitors (e.g., panobinostat), or immunoconjugates (e.g., SGN-35), as reviewed in Chap. 20.

## 18.6 Therapy

### 18.6.1 Early Stages

Early stages comprise the early favorable and the early unfavorable stages. In young patients, standard of care is a combined modality treatment using two to six cycles of ABVD plus involved field radiotherapy. In older patients though, current data are not sufficient to discriminate the early stages, but one smaller study has shown the advantage of a combined modality treatment approach also for older patients. Kim et al. report on 52 early stage HL patients over 60 years, who have been treated between 1969 and 1995. Thirty-seven of them received radiotherapy only, nine received chemotherapy only, and six combined chemo-radiotherapy. Although these patient numbers are too small to reach statistical significance, the relapse rate was low for the combined modality approach (20%), higher for chemotherapy alone (33%), and highest for the radiotherapy alone group (46%) [42].

In the GHSG HD 8 trial, patients in early unfavorable stage were randomized to four courses of chemotherapy (COPP/ABVD – cyclophosphamide, vincristine, procarbazine, prednisone, doxorubicin, bleomycin, vinblastine, dacarbazine) and either involved field or extended field radiotherapy [54]. The recent analysis of the elderly patients in this study, compared with younger patients, demonstrated lower 5-year freedom from treatment failure (FFTF) and OS in elderly patients (FFTF 64 vs. 87%; $p<0.001$ and OS 70 vs. 94%; $p<0.001$). Importantly, elderly patients had a poorer outcome when treated with extended field radiation compared with involved field radiotherapy, 5-year FFTF (58 vs. 70%; $p=0.034$), and OS (59 vs. 81%; $p=0.008$). In addition, increased toxicity was also observed when receiving extended field radiotherapy. Thus, EF radiotherapy should be avoided in older patients.

In the study by Levis et al. utilizing the specifically designed VEPEMB schedule, 48 patients were in stages IA–IIA, thus matching the early favorable risk group [25]. The therapeutic approach was to administer three courses of VEPEMB chemotherapy plus involved field radiotherapy. The CR rate was 98% and 5-year failure-free survival (FFS) and OS were 79 and 94%, respectively. However, this FFS would be unacceptably low for early favorable stage HL in younger patients.

A recent small study by a Norwegian group has investigated the well-known CHOP-21 schedule (cyclophosphamide, vincristine, prednisone, and adriamycin) in elderly HL patients [55]. Among 29 patients, 11 patients were in stages I–IIA and 18 patients in stages IIB–IV. Patients in early stages received two or four cycles of CHOP-21 (depending on presence of risk factors) followed by involved field radiotherapy. The complete remission (CR) rate for early stages was 91%; 3-year OS and PFS were 91 and 82%, respectively. Obviously, the number of patients is again much too small to judge on this NHL regimen for the treatment of HL.

So far, outside clinical studies the GHSG recommends treatment of early favorable stage disease in analogy to younger patients with two cycles of ABVD followed by 20 Gy involved field radiotherapy. Accordingly, four cycles ABVD plus 30 Gy IF radiotherapy is recommended for early unfavorable stage HL. Outside clinical studies also the use of bleomycin in the ABVD regimen might be questioned. So far, only retrospective data are available, but these do not suggest a substantial impact of bleomycin [56]. Thus, in case of preexisting pulmonary comorbidity in an older patient, omitting bleomycin could be justified.

While there are no specific therapy guidelines that can be categorically stated it is clear that for favorable early stage disease two to three courses of chemotherapy (ABVD, VEPEMB) and involved field radiotherapy

can be recommended as a curative approach in the vast majority of patients [5, 10, 25]. Clearly the form of chemotherapy chosen will depend on the overall clinical status of the patient, but in the future studies on the use of routine FDG PET scanning postchemotherapy in early stage elderly patients is likely to dictate whether radiotherapy is necessary in all cases.

## 18.6.2 Advanced Stages

Six to eight cycles ABVD can be regarded as the gold standard for advanced stage HL, though a superior outcome of younger HL patients can be reached by intensification of chemotherapy, as it was shown by the GHSG [57, 58]. However, in elderly HL patients these aggressive schedules are often too toxic and cannot be recommended for patients over 60 years. Especially the use of anthracyclines can be complicated in older patients suffering from impaired cardiac function or cardiac arrhythmias. Therefore, some studies investigated the need of anthracyclines in older patients.

The Nebraska Group compared ChlVPP (chlorambucil, vinblastine, procarbazine, and prednisone) with the hybrid ChlVPP/ABV (added adriamycin, bleomycin, and vincristine) in a non-randomized study including 262 previously untreated patients with HL (see Table 18.1) [59]. Fifty-six patients were ≥60 years old and 205 younger than 60 years. Among the older patients, 31 patients were treated with ChlVPP and 25 patients with hybrid. This trial showed a very poor outcome for older patients with 31% 5-year event-free survival (EFS) and 39% (OS) at 5 years, compared with 75% (EFS) and 87% (OS) for younger patients. Importantly, older patients treated with ChlVPP had a poorer outcome as those treated with ChlVPP/ABV. The 5-year EFS was 24 vs. 52%, respectively ($p=0.011$), and 5-year OS 30 vs. 67%, respectively ($p=0.0086$). Though the numbers are again small, these differences were statistically significant favoring the use of anthracyclines.

The Swedish study by Landgren et al. assessed the impact of relative dose intensity (RDI) and type of chemotherapy comparing ABVD-like with MOPP-like (mechlorethamine, vincristine, procarbazine, and prednisone) regimens among 88 patients with advance HL [19]. The 5-year cause specific survival (CSS) and OS for entire population was 51 and 39%, respectively.

**Table 18.1** Selected studies for elderly HL patients in advanced stages

| Author, year | N | Therapy | Outcome | Therapy-associated death rate (%) |
|---|---|---|---|---|
| Levis, 1994 [41] | 26 | ABVD, MOPP/ABVD | CR rate=61%<br>8-year OS=48%<br>8-year RFS=75%<br>8-year EFS=36% | 23 |
| Levis, 1996 [46] | 25 | CVP/CEB | CR rate=73%<br>5-year OS=65%<br>5-year RFS=47% | 4 |
| Weeks, 2002 [6] | 31 | ChlVPP | 5-year OS=30%<br>5-year EFS=24% | 13 |
| | 25 | ChlVPP/ABV | 5-year OS=67%<br>5-year EFS=52% | 16 |
| Macpherson, 2002 [49] | 38 | ODBEP | 5-year OS=42%<br>5-year DFS=49% | 0 |
| Levis, 2004 [25] | 57 | VEPEMB | CR rate=58%<br>5-year OS=32%<br>5-year RFS=66% | 3 |
| Ballova, 2005 [44] | 26 | COPP/ABVD | CR rate=77%<br>5-year OS=50%<br>5-year HD-FFTF=55%<br>Relapse rate=23% | 8 |
| | 42 | BEACOPP basis | CR rate=76%<br>5-year OS=50%<br>5-year HD-FFTF=74%<br>Relapse rate=12% | 21 |
| Levis, 2007 [47] | 26 | ABVD | CR rate=86%<br>3-year OS=79%<br>3-year RFS=57% | 0 |
| | 28 | VEPEMB | CR rate=77%<br>3-year OS=60%<br>3-year RFS=50% | 0 |
| Kolstad, 2007[a] [55] | 18 | CHOP-21 | CR rate=72%<br>3-year OS=67%<br>3-year PFS=72% | 5, 6 |
| Mueller, 2008 [60] | 60 | BACOPP | CR rate=85%<br>2-year OS=76%<br>2-year PFS=71%<br>Relapse rate=13% | 12 |

[a]Results are reported for advanced stage HL; total number of therapy-associated deaths 7%

Patients with a RDI >65% had a significantly better CCS and OS than those with RDI ≤65% ($p$=0.024 and 0.029, respectively). Additionally, patients treated with anthracycline-based chemotherapy with RDI >65% had statistically significant better OS as compared with those with RDI ≤65% and those given MOPP-like regimen regardless of the RDI ($p$=0.001). Importantly, RDI was >65% in the majority (92%) of patients given ABVD-like chemotherapy and in 24% of patients given MOPP-like chemotherapy only. To summarize this study, anthracyclines and dose intensity seem to improve the outcome also in older patients.

However, the GHSG has extensively studied the intensification of ABVD also in older patients without meaningful benefit for these patients. The GHSG sub-trial HD9-elderly was designed for patients aged 66–75 years in stages IIB–IV who were randomized between eight cycles of COPP/ABVD (26 patients) and eight cycles of BEACOPP baseline (42 patients); 18 patients with bulky disease or with residual disease after che-motherapy received consolidating radiotherapy (see Table 18.1). The full-planned number of treatment cycles was given to 18 patients (69%) in COPP/ABVD group and to 23 patients (55%) in BEACOPP baseline

group only. The complete remissions (CR) rate was the same in both treatment arms (76%), and there was also no difference for patients with progressive disease (8% for COPP/ABVD and 7% for BEACOPP). The disease-specific FFTF at 5 years was better for the more aggressive BEACOPP regimen than for COPP/ABVD (74 vs. 55%, $p=0.13$), but this did not translate into a superior OS at 5 years (see Fig. 18.2a, b). This was due to more therapy-associated fatal events in the BEACOPP arm (21 vs. 8% for COPP/ABVD) [44].

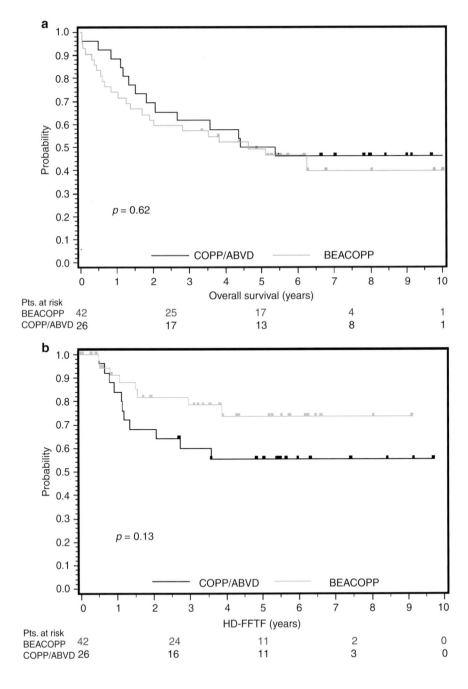

**Fig. 18.2** (**a**) Overall survival (OS) in the HD9-elderly study (modified from Ballova et al. [44]) (**b**) HL-specific FFTF in the HD9-elderly study. (Modified from [44])

Since etoposide was thought to contribute to the poor tolerability of BEACOPP in older patients, the GHSG then developed a new BEACOPP variant especially for this patient cohort (see Table 18.1). This was the BACOPP schedule, in which etoposide was omitted whereas the dose of adriamycin was increased (from 25 to 50 mg/m² [60]. Sixty patients (92%) were eligible for the final analysis. The majority of treatment courses (75%) were administered according to protocol. However, there was a tendency toward reduced dosing in cycles five to eight, especially for patients who had reached CR after four cycles of BACOPP. In total, 51 patients showed CR/CRu (85%), 2 PR (3%) and 4 progression of disease (7%). WHO grade III–IV toxicities were documented in 52 patients (87%). With a median observation time of 33 months, 18 deaths (30%) have been observed including seven therapy-associated fatal outcomes. Thus, with a therapy-associated death rate > 10%, this regimen also requires modification.

Another phase II study from the GHSG investigated the incorporation of gemcitabine into the first-line treatment of older patients. Bleomycin and dacarbazine in the ABVD schedule were replaced by gemcitabine and prednisone, resulting in the PVAG regimen. Fifty patients have been included and the final analysis is planned for 2010.

The Vancouver Group tried to intensify the treatment for older patients [49]. They used a 5-drug chemotherapy regimen called ODBEP (vincristine, doxorubicin, bleomycin, etoposide, and prednisone) from 1986 to 1995. This regimen tested the increase of dose intensity through delivery of treatment without delays, and increasing the number of non-cross-resistant chemotherapeutic drugs that were selected for minimal cumulative myelotoxicity (see Table 18.1). Comparison was made with a similar group of patients treated from 1981 to 1986 with MOPP/ABV-variant chemotherapy. Ninety-nine patients who were 65 years or older were diagnosed with HL from 1981 to 1995. Seventy-one patients had advanced disease and 55 of this group were treated with curative intent using multi-agent chemotherapy (ODBEP=38; MOPP/ABV-variant=17). The 5-year disease-free survival and OS were higher in patients treated with ODBEP as compared with patients treated with MOPP/ABV; however, the differences were not significant (DFS: 49 vs. 37% and OS: 42 vs. 32%, respectively). Both treatments were well tolerated but ODBEP was less myelotoxic.

The Italian group with Levis et al. has followed another strategy by developing less-intensive polychemotherapy regimens specifically for older patients (see Table 18.1). They started in the early 1990s with CVP/CEB regimen (chlorambucil, vinblastine, procarbazine, prednisone, cyclophosphamide, etoposide, bleomycin), and subsequently VEPEMB [46, 47]. CVP/CEB, a low-toxicity regimen, was administered to 25 patients and well tolerated. The CR rate at the end of treatment was 73%. However, the 5-year EFS and OS with 32 and 55%, respectively, was rather poor. This disappointing result was due to the high relapse rate in the CVP/CEB group.

The subsequent study investigated the VEPEMB regimen (see Table 18.1). Among 105 patients, 57 patients were in advanced stages of disease and were treated with six cycles of the regimen and with additional radiotherapy on bulky disease or residual mass. The regimen was well tolerated, could be administrated to most patients, and only one patient died during treatment. After the end of treatment, 58% of patients were in CR; the 5-year FFS was 34% and OS 32% [25]. In an interim analysis of a prospectively randomized phase III study comparing this regimen with ABVD, the final CR rate was slightly better in the ABVD than in the VEPEMB arm, even if this difference was not statistically significant with 86 vs. 77%. The 3-year relapse-free survival rates were 57 and 50% ($p$=ns) for the ABVD and VEPEMB arms, respectively. The 3-year OS and the EFS rates for ABVD and VEPEMB were 79 vs. 60% ($p$=ns) and 52 vs. 24% ($p$=0.08), respectively [47]. Though this is not the final analysis, the data obviously do not support the use of VEPEMB outside clinical studies, since superiority to ABVD cannot be seen so far and only a minority of patients with advanced stage disease might be cured using this schedule.

Another very well-tolerated regimen containing an anthracycline, an alkylating agent, and a vinca alkaloid is the well known CHOP schedule (cyclophosphamide, doxorubicin, vincristine, and prednisone). Compared to the ABVD regimen, the dose density of the anthracycline is somewhat higher, and myelotoxicity is no major problem in elderly NHL patients, at least. In a Norwegian study evaluating CHOP-21 in elderly patients with HL, among 29 patients 18 patients were in the advanced stage of disease and received six to eight cycles of CHOP-21 with subsequent radiotherapy to any residual mass (see Table 18.1) [55]. The CR rate at final staging was 72%, 3-year OS 67%, and 3-year PFS 72%. Twenty-seven (93%) patients completed the planned therapy, and there was only one therapy-associated fatal outcome. A larger study is warranted before any conclusion can be drawn to ensure results are robust, bearing in mind the more-intensive BEACOPP schedule cannot deliver such outcomes. However, the CHOP-21 regimen can be safely administered in a 14 days schedule using growth factor support in older patients [61]. This approach could even increase the dose density and might even improve the RR and outcome with acceptable toxicity.

In conclusion, the use of anthracycline-based chemotherapy for treatment of elderly patients with advanced HL is of great value. Though no randomized studies for this special cohort of elderly patients are available, six to eight cycles ABVD followed by radiotherapy to residual disease are regarded as standard of care [9, 11]. The data for the importance of bleomycin in the ABVD regimen with regard to efficacy are not convincing, thus bleomycin might be omitted in case of any preexisting pulmonary disease [56]. Dose intensification approaches including BEACOPP variants have not been successful, mainly due to an unacceptable increase in toxicity. The most important issue remains to find a balance between the intensity of chemotherapy and acceptable toxicities in older patients.

Future developments addressing this important issue might include an individual response-adapted treatment strategy. This approach is supported by the use of functional imaging. It is known for a long time already that response to chemotherapy has an impact on the final outcome [62, 63]. However, response as defined by the lymph node size and measured by computed tomography scan might occur with remarkable delay in advanced HL. This is likely due to the fibrotic tissue infiltrating the malignant lymph nodes, which often remains visible for several months after therapy especially in case of bulky disease at baseline. For example, in the GHSG HD15 trial, 311 out of 817 patients (38%) showed residual disease >2, 5 cm as determined by CT scan after the completion of chemotherapy [64]. However, 79% ($n = 245$) of these patients then had a negative FDG-PET scan. These patients did not receive any additional radiotherapy and, with a rather short median observation time of 18 months, their outcome was not inferior compared to patients reaching a complete remission after chemotherapy. These data indicate that the biologic response determined by FDG-PET is superior to the morphologic response in terms of its negative predictive value, at least. For more detailed information, please see Chap. 6. The work by Gallamini, Hutchings, and their coworkers should be mentioned in this context, though. They showed that the early PET response (after two cycles of ABVD) overshadows the prognostic value of the International Prognostic Score and thus is an important tool for planning a risk-adapted treatment in advanced HL [65, 66].

Taken together, this new response-adapted strategy might help to tailor the treatment according to the patients' need, thereby reducing the toxicity to a minimum amount. Data for older HL patients still have to be generated, though.

### 18.6.3  Relapsed Patients

In patients with refractory disease to first-line therapy, salvage is virtually impossible and usually palliative chemotherapy/radiotherapy is all that is available. In relapsing patients, following chemotherapy or relapsing after treatment of localized disease, alternative second-line treatments are possible, though again usually in a palliative intent. Of course, no studies specifically evaluating the treatment of relapsed elderly HL patients are available. Thus, any conclusions must be drawn either from few old studies, or in analogy to results from studies in younger HL patients or elderly NHL patients. Since treatment decisions in relapsed elderly patients are depending on several highly individual factors, no general recommendations can be given. Of course, the treatment goal has to be defined before starting any therapy. And, of course, whenever the relapse is diagnosed in a limited stage, the option of radiotherapy should be explored. For all remaining patients with the need for systemic therapy, treatment decisions can be guided by the duration of response to first-line therapy.

If there was a long-lasting remission after first-line therapy (i.e., >1 year) and the patient is in good general condition, a second-line therapy with a polychemotherapy regimen might be justified. Usually, anthracyclines cannot be given anymore due to their cumulative cardiotoxicity. Drugs with known single-agent activity in HL include alkylating agents (e.g., ifosfamide, trofosfamide, and procarbazine), gemcitabine, vinca alkaloids, and platinum derivates. Promising results in elderly NHL patients have been reported for the combination of gemcitabine and oxaliplatin (GemOx) [67]. This schedule has limited hematotoxicity and is safe in this elderly patient cohort. However, no reports on its use in HL patients have been published so far. There is another polychemotherapy regimen that has been developed many years ago and utilized by the SNLG as a palliative therapy over a prolonged period. This regimen is a very well-tolerated all oral schedule (prednisolone, etoposide, chlorambucil, and CCNU (PECC)) [68]. Recently, an update on the use of the schedule in relapsed HL from the SNLG database demonstrated that in 92 patients 12 were >60 years and PECC induced CR in 7/12 (58%) suggesting CCNU-containing combinations might have a useful role in this relapse situation [69].

If the duration of remission after first-line therapy was less than 1 year or the patient cannot tolerate polychemotherapy for any reasons, then single-agent chemotherapy should be considered as an option. After first promising reports in a palliative setting in young HL patients with refractory and progressive disease, gemcitabine has been used extensively in this situation [70]. Dose reductions may be necessary though especially in elderly patients due to thrombocytopenia that is the most prominent side effect. Also oral alkylating agents like trofosfamide can induce remissions in HL patients without causing relevant side effects [71, 72].

### 18.6.4 SHIELD Study

In order to resolve some of the most important questions in elderly patients with HL the SNLG is currently running the SHIELD study. SHIELD is a phase II, multi-center, international study, which has two elements: a VEPEMB treatment regimen and a registration arm where details of eligible patients (who do not receive the VEPEMB treatment) are recorded. Data collection utilizes an electronic Web-based Clinical Report Form (www.shieldstudy.co.uk). Recruitment to this study closed in September 2009 with 232 patients recruited including 57 registration patients on the GHSG BACOPP study and 175 from the UK (103 VEPEMB patients and 72 registration). The objectives of the study were to evaluate the efficacy and toxicity of VEPEMB therapy in older patients with HL, adapted to patients' performance. By collecting data on all patients with HL in this age group, regardless of treatment, the study will provide a clearer overall clinical picture of outcome in this patient cohort. The primary endpoints

of the study are (a) complete RR, (b) time to treatment failure, and (c) OS following the VEPEMB treatment schedule and the comparative treatment schedules undertaken by registration-only patients [73].

Sub-division by age (66–70, 71–75, and >75) predicted for outcome in the Levis study but it was apparent that there was a need for a methodology to assess fragility and toleration of aggressive treatments. A CGA is achieved in the SHIELD study by using a Co-morbidity Rating Scale, Activities of Daily Living Score, Instrumental Activities of Daily Living, and Quality of Life Assessment, which are recorded by the VEPEMB patients pre-treatment, post-treatment, and at years 2 and 5 [74]. Patients who are deemed "fragile" have been excluded from the phase II VEPEMB regimen but included as registration-only patients. It is hoped to identify alternative treatments for "frail" patients by assessing prospectively if it is possible to predict their inability to tolerate chemotherapy and for whom other treatment options would be more suitable [75].

### 18.7 Conclusions and Perspectives

Currently, it is not possible to provide evidence-based recommendations for the treatment of older HL patients due to a lack of definitive prospective randomized studies. Of course, HL should be potentially curable in all age groups; however, the results for the elderly remain disappointing, particularly in patients presenting with advanced stage disease. The poor clinical outcome has been related to the fact that there are more patients who present with advanced stages in this age group. In addition, most analyses indicate that delivery of appropriate drugs at optimal dose intensity is compromised in patients over 65 years and this has a major effect on their outcome. Additionally, there remains the possibility that additional chemoresistance mechanisms are operating in a proportion of HL cases in this age group.

From available existing data it seems clear that elderly patients with early stage HL (stages I and II) should be treated with short-course chemotherapy followed by involved field radiotherapy. Though ABVD has some toxicity in elderly patients and no prospective studies of ABVD in elderly patients are available, this regimen is considered standard of care also for older patients. Most recent results from the GHSG

HD10 trial support the administration of only two cycles ABVD followed by only 20 Gy involved field radiotherapy. It will be very interesting to compare these data with the results from the SHIELD study once those are available. In advanced stage disease, again six to eight cycles of ABVD are regarded as standard of care, though dose density is often under a critical limit of 65% in elderly patients and the outcome, therefore, is poor as compared to younger patients. Thus, the best approach would be to enter the patients on study protocols whenever possible so that clear treatment strategies can be developed and evaluated. Due to the obvious limitations of conventional chemotherapy in elderly HL patients, these new protocols should incorporate new therapeutic approaches. The GHSG has initiated a study in which bleomycin is replaced by lenalidomide, an immunomodulatory drug with single-agent activity in HL, in the ABVD regimen (AVD-Rev). But more alternative approaches are currently being investigated in HL (see Chap. 20) and hopefully will also be made available for elderly patients.

# References

1. Diehl V, Franklin J, Pfreundschuh M, et al. Standard and increased-dose BEACOPP chemotherapy compared with COPP-ABVD for advanced Hodgkin's disease. N Engl J Med. 2003;348:2386–95.
2. Horning SJ, Hoppe RT, Breslin S, Bartlett NL, Brown BW, Rosenberg SA. Stanford V and radiotherapy for locally extensive and advanced Hodgkin's disease: mature results of a prospective clinical trial. J Clin Oncol. 2002;20:630–7.
3. Radford JA, Rohatiner AZ, Ryder WD, et al. ChlVPP/EVA hybrid versus the weekly VAPEC-B regimen for previously untreated Hodgkin's disease. J Clin Oncol. 2002;20:2988–94.
4. Austin-Seymour MM, Hoppe RT, Cox RS, Rosenberg SA, Kaplan HS. Hodgkin's disease in patients over sixty years old. Ann Intern Med. 1984;100:13–8.
5. Engert A, Ballova V, Haverkamp H, et al. Hodgkin's lymphoma in elderly patients: a comprehensive retrospective analysis from the German Hodgkin's Study Group. J Clin Oncol. 2005;23:5052–60.
6. Weekes CD, Vose JM, Lynch JC, et al. Hodgkin's disease in the elderly: improved treatment outcome with a doxorubicin-containing regimen. J Clin Oncol. 2002;20:1087–93.
7. Enblad G, Glimelius B, Sundstrom C. Treatment outcome in Hodgkin's disease in patients above the age of 60: a population-based study. Ann Oncol. 1991;2:297–302.

8. Erdkamp FL, Breed WP, Bosch LJ, Wijnen JT, Blijham GB. Hodgkin disease in the elderly. A registry-based analysis. Cancer. 1992;70:830–4.
9. Evens AM, Sweetenham JW, Horning SJ. Hodgkin lymphoma in older patients: an uncommon disease in need of study. Oncology (Williston Park). 2008;22:1369–79.
10. Stark GL, Wood KM, Jack F, Angus B, Proctor SJ, Taylor PR. Hodgkin's disease in the elderly: a population-based study. Br J Haematol. 2002;119:432–40.
11. Proctor SJ, Rueffer JU, Angus B, et al. Hodgkin's disease in the elderly: current status and future directions. Ann Oncol. 2002;13 Suppl 1:133–7.
12. Hamlin PA. Treatment of aggressive non-hodgkin's and Hodgkin's lymphoma in older patients. American Society of Clinical Oncology: Educational Book. 2007;295–299.
13. Hurria A, Gupta S, Zauderer M, et al. Developing a cancer-specific geriatric assessment: a feasibility study. Cancer. 2005;104:1998–2005.
14. Parkin DM, Muir CS. Cancer Incidence in Five Continents. Comparability and quality of data. IARC Sci Publ. 1992; 45–173.
15. Taylor PR, Angus B, Owen JP, Proctor SJ. Hodgkin's disease: a population-adjusted clinical epidemiology study (PACE) of management at presentation. Northern Region Lymphoma Group. QJM. 1998;91:131–9.
16. Miller T, LeBlanc M, Braziel R, et al. Was the bimodal age incidence of Hodgkin's lymphoma a result of mistaken diagnosis of non-Hodgkin's lymphoma? Blood. 2002;100:771a. abstract 3048.
17. Mir R, Anderson J, Strauchen J, et al. Hodgkin disease in patients 60 years of age or older. Histologic and clinical features of advanced-stage disease. The Cancer and Leukemia Group B. Cancer. 1993;71:1857–66.
18. Roy P, Vaughan Hudson G, Vaughan Hudson B, Esteve J, Swerdlow AJ. Long-term survival in Hodgkin's disease patients. A comparison of relative survival in patients in trials and those recorded in population-based cancer registries. Eur J Cancer. 2000;36:384–9.
19. Landgren O, Algernon C, Axdorph U, et al. Hodgkin's lymphoma in the elderly with special reference to type and intensity of chemotherapy in relation to prognosis. Haematologica. 2003;88:438–44.
20. Proctor SJ, White J, Jones GL. An international approach to the treatment of Hodgkin's disease in the elderly: launch of the SHIELD study programme. Eur J Haematol Suppl. 2005;63–67.
21. Guinee VF, Giacco GG, Durand M, et al. The prognosis of Hodgkin's disease in older adults. J Clin Oncol. 1991;9:947–53.
22. Jarrett RF, Stark GL, White J, et al. Impact of tumor Epstein-Barr virus status on presenting features and outcome in age-defined subgroups of patients with classic Hodgkin lymphoma: a population-based study. Blood. 2005;106:2444–51.
23. Asano N, Yamamoto K, Tamaru J, et al. Age-related Epstein-Barr virus (EBV)-associated B-cell lymphoproliferative disorders: comparison with EBV-positive classic Hodgkin lymphoma in elderly patients. Blood. 2009;113:2629–36.
24. van Spronsen DJ, Janssen-Heijnen ML, Breed WP, Coebergh JW. Prevalence of co-morbidity and its relationship to treatment among unselected patients with Hodgkin's disease and non-Hodgkin's lymphoma, 1993–1996. Ann Hematol. 1999;78:315–9.

25. Levis A, Anselmo AP, Ambrosetti A, et al. VEPEMB in elderly Hodgkin's lymphoma patients. Results from an Intergruppo Italiano Linfomi (IIL) study. Ann Oncol. 2004; 15:123–8.

26. Yancik R, Wesley MN, Ries LA, et al. Comorbidity and age as predictors of risk for early mortality of male and female colon carcinoma patients: a population-based study. Cancer. 1998;82:2123–34.

27. Janssen-Heijnen ML, van Spronsen DJ, Lemmens VE, Houterman S, Verheij KD, Coebergh JW. A population-based study of severity of comorbidity among patients with non-Hodgkin's lymphoma: prognostic impact independent of International Prognostic Index. Br J Haematol. 2005; 129:597–606.

28. van Spronsen DJ, Janssen-Heijnen ML, Lemmens VE, Peters WG, Coebergh JW. Independent prognostic effect of co-morbidity in lymphoma patients: results of the population-based Eindhoven Cancer Registry. Eur J Cancer. 2005; 41:1051–7.

29. Balducci L, Beghe C. The application of the principles of geriatrics to the management of the older person with cancer. Crit Rev Oncol Hematol. 2000;35:147–54.

30. Extermann M. Measuring comorbidity in older cancer patients. Eur J Cancer. 2000;36:453–71.

31. Proctor SJ, Wilkinson J. A web-based study concept designed to progress clinical research for "orphan" disease areas in haematological oncology in the elderly: the SHIELD programme. Crit Rev Oncol Hematol. 2007;61:79–83.

32. Extermann M, Aapro M, Bernabei R, et al. Use of comprehensive geriatric assessment in older cancer patients: recommendations from the task force on CGA of the International Society of Geriatric Oncology (SIOG). Crit Rev Oncol Hematol. 2005;55:241–52.

33. Dittus K, Muss HB. Management of the frail elderly with breast cancer. Oncology (Williston Park). 2007;21:1727–34. discussion 1737, 1740.

34. Bergner M. Quality of life, health status, and clinical research. Med Care. 1989;27:S148–56.

35. Hjermstad MJ, Oldervoll L, Fossa SD, Holte H, Jacobsen AB, Loge JH. Quality of life in long-term Hodgkin's disease survivors with chronic fatigue. Eur J Cancer. 2006;42: 327–33.

36. Kawiecka-Dziembowska B, Borkowska A, Zurawski B, Palaszynska R, Makarewicz R. The assessment of temperament, quality of life and intensity of depressive symptoms in patients with Hodgkin's disease in different stages of the illness. Psychiatr Pol. 2005;39:679–90.

37. Mols F, Aaronson NK, Vingerhoets AJ, et al. Quality of life among long-term non-Hodgkin lymphoma survivors: a population-based study. Cancer. 2007;109:1659–67.

38. van Tulder MW, Aaronson NK, Bruning PF. The quality of life of long-term survivors of Hodgkin's disease. Ann Oncol. 1994;5:153–8.

39. Ruffer JU, Flechtner H, Tralls P, et al. Fatigue in long-term survivors of Hodgkin's lymphoma; a report from the German Hodgkin Lymphoma Study Group (GHSG). Eur J Cancer. 2003;39:2179–86.

40. Wettergren L, Bjorkholm M, Axdorph U, Langius-Eklof A. Determinants of health-related quality of life in long-term survivors of Hodgkin's lymphoma. Qual Life Res. 2004;13: 1369–79.

41. Levis A, Depaoli L, Urgesi A, et al. Probability of cure in elderly Hodgkin's disease patients. Haematologica. 1994;79: 46–54.

42. Kim HK, Silver B, Li S, Neuberg D, Mauch P. Hodgkin's disease in elderly patients (> or =60): clinical outcome and treatment strategies. Int J Radiat Oncol Biol Phys. 2003;56: 556–60.

43. Specht L, Nissen NI. Hodgkin's disease and age. Eur J Haematol. 1989;43:127–35.

44. Ballova V, Ruffer JU, Haverkamp H, et al. A prospectively randomized trial carried out by the German Hodgkin Study Group (GHSG) for elderly patients with advanced Hodgkin's disease comparing BEACOPP baseline and COPP-ABVD (study HD9elderly). Ann Oncol. 2005;16:124–31.

45. Enblad G, Gustavsson A, Sundstrom C, Glimelius B. Patients above sixty years of age with Hodgkin's lymphoma treated with a new strategy. Acta Oncol. 2002;41:659–67.

46. Levis A, Depaoli L, Bertini M, et al. Results of a low aggressivity chemotherapy regimen (CVP/CEB) in elderly Hodgkin's disease patients. Haematologica. 1996;81:450–6.

47. Levis A, Merli F, Tamiazzo S, et al. ABVD versus VEPEMB in elderly hodgkin's lymphoma patients. Blood. 2007;110. abstract 2322.

48. Zinzani PL, Magagnoli M, Bendandi M, et al. Efficacy of the VBM regimen in the treatment of elderly patients with Hodgkin's disease. Haematologica. 2000;85:729–32.

49. Macpherson N, Klasa RJ, Gascoyne R, O'Reilly SE, Voss N, Connors JM. Treatment of elderly Hodgkin's lymphoma patients with a novel 5-drug regimen (ODBEP): a phase II study. Leuk Lymphoma. 2002;43:1395–402.

50. Brusamolino E, Bacigalupo A, Barosi G, et al. Classical Hodgkin's lymphoma in adults: guidelines of the Italian Society of Hematology, the Italian Society of Experimental Hematology, and the Italian Group for Bone Marrow Transplantation on initial work-up, management, and follow-up. Haematologica. 2009;94:550–65.

51. Repetto L, Biganzoli L, Koehne CH, et al. EORTC Cancer in the Elderly Task Force guidelines for the use of colony-stimulating factors in elderly patients with cancer. Eur J Cancer. 2003;39:2264–72.

52. Doorduijn JK, van der Holt B, van Imhoff GW, et al. CHOP compared with CHOP plus granulocyte colony-stimulating factor in elderly patients with aggressive non-Hodgkin's lymphoma. J Clin Oncol. 2003;21:3041–50.

53. Bohlius J, Reiser M, Schwarzer G, Engert A. Impact of granulocyte colony-stimulating factor (CSF) and granulocyte-macrophage CSF in patients with malignant lymphoma: a systematic review. Br J Haematol. 2003;122:413–23.

54. Klimm B, Eich HT, Haverkamp H, et al. Poorer outcome of elderly patients treated with extended-field radiotherapy compared with involved-field radiotherapy after chemotherapy for Hodgkin's lymphoma: an analysis from the German Hodgkin Study Group. Ann Oncol. 2007;18:357–63.

55. Kolstad A, Nome O, Delabie J, Lauritzsen GF, Fossa A, Holte H. Standard CHOP-21 as first line therapy for elderly patients with Hodgkin's lymphoma. Leuk Lymphoma. 2007;48:570–6.

56. Canellos GP, Duggan D, Johnson J, Niedzwiecki D. How important is bleomycin in the adriamycin + bleomycin + vinblastine + dacarbazine regimen? J Clin Oncol. 2004;22: 1532–3.

57. Hagemeister FB. Hodgkin's lymphoma in younger patients: lessons learned on the road to success. Oncology (Williston Park). 2007;21:434–40. discussion 441-432, 445-436.

58. Engert A, Diehl V, Franklin J, et al. Escalated-dose BEACOPP in the treatment of patients with advanced-stage Hodgkin's lymphoma: 10 years of follow-up of the GHSG HD9 study. J Clin Oncol. 2009;27:4548–54.

59. Walker A, Schoenfeld ER, Lowman JT, Mettlin CJ, MacMillan J, Grufferman S. Survival of the older patient compared with the younger patient with Hodgkin's disease. Influence of histologic type, staging, and treatment. Cancer. 1990;65:1635–40.

60. Mueller H, Nogova L, Eichenauer DA, et al. The newly developed modified BEACOPP-regimen (BACOPP) is active and feasible in elderly patients with Hodgkin lymphoma: Results of a Phase II Study of the German Hodgkin Study Group (GHSG). Blood. 2008;112. abstract 2600.

61. Pfreundschuh M, Schubert J, Ziepert M, et al. Six versus eight cycles of bi-weekly CHOP-14 with or without rituximab in elderly patients with aggressive CD20+ B-cell lymphomas: a randomised controlled trial (RICOVER-60). Lancet Oncol. 2008;9:105–16.

62. Carde P, Koscielny S, Franklin J, et al. Early response to chemotherapy: a surrogate for final outcome of Hodgkin's disease patients that should influence initial treatment length and intensity? Ann Oncol. 2002;13 Suppl 1:86–91.

63. Colonna P, Jais JP, Desablens B, et al. Mediastinal tumor size and response to chemotherapy are the only prognostic factors in supradiaphragmatic Hodgkin's disease treated by ABVD plus radiotherapy: ten-year results of the Paris-Ouest-France 81/12 trial, including 262 patients. J Clin Oncol. 1996;14:1928–35.

64. Kobe C, Dietlein M, Franklin J, et al. Positron emission tomography has a high negative predictive value for progression or early relapse for patients with residual disease after first-line chemotherapy in advanced-stage Hodgkin lymphoma. Blood. 2008;112:3989–94.

65. Gallamini A, Hutchings M, Rigacci L, et al. Early interim 2-[18F]fluoro-2-deoxy-D-glucose positron emission tomography is prognostically superior to international prognostic score in advanced-stage Hodgkin's lymphoma: a report from a joint Italian-Danish study. J Clin Oncol. 2007;25:3746–52.

66. Hutchings M, Loft A, Hansen M, et al. FDG-PET after two cycles of chemotherapy predicts treatment failure and progression-free survival in Hodgkin lymphoma. Blood. 2006;107:52–9.

67. Lopez A, Gutierrez A, Palacios A, et al. GEMOX-R regimen is a highly effective salvage regimen in patients with refractory/relapsing diffuse large-cell lymphoma: a phase II study. Eur J Haematol. 2008;80:127–32.

68. Lennard AL, Carey PJ, Jackson GH, Proctor SJ. An effective oral combination in advanced relapsed Hodgkin's disease prednisolone, etoposide, chlorambucil and CCNU. Cancer Chemother Pharmacol. 1990;26:301–5.

69. Proctor SJ, Lennard AL, Jackson GH, et al. The role of an all-oral chemotherapy containing lomustine (CCNU) in advanced, fs progressive Hodgkin lymphoma: a patient-friendly palliative option which can result in long-term disease control. Ann Oncol. 2010;21:426–8.

70. Santoro A, Bredenfeld H, Devizzi L, et al. Gemcitabine in the treatment of refractory Hodgkin's disease: results of a multicenter phase II study. J Clin Oncol. 2000;18:2615–9.

71. Andersson PO, Braide I, Nilsson-Ehle H. Trofosfamide as salvage therapy for anaplastic large cell lymphoma relapsing after high-dose chemotherapy. Leuk Lymphoma. 2002;43:2351–3.

72. Latz D, Nassar N, Frank R. Trofosfamide in the palliative treatment of cancer: a review of the literature. Onkologie. 2004;27:572–6.

73. Lawton MP, Brody EM. Assessment of older people: self-maintaining and instrumental activities of daily living. Gerontologist. 1969;9:179–86.

74. Katz S, Akpom CA. A measure of primary sociobiological functions. Int J Health Serv. 1976;6:493–508.

75. Ferrucci L, Guralnik JM, Cavazzini C, et al. The frailty syndrome: a critical issue in geriatric oncology. Crit Rev Oncol Hematol. 2003;46:127–37.

## Contents

Hodgkin lymphoma (HL) is highly responsive to conventional chemotherapy (CT). Close to 90% of patients even with advanced disease are cured with modern CT sometimes followed by irradiation [1, 2]. Patients who prove refractory to or relapse after first-line therapy, do significantly worse. High-dose therapy (HDT) followed by autologous stem cell transplantation (ASCT) is the standard of care for medically fit patients with relapsed HL [3, 4]. The results of ASCT, however, vary significantly depending on a number of prognostic factors the most important of which are the time interval between first-line treatment and relapse, the clinical stage at relapse, and the sensitivity of the tumor to salvage chemotherapy [5–9]. For example, approximately 70% of patients with late first relapse can be salvaged by HDT/ASCT whereas not more than 40% of patients suffering from early first relapse are rescued by this modality [4]. Only 20–35% of patients with refractory HL may achieve long-term survival after ASCT [10–13]. In addition, a significant proportion of patients with HL still relapse after an ASCT. Therefore, although HDT/ASCT may cure a significant proportion of patients with relapsed or refractory HL, subsets of patients carry a high risk of failure and are candidates for more experimental procedures such as allo-SCT.

## 19.1 Myeloablative Allogeneic Stem Cell Transplantation in Hodgkin Lymphoma: A Historical Perspective

The first reports on allogeneic stem cell transplantation (allo-SCT) in patients with HL appeared in the mid-1980s [14, 15]. Patient numbers were low and a realistic evaluation of the therapeutic potential of allo-SCT

A. Sureda (✉)
Clinical Haematology Division, Hospital de la Santa Creu I Sant Pau, Antoni Maria I Claret, 167, Barcelona 08025, Spain
e-mail: asureda@santpau.cat

S. Mackinnon
Department of Haematology, Institute of Cancer Sciences, University College London, Pond Street, London NW3 2QG, UK

A. Engert and S.J. Horning (eds.), *Hodgkin Lymphoma*,
DOI: 10.1007/978-3-642-12780-9_19, © Springer-Verlag Berlin Heidelberg 2011

was not possible. Two larger registry-based studies published in 1996 gave disappointing results. Gajewski et al. analyzed 100 HL patients allografted from HLA-identical siblings and reported to the International Bone Marrow Transplant Registry (IBMTR) [16]. A significant proportion of these patients were not in remission before transplant, and had a poor performance status and active infections before transplantation. Almost 50% of the patients received total body irradiation (TBI) containing regimens. The 3-year-rates for overall survival (OS), disease-free survival (DFS), and the probability of relapse were 21, 15, and 65%, respectively. The major problems after transplantation were persistent or recurrent disease or respiratory complications, which accounted for 35–51% of deaths. Acute and/or chronic graft vs. host disease (GVHD) did not significantly reduce the risk of relapse. At the same time, a case-matched analysis including 45 allografts and 45 autografts reported to the European Group for Blood and Marrow Transplantation (EBMT) was performed by Milpied et al. [17]. The matching criteria were sex, age at time of transplantation, stage of disease at diagnosis, bone marrow involvement at diagnosis and at transplantation, year of transplantation, disease status at time of transplantation, time from diagnosis to transplantation, and conditioning regimen with or without total-body irradiation (TBI). The 4-year actuarial probabilities of survival, progression-free survival (PFS), relapse, and nonrelapse mortality (NRM) were 25, 15, 61, and 48%, and 37, 24, 61, and 27% after allo-SCT and ASCT, respectively. The toxic death rate at 4 years was significantly higher for allo-SCT patients ($p=0.04$). Even for patients with sensitive disease at the time of transplantation, the 4-year actuarial probability of survival was 30% after allo-SCT and 64% after ASCT ($p=0.007$). This difference was mainly due to a higher transplant-related mortality rate after allo-SCT (65 vs. 12%, $p=0.005$) that was basically associated with the development of acute GVHD after transplantation and/or concomitant infectious episodes. Although a GVHD $>$ or $=$ grade II was associated with a significantly lower risk of relapse, it was also associated with a lower OS rate.

A number of reports confirmed the registry data: allo-SCT resulted in lower relapse rates but significantly higher toxicity with no improvement over ASCT when PFS or OS were considered [18–20]. Although the poor results after myeloablative conditioning could at least partly be explained by the very poor-risk features of many individuals included in these early studies, the high procedure-related morbidity and mortality prevented the widespread use of allo-SCT.

## 19.2  Reduced Intensity Regimens

Given the high NRM seen in adults with HL following myeloablative allo-SCT, the use of reduced intensity or non-myeloablative conditioning regimens would appear to be a potentially attractive option. The goal of these therapies is to reduce regimen-related toxicity while still providing sufficient immunosuppression to facilitate donor engraftment and a subsequent graft vs. lymphoma (GVL) effect. There are many published regimens ranging from the truly non-myeloablative single-fraction 2 Gy TBI to moderately myelosuppressive chemotherapy-based regimens that often combine fludarabine with an alkylator agent such as melphalan or busulfan. The aim of all of these regimens is to shift the balance from the antilymphoma activity of the conditioning regimen to the immune cells transferred with the donor graft, which may mediate a GVL response. The marked reduction in upfront toxicity of these regimens has extended the applicability of allo-SCT to older patients, those with comorbidities, and to patients who had previously failed a prior ASCT.

The literature now contains several reports detailing the outcomes of reduced intensity transplants for patients with relapsed HL (Table 19.1). These results can be difficult to compare due to the differing patient populations and conditioning regimens; however, in general, the transplant related mortality has been impressively reduced when compared to myeloablative conditioning regimens. This reduction in transplant mortality was confirmed by the Lymphoma Working Party (LWP) of the EBMT that compared Hodgkin patients having standard myeloablative conditioning to those having reduced intensity regimens between 1997 and 2002 [21]. Transplant-related mortality was 48% at 3 years in the myeloablative group and 24% in the reduced intensity group ($p=0.003$; Fig. 19.1).

Although reduced intensity conditioning has allowed allo-SCT to be performed more safely, relapse is now the commonest cause of treatment failure. Conditioning intensity/antilymphoma activity may be an important factor in determining relapse rates [22].

**Table 19.1** Conditioning regimens

| Study and regimen | Reference | Patient number | Median age (years) | TRM (%) | Relapse (%) | OS (%) | PFS (years) |
|---|---|---|---|---|---|---|---|
| EBMT various | [21] | 89 | 30 | 24 | 57 | 27 | 18% at 5 |
| UK AMF | [27] | 49 | 32 | 16 | 45 | 56 | 39% at 4 |
| Spain MF ± ATG | [28] | 40 | 31 | 25 | 44 | 48 | 32% at 2 |
| Seattle F + TBI | [24] | 90 | 28–33 | 0–18 | 40–63 | 53–58 | 23–51% at 2 |
| Houston MF | [30] | 58 | 32 | 15 | 55 | 64 | 32% at 2 |
| GITMO CFT | [23] | 32 | – | 3 | 81 | 32 | 16% at 3 |

*TRM* transplant-related mortality; *OS* overall survival; *PFS* progression-free survival; *EBMT* European Group for Blood and Marrow Transplantation; *A* alemtuzumab; *M* melphalan; *F* fludarabine; *ATG* antithymocyte globulin; *TBI* total body irradiation; *GITMO* Gruppo Italiano Trapianto di Midollo Osseo; *C* cyclophosphamide; *T* thiotepa

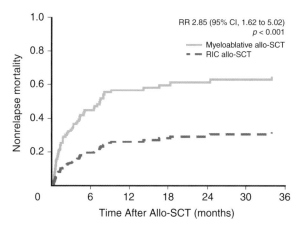

RR 2.85 (95% CI, 1.62 to 5.02)
$p < 0.001$

— Myeloablative allo-SCT
- - - RIC allo-SCT

**Fig. 19.1** Non-relapse mortality after allo-SCT for Hodgkin lymphoma, according to the type of conditioning regimen (Sureda et al. [21])

This may be secondary to a requirement for a lengthy period of clinical remission to allow the incoming donor immune system to eradicate residual disease. An early GVL response is often delayed by the use of immunosuppressive drugs to prevent GVHD following T cell replete transplantation or by the use of a T-cell-depleted graft, which often necessitates the use of post-transplant donor lymphocyte infusions (DLI). Some of the truly non-myeloablative regimens have been associated with particularly high relapse rates [23, 24]. This concept of regimen intensity being important is also supported by the EBMT analysis that showed a 32% relapse rate following myeloablative conditioning compared to 58% with reduced intensity regimens [21]. Furthermore, within the reduced intensity group, there was a higher relapse and lower OS rate in patients who were conditioned with low-dose TBI, which is one of the regimens with the least toxicity ($p < 0.04$). Other studies have also shown a better outcome using more intensive regimens like the combination of fludarabine and melphalan when compared to less intensive regimens [22] and the BEAM–alemtuzumab regimen has also been demonstrated to give good disease control in the medium term [25].

There is mounting evidence that successful allogeneic transplantation for HL needs a combination of effective salvage chemotherapy and a moderately intensive pre-transplant conditioning regimen to keep the disease under control for several months to allow the withdrawal of immunosuppression and/or the use of DLI sufficient time to mount an effective GVL response.

## 19.3 Prognostic Factors of Long-Term Outcome for Allogeneic SCT

The introduction of reduced intensity conditioning regimens in the allogeneic field has allowed a significant reduction in the NRM associated with the procedure in the population of HL patients [21]. The identification of independent prognostic factors may help to guide physicians in the choice of therapy for individual patients. However, the reported experience of RIC-Allo in HL is still limited in terms of number of patients included [22, 24, 26–28], making it difficult to identify independent predictors of outcome.

The LWP of the EBMT performed a retrospective analysis comprising a population of 285 patients with relapsed or refractory HL treated with a reduced intensity allo-SCT in order to try to identify prognostic factors for long-term outcome [29]. Sixty patients died of NRM at a median of 91 days (range 1 day to 20 months) following transplantation. The cumulative incidence estimate of NRM at 100 days, and 1 and 3 years post-transplant were 10.9, 19.5, and 21.1% respectively. In multivariate analysis, NRM was associated with poor performance status, chemorefractory disease at transplantation, age greater than 45, and transplantation before 2002. Identifying poor PS, chemorefractory disease, and older age as adverse risk factors for NRM, patients with no adverse risk factors had a 3-year NRM rate of 12.5% compared with 46.2% for those with two or three risk factors. Interestingly, the use of an unrelated donor and a single prior high-dose procedure had no impact on the NRM.

With a median follow-up of 26 months (range 3–94 months), 126 patients remained alive and 159 have died. The Kaplan–Meier estimates of OS and PFS at 1, 2, and 3 years were 67 and 52%, 43 and 39%, 29 and 25% respectively. In multivariate analysis, patients in complete remission (CR) or with chemosensitive disease, those with a good performance status, transplants other than sex mismatched male recipients, and CMV –/– transplants had a significantly better OS. For PFS good performance status, CR or chemosensitive disease at transplantation and transplants other than male recipients from female donors were associated with a significantly better PFS in the multivariate analysis. Considering chemorefractory disease and poor performance status as risk factors for a poor OS and PFS, patients with neither of these risk factors have a 3-year PFS and OS of 42 and 56% compared to 8 and 25% for patients with 1 or 2 of these risk factors. In an analysis restricted to patients who had relapsed after a prior ASCT, relapse within 6 months of the autograft was associated with a significantly worse disease progression rate (RR = 1.9 (1.2–3.1) $p$ = 0.01) and PFS (RR = 1.9 (1.2–2.9) $p$ = 0.003) following reduced intensity allo-SCT. Reduced intensity allo-SCT may be an effective salvage strategy for patients with good risk features who relapse after an ASCT (Fig. 19.2) and that outcomes are similar for both sibling and MUD transplants. Conversely for patients with chemorefractory disease or a poor performance status, the overall outcome is poor, and it is difficult to recommend reduced intensity conditioning allo-SCT for these patients.

These results are in agreement with what has already been published in smaller series of patients. The UK Cooperative Group reported that disease status before allo-SCT was the strongest prognostic factor for PFS and OS, the results being significantly better for those patients allografted in CR [27]. Disease status was also

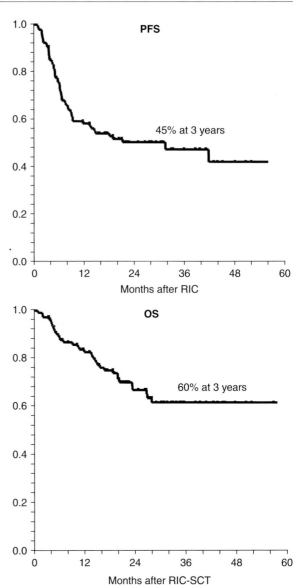

**Fig. 19.2** Progression-free survival (PFS) and overall survival (OS) in patients with HL treated with a reduced intensity conditioning regimen allogeneic transplantation and showing good prognostic factors at the time of allo-SCT. Patients with chemosensitive disease and good performance status at SCT treated with a RIC SCT in the period 2002–2005 ($n$ = 104) (Robinson 2009 [29] et al.)

the strongest factor predicting for survival in the Spanish series [28] as well as in the updated MDACC [30], although both studies include small number of patients that preclude more specific studies.

In summary, disease status seems to be the strongest prognostic factor for long-term outcome of these patients. In the vast majority of the patients included in these studies, disease status was evaluated using CT scans; no metabolic responses using positron emission tomography (PET) were evaluated. Future prospective trials should eventually include PET/CT before allo-SCT in order to define the role of metabolic techniques in the allogeneic setting.

## 19.4  Evidence for Graft vs. Hodgkin Lymphoma

Despite the theoretical reliance of reduced intensity transplantation on a GVL effect, there are relatively few studies that convincingly demonstrate this activity in HL. Many of the myeloablative transplants done in adults had such a high TRM that it would have been almost impossible to see a GVL effect if one had existed. In the context of reduced intensity transplantation, there is some evidence of a reduction in relapse in association with GVHD. Conversely, the apparent lack of impact of T cell depletion on relapse risk is unexpected. This finding might simply be a function of the relatively small numbers of patients reported or it is possible that the in vivo monoclonal antibody used to facilitate T cell depletion may have anti-HL activity.

The most convincing evidence of GVL activity in HL comes from the use of DLI to treat patients who relapse following allogeneic SCT (Table 19.2). Response rates to DLI have been reported to be between 15 and 54%, with complete responses seen in around 30% of patients. Many of these patients had received concurrent CT or radiotherapy but responses have been seen to DLI alone and some of these have been durable. There appears to be a higher response rate in the UK series, and it is not known whether the high incidence of mixed chimerism seen in patients who received alemtuzumab promotes GVL responses as it does in some animal models. The optimal T cell dose for GVL remains unclear, although many groups use an escalating dose schedule to try and

**Table 19.2**  Donor leukocyte infusions

| Study and regimen | Reference | Patient number | CR/PR | Response at last follow-up |
| --- | --- | --- | --- | --- |
| UK | [27] | 16 | 8/1 | 5 CR at 4+ years |
| Spain | [28] | 11 | 3/3 | None ongoing |
| Houston | [30] | 14 | 3/3 | 1 PR at 8+ months |
| Total | | 31 | 14/7 | 5/1 |

*CR* complete remission; *PR* partial remission

reduce the risk of severe GVHD. Unlike follicular lymphoma, there is preliminary evidence that in overt clinical relapse of HL, GVL responses are less common in the absence of GVHD. There are a number of factors that may increase the toxicity of DLI including increasing age of the patient, HLA mismatching, use of unrelated donors, and short time interval from transplant to DLI infusion. Although the DLI responses are impressive in some patients, the majority of patients will not achieve long-term benefit from DLI and further study is needed to optimize this potential effect.

## 19.5  Role of Allogeneic SCT in Autograft Failures

It has been demonstrated that HDT with autologous stem cell rescue can successfully salvage many of these relapsed/refractory patients, with two randomized studies demonstrating the superiority of such treatment over conventional dose salvage chemotherapy [3, 4].

In contrast, results with myeloablative allogeneic transplantation in adults with HL have been disappointing. No randomized studies comparing autologous transplantation and allogeneic transplantation exist, but a retrospective EBMT registry study reported improved outcome post-autograft, and this has become the consolidation of choice in relapsed or refractory disease [17]. Despite the success of autologous transplantation, there remains a cohort of patients whose disease progresses/relapses following transplant, and the outcome in this group is extremely poor, with a median survival post-relapse of less than 1 year [31, 32].

Although some patients achieve good outcomes following a second autologous transplant, these have generally represented a highly selected group who relapsed more than 3 years post first autologous transplant [33]. In addition to the small group of patients who may benefit from a second autograft, there are a number of patients who relapse following autologous transplantation who may not be suitable candidates for a reduced intensity allogeneic transplant. These might include patients with poorly controlled aggressive relapse and patients who have multiple comorbidities who have either a high relapse rate or treatment-related mortality with allogeneic transplantation.

With the advent of reduced intensity conditioning regimens, there has been renewed interest in allogeneic transplantation for patients who relapse following

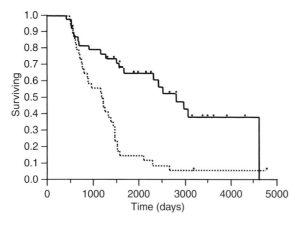

**Fig. 19.3** Overall survival from autograft for the allogeneic transplant group (n=38; solid line) and the control group (n=34; dotted line). Estimated OS for the allogeneic group at 5 years is 65% and the control group 15%, p=<0.0001 (Thomson et al. [35])

an autograft [22, 34]. This is because of the introduction of reduced intensity conditioning regimens that have dramatically reduced transplant-related mortality [27]. Although there are no randomized trials comparing the results of chemotherapy±radiotherapy in patients who relapse post-autograft, comparisons have been made with the outcomes of historical controls. The UK group identified a group of patients who had relapsed following a BEAM autograft who were chemosensitive at relapse and had survived at least 12 months from relapse and who would therefore have been eligible for a reduced intensity transplant [35]. This was a highly selected group representing 44% of all relapses who were predicted to have the best survival. These conventionally treated patients were compared to more recently treated patients who received a reduced intensity allograft. The groups did not differ significantly in age, number of lines of prior therapy, or in time from diagnosis to autograft but there was a small difference in time from relapse to autograft (13 months for the allograft group vs. 10 months in the chemotherapy ± radiotherapy group). Conversely, 34% of the allograft group were chemorefractory following salvage. Despite the selection of a control group with a relatively good prognosis, both OS from time of diagnosis and time of autograft were significantly improved following allogeneic transplant, when compared to the historical control group. The estimated current PFS for the allografted patients was 34% at 5 years and 42% if in chemosensitive relapse at the time of transplant, suggesting the early promising

results might translate into a favorable long-term outcome (Fig. 19.3). A recently published study had similar outcomes and showed an advantage for allogeneic transplant over chemotherapy alone in patients with poor risk HL [36].

## 19.6 Role of Allogeneic SCT in the Pediatric Population

Information regarding the role of allogeneic HSCT for HL in the pediatric population is very limited. Children undergoing allogeneic HSCT have been occasionally included in series of adult patients [18–21], whereas exclusively pediatric series were limited to fewer than ten patients [37].

The most extensive analysis of allo-SCT in the pediatric population comes from the LWP of the EBMT, and it comprises a group of 91 children and adolescents 18 years or younger treated with an allograft (myeloablative, n=40; reduced intensity, n=51) for relapsed or refractory HL [38]. Comparing patients who received MAC with RIC, the latter group had a longer time interval between diagnosis and allo-SCT, had failed more lines of therapy including HDT and ASCT, and was significantly older than patients who underwent transplantation after conventional conditioning. No significant differences existed in the percentages of patients grafted in CR, partial remission (PR), refractory disease, or untreated relapse and the performance status at the time of transplantation. In addition, the percentages of patients with HLA-identical sibling donors, other matched related or unrelated donors, as well as mismatched donors were not significantly different. Not surprisingly, patients with reduced intensity conditioning underwent transplantation more recently and preferentially received mobilized peripheral blood stem cells. NRM at 1 year was 21%, with comparable results after reduced intensity or myeloablative allo-SCT. Probabilities of relapse at 2 and 5 years were 36 and 44%, respectively. Reduced intensity conditioning allo-SCT was associated with an increased relapse risk compared with myeloablative transplantation, which was most apparent beginning 9 months after allo-SCT (p=0.01). PFS was 40 and 30%, and OS was 54 and 45% at 2 and 5 years, respectively. Beyond 9 months, PFS after reduced intensity allograft was lower compared with myeloablative protocols

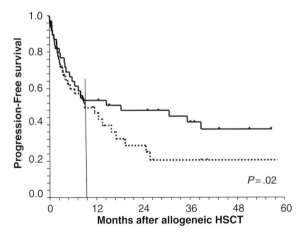

**Fig. 19.4** Outcome after allo-SCT for pediatric patients with HL according to conditioning regimen intensity (MAC vs. RIC). PFS is lower (*p*=0.02) from 9 months on after RIC (Claviez et al. [38])

(*p*=0.02) (Fig. 19.4). The development of GVHD did not have any impact on PFS after allo-SCT. Of note, the 26 patients with sensitive disease and good performance status who underwent transplantation between 2002 and 2005 showed a PFS of 60% (95% CI: 33–87%) and OS of 83% (95% CI: 67–98%), respectively, at 3 years. Fifteen of these patients (58% of the group) had previously failed ASCT. This retrospective analysis in a pediatric population of patients raises again the question of the exact dose intensity needed in HL patients. Because relapse now is the major problem after allogeneic transplantation for HL in pediatric as well as in adult patients, whereas NRM was no worse after myeloablative allo-SCT in these younger patients, it may be wise to use myeloablative or "intermediate" conditioning at least in those children and adolescents who arrive at the transplantation center in good performance status but with multiply relapsed or refractory disease. Alternatively, other attempts to debulk the tumor before SCT – using aggressive salvage therapy or HDT – should be considered.

## 19.7 Alternative Donor Transplants

In Europe and North America, only around a third of patients will have an HLA-matched sibling donor; therefore, the use of alternative donors is essential to expand the number of patients eligible for the procedure. The advent of molecular techniques has improved the accuracy of tissue typing reports but the associated increase in HLA polymorphism has made finding an exact molecularly matched donor more difficult. However, the continual increase in unrelated donor numbers, the availability of cord blood, and the use of T cell depletion has allowed a rise in the number of alternative donor transplants to be performed.

Although the number of published studies using unrelated donors remains limited at present, the transplant outcomes appear similar to those using sibling donors [21, 27, 29, 39]. Not surprisingly, rates of GVHD may be higher and many groups have used T cell depletion strategies with either alemtuzumab or ATG to reduce the incidence of this complication. Interestingly, unrelated donor transplants in patients with HL appear to have a similar OS and PFS to sibling donor transplants [21, 27]. Therefore, given the lack of effective therapeutic options for patients who relapse post-autologous transplantation, consideration of an unrelated allogeneic transplant may be an appropriate option for these patients.

The published experience with cord blood donors in HL is much more limited but may be feasible [40]. While cord blood may have a GVL effect on its own, the high relapse rate seen with reduced intensity regimens may restrict the use of this donor source where there is no opportunity to use DLI. A recently published Eurocord–Netcord study showed a 30% progression-free survival at 1 year in patients with relapsed HL [41]. Longer-term follow-up of these patients will obviously be necessary to determine whether the GVL activity of the cord blood obviates the need for post-transplant DLI. Finally, haploidentical donors have been used in a small series indicating that this may also be a useful donor source although follow-up is too short to determine the long-term impact of this approach [24].

## References

1. Horning SJ, Hoppe RT, Breslin S, Bartlett NL, Brown BW, Rosenberg SA. Stanford V and radiotherapy for locally extensive and advanced Hodgkin disease: mature results of a prospective clinical trial. J Clin Oncol. 2002;20:630–7.
2. Diehl V, Franklin J, Pfreundschuh M, et al. Standard and increased-dose BEACOPP chemotherapy compared with COPP-ABVD for advanced Hodgkin disease. N Engl J Med. 2003;348:2386–95.

3. Linch DC, Winfield D, Goldstone AH, et al. Dose intensification with autologous bone-marrow transplantation in relapsed and resistant Hodgkin disease: results of a BNLI randomised trial. Lancet. 1993;341:1050–4.

4. Schmitz N, Pfistner B, Sextro M, et al. Aggressive conventional chemotherapy compared with high dose chemotherapy with autologous haematopoietic stem cell transplantation for relapsed chemosensitive Hodgkin disease: a randomised trial. Lancet. 2002;359:2065–71.

5. Sureda A, Arranz R, Iriondo A, et al. Autologous stem cell transplantation for Hodgkin disease: results and prognostic factors in 494 patients from the Grupo Español de Linfomas/Transplante Autólogo de Médula Ósea Spanish Cooperative Group. J Clin Oncol. 2001;19:1395–404.

6. Lazarus HM, Loberiza FR, Zhang M-J, et al. Autotransplants for Hodgkin disease in first relapse or second remission: a report from the autologous blood and marrow transplant registry (ABMTR). Bone Marrow Transplant. 2001;27: 387–96.

7. Horning SJ, Chao NJ, Negrin RS, et al. High-dose therapy and autologous hematopoietic progenitor cell transplantation for recurrent or refractory Hodgkin disease: analysis of the Stanford University results and prognostic indices. Blood. 1997;89:801–13.

8. Brice P, Bouabdallah R, Moreau P, et al. Prognostic factors for survival after high-dose therapy and autologous stem cell transplantation for patients with relapsing Hodgkin disease: analysis of 280 patients from the French registry. Bone Marrow Transplant. 1997;20:21–6.

9. Sweetenham JW, Taghipour G, Milligan D, The Lymphoma Working Party of the European Group for Blood and Marrow Transplantation, et al. High-dose therapy and autologous stem cell rescue for patients with Hodgkin disease in first relapse after chemotherapy: results from the EBMT. Bone Marrow Transplant. 1997;20:745–52.

10. Josting A, Reiser M, Rueffer U, Salzberger B, Diehl V, Engert A. Treatment of primary progressive Hodgkin and aggressive non-Hodgkin lymphoma: is there a chance for cure? J Clin Oncol. 2000;18:332–9.

11. Sweetenham JW, Carella AM, Taghipour, et al. High-dose therapy and autologous stem-cell transplantation for adult patients with Hodgkin disease who do not enter remission after induction chemotherapy: results in 175 patients reported to the European Group for Blood and Marrow Transplantation. J Clin Oncol. 1999;17:3101–9.

12. Lazarus HM, Rowlings PhA, Zhang M-J, et al. Autotransplants for Hodgkin disease in patients never achieving remission: a report from the autologous blood and marrow transplant registry. J Clin Oncol. 1999;17:534–45.

13. Josting A, Rueffer U, Franklin J, Sieber M, Diehl V, Engert A. Prognostic factors and treatment outcome in primary progressive Hodgkin lymphoma: a report from the German Hodgkin Lymphoma Study Group. Blood. 2000;96: 1280–6.

14. Appelbaum FR, Sullivan KM, Thomas ED, et al. Allogeneic marrow transplantation in the treatment of MOPP-resistant Hodgkin disease. J Clin Oncol. 1985;3:1490–4.

15. Phillips GL, Reece DE, Barnett MJ, et al. Allogeneic marrow transplantation for refractory Hodgkin's disease. J Clin Oncol. 1989;7:1039–45.

16. Gajewski JL, Phillips GL, Sobocinski KA, et al. Bone marrow transplants from HLA-identical siblings in advanced Hodgkin disease. J Clin Oncol. 1996;14:572–8.

17. Milpied N, Fielding AK, Pearce RM, Ernst P, Goldstone AH. Allogeneic bone marrow transplant is not better than autologous transplant for patients with relapsed Hodgkin disease. J Clin Oncol. 1996;14:1291–6.

18. Anderson JE, Litzow MR, Appelbaum FR, et al. Allogeneic, syngeneic, and autologous marrow transplantation for Hodgkin disease: the 21-year Seattle experience. J Clin Oncol. 1993;11:2342–50.

19. Jones RJ, Ambinder RF, Piantadosi S, Santos GW. Evidence of a graft-versus-lymphoma effect associated with allogeneic bone marrow transplantation. Blood. 1991;77:649–53.

20. Akpek G, Ambinder RF, Piantadosi S, et al. Long-term results of blood and marrow transplantation for Hodgkin disease. J Clin Oncol. 2001;19:4314–21.

21. Sureda A, Robinson S, Canals C, et al. Reduced-intensity conditioning compared with conventional allogeneic stem-cell transplantation in relapsed or refractory Hodgkin lymphoma: an analysis from the Lymphoma Working Party of the European Group for Blood and Marrow Transplantation. J Clin Oncol. 2008;26:455–62.

22. Anderlini P, Saliba R, Acholonu S, et al. Reduced-intensity allogeneic stem cell transplantation in relapsed and refractory Hodgkin disease: low transplant-related mortality and impact of intensity of conditioning regimen. Bone Marrow Transplant. 2005;35:943–51.

23. Corradini P, Dodero A, Farina L, et al. Allogeneic stem cell transplantation following reduced-intensity conditioning can induce durable clinical and molecular remissions in relapsed lymphomas: pre-transplant disease status and histotype heavily influence outcome. Leukemia. 2007;21:2316–23.

24. Burroughs LM, O'Donnell PV, Sandmaier BM, et al. Comparison of outcomes of HLA-matched related, unrelated, or HLA-haploidentical related hematopoietic cell transplantation following nonmyeloablative conditioning for relapsed or refractory Hodgkin lymphoma. Biol Blood Marrow Transplant. 2008;14:1279–87.

25. Faulkner RD, Craddock C, Byrne JL, et al. BEAM-alemtuzumab reduced-intensity allogeneic stem cell transplantation for lymphoproliferative diseases: GVHD, toxicity, and survival in 65 patients. Blood. 2004;103:428–34.

26. Robinson SP, Goldstone AH, Mackinnon S, et al. Chemoresistant or aggressive lymphoma predicts for a poor outcome following reduced intensity allogeneic progenitor cell transplantation: an analysis from the Lymphoma Working Party of the European Group for Blood and Bone Marrow Transplantation. Blood. 2002;100:4310–6.

27. Peggs KS, Hunter A, Chopra R, et al. Clinical evidence of a graft-versus lymphoma effect after reduced intensity allogeneic transplantation. Lancet. 2005;365:1906–8.

28. Alvarez I, Sureda A, Caballero D, et al. Nonmyeloablative stem cell transplantation is an effective therapy for refractory or relapsed Hodgkin lymphoma: results of a Spanish Prospective Cooperative Protocol. Biol Blood Marrow Transplant. 2006;12:172–83.

29. Robinson SP, Sureda A, Canals C, et al. Reduced intensity conditioning allogeneic stem cell transplantation for Hodgkin lymphoma: identification of prognostic factors predicting outcome. Haematologica. 2009;94:230–8.

30. Anderlini P, Saliba R, Acholonu S, et al. Fludarabine-melphalan as a preparative regimen for reduced-intensity conditioning allogeneic stem cell transplantation in relapsed and refractory Hodgkin lymphoma: the updated M.D. Anderson Cancer Center experience. Haematologica. 2008;93:257–64.

31. Vose JM, Bierman PJ, Anderson JR, et al. Progressive disease after high-dose therapy and autologous transplantation for lymphoid malignancy: clinical course and patient follow-up. Blood. 1992;80:2142–8.

32. Varterasian M, Ratanatharathorn V, Uberti JP, et al. Clinical course and outcome of patients with Hodgkin disease who progress after autologous transplantation. Leuk Lymphoma. 1995;20:59–65.

33. Smith SM, van BK, Carreras J, et al. Second autologous stem cell transplantation for relapsed lymphoma after a prior autologous transplant. Biol Blood Marrow Transplant. 2008;14:904–12.

34. Carella AM, Beltrami G, Carella Jr M, et al. Immunosuppressive non-myeloablative allografting as salvage therapy in advanced Hodgkin disease. Haematologica. 2001;86:1121–3.

35. Thomson KJ, Peggs KS, Smith P, et al. Superiority of reduced-intensity allogeneic transplantation over conventional treatment for relapse of Hodgkin lymphoma following autologous stem cell transplantation. Bone Marrow Transplant. 2008; 41:765–70.

36. Castagna L, Sarina B, Todisco E, et al. Allogeneic stem cell transplantation compared with chemotherapy for poor-risk Hodgkin lymphoma. Biol Blood Marrow Transplant. 2009; 15:432–8.

37. Claviez A, Klingebiel T, Beyer J, et al. Allogeneic peripheral blood stem cell transplantation following fludarabine-based conditioning in six children with advanced Hodgkin disease. Ann Hematol. 2004;83:237–41.

38. Claviez A, Canals C, Dierickx D, et al. Allogeneic hematopoietic stem cell transplantation in children and adolescents with recurrent and refractory Hodgkin lymphoma: an analysis of the European Group for Blood and Marrow Transplantation. Blood. 2009;114:2060–7.

39. Devetten MP, Hari PN, Carreras J, et al. Unrelated donor reduced-intensity allogeneic hematopoietic stem cell transplantation for relapsed and refractory Hodgkin lymphoma. Biol Blood Marrow Transplant. 2009;15:109–17.

40. Majhail NS, Weisdorf DJ, Wagner JE, et al. Comparable results of umbilical cord blood and HLA-matched sibling donor hematopoietic stem cell transplantation after reduced-intensity preparative regimen for advanced Hodgkin lymphoma. Blood. 2006;107:3804–7.

41. Rodrigues CA, Sanz G, Brunstein CG, et al. Analysis of risk factors for outcomes after unrelated cord blood transplantation in adults with lymphoid malignancies: a study by the Eurocord-Netcord and lymphoma working party of the European group for blood and marrow transplantation. J Clin Oncol. 2009;27:256–63.

# New Agents for Patients with Hodgkin Lymphoma

# 20

Anas Younes and Andreas Engert

## Contents

## 20.1 Introduction

Hodgkin lymphoma (HL) is a rare human cancer with about 8,500 new cases in the United States [1]. It is estimated that 1,290 patients will die of this malignancy in 2009, making HL one of the best curable human cancers. Despite the success of initial therapy, the treatment of patients with relapsed and refractory disease, especially those who relapse after autologous stem cell transplantation, remains challenging with an estimated median survival of less than 3 years [2]. Furthermore, because the median age of the patients is in the mid-30s, the impact of early mortality on the number of years lost from productive life is remarkable. Drug development in this area will, therefore, address a significant unmet medical need [3]. Over the past decade, several potential therapeutic targets in HL have been identified, and are currently under preclinical and clinical investigation [3, 4]. This chapter will focus on promising new monoclonal antibodies and small molecules that are currently in clinical trials for the treatment of patients with relapsed HL.

## 20.2 Monoclonal Antibodies

### 20.2.1 CD30

CD30 is considered an ideal target for monoclonal antibody therapy because it is highly restricted to the malignant Hodgkin and Reed–Sternberg (HRS) cells and is rarely expressed by nonmalignant T-cells [7, 8]. CD30 is primarily expressed as a transmembrane protein, which can be shed in a soluble form [9–11]. Early, first-generation naked monoclonal antibodies

A. Younes (✉)
Department of Lymphoma and Myeloma, M.D. Anderson Cancer Center, 1515 Holcombe Boulevard, Houston, TX 77030, USA
e-mail: ayounes@mdanderson.org

A. Engert
Department of Hematology and Oncology, University Hospital of Cologne, Kerpener Straße 62, 50924 Köln, Germany

A. Engert and S.J. Horning (eds.), *Hodgkin Lymphoma*,
DOI: 10.1007/978-3-642-12780-9_20, © Springer-Verlag Berlin Heidelberg 2011

targeting CD30 were examined in phase I and II clinical trials in patients with relapsed HL, with disappointing results possibly due to their poor antigen-binding properties, ineffective activation of effector cells, and neutralization by soluble CD30 [12, 13]. A second-generation anti-CD30 antibody was recently developed that has an improved antigen binding and Fcγ receptor IIIA affinity and specificity by optimizing human string content [14, 15]. This second-generation anti-CD30 humanized antibody, XmAb2513, demonstrated approximately threefold higher preclinical efficacy than that of cAC10-IgG1 and tenfold higher than 5F11. A phase I study of Xmab2513 is currently enrolling patients in the United States, and preliminary results were recently reported [16]. To date, 17 patients received escalating doses ranging between 0.3 and 12 mg/kg, given every 2 weeks. The study is ongoing, and the maximum tolerated dose (MTD) has not yet been reached. One patient treated at the 9 mg/kg dose level achieved a partial remission, suggesting that this novel antibody may indeed be effective.

The anti-CD30 antibody cAC10 was recently conjugated to monomethylauristatin E (MMAE), a synthetic antimicrotubule agent, resulting in a novel antibody drug conjugate called SGN-35 (brentuximab vedotin) [17]. Two phase I clinical trials were recently conducted using SGN-35 every 3 weeks and weekly schedules. In the first study, 45 patients with relapsed HL ($n = 42$) and ALCL ($n = 3$) were treated with escalating doses of SGN-35 (0.1–3.6 mg/kg) by intravenous infusions every 3 weeks [18]. Dose-limiting toxicities were observed at doses higher than 1.8 mg/kg. SGN-35 demonstrated a significant single-agent activity, with 37% of patients achieving partial or complete remissions and 88% tumor reductions [18]. A second phase I study used SGN-35 on a weekly schedule for 3 weeks in 4-week cycles. Preliminary results demonstrated that doses up to 1.2 mg/kg could be administered safely. Of 17 evaluable patients, 7 achieved CR and 1 PR. A phase II study in patients with relapsed HL recently completed enrollment of 102 patients, and results will be used to seek FDA approval in patients with relapsed HL.

Other interesting and promising approaches that target CD30 are currently being explored, including radio-immunoconjugation and diabody drug-conjugates [19–21].

## 20.2.2 CD40

The CD40 receptor is physiologically expressed on hematopoietic (B- and T-cells, monocytes, dendritic cells), epithelial, and endothelial cells [7, 8]. CD40 is also expressed on malignant T-cells originating from CD40-expressing benign cell, including B-cell lymphoma, HRS cells of HL, and breast carcinoma [7, 22, 23]. Activation of the CD40 receptor in HRS cells induces NF-κB, cytokine and chemokine secretion, and possibly survival. Although HRS cells do not express CD40L (CD154), they receive CD40L signals from the surrounding reactive cells, including B-cells, T-cells, and eosinophils [24, 25]. Thus, CD40 is more widely expressed than CD30 or CD20. However, despite this, it remains interesting as a therapeutic target. To date, two anti-CD40 antibodies (SGN-40 and HCD122) are being evaluated in patients with CD40-expressing lymphoid malignancies, but only the HCD122 study is enrolling patients with HL [26–30].

## 20.2.3 TRAIL (Apo2L) and Its Receptors

Tumor necrosis factor apoptosis inducing ligand (TRAIL) is a death protein that is primarily expressed by activated T-cells and NK cells [8]. TRAIL has four exclusive receptors: TRAIL-R1 (DR4), TRAIL-R2 (DR5, KILLER, TRICK2), TRAIL-R3 (DcR1, TRID, LIT), and TRAIL-R4 (DcR2 (TRAIL-R4, TRUNDD) [31]. TRAIL-R1 and TRAIL-R2 are death receptors that primarily recruit the death domain-containing adaptor protein FADD (Fas-associated death domain), which then activates the apical caspases eight and ten to initiate apoptosis. TRAIL-R3 and TRAIL-R4 are decoy receptors [32]. TRAIL has a wide range of activity against primary and cultured tumor cells [33]. HL cell lines express TRAIL receptors R1, R2, and R4, but not R3 [6]. Both APO2L/TRAIL protein and agonistic anti-TRAIL-R1 and TRAIL-R2 antibodies can induce cell death in selected HL cell lines [6, 34]. Results from a phase II study using an agonistic anti-TRAIL-R1 monoclonal antibody in patients with relapsed NHL demonstrated excellent safety profile and a promising clinical activity, especially in patients with follicular lymphoma [35]. Although there is currently no single agent activity for TRAIL or agonistic antibodies to TRAIL-R1/R2 in patients with HL, an ongoing phase I clinical trial combining the agonistic anti-TRAIL-R2 (AMG655) with vorinostat or bortezomib is currently enrolling patients with both HL and NHL. The rationale for this combination is based on preclinical data demonstrating synergy between TRAIL receptor agonistic antibodies with histone deacetylase (HDAC) inhibitors and proteasome inhibitors.

### 20.2.4 IL-13 and IL-13 Receptor

The rationale for targeting IL-13/IL-13R pathway is based on data demonstrating that cultured and primary HRS cells express both IL-13 and IL-13Rα-1. Neutralizing antibodies to IL-13 inhibited the growth of HL cell lines in vitro [36, 37]. IL-13 and IL-13Rα-1 are expressed in more than 70% of classical HL lymph nodes, and approximately 10% of newly diagnosed patients with HL and 16% of patients with relapsed HL have detectable levels of IL-13 in their sera [38]. With this background, a phase I clinical trial using a fully human anti-IL13 monoclonal antibody (TNX-650) has recently completed enrollment in patients with relapsed HL, and the results should become available shortly.

### 20.2.5 CD25 (Daclizumab)

CD25 is the interleukin-2 receptor (IL-2R) alpha subunit that is expressed on only few normal cells, such as activated T-cells, activated B-cells, but also expressed in T-cell and B-cell malignancies such as adult T-cell leukemia, cutaneous T-cell lymphoma, anaplastic large cell lymphoma, hairy cell leukemia, and also on Reed–Sternberg and associated polyclonal T-cells in HL. Daclizumab is a humanized anti-CD25 monoclonal antibody that is approved by the FDA for prevention of renal allograft rejection. A phase I/II trial of daclizumab conjugated to the *Pseudomonas aeruginosa* toxin PE38 was recently conducted in 59 patients with leukemia and lymphoma expressing IL-2R alpha. Eight patients showed objective responses (one patient had relapsed HL). In a follow-up phase II trial (56), daclizumab conjugated with the radionuclide yttrium-90 ($^{90}$Y-daclizumab) was investigated in 30 relapsed/ refractory HL patients (57). Radioimmunotherapy with $^{90}$Y-daclizumab was given once every 6 weeks at doses of 15 mCi, for a maximum of seven cycles. Twelve patients achieved CR, seven had PR, and five stable disease (SD). The main side effects were hematologic with prolonged thrombopenia. Three patients developed a myelodysplastic syndrome following treatment.

## 20.3 Small Molecules

Another treatment strategy is to target intracellular survival pathways that are activated in HRS cells, such as NF-κB, Jak/STAT, Akt/mTOR, Notch-1, and ERK [5, 6, 41]. These pathways can be targeted with small molecules that selectively inhibit a specific signaling molecule (Jak2 inhibitors, mTOR inhibitors, Bcl2 family inhibitors), or may inhibit several molecules (HDAC inhibitors, proteasome inhibitors, heat shock protein (HSP)-90 inhibitors) (Fig. 20.1).

### 20.3.1 Histone Deacetylases (HDAC) Inhibitors

HDACs are a family of enzymes that have diverse biologic activities, including cell proliferation, survival, angiogenesis, and immunity [42–46]. To date, 18 HDACs have been identified in humans, and are grouped in two major categories: zinc-dependent HDACs and NAD-dependent HDACs [47, 48]. Furthermore, HDACs are classified into four major classes: Class I (HDAC 1, 2, 3, 8, and 11), class II (HDAC 4, 5, 6, 7, 9, and 10), class III (SIRT 1–7), and class IV (HDAC 11) (Fig. 20.2). Class III is NAD-dependent, whereas classes I, II, and IV are zinc-dependent. At the present time, clinical grade pharmacologic inhibitors of zinc-dependent HDACs are available for clinical trials. Two inhibitors (vorinostat and romidepsin) have already been approved by the FDA for the treatment of patients with relapsed cutaneous T-cell lymphoma. Vorinostat and panobinostat (LBH589) inhibit HDAC classes I and II, and, therefore, are referred to as pan-HDAC inhibitors. MGCD0103 and etinostat (SNDX-275, formerly MS-275) preferentially inhibit

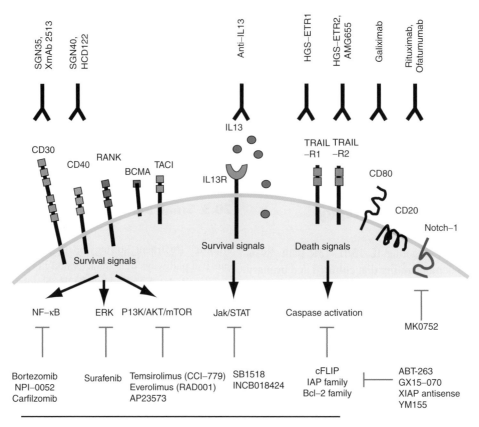

**Fig. 20.1** Targeted therapy of HRS cells. HRS cells express a variety of receptors and antigens that can be targeted by monoclonal antibodies. Many of these receptors trigger well-defined signaling pathways that promote HRS cell survival. These signaling pathways can be targeted by a variety of small molecules

HDAC class I, and frequently are referred to as isotype-selective HDACi (Fig. 20.2).

Interest in the potential use of epigenetic modulating therapy in HL is driven by the fact that although HRS cells are of B-cell origin, they infrequently express B-cell antigens [49]. This loss of B-cell phenotype has been reported as epigenetically regulated. Importantly, the expression of the B-cell silenced genes could be reinduced by the DNA hypomethylating agent 5-aza-deoxycytidine [50, 51]. Several HDACi have antiproliferative activity in HL-derived cell lines in vitro. In a recent study, vorinostat was shown to induce cell cycle arrest and apoptosis in HL cell lines and to synergize with chemotherapy [52]. Furthermore, vorinostat inhibited STAT6 phosphorylation and transcription in HL cell lines, an effect that was associated with a decrease in the expression and secretion of $T_h2$-type cytokines and chemokines, including thymus and activation-regulated chemokine (TARC/CCL17) and interleukin (IL)-5, and an increase in $T_h1$-type cytokines/chemokines, including a profound increase in IP-10 levels [52]. Finally, both HDAC inhibitors, alone or in combination with hypomethylating agents, have been shown to induce cancer testis antigen (CTA) expression, including MAGE, SSX, and NY-ESO-1 family members in a variety of tumors, and therefore may induce favorable antitumor immune response in vivo [53].

Several HDAC inhibitors are currently being evaluated for the treatment of HL. Clinical responses have been observed with MGCD0103, panobinostat, and vorinostat (Table 20.1). MGCD0103 is a novel nonhydroxymatebenzamide-based HDAC inhibitor that selectively inhibits HDAC 1 and 2 (and to a lesser extent, 3 and 11) isoforms [54]. It has a reported $IC_{50}$ inhibition of recombinant HDAC1 activity of 0.082 μM

**Fig. 20.2** Human zinc-dependent HDACs and their inhibitors

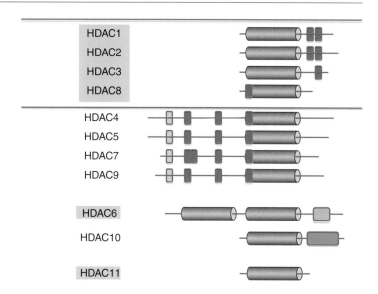

**Table 20.1** Summary results of novel agents for relapsed HL

| Agent | Target | Route | Phase | Number of evaluable patients | PR | CR | PR+CR | First author |
|-------|--------|-------|-------|------------------------------|----|----|-------|--------------|
| SGN35 [39] | CD30 | IV | I (q3 weeks) | 42 | 7 | 10 | 17 (40%) | Younes |
| SGN35 [40] | CD30 | IV | I (weekly) | 17 | 1 | 7 | 8 (47%) | Bartlett |
| Y-90 Daclizumab [47] | CD25 | IV | II | 30 | 7 | 12 | 19 (63%) | O'Mahony |
| MGCD0103 [66] | HDACs | Oral | II | 21 | 6 | 2 | 8 (38%) | Younes |
| ITF 2357 [72] | HDACs | Oral | II | 13 | 0 | 0 | 0 | Viviani |
| Panobinostat [68] | HDACs | Oral | I | 20 | 8 | 0 | 5 (40%) | DeAngelo |
| Panobinostat [69] | HDACs | Oral | II | 27 | 4 | 1 | 5 (18%) | Younes |
| Vorinostat [70] | HDACs | Oral | II | 25 | 1 | 0 | 1 (4%) | Kirschbaum |
| Lenalidomide [95] | Multiple | Oral | II | 12 | 3 | 1 | 4 (33%) | Fehniger |
| Lenalidomide [96] | Multiple | Oral | II | 12 | 6 | 0 | 6 (50%) | Böll |
| Lenalidomide [97] | Multiple | Oral | II | 15 | 2 | 0 | 2 (13%) | Kuruvilla |
| Everolimus [81] | mTOR | Oral | II | 17 | 8 | 1 | 9 (53%) | Witzig |

compared with $IC_{50} > 30$ μM for HDAC6 [55, 56]. It is orally available with a relatively long half-life of 9 h. The safety and efficacy of MGCD0103 was recently evaluated in a phase II study in patients with relapsed and refractory HL [57]. In the absence of disease progression or prohibitive toxicity, patients were allowed to continue therapy for a maximum of 12 months. Initially, 20 patients were treated with 110 mg orally given three times per week. Seven (35%) patients achieved partial and complete remissions. However, treatment was discontinued after a median of 4.5 months due to grade 3 or 4 toxicity. Subsequently, the study was revised to allow a lower starting dose of 85 mg at the same schedule. Three of the ten patients enrolled on the reduced dose achieved partial remissions. Furthermore, grade 3 and 4 toxicity was reduced to 20%. Overall, 80% of the 30 evaluable patients had some decrease in their tumor measurements. Although none of the patients developed significant EKG abnormalities, two patients developed pericardial effusions requiring discontinuation of therapy. In a second trial, panobinostat, a potent pan-DAC inhibitor, was recently evaluated in a phase I study in patients with hematologic malignancies that also included patients with HL [58]. Five of 13 (38%) patients achieved partial remissions. The most common side effects were fatigue, nausea, and diarrhea. Furthermore, 38% of patients developed grade 4 thrombopenia. However, no clinically significant cardiac toxicity was reported. Based on this promising clinical activity, a large international phase II study of panobinostat in relapsed HL is now enrolling patients to confirm these results. Finally, the Southwest Oncology Group (SWOG) conducted a phase II study of vorinostat in patients with relapsed HL [59]. Twenty-five patients were treated with 200 mg vorinostat given orally twice per day for 14 days every 21 day cycle. Unlike MGCD0103 and panobinostat, vorinostat produced modest clinical activity, as only one patient (4%) achieved a partial remission.

ITF 2357 is a pan-HDAC inhibitor that was recently evaluated in a phase II study in patients with relapsed HL. Fifteen patients were treated with daily doses of 100 mg, of whom 13 were evaluable for response. Seven patients (54%) had a stable disease, with a reduction in FDG-PET uptake in six patients (46%) lasting at least 3 months; six patients had disease progression. Interestingly, a correlation was found between a decrease in serum TARC levels and the response to treatment in this study [6]. In a follow-up study, ITF 2357 was combined with mechlorethamine. Preliminary data in 17 evaluable patients reported two CR (12%), three PR (18%), and five SD (29%). The main toxicity was hematologic, with seven patients experiencing grade III/IV neutropenia and eight thrombopenia; four patients had infections during treatment [73]. Taken together, these data suggest that ITF 2357 has a modest clinical activity in relapsed/refractory HL.

## 20.3.2 PI3K/Akt/mTOR

The phosphatidylinositol-3-kinase (PI3K)/Akt/mTOR signaling pathway is one of the most aberrantly activated survival pathway in cancer, making it an important target for drug development [60, 61]. This pathway is aberrantly activated in cultured and primary HRS cells by several mechanisms, including activation of CD30, CD40, and RANK receptors, presence of mutations in the p85α subunit of PI3K, and inactivation of PTEN function by phosphorylation [62–67]. Inhibition

of PI3K, Akt, or mTOR by various small molecules have reported to induce cell cycle arrest, autophagy, and apoptosis in HRS-derived cell lines in vitro [68–70]. To date, only the mTOR inhibitor everolimus has been evaluated in patients with relapsed HL. Johnston et al recently reported results from an ongoing phase II study using the oral mTOR inhibitor everolimus (RAD001) [71]. Fifteen evaluable patients with relapsed HL were treated with daily doses of 10 mg everolimus for up to 1 year. Seven patients (47%) achieved partial responses (Table 20.1). Grade 3 adverse events included thrombopenia and anemia. Despite the small number of patients treated on this ongoing study, this data generated excitement for the potential role of mTOR inhibitors, and potentially Akt and PI3K inhibitors for the treatment of HL. It is important to note that response to mTOR inhibitors might be augmented by modulating immune response and inhibiting angiogenesis. These mechanisms should be explored in future clinical trials [72, 73].

Because HRS cells frequently demonstrate aberrant and simultaneous activation of several survival pathways, including NF-κB, ERK, PI3K/Akt, rationally designed combination strategies will be required to improve response rates and to prolong response duration of mTOR inhibitors. In vitro experiments suggested that mTOR inhibitors synergize with chemotherapy, PI3K inhibitors, and HDAC inhibitors in a variety of tumor models, including HL [68, 74]. A phase I clinical trial combining the HDAC inhibitor panobinostat with the mTOR inhibitor everolimus is currently enrolling patients with NHL and HL.

## 20.3.3 NF-κB

NF-κB plays a central role in regulating the expression of various genes involved in cell survival, apoptosis, carcinogenesis, and inflammation, making it a potential therapeutic target [75]. The NF-κB family is composed of five proteins: NF-κB1 (p50/p105), NF-κB2 (p52/p100), RelA (p65), RelB, and c-Rel. These proteins are homodimers and heterodimers that are organized into two distinctive pathways: the classical (or canonical) and the alternative (noncanonical) pathways. At the center of the classical pathway is the p50/p65 heterodimer. In unstimulated cells, p50/p56 is present in the cytoplasm in an inactive form, bound to inhibitors of NF-κB (IκBα, IκBβ, and IκBε). Upon activation, IκB is rapidly phosphorylated, ubiquitinated and subsequently degraded by the proteasome. Consequently, the active p50/p65 heterodimer is translocated to the nucleus to induce transcription of target genes [76]. Activation of the alternative pathway results in the RelB/p52 and RelB/p50 dimers that also translocate to the nucleus and induce gene transcription. Both pathways have shown to be activated in primary and cultured HRS cells, and to be involved in promoting HRS cell survival [4, 5, 77–79]. In addition to autocrine and paracrine cytokine loops that can activate NF-κB in HRS cells, mutations in the I-κB and A20 genes were also reported to be involved in the aberrant activation of NF-κB in HRS cells [4, 80, 81]. The first attempt to therapeutically inhibit NF-κB activation in HL used the proteasome inhibitor bortezomib. By inhibiting the degradation of cytoplasmic IκBα, bortezomib inhibits the activation of NF-κB. Furthermore, bortezomib has been reported to alter the levels of p21, p27, Bcl-2, Bax, XIAP, survivin, and p53, leading to cell cycle arrest and apoptosis in several tumor types [82]. In preclinical studies, bortezomib inhibited HL cell line proliferation and induced cell apoptosis and cycle arrest at the $G_2/M$ phase and in a time- and dose-dependent manner. Bortezomib was effective even in HL cell lines that harbored mutations in the Iκ-Bα gene [83]. Furthermore, bortezomib enhanced the effects of gemcitabine, and potentiated treatment with anti-CD30 antibodies and TRAIL/APO2L [83, 84]. Despite these promising preclinical results, bortezomib demonstrated no significant clinical activity in patients with relapsed HL [85–87].

Based on preclinical experiments that demonstrated synergy between bortezomib and chemotherapy, a phase I study was recently conducted to evaluate the combination of bortezomib with ICE chemotherapy in patients with relapsed/refractory HL [88]. Bortezomib was given at doses 1, 1.3, or 1.5 mg/m² on day 1 and 4 of each ICE cycle. Twelve patients were enrolled, of whom six achieved PR and three achieved CR, for an overall response rate of 75%. Treatment was well tolerated and was associated with reversible grade 4 neutropenia and thrombopenia in 33 and 50% of patients, respectively. Based on these encouraging data, a randomized phase II study is planned and will open for patient enrollment soon. In a second study, bortezomib was combined with gemcitabine for the treatment of patients with relapsed HL [89]. Bortezomib 1 mg/m² was given on days 1, 4, 8, and 11, and gemcitabine 800 mg/m² was given on days 1 and 8. Treatment was repeated every 21 days. The overall response rate in 18 patients who were enrolled on study was 22%. Because of the relatively low response rate, coupled with treatment-related liver toxicity, the authors concluded that this regimen should not be further developed in HL.

### 20.3.4 Heat Shock Protein 90 (HSP90)

Heat shock proteins (HSPs) are cellular chaperone proteins that are required for essential housekeeping functions such as protein folding, assembly, and transportation across different T-cell compartments. HSPs also promote cell survival by maintaining the structural and functional integrity of several client proteins that regulate cell survival, proliferation, and apoptosis [90, 91]. Although HSPs are expressed in both normal and malignant T-cells, they are frequently overexpressed in cancer cells, raising the possibility that they play a role in maintaining malignant transformation. HSP90 is the most abundant proteins in eukaryotic cells, and it selectively interacts with and stabilizes several key signaling proteins, protein kinases, and oncogenic signal transduction proteins, making it an attractive target for cancer therapy.

Several new targets have recently been identified for potential treatment of HL, including ERK, Akt, and NF-κB, all of which are chaperoned by HSP90 [6, 83, 92]. Furthermore, HSP90 is overexpressed in primary and cultured HL cells [93, 94]. Preclinical experiments indicated potential therapeutic value for inhibition of HSP90 function by the small molecule 17-AAG in HL cell lines, as it downregulated several survival proteins and induced apoptosis in a dose- and time-dependent manner [93]. Furthermore, 17-AAG depleted cellular contents of Akt, reduced cFLIP levels, and synergized with doxorubicin and agonistic anti-TRAIL death receptor antibodies [94]. With this background, a phase II study to explore the potential clinical efficacy of 17-AAG in patients with relapsed HL was initiated, and the results are expected to be available in the near future.

### 20.3.5 Lenalidomide

Three independent groups recently evaluated the safety and efficacy of lenalidomide in patients with relapsed HL. Fehnigeret al reported their experience with 25 mg/day of lenalidomide on days 1–21 of a 28-day cycle [95]. Treatment continued until disease progression or unacceptable adverse events. Despite the liberal dose reductions that were allowed for hematologic and nonhematologic toxicity, four of 12 evaluable patients responded (1 CR and 3 PR). Most common adverse events (grade III/IV) included neutropenia (47%), leukopenia (33%), thrombopenia (27%), and anemia (20%). The same regimen was used by the GHSG in a named-patient-program [96]. Twelve patients with relapsed or refractory HL were included of whom ten had not responded to their last treatment. Lenalidomide was generally well tolerated. Six of the 12 patients achieved remission (1CR and 5 PR); six patients had stable disease. One patient continued treatment for more than 24 months in ongoing CR. In another study, Kuruvilla and colleagues treated 15 patients with relapsed HL using the same dose and schedule of lenalidomide as in the previous study [97]. Two patients achieved PR and seven achieved stable disease, with a median time to progression of 3.2 months. Six patients discontinued therapy due to disease progression and five due to toxicity. Four patients developed grade III/IV neutropenia and thrombopenia and five patients developed skin rash (grade 1–2).Taken together, these data suggest that lenalidomide has promising single-agent activity in relapsed HL.

## 20.4 Other Emerging Novel Therapies

### 20.4.1 Autologous LMP2-Specific Cytotoxic T Lymphocytes (CTL) for the Treatment of Relapsed EBV-Positive HL

HRS cells that are infected with EBV virus express several viral antigens that may serve as targets for T-cell therapy [98]. Initial clinical studies using polyclonal EBV-specific CTLs had clinical remissions in patients with relapsed EBV+ HL [99]. Analyses of EBV-CTL lines also indicated that small populations of T-cells reactive against the tumor-associated antigen LMP2 were present in the majority of the infused lines. There was some expansion in the peripheral blood following infusion, suggesting that CTLs specifically targeting LMP2 might have greater efficacy in these patients. In a recent study, LMP2-CTLs were generated from 14 patients with EBV+ lymphomas (HL and NHL) [100]. Polyclonal LMP2-CTL lines recognized 1–7 LMP2 epitopes. Using this approach, five out of six patients who received LMP2-CTL as adjuvant therapy post-stem-cell transplant or chemotherapy remained in remission up to 22 months post-LMP2-CTL infusion. To improve the efficacy of this approach, Bollard and colleagues used gene transfer into antigen-presenting cells (APCs) to augment the expression and immunogenicity of LMP2 [101]. These modified APCs increased the frequency of LMP2-specific CTLs by up to 100-fold compared with unmodified LCL-APCs. The LMP2-specific population expanded and persisted in vivo without adverse effects. Nine of ten patients treated in remission of high-risk disease remained in remission, and five of six patients with active relapsed disease had a tumor response, which was sustained for more than 9 months. In a different approach, Di Stasi and colleagues hypothesized that for the adoptive transfer of tumor-directed T-lymphocytes to be effective, a match between HRS-cell-produced chemokines and chemokine receptors expressed by effector T-cells will be needed. Taking advantage of the fact that HRS cells produce thymus- and activation-regulated chemokine/CC chemokine ligand 17 (TARC/CCL17) and macrophage-derived chemokine (MDC/CCL22), effector cells were transfected with the TARC receptor CCR4, which enhanced their migration to the HRS environment [102]. Furthermore, T-lymphocytes expressing both CCR4 and a chimeric antigen receptor directed to CD30 sustain their cytotoxic function and cytokine secretion in vitro, and produce enhanced tumor control when infused intravenously in mice engrafted with human HL. These proof-of-principle experiments provide very encouraging results for an improved efficacy of T-cell therapy in patients with HL, and will soon be examined in clinical trials in patients with relapsed HL.

## 20.4.2 Future Directions: New Targets, Combination Therapy, and Predictive Molecular Markers

Notch1, JAK/STAT, MAPK/ERK, cIAP2, and cFLIP activation or overexpression have all been shown to promote HRS cell survival and resistance to therapy. Inhibition of these pathways by small molecules or siRNA have been reported to induce cell death of HRS cells in vitro, and in some cases enhanced the efficacy of other treatment modalities. Clinical trials targeting these pathways are likely to be initiated in the near future. As more targets are being identified, it will be necessary to prioritize clinical trials with these novel agents, especially with the relatively small pool of patients eligible for these studies. Furthermore, as many of these agents are expected to produce low response rates, it will be important to perform correlative studies on patients' biospecimens to prospectively identify those who are likely to respond to therapy. Finally, it will be important to prioritize combination regimens to be evaluated in future randomized studies in order to improve long-term remission rates while reducing treatment-related toxicity.

## References

1. Jemal A, Center MM, Ward E, Thun MJ. Cancer occurrence. Methods Mol Biol. 2009;471:3–29.
2. Horning S, Fanale M, deVos S, et al. Defining a population of Hodgkin lymphoma patients for novel therapeutics: an international effort. Ann Oncol. 2008;20:Abstract 118.
3. Buglio D, Georgakis G, Younes A. Novel small-molecule therapy of Hodgkin lymphoma. Expert Rev Anticancer Ther. 2007;7:735–40.
4. Kuppers R. The biology of Hodgkin's lymphoma. Nat Rev Cancer. 2009;9:15–27.
5. Younes A, Garg A, Aggarwal BB. Nuclear transcription factor-kappa B in Hodgkin's disease. Leuk Lymphoma. 2003;44:929–35.
6. Zheng B, Fiumara P, Li YV, et al. MEK/ERK pathway is aberrantly active in Hodgkin disease: a signaling pathway shared by CD30, CD40, and RANK that regulates cell proliferation and survival. Blood. 2003;102:1019–27.
7. Younes A, Carbone A. CD30/CD30 ligand and CD40/CD40 ligand in malignant lymphoid disorders. Int J Biol Markers. 1999;14:135–43.
8. Younes A, Aggarwall BB. Clinical implications of the tumor necrosis factor family in benign and malignant hematologic disorders. Cancer. 2003;98:458–67.
9. Pizzolo G, Vinante F, Morosato L, et al. High serum level of the soluble form of CD30 molecule in the early phase of HIV-1 infection as an independent predictor of progression to AIDS. Aids. 1994;8:741–5.
10. Fattovich G, Vinante F, Giustina G, et al. Serum levels of soluble CD30 in chronic hepatitis B virus infection. Clin Exp Immunol. 1996;103:105–10.
11. Giacomelli R, Cipriani P, Lattanzio R, et al. Circulating levels of soluble CD30 are increased in patients with systemic sclerosis (SSc) and correlate with serological and clinical features of the disease. Clin Exp Immunol. 1997;108:42–6.
12. Bartlett NL, Younes A, Carabasi MH, et al. A phase 1 multi-dose study of SGN-30 immunotherapy in patients with refractory or recurrent CD30+ hematologic malignancies. Blood. 2008;111:1848–54.
13. Ansell SM, Horwitz SM, Engert A, et al. Phase I/II study of an anti-CD30 monoclonal antibody (MDX-060) in Hodgkin's lymphoma and anaplastic large-cell lymphoma. J Clin Oncol. 2007;25:2764–9.
14. Hammond PW, Vafa O, Jacinto J, et al. A humanized anti-CD30 monoclonal antibody, XmAbTM2513, with enhanced in vitro potency against CD30-positive lymphomas mediated by high affinity Fc-receptor binding. Blood (ASH Annual Meeting Abstracts). 2005;106:1470.
15. Lawrence CE, Hammond PW, Zalevsky J, et al. XmAbTM2513, an Fc engineered humanized anti-CD30 monoclonal antibody, has potent in vitro and in vivo activities, and has the potential for treating hematologic malignancies. Blood (ASH Annual Meeting Abstracts). 2007;110:2340.
16. Younes A, Zalevsky J, Blum KA, et al. Evaluation of the pharmacokinetics, immunogenicity, and safety of XmAb(R)2513 in the ongoing study XmAb2513-01: a phase 1 study of every other week XmAb2513 to evaluate the safety, tolerability, and pharmacokinetics in patients with hodgkin lymphoma or anaplastic large cell lymphoma. Blood (ASH Annual Meeting Abstracts). 2008;112:5012.
17. Oflazoglu E, Kissler KM, Sievers EL, Grewal IS, Gerber HP. Combination of the anti-CD30-auristatin-E antibody-drug conjugate (SGN-35) with chemotherapy improves antitumour activity in Hodgkin lymphoma. Br J Haematol. 2008;142:69–73.
18. Younes A, Forero-Torres A, Bartlett NL, et al. Multiple complete responses in a phase 1 dose-escalation study of the antibody-drug conjugate SGN-35 in patients with relapsed or refractory CD30-positive lymphomas. Blood (ASH Annual Meeting Abstracts). 2008;112:1006.
19. Schnell R, Dietlein M, Staak JO, et al. Treatment of refractory Hodgkin's lymphoma patients with an iodine-131-labeled murine anti-CD30 monoclonal antibody. J Clin Oncol. 2005;23:4669–78.
20. Zhang M, Yao Z, Patel H, et al. Effective therapy of murine models of human leukemia and lymphoma with radiolabeled anti-CD30 antibody, HeFi-1. Proc Natl Acad Sci U S A. 2007;104:8444–8.
21. Kim KM, McDonagh CF, Westendorf L, et al. Anti-CD30 diabody-drug conjugates with potent antitumor activity. Mol Cancer Ther. 2008;7:2486–97.

22. Carbone A, Gloghini A. Diagnostic significance of CD40, CD40L, and CD26 expression in Hodgkin's disease and other lymphomas. Am J Clin Pathol. 1996;105:522–3.

23. Carbone A, Gloghini A, Gruss HJ, Pinto A. CD40 antigen expression on Reed-Sternberg cells. A reliable diagnostic tool for Hodgkin's disease [letter; comment]. Am J Pathol. 1995;146:780–1.

24. Clodi K, Asgari Z, Younes M, et al. Expression of CD40 ligand (CD154) in B and T lymphocytes of Hodgkin disease: potential therapeutic significance. Cancer. 2002;94:1–5.

25. Carbone A, Gloghini A, Gruss HJ, Pinto A. CD40 ligand is constitutively expressed in a subset of T-cell lymphomas and on the microenvironmental reactive T-cells of follicular lymphomas and Hodgkin's disease. Am J Pathol. 1995; 147:912–22.

26. Advani R, Forero-Torres A, Furman RR, et al. SGN-40 (anti-huCD40 mAb) monotherapy induces durable objective responses in patients with relapsed aggressive non-Hodgkin's lymphoma: evidence of antitumor activity from a Phase I Study. ASH Annu Meet Abstr. 2006;108:695.

27. Luqman M, Klabunde S, Lin K, et al. The antileukemia activity of a human anti-CD40 antagonist antibody, HCD122, on human chronic lymphocytic leukemia cells. Blood. 2008;112:711–20.

28. Advani R, De Vos S, Ansell SM, et al. A phase 2 clinical trial of SGN-40 monotherapy in relapsed diffuse large B-cell lymphoma. Blood (ASH Annual Meeting Abstracts). 2008; 112:1000.

29. Advani RH, Furman RR, Rosenblatt JD, et al. A phase I study of humanized anti-CD40 immunotherapy with SGN-40 in non-Hodgkin's lymphoma. Blood (ASH Annual Meeting Abstracts). 2005;106:1504.

30. Law C-L, McEarchern JA, Cerveny CG, et al. The humanized anti-CD40 monoclonal antibody SGN-40 targets Hodgkin's disease cells through multiple mechanisms. Blood (ASH Annual Meeting Abstracts). 2005;106:1476.

31. Ashkenazi A. Targeting death and decoy receptors of the tumour-necrosis factor superfamily. Nat Rev Cancer. 2002; 2:420–30.

32. Wilson NS, Dixit V, Ashkenazi A. Death receptor signal transducers: nodes of coordination in immune signaling networks. Nat Immunol. 2009;10:348–55.

33. Fiumara P, Younes A. CD40 ligand (CD154) and tumour necrosis factor-related apoptosis inducing ligand (Apo-2L) in haematological malignancies. Br J Haematol. 2001;113: 265–74.

34. Georgakis GV, Li Y, Humphreys R, et al. Activity of selective fully human agonistic antibodies to the TRAIL death receptors TRAIL-R1 and TRAIL-R2 in primary and cultured lymphoma cells: induction of apoptosis and enhancement of doxorubicin- and bortezomib-induced cell death. Br J Haematol. 2005;130:501–10.

35. Younes A, Vose JM, Zelenetz AD, et al. Results of a phase 2 trial of HGS-ETR1 (agonistic human monoclonal antibody to TRAIL receptor 1) in subjects with relapsed/refractory non-Hodgkin's lymphoma (NHL). Blood (ASH Annual Meeting Abstracts). 2005;106:489.

36. Skinnider BF, Elia AJ, Gascoyne RD, et al. Interleukin 13 and interleukin 13 receptor are frequently expressed by Hodgkin and Reed-Sternberg cells of Hodgkin lymphoma. Blood. 2001;97:250–5.

37. Kapp U, Yeh WC, Patterson B, et al. Interleukin 13 is secreted by and stimulates the growth of Hodgkin and Reed-Sternberg cells. J Exp Med. 1999;189:1939–46.

38. Fiumara P, Cabanillas F, Younes A. Interleukin-13 levels in serum from patients with Hodgkin disease and healthy volunteers. Blood. 2001;98:2877–8.

39. June CH, Bluestone JA, Nadler LM, Thompson CB. The B7 and CD28 receptor families. Immunol Today. 1994;15: 321–31.

40. Vyth-Dreese FA, Dellemijn TA, Majoor D, de Jong D. Localization in situ of the co-stimulatory molecules B7.1, B7.2, CD40 and their ligands in normal human lymphoid tissue. Eur J Immunol. 1995;25:3023–9.

41. Skinnider BF, Elia AJ, Gascoyne RD, et al. Signal transducer and activator of transcription 6 is frequently activated in Hodgkin and Reed-Sternberg cells of Hodgkin lymphoma. Blood. 2002;99:618–26.

42. Glozak MA, Seto E. Histone deacetylases and cancer. Oncogene. 2007;26:5420–32.

43. Glozak MA, Sengupta N, Zhang X, Seto E. Acetylation and deacetylation of non-histone proteins. Gene. 2005;363:15–23.

44. Heider U, Kaiser M, Sterz J, et al. Histone deacetylase inhibitors reduce VEGF production and induce growth suppression and apoptosis in human mantle cell lymphoma. Eur J Haematol. 2006;76:42–50.

45. Wang S, Yan-Neale Y, Cai R, Alimov I, Cohen D. Activation of mitochondrial pathway is crucial for tumor selective induction of apoptosis by LAQ824. Cell Cycle. 2006;5: 1662–8.

46. Brogdon JL, Xu Y, Szabo SJ, et al. Histone deacetylase activities are required for innate immune cell control of Th1 but not Th2 effector cell function. Blood. 2007;109: 1123–30.

47. Bolden JE, Peart MJ, Johnstone RW. Anticancer activities of histone deacetylase inhibitors. Nat Rev Drug Discov. 2006;5:769–84.

48. Minucci S, Pelicci PG. Histone deacetylase inhibitors and the promise of epigenetic (and more) treatments for cancer. Nat Rev Cancer. 2006;6:38–51.

49. Schwering I, Brauninger A, Klein U, et al. Loss of the B-lineage-specific gene expression program in Hodgkin and Reed-Sternberg cells of Hodgkin lymphoma. Blood. 2003; 101:1505–12.

50. Ushmorov A, Ritz O, Hummel M, et al. Epigenetic silencing of the immunoglobulin heavy-chain gene in classical Hodgkin lymphoma-derived cell lines contributes to the loss of immunoglobulin expression. Blood. 2004;104:3326–34.

51. Ushmorov A, Leithauser F, Sakk O, et al. Epigenetic processes play a major role in B-cell-specific gene silencing in classical Hodgkin lymphoma. Blood. 2006;107: 2493–500.

52. Buglio D, Georgiakis GV, Hanabuchi S, et al. Vorinostat inhibits STAT6-mediated TH2 cytokine and TARC production and induces cell death in Hodgkin lymphoma cell lines. Blood. 2008;112(4):1424–33.

53. Shichijo S, Yamada A, Sagawa K, et al. Induction of MAGE genes in lymphoid cells by the demethylating agent 5-aza-2'-deoxycytidine. Jpn J Cancer Res. 1996;87:751–6.

54. Khan N, Jeffers M, Kumar S, et al. Determination of the class and isoform selectivity of small-molecule histone deacetylase inhibitors. Biochem J. 2008;409:581–9.

55. Beckers T, Burkhardt C, Wieland H, et al. Distinct pharmacological properties of second generation HDAC inhibitors with the benzamide or hydroxamate head group. Int J Cancer. 2007;121(5):1138–48.

56. Riester D, Hildmann C, Grunewald S, Beckers T, Schwienhorst A. Factors affecting the substrate specificity of histone deacetylases. Biochem Biophys Res Commun. 2007;357:439–45.

57. Younes A, Pro B, Fanale M, et al. Isotype-selective HDAC inhibitor MGCD0103 decreases serum TARC concentrations and produces clinical responses in heavily pretreated patients with relapsed classical Hodgkin lymphoma (HL). Blood (ASH Annual Meeting Abstracts). 2007;110:2566.

58. Prince HM, George D, Patnaik A, et al. Phase I study of oral LBH589, a novel deacetylase (DAC) inhibitor in advanced solid tumors and non-Hodgkin's lymphoma. J Clin Oncol (Meeting Abstracts). 2007;25:3500.

59. Kirschbaum MH, Goldman BH, Zain JM, et al. Vorinostat (suberoylanilide hydroxamic acid) in relapsed or refractory Hodgkin lymphoma: SWOG 0517. Blood (ASH Annual Meeting Abstracts). 2007;110:2574.

60. Ihle NT, Powis G. Take your PIK: phosphatidylinositol 3-kinase inhibitors race through the clinic and toward cancer therapy. Mol Cancer Ther. 2009;8:1–9.

61. Franke TF. PI3K/Akt: getting it right matters. Oncogene. 2008;27:6473–88.

62. Georgakis GV, Yazbeck VY, Li Y, Younes A. Preclinical rationale for therapeutic targeting of mTOR by CC-I779 and rapamycin in Hodgkin lymphoma. ASCO Meet Abstr. 2006;24:10070.

63. Jucker M, Sudel K, Horn S, et al. Expression of a mutated form of the p85alpha regulatory subunit of phosphatidylinositol 3-kinase in a Hodgkin's lymphoma-derived cell line (CO). Leukemia. 2002;16:894–901.

64. Morrison JA, Gulley ML, Pathmanathan R, Raab-Traub N. Differential signaling pathways are activated in the Epstein-Barr virus-associated malignancies nasopharyngeal carcinoma and Hodgkin lymphoma. Cancer Res. 2004;64: 5251–60.

65. Nagel S, Scherr M, Quentmeier H, et al. HLXB9 activates IL6 in Hodgkin lymphoma cell lines and is regulated by PI3K signalling involving E2F3. Leukemia. 2005;19:841–6.

66. Renne C, Willenbrock K, Martin-Subero JI, et al. High expression of several tyrosine kinases and activation of the PI3K/AKT pathway in mediastinal large B-cell lymphoma reveals further similarities to Hodgkin lymphoma. Leukemia. 2007;21:780–7.

67. Dutton A, Reynolds GM, Dawson CW, Young LS, Murray PG. Constitutive activation of phosphatidyl-inositide 3 kinase contributes to the survival of Hodgkin's lymphoma cells through a mechanism involving Akt kinase and mTOR. J Pathol. 2005;205:498–506.

68. Georgakis GV, Yazbeck VY, Li Y, Younes A. The mTOR inhibitor temsirolimus (CCI-779) induces cell cycle arrest and autophagy in Hodgkin lymphoma (HL) cell lines and enhances the effect of the PI3-kinase inhibitor LY294002. ASH Annu Meet Abstr. 2006;108:2259.

69. Georgakis GV, Li Y, Rassidakis GZ, Medeiros LJ, Mills GB, Younes A. Inhibition of the phosphatidylinositol-3 kinase/Akt promotes G1 cell cycle arrest and apoptosis in Hodgkin lymphoma. Br J Haematol. 2006;132:503–11.

70. Jundt F, Raetzel N, Muller C, et al. A rapamycin derivative (everolimus) controls proliferation through down-regulation of truncated CCAAT enhancer binding protein beta and NF-{kappa}B activity in Hodgkin and anaplastic large cell lymphomas. Blood. 2005;106:1801–7.

71. Johnston PB, Ansell SM, Colgan JP, et al. mTOR inhibition for relapsed or refractory Hodgkin lymphoma: promising single agent activity with everolimus (RAD001). Blood (ASH Annual Meeting Abstracts). 2007;110:2555.

72. Zheng Y, Collins SL, Lutz MA, et al. A role for mammalian target of rapamycin in regulating T-cell activation versus anergy. J Immunol. 2007;178:2163–70.

73. Del Bufalo D, Ciuffreda L, Trisciuoglio D, et al. Antiangiogenic potential of the Mammalian target of rapamycin inhibitor temsirolimus. Cancer Res. 2006;66:5549–54.

74. Yazbeck VY, Buglio D, Georgakis GV, et al. Temsirolimus downregulates p21 without altering cyclin D1 expression and induces autophagy and synergizes with vorinostat in mantle cell lymphoma. Exp Hematol. 2008;36:443–50.

75. Baud V, Karin M. Is NF-kappaB a good target for cancer therapy? Hopes and pitfalls. Nat Rev Drug Discov. 2009; 8:33–40.

76. Karin M, Lin A. NF-kappaB at the crossroads of life and death. Nat Immunol. 2002;3:221–7.

77. Staudt LM. The molecular and cellular origins of Hodgkin's disease. J Exp Med. 2000;191:207–12.

78. Bargou RC, Leng C, Krappmann D, et al. High-level nuclear NF-kappa B and Oct-2 is a common feature of cultured Hodgkin/Reed-Sternberg cells. Blood. 1996;87:4340–7.

79. Bargou RC, Emmerich F, Krappmann D, et al. Constitutive nuclear factor-kappaB-RelA activation is required for proliferation and survival of Hodgkin's disease tumor cells. J Clin Invest. 1997;100:2961–9.

80. Kato M, Sanada M, Kato I, et al. Frequent inactivation of A20 in B-cell lymphomas. Nature. 2009;459(7247):712–6.

81. Schmitz R, Hansmann ML, Bohle V, et al. TNFAIP3 (A20) is a tumor suppressor gene in Hodgkin lymphoma and primary mediastinal B-cell lymphoma. J Exp Med. 2009;206:981–9.

82. Adams J. Potential for proteasome inhibition in the treatment of cancer. Drug Discov Today. 2003;8:307–15.

83. Zheng B, Georgakis GV, Li Y, et al. Induction of cell cycle arrest and apoptosis by the proteasome inhibitor PS-341 in Hodgkin disease cell lines is independent of inhibitor of nuclear factor-kappaB mutations or activation of the CD30, CD40, and RANK receptors. Clin Cancer Res. 2004;10:3207–15.

84. Boll B, Hansen H, Heuck F, et al. The fully human anti-CD30 antibody 5F11 activates NF-{kappa}B and sensitizes lymphoma cells to bortezomib-induced apoptosis. Blood. 2005;106:1839–42.

85. Younes A, Pro B, Fayad L. Experience with bortezomib for the treatment of patients with relapsed classical Hodgkin lymphoma. Blood. 2006;107:1731–2.

86. Blum KA, Johnson JL, Niedzwiecki D, Canellos GP, Cheson BD, Bartlett NL. Single agent bortezomib in the treatment of relapsed and refractory Hodgkin lymphoma: cancer and leukemia Group B protocol 50206. Leuk Lymphoma. 2007; 48:1313–9.

87. Trelle S, Sezer O, Naumann R, et al. Bortezomib in combination with dexamethasone for patients with relapsed Hodgkin's lymphoma: results of a prematurely closed phase II study (NCT00148018). Haematologica. 2007;92:568–9.

# Quality of Life in Hodgkin Lymphoma

21

Hans-Henning Flechtner and Peter Borchmann

## Contents

H.-H. Flechtner
Department of Child and Adolescent Psychiatry,
Otto-von-Guericke-University, Magdeburg, Germany

P. Borchmann (✉)
Department of Internal Medicine I, University of Cologne,
Kerpener Strasse 64, 50924 Köln, Germany
e-mail: peter.borchmann@uni-koeln.de

## 21.1 Quality of Life in Hodgkin Lymphoma

The long-term cure rates for Hodgkin lymphoma (HL) patients are above 80% for all stages. Given this impressive long-term outcome for a patient population with a median age of about 30 years at diagnosis, the quality of survivorship has become more and more important. Organ dysfunctions including hypothyroidism, hypogonadism, cardiopulmonary complications, and secondary neoplasia as well as health-related quality of life (HRQoL) are major factors contributing to the patient´s general well-being.

Accordingly, we have experienced an increasing amount of research over the past 10–20 years focusing on HRQoL in HL survivors. Most HL-related HRQoL research has been limited by the use of cross-sectional approaches and small patient numbers, with inadequate patient and treatment history and variable follow-up. So far, only two prospectively planned HRQoL studies in HL are available: one from the SWOG (Southwest Oncology Group) and the other from the EORTC (European Organisation for Research and Treatment of Cancer) [1, 2]. Both studies included only early-stage disease patients, and only in the SWOG-study pretreatment baseline values were documented. Taken together, there is only very limited validated knowledge on HRQoL in HL patients.

Impaired HRQoL is a major problem for many HL survivors, often related to high levels of fatigue and persisting cognitive and gonadal dysfunction. Very little is known on factors contributing to this poor long-term outcome of the affected patients. Treatment-induced organic dysfunctions, like endocrine, immunological, and cardiopulmonary changes, have been discussed but were not confirmed in more recent

A. Engert and S.J. Horning (eds.), *Hodgkin Lymphoma*,
DOI: 10.1007/978-3-642-12780-9_21, © Springer-Verlag Berlin Heidelberg 2011

studies. Also, psychological consequences might play a role. These include emotional distress, especially depression and anxiety. In addition, social or role-functioning difficulties might influence HRQoL, including inability to return to work and adjustment to the workplace environment secondary to diminished capacity to complete work tasks. Finally, the long-term outcome in terms of HRQoL might only reflect patients' coping capacity facing the existential crisis of a malignant disease. Another factor is the patients' spirituality that might help to get back to "normal" life after the end of cancer treatment.

Thus, many very different factors contribute to the complexity of HRQoL. Most of them are difficult to measure and render research in this field challenging. Fortunately, there is increasing recognition that the survivorship experience among young adults needs to be better understood in order to develop intervention strategies. Currently, large study groups including EORTC and GHSG (German Hodgkin Study Group) have focused their research on HRQoL, and new perspectives are evolving. As a result from these studies, we will hopefully learn to better understand the patient and his or her well-being and not only to treat the lymphoma successfully. In this chapter, we describe the methods to determine HRQoL and then summarize the currently available results from cross-sectional and longitudinal studies in HL.

## 21.2  Health-Related Quality of Life Assessment

As indicated above, a major problem is to assess HRQoL due to its multiple dimensions. HRQoL includes many aspects of physical, psychological, and social functioning. It therefore mirrors the physical, psychological, and social health of patients after treatment for cancer. The determination of HRQoL relies on the patient-reported outcomes (PRO) – a term which is used for health-status measurement that comes directly from the patient. According to the FDA (US Food and Drug Administration), PRO measures include "such extremely complex concepts as HRQoL, which is widely understood to be a multidomain concept with physical, psychological, and social components" [3].

### 21.2.1  HRQoL Instruments

To obtain information from the patients' point of view, validated instruments are needed. Until recently, HRQoL assessment was predominantly conducted in palliative settings, and questionnaires such as the EORTC QLQ-C30 were developed for patient groups in palliative settings, more focusing on short-term effects of treatment and disease. Accepting this limitation, the most suitable cancer-specific core instruments for international assessment are EORTC QLQ-C30 and FACT that are both available in different languages, and are brief and economical to administer [4, 5]. One of the difficulties in designing HL-specific HRQoL modules is that, unlike other cancers, the particular problems are not easily identified. The general disadvantage of all available standard instruments is the lack of a HL-specific module. The wide range of key interval times (treatment period, follow-up, long-term surveillance) is not adequately reflected in available instruments. Most published trials in HL addressing late effects and HRQoL use different instruments (mainly questionnaires, but also mixed questionnaire-interview approaches) that focus on psychological outcome including mood, depression, psychosocial adaptation, and psychiatric symptoms. Besides this complex of psychological outcomes, the socioeconomic impact of the disease is also evaluated. This includes living circumstances, occupational situation, leisure activities, family life, drinking, and smoking habits. Infertility and sexual problems as a consequence of treatment have received particular attention. As outlined above, these instruments derived from the general assessment of late effects and came from a variety of research fields and illnesses. Only recently, explicit HRQoL instruments such as the EORTC QLQ-C30 have been included in cross-sectional studies. Few published reports addressed both late effects and longitudinal HRQoL assessment. Most newer instruments use patient self-reporting of the perceived HRQoL. Apart from the broader and general domains of HRQoL, there is agreement on the necessity of assessing specific disease- and treatment-related problems such as body image, sexuality, fatigue, spirituality, and gender issues, as well as issues pertaining to very old or very young patients. To accomplish this, a number of groups followed the modular approach in the development of questionnaires (FACT-G and the QLQ-C30 represent core instruments) and supplemented the core instrument with specific tumor- or treatment-related modules. A major challenge to prospective multicenter trials using longitudinal data on HRQoL is the completeness of data sets, as missing data limit the value of the results. A high standard of data collection is essential for a given trial to be successful, and HRQoL assessments have to be a mandatory component of the clinical trial design and part of the inclusion criteria.

### 21.2.2 HRQoL Assessment in European Cooperative Study Groups

Since no HL-specific modules for the assessment of HRQoL and fatigue were available, the EORTC Lymphoma Group (EORTC LG) together with the French Groupe D'Etude des Lymphomes de L'Adulte (GELA) and the GHSG, in close collaboration with the EORTC QL Group (EORTC QLG), devised an alternative way to measure HRQoL and fatigue in patients with HL [6]. The main elements of the EORTC QLQ C30 core instrument were supplemented by already-existing instruments or modules addressing particularly fatigue, sexuality, and fear of childlessness, and, as single questions, special side effects of chemotherapy and radiotherapy. The first use of this so-called EORTC H8-QL questionnaire, developed for repeated measurements and extensively tested within the trial groups, has yielded promising results on psychometrics, applicability, and appropriateness of content. The H8-QL questionnaire to date is available in ten European languages and is complemented by the Life Situation Questionnaire (LSQ), developed originally in Caen, France. The LSQ is currently available in French, German, and English and is being prepared for further international evaluation. It addresses the following areas: general living circumstances (e.g., housing), work history and current occupational status, marital status and family relationships, health records, family medical history, current health status, leisure activities, and economic and insurance problems related to HL.

### 21.2.3 HRQoL as Study Endpoint

HRQoL assessment in HL patients is not yet established as a standard procedure in clinical trials. It remains thus unclear whether HRQoL scales can detect clinically relevant differences between defined patient subgroups. Furthermore, the question of which score difference constitutes a clinically relevant difference for the patient has gained considerable attention [2, 7]. Data are available from a number of HRQoL studies that suggest that score differences of at least 8/100 but preferably above 15/100 would mean a clinically relevant change for a given patient. Considering that it is unknown how much time is required before long-term disadvantages in HRQoL become obvious, the length of time during which patients should be evaluated cannot be anticipated. The EORTC, GELA, and GHSG are including longitudinal HRQoL assessment in ongoing trials. Preliminary analyses suggest that 2–3 years after completion of therapy is a crucial time period and a possible turning point for either recovery or long-term limitations [2]. HRQoL assessment is usually regarded as a secondary outcome endpoint. Before it can be used as a primary endpoint, HRQoL assessment must fulfill various requirements, and the method of assessment must clearly be applicable in a multicenter setting. Since these instruments are available (e.g., QLQ-C30), assessment of HRQoL should be mandatory in any clinical trial in HL patients as the secondary endpoint. As long as no model of HRQoL impairment in HL has been established, no evidence-based intervention strategies can be developed and, therefore, HRQoL is not suited as a primary endpoint in randomized clinical trials.

### 21.2.4 Measuring Fatigue

A frequently reported problem in the aftermath of treatment for HL is fatigue. Although certainly not restricted to HL, fatigue seems to occur in a high proportion of patients successfully treated for HL. Over the last years, research activities on fatigue have established instruments that are now available to measure the different aspects of this symptom [8]. As with HRQoL in general, current opinion perceives fatigue as a combined construct with a number of dimensions. One dimension refers to physical and mental fatigue in accordance with what would be seen after intensive exercise or work. Other aspects include motivation, activity, and cognition, and the connection with mood states such as depression. Interestingly, available data suggest that a substantial proportion of fatigue reported by patients is not primarily due to their physical condition. Particularly in surviving patients after HL or breast cancer, high levels of fatigue occur with normal levels of physical functioning. An example of an instrument that assesses fatigue is the Multidimensional Fatigue Inventory (MFI-20), which uses 20 items on five subscales.

### 21.2.5 HRQoL in Special Patient Groups

Only recently there has been progress in the development of instruments to measure HRQoL and late effects in pediatric oncology [9]. HRQoL assessment in children must address normal developmental issues in areas such as peer relations, school, family, and play, which differ from the topics addressed in adult instruments. Questionnaires must also be suitably administered. In children under the age of 10 or 11, self-reporting is neither reliable nor feasible; proxy ratings by the parents or caregivers are necessary. A number of proxy and self-rating tools are already available from pediatric psychology and psychiatry but no established and tested instruments exist for HRQoL research in children and adolescents with HL.

As with the HRQoL assessment in pediatric oncology, only in the last few years the problems of elderly patients have been noticed. HRQoL assessment in elderly patients must address the aspects of daily living and the adjustment to physical and mental disabilities. Questionnaires must be suitably devised and administered and the patients may need assistance in filling out forms. For a subgroup of patients, self-reporting is no longer reliable or feasible; proxy ratings by caregivers are necessary. Some proxy and self-rating tools are meanwhile available from geriatrics but no validated instruments exist for HRQoL research in elderly HL patients.

## 21.3 HRQoL in Clinical Trials for Hodgkin Lymphoma

### 21.3.1 Lessons from Retrospective and Cross-Sectional Studies

More than 30 studies can be identified since 1986 dealing with HRQoL in HL as reviewed recently [10]. In brief, mainly cross-sectional studies in HL survivors have been performed over the last two decades including some retrospective studies. A variety of HRQoL instruments were employed in these studies and some trials used a matched control design or compared patient data with data from general population surveys. Follow-up periods ranged from 0 to 40 years after end of treatment. These analyses have shown that a substantial number of patients still carry a substantial burden even many years after the end of therapy. To illustrate these findings, the work by Fobair and colleagues is well suited [11]. They reported that ongoing fatigue was a major concern for 37% of 403 survivors. This was influenced by age, time after diagnosis, stage of disease, and type of treatment. Factors associated with better outcome were younger age, longer time since diagnosis, earlier stage, and radiation therapy without chemotherapy. Fatigued survivors also reported higher rates of depression. Other concerns identified were marital disruption, problems with infertility, and low sexual activity. In addition, 29% of patients in this sample was unemployed, with 18% currently looking for a job. It was also noted that HL survivors performed more poorly on measures of physical and psychosocial function when compared with either patients having acute leukemia, testicular cancer, or healthy population samples. These studies suggested a relationship between outcomes and the intensity of treatment; however, their retrospective and uncontrolled design limits the chance to determine causality.

Some relevant findings from case-control studies, which deliver somewhat better evidence, performed in HL survivors are listed in Table 21.1. All but one study involved healthy controls from regional population registries or from the general population. In summary, results of these studies are related to a variety of areas but consistently report on emotional strain and fatigue even years after the end of treatment. To summarize, these cross-sectional studies have shown persisting impaired HRQoL especially with regard to fatigue for a substantial number (up to 40%) of HL patients but besides age no risk factor was consistently reported. Although these studies used control groups, their design neither allows firm conclusions on the etiology of persisting impaired HRQoL nor to develop a model for a persisting defective HRQoL in HL.

### 21.3.2 Results from Prospective Trials

The first study reporting a longitudinal prospectively designed investigation on HRQoL in HL was conducted

**Table 21.1** Selected results from HRQoL studies in long-term survivors of HL

| Study | Cases (patients) | Controls | Main results |
|---|---|---|---|
| Joly et al. [12] | 93 patients issued from the regional cancer registry | 186 matched controls (age and sex) from the regional population registry | More physical, role, and cognitive impairments among cases<br>Major limitation in borrowing from banks remained the major problem in cases |
| Loge et al. [13] | 459 patients (1971–1991) treated at the Norwegian Radium Hospital | General Norwegian population | Higher levels and longer lasting of fatigue among cases<br>Disease stage predicted fatigue<br>No association with treatment characteristics |
| Wettergren et al. [14–16] | 121 patients treated in Stockholm County (1972–1991) | 236 matched controls (age and sex) from the regional population registry | Most important reported life areas were family, personal health, work, relations to other people<br>Lower physical health in patients |
| Rüffer et al. [17] | 836 patients from the GHSG trials HL1-6 (1981–1993) | 935 matched controls (age, sex, living area) from regional population registries | Higher levels of fatigue in cases<br>Fatigue associated with systemic symptoms, Karnofsky, occurrence of relapse<br>Time since end of treatment had no influence on the reported fatigue levels |
| Holzner et al. [18] | 126 patients treated at a single institution (1969–1994) | 926 controls from the general Austrian population | Higher functional, social well-being, and total scores in cases compared to controls |
| Hjermstad et al. [19] | 475 patients (1971–1997) treated at the Norwegian Radium Hospital | General Norwegian population | Higher levels of total fatigue (TF) in cases<br>Persisting chronic fatigue (CF) was associated with B-symptoms at diagnosis and treatment period<br>50% of patients reporting CF in 1994 did not report CF 8 years later<br>No correlation of fatigue levels with treatment variables (e.g., radiation fields) |

by the SWOG [1]. In the early 1990s, there was considerable debate about the necessity for staging laparotomy in early-stage HL (clinical stage IA and IIA), which was driven by the morbidity of the procedure. Thus, there was increasing interest in using short courses of chemotherapy with more limited radiotherapy to maximize cure and minimize toxicity. The SWOG designed a treatment protocol (SWOG 9133) to investigate alternative strategies for the management of early-stage HL, investigating subtotal lymphoid irradiation (STLI) vs. three cycles of doxorubicin and vinblastine followed by STLI (combined-modality therapy (CMT)) in early-stage HL patients. This study was accompanied by a prospective quality-of-life study termed SWOG 9208. The objectives of this study were to evaluate prospectively the health status and HRQoL of early-stage HL patients receiving either STLI or CMT, to describe the short-term effects of the treatments on

symptoms and QoL, and to evaluate the intermediate and long-term effects of the two treatments on HRQoL. Short-term and intermediate outcomes during the first 2 years after random assignment were reported. Both treatment groups experienced a short-term increase in symptoms, fatigue, and poorer QoL as a result of the treatment, which was more severe in the CMT group at 6 months after diagnosis due to more prolonged treatment. However, 1 year after random assignment, outcomes in the two treatment groups were indistinguishable. In this study, increased fatigue was identified in favorable HL patients before treatment that persisted after successful curative treatment. Importantly, fatigue levels for both study groups (CMT 45.9 and STLI 49.7) were increased at baseline. These scores were lower than scores for the general population. Before any treatment, these early-stage HL patients reported scores that were about a half SD below normal and were more consistent with scores from older patients with ischemic heart disease. While fatigue is a known symptom for HL, it was unexpectedly prominent in this patient cohort having a favorable prognosis and without B-symptoms. It was expected to improve subsequent to treatment and induction of remission. However, the fatigue level did not improve to normal values. The Vitality Scale scores at 1 and 2 years were slightly below the baseline score, and were substantially lower than comparative data from a breast cancer survivor sample after adjuvant treatment and radiotherapy. Though this is one of the most important studies on HRQoL in HL, no conclusions can be drawn with regard to tumor stage at baseline or aggressiveness of the chemotherapy being a risk factor for HRQoL impairment, since only early-stage low-risk patients were included.

The second study was recently published by Huette and colleagues [2]. They reported the results of their longitudinal HRQoL study examining short-term and long-term HRQoL among HL survivors from a large phase 3 trial (EORTC-H8). The study included early favorable HL patients and compared chemotherapy plus radiotherapy with radiotherapy alone; in patients with early unfavorable disease different chemotherapy–radiotherapy combinations were compared. Of 1,577 patients recruited to the trial throughout Europe, 2,666 assessments from 935 patients were available for the analysis with median follow-up of 92 months. Interestingly, therapeutic modality (radiotherapy vs. chemotherapy) did not have significant effects on HRQoL, and many patients experienced recovery within 18 months of completing treatment. However, high-level fatigue more than 2 years after therapy was common. The only factor that predicted long-term fatigue was fatigue at the end of treatment. Factors associated with significantly impaired HRQoL were older age and female sex. Furthermore, age affected all functioning and symptom scores. Also, of note, emotional domains did not show the same magnitude of improvement after treatment as physical domains.

Strengths of this report were the longitudinal design, large cohort size, homogeneous patient population, and long-term follow-up. These aspects allowed a sufficient analysis of clinically relevant patient-based and disease-based subgroups. A major limitation was the fact that the authors did not capture HRQoL data before treatment, which would have shed light on the potential role of pretreatment fatigue in predicting long-term outcomes. In addition, the number of patients at a given time point within defined treatment arms is rather small and advanced stage patients were not included. Thus, again only a subgroup of patients was evaluated in this study and, without baseline (i.e., pretreatment) values for HRQoL, the findings cannot be used to develop a model of HRQoL outcome in HL.

With regard to this limited knowledge on quality of life in HL patients, the results of the GHSG G4 (HD10–12) analysis are eagerly awaited. In this study generation, more than 4,000 patients were included and the same instruments as in the EORTC trial were used to assess the patients' HRQoL.

## 21.4 Conclusions

The number of clinical trials evaluating HRQoL assessment is increasing. It has become widely accepted that the multidimensional approach of HRQoL assessment reflects the patients situation and presents very important information for the process of treatment evaluation. With the constantly growing cohort of long-term survivors indicating the progress of cancer therapy in different subgroups, there is a need of new approaches in HRQoL assessment dealing with the particular problems of these long-term survivors. Several studies have highlighted the difficulties that survivors may experience long after treatment ends, such as general fatigue, health fragility, and social and financial problems. These findings have been demonstrated in studies where a HRQoL approach has been used. Since these studies mostly were using a cross-sectional design, there is a need for new approaches to describe more precisely the patients' situation, to detect reasons for maladaptation, and to identify patients at high risk.

Combined comprehensive approaches like the one by the EORTC/GELA and the GHSG using a HRQoL questionnaire for survivors and a life situation evaluation could help overcome the difficulties in assessing HRQoL in long-term survivors. Furthermore, this approach can be used with few modifications in the assessment of normal control persons from population registries. It seems plausible that many years after treatment the daily living circumstances have a stronger impact on patients' HRQoL. Therefore, it is essential to also have reference data from age- and gender-matched healthy population for the interpretation of HRQoL results. In addition, a more comprehensive approach that accounts for the patients' life situation is necessary to represent the complexity of HRQoL. The results from the studies by the EORTC/GELA and the GHSG within the next few years will reveal whether this approach proves successful. Quality-of-life assessment should benefit patients by defining relevant issues, even long after initial treatment. Disease- and therapy-independent predisposing factors for long-term HRQoL functions on one hand and those factors associated with therapy or the lymphoma itself on the other hand must be evaluated in well-designed prospective studies.

Results of the GHSG-G4 HRQoL evaluation will be published 2010 and might provide more information to understand how persisting impaired HRQoL develops and which factors contribute to a poor outcome. This will give us the opportunity to develop prevention strategies, to improve our study designs, and to better accompany and support our patients back on their way to a "normal" life.

# References

1. Ganz PA, Moinpour CM, Pauler DK, et al. Health status and quality of life in patients with early-stage Hodgkin's disease treated on Southwest Oncology Group Study 9133. J Clin Oncol. 2003;21:3512–9.
2. Heutte N, Flechtner HH, Mounier N, et al. Quality of life after successful treatment of early-stage Hodgkin's lymphoma: 10-year follow-up of the EORTC-GELA H8 randomised controlled trial. Lancet Oncol. 2009;10:1160–70.
3. Administration. USDoHaHSFaD. Guidance for industry. Patient-reported outcome measures: use in medical product development to support labeling claims. Draft guidance. 2006.
4. Aaronson NK, Ahmedzai S, Bergman B, et al. The European Organization for Research and Treatment of Cancer QLQ-C30: a quality-of-life instrument for use in international clinical trials in oncology. J Natl Cancer Inst. 1993;85:365–76.
5. Cella DF, Tulsky DS, Gray G, et al. The Functional Assessment of Cancer Therapy scale: development and validation of the general measure. J Clin Oncol. 1993;11:570–9.
6. Flechtner H, Ruffer JU, Henry-Amar M, et al. Quality of life assessment in Hodgkin's disease: a new comprehensive approach. First experiences from the EORTC/GELA and GHSG trials. EORTC Lymphoma Cooperative Group. Groupe D'Etude des Lymphomes de L'Adulte and German Hodgkin Study Group. Ann Oncol. 1998;9 Suppl 5:S147–54.
7. Guyatt GH, Osoba D, Wu AW, Wyrwich KW, Norman GR. Methods to explain the clinical significance of health status measures. Mayo Clin Proc. 2002;77:371–83.
8. Bottomley A, Flechtner H, Efficace F, et al. Health related quality of life outcomes in cancer clinical trials. Eur J Cancer. 2005;41:1697–709.
9. Cremeens J, Eiser C, Blades M. Characteristics of health-related self-report measures for children aged three to eight years: a review of the literature. Qual Life Res. 2006;15:739–54.
10. Roper K, McDermott K, Cooley ME, Daley K, Fawcett J. Health-related quality of life in adults with Hodgkin's disease: the state of the science. Cancer Nurs. 2009;32:E1–17; quiz E18–19.
11. Fobair P, Hoppe RT, Bloom J, Cox R, Varghese A, Spiegel D. Psychosocial problems among survivors of Hodgkin's disease. J Clin Oncol. 1986;4:805–14.
12. Joly F, Henry-Amar M, Arveux P, et al. Late psychosocial sequelae in Hodgkin's disease survivors: a French population-based case-control study. J Clin Oncol. 1996;14:2444–53.
13. Loge JH, Abrahamsen AF, Ekeberg O, Kaasa S. Hodgkin's disease survivors more fatigued than the general population. J Clin Oncol. 1999;17:253–61.
14. Wettergren L, Bjorkholm M, Axdorph U, Bowling A, Langius-Eklof A. Individual quality of life in long-term survivors of Hodgkin's lymphoma – a comparative study. Qual Life Res. 2003;12:545–54.
15. Wettergren L, Bjorkholm M, Axdorph U, Langius-Eklof A. Determinants of health-related quality of life in long-term survivors of Hodgkin's lymphoma. Qual Life Res. 2004;13:1369–79.
16. Wettergren L, Bjorkholm M, Langius-Eklof A. Validation of an extended version of the SEIQoL-DW in a cohort of Hodgkin lymphoma survivors. Qual Life Res. 2005;14:2329–33.
17. Ruffer JU, Flechtner H, Tralls P, et al. Fatigue in long-term survivors of Hodgkin's lymphoma; a report from the German Hodgkin Lymphoma Study Group (GHSG). Eur J Cancer. 2003;39:2179–86.
18. Holzner B, Kemmler G, Cella D, et al. Normative data for functional assessment of cancer therapy – general scale and its use for the interpretation of quality of life scores in cancer survivors. Acta Oncol. 2004;43:153–60.
19. Hjermstad MJ, Oldervoll L, Fossa SD, Holte H, Jacobsen AB, Loge JH. Quality of life in long-term Hodgkin's disease survivors with chronic fatigue. Eur J Cancer. 2006;42:327–33.

# Second Malignancy Risk After Treatment of Hodgkin Lymphoma

**22**

David C. Hodgson and Flora E. van Leeuwen

## Contents

D.C. Hodgson
Department of Radiation Oncology,
Princess Margaret Hospital, 610 University Ave,
Toronto, ON, M5G 2M9, Canada
e-mail: david.hodgson@rmp.uhn.on.ca

F.E. van Leeuwen (✉)
Department of Epidemiology, Netherlands Cancer Institute,
Plesmanlaan 121, 1066 CX, Amsterdam, The Netherlands
e-mail: f.v.leeuwen@nki.nl

## 22.1 Introduction

In view of the excellent cure rates that are currently achieved in the relatively young population of patients with Hodgkin Lymphoma (HL), it has become increasingly important to evaluate and limit the long-term complications of treatment. Research conducted over the last three decades has clearly demonstrated that, paradoxically, some treatments used to treat cancer have the potential to induce new (second) primary malignancies. Of all late complications of treatment, second malignant neoplasms (SMNs) are considered to be among the most serious because they cause not only substantial morbidity but also considerable mortality. Among long-term survivors of HL, second cancer deaths have been reported to be the largest contributor to the substantial excess mortality that these patients experience [1–4].

Increased risk of SMNs has been observed after both radiotherapy (RT) and chemotherapy (CT). In 1972, Arsenau [2] and colleagues were the first to report an increased risk of second cancer after HL treatment. Based on 12 second malignancies in 425 patients treated at the U.S. National Institutes of Health from 1953 to 1971, they estimated a 3.5-fold risk increase compared to the general population. MOPP combination CT (mechlorethamine, vincristine, procarbazine, and prednisone) for HL was introduced in 1967; the leukemogenic potential of this regimen and similar ones became evident in reports published in 1973 [5], 1975 [6], and 1977 [7]. In the 1980s, several studies showed that, after an introduction period of 5–10 years, RT for HL increased the risk of solid malignancies, especially lung cancer [8–11].

It is important to recognize that not all SMNs are caused by treatment. The occurrence of two primary

A. Engert and S.J. Horning (eds.), *Hodgkin Lymphoma*,
DOI: 10.1007/978-3-642-12780-9_22, © Springer-Verlag Berlin Heidelberg 2011

malignancies in the same individual may have several causes. It may represent a chance occurrence (in which case the two cancers developed as a result of unrelated factors), it may result from host susceptibility factors (e.g., genetic predisposition or immunodeficiency), it may be linked to carcinogenic influences in common, or a clustering of different risk factors in the same individual, or it may represent an effect of treatment for the first tumor [12, 13]. In view of the high prevalence of cancer in the general population and the increasing incidence of most cancers with age, background etiological factors other than treatment are likely to be responsible for a substantial proportion of second cancer, especially in older populations. Therefore, whenever a clinical impression arises that a specific combination of two distinct primary malignancies occurs more frequently than expected, comparison with cancer risk in the general population is imperative. If a SMN has been demonstrated to occur in excess, the contributions of other risk factors and the role of host susceptibility factors should be ruled out convincingly before the risk increase can be attributed to treatment. Even then, host factors may modify treatment effects, so that the risk associated with a given treatment will vary among individuals. The evaluation of the carcinogenic effects of therapy is further complicated by the fact that therapeutic agents are frequently given in combination. Appropriate epidemiologic and statistical methods are required to quantify the excess risk and to unravel treatment factors responsible for it.

In this chapter we address major aspects of SMN risk following treatment for HL. After a brief overview of the carcinogenic effects of RT and CT, we first discuss the methods used for assessing second cancer risk. Subsequently, a review is given of the risks of leukemia, non-Hodgkin lymphoma (NHL), and selected solid tumors in patients treated for HL. Emphasis is on large studies that were published recently. Clinical implications of the most important findings are discussed, and, finally, we suggest some directions for future research.

## 22.2 Methods of Assessing Second Cancer Risk

Estimates of second cancer risk after treatment for HL derive from several sources, including population-based cancer registries, hospital-based cancer registries, or clinical trial series. The cohort study and the nested case–control study are the epidemiologic study designs generally used in second cancer research [14]. Case reports have an important role in the early recognition of potential associations between different malignancies [15, 16]. However, because of lack of information on the underlying population at risk, they are not useful in quantifying risks.

In a *cohort study*, a large group of patients (the cohort) with a specified first malignancy is followed up for a number of years to determine the incidence of second (and subsequent) malignancies. Because most cohort studies of second cancer risk have been conducted retrospectively, follow-up of all patients in such studies is completed up to some point in the recent past. To evaluate whether second cancer risk in the cohort is increased compared with cancer risk in the general population, the observed number of SMNs in the cohort is compared with the number expected on the basis of age-, gender-, and calendar year-specific cancer incidence rates in the general population. This can be done in a so-called "person-years" type of analysis. In this approach, adjustment is made for the distribution of the cohort according to age, sex, and calendar period, while the observation period of individual patients (person-years at risk) is also taken into account. The *relative risk* (RR) of developing a SMN is estimated by the ratio of the observed number of SMNs in the cohort to the number expected. In epidemiologic terminology, the *observed-to-expected ratio* is often called the *standardized incidence ratio* (SIR). For cancer deaths, the equivalent measure is the *standardized mortality ratio*, in which observed second malignancy deaths are compared with expected numbers of deaths.

A disadvantage of the person-years method as applied in its simplest form is that it assumes the risk of SMN development to be constant over time; that is, it assumes the second cancer experience of 1,000 patients followed for 1 year to be comparable to that of 100 patients followed for 10 years. When this assumption is inappropriate (as with treatment-related cancers developing after an induction period), it is more informative to calculate SIRs within specified post-treatment intervals (usually 5-year periods) [17, 18]. A temporal trend of excess SMN risk may in itself provide an important initial clue to treatment-related causes; for example, the SIR of solid malignancy following RT for HL generally increases with time since exposure.

When the observed-to-expected ratio is increased, the question arises whether the risk increase is caused by the treatment. This can be evaluated by comparing SIRs between treatment groups, preferably with a reference group of patients not treated with RT or CT. Such a comparison group is available when second cancer risk is examined in patients with breast or testicular cancer, who may be treated with surgery alone, but, unfortunately, not for patients with HL. When the observation period (or survival rate) differs between treatments, their overall observed-to-expected ratios cannot be validly compared. Poisson regression analysis can be used to adjust treatment-specific observed-to-expected ratios for differences in age and time since treatment (see below).

Second cancer risk in the cohort (and in different treatment groups) can also be expressed by the *cumulative* (actuarial estimated) *risk* [19], which gives the proportion of patients expected to develop a SMN by time *t* (e.g., 5 years from diagnosis) if they do not die before then. When the cohort's death rate from causes other than SMNs is high, the assumption of "noninformative censoring" underlying the actuarial method is often not valid. In particular, the assumption that patients who died due to other causes would have the same temporal pattern of SMN risk as those who survived is incorrect. In such cases, actuarial risk tends to overestimate the true risk and *competing-risk techniques* should be used to estimate cumulative risk [20–23]. In comparing estimates of cumulative risk across studies, it is important to keep in mind that this measure of risk depends strongly on the age distribution of a specific cohort; because of the low background incidence of cancer at young ages, cohorts of HL patients including childhood HL will report much lower cumulative risks than cohorts including adults only.

Most studies reporting cumulative risks make no comparison with cancer risk in the general population, yet population-expected cumulative risks over time can be easily calculated on the basis of cancer incidence rates from a population-based registry [24].

Because certain treatment-related cancers are rare in the general population (e.g., leukemia, sarcoma), a high SIR (compared to the population) may still translate into a rather low cumulative risk. *Absolute excess risk* (AER), which estimates the excess number of SMNs occurring per 10,000 patients per year (beyond those expected from rates in the general population), best reflects the clinical burden of SMN in a cohort. Consequently, this risk measure is also the most appropriate one to judge which second malignancies contribute most to the excess morbidity or mortality.

The calculation of observed-to-expected ratios on the basis of person-years analysis and the calculation of

cumulative risks using life table analysis involve rather simple statistical methods, which have a strong intuitive appeal. Besides these elementary methods, statistical modeling with Cox proportional hazards model and Poisson regression techniques is increasingly being used to refine the quantification of second cancer RRs (e.g., by estimating dose- and time–response relationships) and to examine the interplay between treatment variables and other factors [25, 26].

Each of the data sources that are commonly used to constitute cohorts has specific advantages and disadvantages. *Population-based cancer registries* have large numbers of patients available, which allows the detection of even small excess risks of second cancers [12, 27, 28]. An additional advantage is that the observed and expected numbers of cancers come from the same reference population. Disadvantages include limited availability of treatment data, underreporting of SMNs [12, 29, 30] (in particular hematologic malignancies), and inconsistent diagnostic criteria for SMNs. Population-based registries differ greatly in these aspects and hence in their usefulness for second cancer studies. If treatment data are not available, it is impossible to know whether excess risk for a SMN is related to treatment or to shared etiology with the first cancer. Underreporting of SMNs clearly leads to an underestimation of second cancer risk. Far higher risks of second leukemia following HL have been found in hospital series [10, 31] than in population-based studies [28, 29]. Part of this difference, however, may be attributable to the more intensive treatments administered in large treatment centers [29]. Despite their disadvantages, population-based registries are well suited to evaluate broadly which SMNs occur in excess following a wide spectrum of different first primary malignancies. They are also a valuable starting point for case–control studies that evaluate treatment effects in detail (see below).

A major advantage of *clinical trial databases* is that detailed treatment data on all patients are available. Comparison of SMN risk between the treatment arms of the trial controls for any intrinsic risk of SMNs associated with the first cancer. However, a limitation of most trials is the small number of patients involved. Although this problem can be overcome by combining data from a number of trials, multicenter trial series pose other problems, such as difficulties in accessing medical records and histologic slides of patients in multiple centers. Further, the main endpoints of interest in most clinical trials are treatment response and survival, and many trials do not routinely collect information on SMNs or on full systematic long-term follow-up, so that follow-up data to a fixed end date may be very incomplete (and biased). Ideally, routine reporting and assessment of SMN risk should become an integral part of clinical trial research [32, 33].

Most *hospital-based tumor registries* have been in existence for decades and collect extensive data on treatment and follow-up. They share the advantages of clinical trial databases without having their disadvantages. Investigators using hospital tumor registries have ready access to the medical records; often a review of the histologic slides of the first and the second malignancy can also be arranged easily. An additional advantage is that, compared with trial data, hospital registries provide a wider range of treatments and dose levels, which may yield important information on drug and radiation carcinogenesis. Most studies of second cancer risk following HL have been based on hospital registries [4, 34–36]. As with trial data, however, loss to follow-up and surveillance bias compared to population-based studies can be problematic.

The cohort study is not an efficient study design for examining detailed treatment factors (e.g., cumulative dose of alkylating agents) in relation to second cancer risk. Large cohorts are required to yield reliable estimates of second cancer risk, rendering the collection of detailed treatment data for all patients prohibitively expensive and time-consuming. In such instances, the so-called nested case–control study within an existing cohort is the preferred approach. The case group consists of all patients identified with the SMN of interest, and the controls are a random sample of all patients in the cohort who did not develop the cancer concerned, although they experienced the same amount of follow-up time. To achieve maximum statistical power, most case–control studies of second cancer risk use a design in which more than one control is individually matched to each second cancer "case." Matching factors employed in most studies include sex, year of birth, and year at diagnosis of the first primary cancer. The most important criterion for control selection is that each control must have survived, without developing the SMN of interest, for at least as long as the interval between the diagnosis of the first and the second malignancy of the corresponding case. Even if the control group is three times as large as the case group, detailed treatment data need to be collected for only a small proportion of the total cohort. It is critical to the validity of the study results that the controls are truly representative of all patients who did not develop the second cancer of interest. For example, biased results may be obtained when controls with untraceable records are replaced by controls with traceable records.

In the analysis of a case–control study of second cancer risk, treatment factors are compared between cases and controls. Treatments that have been administered more often, for a longer duration, or with a higher dose to the case group than to the controls are associated with increased risk of developing the SMN of interest. It is important to understand that in a nested case–control study, the risk associated with specific treatments is estimated relative to the risk in patients receiving other treatment and *not* relative to the risk in the general population. The cumulative risk of developing a SMN cannot be derived using data from a case–control study alone. Estimates of the AERs associated with specific treatments can be derived, however, if the case–control study follows a cohort analysis in which observed-to-expected ratios were calculated for broad treatment groups. Although the case–control methodology has only come into widespread use for the investigation of SMN risk in recent decades, several landmark studies have already demonstrated its strengths [13, 29, 37–45].

## 22.3 Magnitude of the Risk Increase of Second Malignancy, Temporal Patterns, and Age Effects

The largest overall SIR (10- to 15-fold increase) compared to the general population is observed for leukemia (with the greatest risk seen for acute myeloid leukemia (AML) (22-fold), followed by a 6- to 14-fold increased risk for non-Hodgkin lymphoma (NHL), and 4- to 11-fold excesses for connective tissue, bone, and thyroid cancers (Table 22.1). Moderately increased risks (two- to sixfold) are observed for a number of solid tumors, such as cancer of the lung, stomach, esophagus, colon, breast, cervix, mouth and pharynx, and melanoma [36, 46–48] (Table 22.1). Because leukemia and NHL are diseases with a low incidence in the population, even a high RR compared to the population translates into a relatively low cumulative risk.

Many studies show that, over the long-term, the cumulative risk of solid tumors far exceeds that of leukemia and NHL (e.g., 25-year cumulative risks of 23

**Table 22.1** Relative risks of second malignancy after HL for selected sites in large[a] cohort studies published since 2000

| Site | Swerdlow et al. [48] | van Leeuwen et al. [36] | Dores et al. [46] | Foss Abrahamsen et al. [132] | Ng [4] | Metayer et al. [22] | Bhatia et al. [49] | Hodgson et al. [61] |
|---|---|---|---|---|---|---|---|---|
| | Britain | Netherlands | International | Norway | International | International | United States | International |
| | $N=5,519$[b] | $N=1,253$[b] | $N=32,591$[b] | $N=1,024$[b] | $N=32,591$[b] | $N=5,925$[b] | $N=1,380$[b] | $N=18,862$[b] |
| | All ages | Ages <40 | All ages | All ages | All ages | Ages ≤20 | Ages ≤16 | All ages |
| | Med. fup 8.5 years | Med. fup 14.1 years | Med. fup <10 years | Med. fup 14 years | Med. fup 12 years | Med. fup 10.5 years | Med. fup 17 years | Med. fup 12.2 years |
| | Yrs of dx 1963–1993 | Yrs of dx 1966–1986 | Yrs of dx 1935–1994 | Yrs of dx 1968–1985 | Yrs of dx 1935–1994 | Yrs of dx 1935–1994 | Yrs of dx 1955–1986 | Yrs of dx 1970–1997 |
| | SIR (N observed) | SIR (N observed) | SIR (N observed) | SIR (N observed) | SIR (N observed) | SIR (N observed) | SIR (N observed) | RR[c] (N observed) |
| All sites | 2.9[d] (322) | 7.0 (137) | 2.3[d] (2,153) | 3.5[d] (194) | 4.6[d] (181) | 7.7[d] (195) | 18.5[d] (143) | –[e] |
| All solid | 2.2[d] (227) | 6.1[d] (106) | 2.0[d] (1,726) | –[d] | 3.5[d] (131) | 7.0[d] (157) | 18.5[d] (109) | –[e] (1,490) |
| Leukemia | 14.6[d] (45) | 37.5[d] (18) | 9.9[d] (249) | 13.0[d] (14) | 82.5[d] (23) | 20.9[d] (28) | 174.8[d] (27) | –(–)[e] |
| NHL | 14.0[d] (50) | 21.5[d] (16) | 5.5[d] (162) | 24.2[d] (31) | 16.5[d] (24) | 6.9[d] (10) | 11.7[d] (7) | –(–)[e] |
| Female breast | 1.4 (19) | 5.2[d] (27) | 2.0[d] (234) | 3.8[d] (23) | 6.7[d] (39) | 14.1[d] (52) | 55.5[d] (39) | 6.1[g] (–) |
| Lung | 3.4[d] (78) | 7.0[d] (13) | 2.9[d] (377) | 5.1[d] (26) | 4.9[d] (22) | 5.1[d] (6) | 27.3[d] (4) | 6.7[g] (–) |
| Stomach | 2.2[d] (13) | 10.9[d] (7) | 1.9[d] (80) | 4.4[d] (12) | –[e] | 13.8[d] (5) | 63.9[d] (3) | 9.5[g] (–) |
| Colon | 2.3[d] (18) | 2.8 (3) | 1.6[d] (129) | 1.9 (9) | –[e] | 4.7[d] (4) | 36.4[d] (8)[f] | 4.3[g] (–) |
| Pancreas | 1.0[d] (3) | –[e] | 1.5[d] (40) | 1.3 (2) | –[e] | 10.8[d] (2) | –[e] | 4.7[g] (–) |
| Bone | 10.7[d] (4) | –[e] | 3.8[d] (9) | –[e] | –[e] | 9.7[d] (5) | 37.1[d] (8) | –(–)[e] |
| Soft tissue | 3.9[d] (3) | 12.1[d] (3) | 5.1[d] (32) | –[e] | –[e] | 15.1[d] (9) | –[e] | –(–)[e] |
| Bone and soft tissue | –[e] | –[e] | –[e] | –[e] | 26.6[d] (11) | –[e] | –[e] | 11.7[g] (–) |
| Melanoma | 2.3 (6) | 5.5[d] (7) | 1.7[d] (52) | 2.8[d] (8) | 3.3[d] (7) | 1.9 (5) | –[e] | 1.6[g] (–) |
| Cervix | 2.1 (7) | –[e] | 2.0[d] (37) | 1.5 (2) | –[e] | 6.1[d] (10) | –[e] | 2.2[h] (–) |
| Thyroid | 7.6[d] (5) | 15.2[d] (4) | 4.1[d] (47) | –[e] | 5.6[d] (5) | 13.7[d] (22) | 36.4[d] (19) | 3.1[i] (–) |

*NHL* non-Hodgkin lymphoma; *Med. fup* median follow-up; *Yrs of dx* years of diagnosis; *RR* relative risk; *N* number of second malignancies

[a] Only includes studies with ≥100 second malignancies; for cohorts included in several reports, only the paper with the longest follow-up is included

[b] Number of Hodgkin Lymphoma patients included in the study

[c] RRs are for males and females combined and for individuals diagnosed with HL at age 30 years and attained age range 40–60 years

[d] Significantly raised ($p < 0.05$)

[e] Data not published

[f] Excluding nonmelanoma skin cancers

[g] RR is for women diagnosed with HL at age 30 years and attained age 40 years

[h] RR is for all female genital second cancers

[i] RR is for individuals diagnosed with HL at age 30 years and all attained ages

and 3% for solid tumors and leukemia, respectively) [36] (Table 22.2). Several studies [36, 46, 48] show that, compared with the general population, HL patients experience an excess of about 45–80 malignancies per 10,000 person-years of observation (Table 22.2). Solid tumors account for the majority of excess cancers (approximately 30–60 per 10,000 patients per year), with lung cancer contributing 10–12 excess cases per 10,000 person-years. Leukemia and NHL each account for about eight to nine cases per 10,000 person-years.

Although SMN risks are often summarized as a single relative risk (SIR) or AER value for sake of simplicity, it is important to recognize that variation over time is one of the fundamental features of second cancer risk. Further, the nature of this variation is different for different second malignancy sites, and ages at treatment, and additionally relative risks vary over time differently than AERs (Figs. 22.1 and 22.2). Consequently, no single risk value fully describes the SMN risk that patients experience at different times after treatment. Leukemia risk increases approximately 2–4 years following alkylator-based CT, with the SIR peaking 5–9 years after treatment, and decreasing thereafter [36, 40, 46, 48–51]. The SIR of NHL is increased in the first 5 years after treatment, and study findings disagree regarding whether NHL risk increases [10, 51] or remains constant over time [4, 46, 50].

Most studies report that the overall SIR of solid tumors is minimally elevated in the 1–4 year follow-up period, and increases thereafter [4, 10, 31, 36, 46, 48, 50, 52]. In studies that include data on 20-year survivors, the RR of solid tumors continued to increase through the 15–20 year follow-up period [4, 31, 36, 46, 48, 49, 52–55]. A Dutch study of patients diagnosed with HL before age 40 reported a SIR of solid tumors of 8.8 in the 20–24-year interval, and 5.3 among 25-year survivors, suggesting a possible decrease in very long-term survivors. However, Ng et al. [4] reported an increasing RR of solid malignancy throughout follow-up among patients all of whom received RT. A report from the Late Effects Study Group on survivors of pediatric HL reported a stable 20- to 24-fold increased RR from 15 to over 30 years after diagnosis [49]. An international registry-based study of 5-year HL survivors employed Poisson regression methods comparable to those used to evaluate the temporal trends of cancer risk among atomic bomb survivors [47]. Variation in the risk of solid cancer was found to depend strongly on age at exposure, and attained age, with distinctly

different patterns for female breast cancer, thyroid cancer, and other solid tumors (Fig. 22.3). With increasing attained age, the RR of breast cancer declined among females diagnosed at a young age (modeled age 20 years), whereas this decline was much less pronounced among women treated at older ages (30 or 40 years at HL diagnosis) (Fig. 22.2). In contrast, the RR of other solid cancers remained stable with advancing attained age, with a small decline after attained age of 60 years (Fig. 22.1). The AER of breast cancer and nonbreast solid cancers increased with increasing attained age for all age groups [47] (Figs. 22.1 and 22.2). These findings demonstrate the importance of considering both age at exposure and attained age in the evaluation of SMN risk, as well the potential importance of considering different solid cancers separately. Combining different age-at-treatment groups or all solid tumor types together may obscure significant variation in risks over time that can occur among different age groups or different SMN types. Also, the AER of SMNs changes over time differently than the SIR (Figs. 22.1 and 22.2). With increasing time since treatment, the major influence on the AER is the increasing background (i.e., "expected") rate of cancer, which rises rapidly with increasing age. As these baseline risks increase with advancing age, even stable elevations in SIRs translate into rising AER, over time (Fig. 22.1).

## 22.4 Contributors to Second Cancer Risk

### 22.4.1 Radiation Therapy

Increased risks of second cancers following RT for HL have been reported for over two decades [28]. These reports add to a substantial body of evidence demonstrating that radiation is carcinogenic over a broad range of doses, and can increase the risk of a variety of different tumor types [56–60]. Certain tissues, such as the female breast, and thyroid appear to be particularly susceptible to radiation-induced malignancy.

Among HL patients, treatment with mantle RT (involving the axillary, mediastinal, and neck nodes) to doses of 35–45 Gy is associated with a 2- to 20-fold increased RR of breast cancer, with a strong influence of age at exposure, as discussed in detail below [4, 36, 49, 61, 62]. Mantle RT is also associated with an increased RR of lung cancer, although the AER is in

**Table 22.2**  SIR, AER, and cumulative incidence of second malignancy among HL survivors in selected studies

Second malignancy among HL survivors in selected studies

| | van Leeuwen et al. [36] | Dores et al. [46] | Foss Abrahamsen et al. [132] | Ng et al. [4][a] | Forrest et al. [129] | Hodgson et al. [61] |
|---|---|---|---|---|---|---|
| | Netherlands | International | Norway | International | Canada | International |
| | N=1,253 | N=32,591[b] | N=1,024[b] | N=32,591[b] | N=1,732 | N=18,862[b] |
| | Ages <40 | All ages | All ages | All ages | All ages | All ages |
| | Med. fup 14.1 yrs | Med. fup <10 years | Med. fup 14 years | Med. fup 12 years | Med. fup 9.8 years | Med. fup 12.2 years |
| | Yrs of dx 1966–1986 | Yrs of dx 1935–1994 | Yrs of dx 1968–1985 | Yrs of dx 1935–1994 | Yrs of dx 1976–2001 | Yrs of dx 1970–1997 |
| **All cancers** | | | | | | |
| SIR | 7.0 | 2.3 | 3.5 | 4.6 | 3.5 | – |
| AER | 72.3 | 47.2 | 10 | 89.3 | – | – |
| CI | 25 years=27.7% | – | 28 years=18.8% | 15 years=13% | 15 years=9% | – |
| **All solid** | | | | | | |
| SIR | 6.1 | 2.0 | – | 3.5 | 2.8 | 4.6[b], 3.7[c] |
| AER | 54.5 | 33.1 | – | 59.1 | – | – |
| CI | 25 years=23.3% | 25 years=21.9% | 28 years=14.4% | – | 15 years=7.2% | 30 years=18.3% (M)[d]=26.1% (F)[d] |
| **Breast (females)** | | | | | | |
| SIR | 5.2 | 2.0 | 3.8 | 6.7 | – | 6.1 |
| AER | 29.4 | 10.5 | 27[e] | 20.8 | – | 61[f] |
| CI | 25 years=16.3% | 25 years=9.3% | – | – | – | – |
| **Acute leukemia** | | | | | | |
| SIR | 37.5 | 9.9 | 13 | 82.5 | 19.6[j] | – |
| AER | 10.8 | 8.8 | 8[g] | 14.3 | – | – |
| CI | 25 years=3.3% | – | 28 years=1.5% | – | 15 years = 1.4%[l] | – |

(continued)

**Table 22.2** (continued)

Second malignancy among pediatric HL survivors

| | Metayer et al. [62] | Bhatia et al. [49] | Basu et al. [156], Constine et al. [54] |
|---|---|---|---|
| | International | United States | United States |
| | $N=5,925$ | $N=1,380$ | $N=930$ |
| | Ages ≤20 | Ages ≤16 | Ages <19 |
| | Med. fup 10.5 yrs | Med. fup 17 yrs | Med. fup 16.8 years |
| | Yrs of dx 1935–1994 | Yrs of dx 1955–1986 | Yrs of dx 1960–1990 |
| **All cancers** | | | |
| SIR | 7.7 | 18.5 | 14.2 |
| AER | – | 65h | 62.6 |
| CI | – | 30 years=26.3% | 20 years=8% (M)=23% (F) |
| **All solid** | | | |
| SIR | 7.0 | 18.5 | – |
| AER | 48i | 51h | – |
| CI | 25 years=11.7% | 30 years=23.5% | – |
| **Breast (females)** | | | |
| SIR | 14.1 | 55.5 | 37.3 |
| AER | 19j | 53h | 18.6 |
| CI | – | 30 years=16.9% | 30 years=24% |
| **Acute leukemia** | | | |
| SIR | 27.4 | 174.8 | 21.5 |
| AER | 2.0k | 1.3 | 5.7 |
| CI | – | 30 years=2.1% | – |

*SIR* standardized incidence ratio; *AER* absolute excess risk; *CI* cumulative incidence; *Yrs of dx* years of diagnosis; *med. fup* median follow-up; *M* male; *F* female

aAll patients received RT

bSupradiaphragmatic sites

cInfradiaphragmatic sites

dDiagnosed at age 30

eFor women with 10–19 years of follow-up

fAER predicted for a 30-year old female attained age 50

gApplies to patients diagnosed ≤40 years of age

hResults were published per 1,000 person-years. For consistency these have been multiplied by 10 (i.e., 10,000 P–Y)

iFor patients treated at age ≤16 years with attained age 35–39 years

jFor females aged 17–20 at HL diagnosis

kFor patients aged 17–20 at HL diagnosis

lIncludes acute myeloid leukemia and myelodysplasia

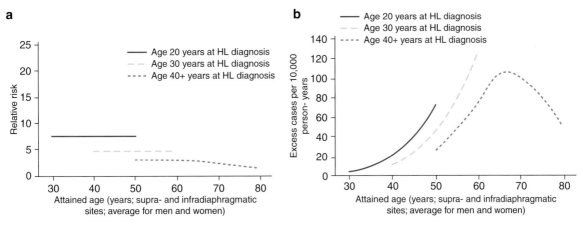

**Fig. 22.1** Relative risk (RR) and absolute excess risk of supra- and infradiaphragmatic solid cancers according to age at HL diagnosis and attained age. (**a**) RR of supra- and infradiaphragmatic solid cancers. (**b**) AER of supra- and infradiaphragmatic solid cancers (Adapted from [61])

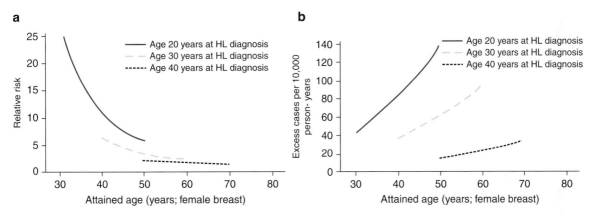

**Fig. 22.2** Relative risk (RR) and absolute excess risk of female breast cancer according to age at HL diagnosis and attained age. (**a**) RR of female breast cancer. (**b**) AER of female breast cancer (Adapted from [61])

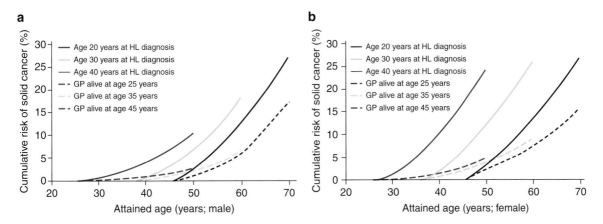

**Fig. 22.3** (**a**) Cumulative incidence of all solid cancers among 10,619 male 5-year survivors of Hodgkin lymphoma (HL) compared with men of the same age in the general population (GP). (**b**) Cumulative incidence for 8,243 female 5-year survivors compared with women of the same age in the GP (Adapted from [61])

fact small in the first 10–20 years after exposure, particularly among those treated at young ages (e.g., ≤0.2 per 10,000 person-years among those treated before age 20 years) [48, 49]. The risks of other solid cancers have also been shown to be elevated after RT.

Much of our current understanding of the relationship between radiation dose and cancer risk has been derived from cohort studies of individuals exposed to low levels of radiation, such as atomic bomb survivors [59, 63–65]. However, extrapolation of the dose–risk relationships seen at low total body doses into the 15–40 Gy ranges used for HL RT cannot be done with certainty, due to differences relating to dose rate, neutron exposure, and the possibility of cell killing at high doses. More recently, studies of SMN risk have evaluated the dose–risk relationship in the radiation dose range commonly used in the treatment of HL.

There appears to be an approximately linear increase in the risk of leukemia with increasing radiation dose to the bone marrow, up to approximately 2–4 Gy [37, 66, 67]. At doses above this, the risk of leukemia per unit radiation dose to the bone marrow appears to decline [37, 66, 67], a finding generally attributed to killing or inactivation of preleukemic cells at the higher radiation doses [37, 68]. One study of leukemia risk in survivors of uterine cancer, however, showed little evidence for such a clear downturn in risk [66].

The "bell-shaped" dose–risk curve for leukemia, with a peak at 2–4 Gy, does not seem to apply to the risk of most solid tumors. Most studies examining the dose–risk relationship for solid tumors suggest a continued increase in risk with doses up to approximately 40 Gy [42, 45, 69, 70]. Two studies have evaluated the relationship between radiation dose and breast cancer risk among adult females treated for HL with mantle RT [42, 45]. The RT dose to the area of the breast where the case's tumor had developed was estimated for each case–control set based on simulation films of the original HL RT and mammograms indicating the position of the breast tumor. Both studies showed increasing risk of breast cancer over the dose range commonly used in the treatment of HL. For example, in a large international collaborative case–control study of women treated for HL at age 30 years or less [42] (105 patients with breast cancer after HL and 266 controls without breast cancer), the risk was eightfold increased (95% confidence interval, 2.6–26.4 ) for the highest dose category (median dose of 42 Gy) compared to the lowest one (<4 Gy) (P trend <0.001, Table 22.3) [42]. Similarly, Inskip et al. [69] conducted a case–control study of

**Table 22.3** Relative risks of breast and lung cancers after Hodgkin Lymphoma, according to radiation dose to affected site in breast/lung and number of cycles of alkylating chemotherapy[a,b]

| Breast cancer[a] | | | Lung cancer[b] | | |
|---|---|---|---|---|---|
| Radiation dose to affected site in breast (Gy) | Relative risk | 95% CI | Radiation dose to affected site in lung (Gy) | Relative risk | 95% CI |
| 0–3.9 | 1.0 | Referent | 0 | 1.0 | Referent |
| 4.0–6.9 | 1.8 | 0.7–4.5 | >0–4.9 | 1.6 | 0.5–5.2 |
| 7.0–23.1 | 4.1 | 1.4–12.3 | 5–14.9 | 4.2 | 0.7–21 |
| 23.2–27.9 | 2.0 | 0.7–5.9 | 15.0–29.9 | 2.7 | 0.2–15 |
| 28.0–37.1 | 6.8 | 2.3–22.3 | 30.0–39.9 | 8.5 | 3.3–24 |
| 37.2–40.4 | 4.0 | 1.3–13.4 | ≥40.0 | 6.3 | 2.2–19 |
| 40.5–61.3 | 8.0 | 2.6–26.4 | | | |
| Number of cycles of alkylating agents | | | Number of cycles of alkylating agents | | |
| 0 | 1.0 | Referent | 0 | 1.0 | Referent |
| 1–4 | 0.7 | 0.3–1.7 | 1–4 | 4.0 | 1.3–12.5 |
| 5–8 | 0.6 | 0.3–1.1 | 5–8 | 6.2 | 2.6–17.1 |
| ≥9 | 0.2 | 0.1–0.7 | ≥9 | 13.0 | 4.3–45 |

[a]Adapted from [42]

[b]Adapted from [71]

breast cancer in a cohort of 6,647 female survivors of childhood cancer participating in the U.S. Childhood Cancer Survivors Study. Radiation dose was estimated to the site of breast cancer for 120 cases (65% treated for HL) and 464 controls (40.5% treated for HL). They reported a linear increase in breast cancer risk with increasing dose, such that, compared to those with no radiation dose to the breast, the odds ratio of breast cancer was 11-fold higher among those with breast exposures of 40 Gy. This dose–risk relationship was modified by ovarian radiation exposure: the slope of the dose–risk curve was significantly less steep among those with ovarian radiation (>5 Gy), presumably due to the impact of hormonal influences on breast cancer risk [69] (Fig. 22.4).

The risk of lung cancer also rises with increasing radiation dose up to 40 Gy and with an increasing volume of lung irradiated [71, 72] (Table 22.3). Similarly, two studies in survivors of childhood cancer [43, 73] suggest that the risk of bone sarcoma increases rapidly with increasing dose above 10 Gy [74]. A recent case–control study found that the risk of stomach cancer also increases linearly with radiation dose to the stomach, with tenfold increased risk for mean stomach doses of >20 Gy compared to less than 11 Gy [75]. Radiation-induced thyroid cancer may be an exception to these general findings for other solid cancers: dose–risk studies have suggested a leveling or decrease in thyroid cancer risk with doses above 10–30 Gy [60, 76, 77] although one study reported increasing risk of

thyroid cancer with increasing dose up to 60 Gy [77].

These dose–risk studies provide a critical component to understanding the potential risk of second cancers associated with contemporary involved field RT (IFRT) for HL. Specifically, they suggest that reduction in normal tissue dose associated with reducing the prescribed dose from 36–40 to 20–30 Gy should produce a lower risk of breast, lung, and (when infradiaphragmantic RT is used) stomach cancers. The risk of thyroid cancer, however, may not be reduced.

In addition to lower prescribed doses, for most patients contemporary IFRT reduces the volume of normal tissue irradiated (and hence the normal tissue dose) compared to historic mantle or extended-field RT. One study found that for patients with mediastinal disease, the transition from mantle fields to mediastinal IFRT resulted in an approximately 65% reduction in breast tissue exposure, largely due to the exclusion of the axillae [78]. Clinical studies provide evidence that that this volume-related reduction in breast exposure appears to translate into a reduced risk of subsequent breast cancer. A recent large Dutch study, including 1,122 female 5-year survivors of HL, examined the effect of radiation fields (volume) on the risk of breast cancer up to more than 30 years after treatment of HL [79]. Mantle field irradiation was associated with a 2.7-fold (95% CI, 1.1–6.9) increased risk of breast cancer compared to similarly dosed (36–44 Gy) radiation to the mediastinum alone [79] (Fig. 22.5). This finding is reassuring since present-day RT for HL employs smaller radiation volumes [79, 80].

### 22.4.2 Chemotherapy

There is a well-established association between exposure to alkylating CT agents and an increased risk of AML in HL survivors. The MOPP-CT regimen was widely employed in the 1970s, as it became evident that it was superior to RT alone in curing high-risk HL. However, it was associated with an increased RR of AML of 20- to 50-fold [10, 31, 51, 81–84]. As described below, there is no consistent evidence that the addition of extended-field RT to MOPP increases AML risk further [40, 86]. Since CT agents are given in combination, it is challenging to disentangle the effects of individual agents and the impact of cumulative dose, duration of use, and dose intensity on the risk of AML.

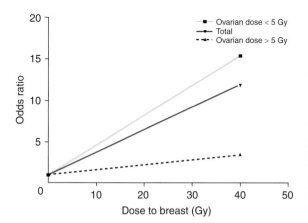

**Fig. 22.4** Fitted breast cancer risk by radiation dose to the breast and ovary, results from the Childhood Cancer Survivor Study, based on 120 breast cancer cases and 464 controls. (Adapted from [68])

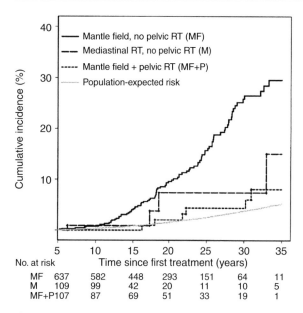

**Fig. 22.5** The cumulative incidence of breast cancer after HL. Cumulative incidence of invasive breast cancer according to radiation fields and population-expected risk (*RT* radiotherapy) (Adapted from [79])

In general, the cumulative alkylator dose appears to be the strongest determinant of risk [39, 51].

Most cases of alkylator-induced AML are preceded by myelodysplasia (MDS), which generally progresses to AML within a year [31, 86, 87]. Cytogenetic studies of alkylator-induced AML/MDS have shown unbalanced chromosome aberrations, primarily with loss of whole chromosomes 5 and/or 7 or various parts of the long arms of these chromosomes [87, 88].

More recently, another class of drugs used in the treatment of HL, topoisomerase II inhibitors, have also been associated with elevated risks of AML. Examples of these drugs used in HL treatment include doxorubicin and etoposide. Early evidence suggests that doxorubicin and 4-epidoxorubicin (epirubicin) may be associated with increased risks of AML [40, 89, 90], but this association is not nearly as well established as it is for alkylating agents, and requires further study. Certainly, ABVD CT (doxorubicin, bleomycin, vinblastine, dacarbazine) is associated with a lesser risk of AML than MOPP CT, although it is not clear that this risk is eliminated altogether [31, 91]. Etoposide, used in newer HL CT regimens such as BEACOPP (bleomycin, etoposide, doxorubicin, cyclophosphamide, vincristine, procarbazine, prednisone), and OEPA (vincristine, etoposide, prednisolone, doxoribicin) is also leukemogenic [92]. As compared with "classical"

alkylating agent-induced AML, etoposide-related AML typically occurs sooner after exposure, generally lacks a preceding myelodysplastic phase, and is characterized by balanced translocations involving chromosome bands 11q23 and 21q22 [93–95].

Much less is known about the solid tumor risks associated with CT. Mechlorethamine and procarbazine are associated with significantly increased risks of lung cancer (RR = 1.5–6.1), with increasing cumulative dose associated with increasing risk [13, 72] (Table 22.3). Alkylating agents have also been associated with increased risks of bone sarcomas [43, 73], bladder cancer [41, 96], and gastrointestinal cancers [75]

### 22.4.3 Genetic Factors

There is increasing interest in identifying the molecular and cellular basis underlying the development of SMNs in HL survivors, and other cancer survivors. Germline mutations in the RB1 tumor suppressor gene, associated with hereditary retinoblastoma, constitute a well-described example of a rare mutation with high penetrance that confers a large risk of developing radiation-related SMNs [97–99]. Although there is evidence that patients with a family history of cancer are more likely to develop radiation-related SMNs [100–105], it is unlikely that a single candidate gene abnormality will account for a significant component of the SMN risk following HL treatment. Currently, there is no uniform evidence that BRCA1 or BRCA2 gene mutations mediate the development of radiation-related breast cancers. Two studies have reported that mammographic radiation exposure does not significantly contribute to the risk seen in BRCA1/2 mutation carriers [106, 107], though two other studies found that young BRCA1/2 mutation carriers had an increased risk of breast cancer if exposed to a significant number of chest X-rays [108, 109]. There have been no studies examining whether carriers of BRCA mutations with HL have an increased risk of RT-associated cancers. Homozygous mutations in the ataxia-telangiectasia (ATM) gene are associated with significant radiation toxicity, although two studies have reported that no ATM mutations were found in women who had developed breast cancer after RT for HL [104, 110]. Moreover, while P53 gene mutations are associated with an increased risk of primary malignancy [111], and increased radiation sensitivity in vitro [112, 113], there is currently no evidence that P53 mutations modify the risk of treatment-related SMNs in HL patients. Remarkably, one study found that breast cancers following RT for HL have a molecular profile distinct from idiopathic breast cancers from age-matched women [114].

Methylating agents (e.g., dacarbazine) produce DNA damage, the repair of which is mediated in part by the MLH1 gene. Worrillow et al. [115] examined the frequency of a common MLH1–93 polymorphism among patients who developed cancer following CT and/or RT, or were diagnosed with de novo myeloid leukemia, or HL, and healthy controls. Carrier frequency of the MLH1–93 variant was higher in patients who developed therapy-related AML or breast cancer after methylating CT for HL compared to patients without previous methylating exposure. The MLH1–93 variant was also associated with a significantly increased risk of developing therapy-related AML in patients previously treated with a methylating agent [115]. Other factors in the development of CT-related leukemias may include interindividual differences in repair of DNA damage [116, 117] and germline mutations in tumor suppressor genes [118, 119].

The development of rapid genotyping, and catalogs of genetic variants now permit genome-wide association studies that compare the entire genomes of patients with and without a given condition to look for allelic variants associated with the outcome of interest. These studies may potentially allow the identification of common low-risk alleles associated with the risk of SMNs following cancer treatment. One major issue is the large sample size required to identify such genetic variants, and there are emerging efforts to create large consortia to conduct such studies [120].

## 22.5 Risk of Selected Second Malignancies

### 22.5.1 Risk Factors for Leukemia

Leukemia following HL is certainly the most studied treatment-induced malignancy, and thus extensive knowledge of its risk factors has emerged [85]. Leukemia was the first malignancy for which elevated

risk after treatment for HL was observed, probably because of the relatively short latency period, the rarity of acute leukemia in the general population, and the large SIR.

Overall, risks compared with the general population have been reported to be 10- to over 80-fold increased (Table 22.1). Nearly all studies show that the SIR of leukemia is higher than that of NHL and much greater than that of solid tumors overall (Table 22.1). Because the background risk of leukemia in the population is low, however, this strongly increased SIR translates into a relatively low cumulative risk, ranging between 1.4 and 4.1% at 15 years [10, 31, 36, 48, 49, 52, 91]. Overall, the AER has varied between 8 and 30 excess cases per 10,000 patients per year (Table 22.2) [46, 48, 121].

RT alone is associated with a small, or no, increased risk of leukemia compared with the risk in the general population [10, 36, 48, 51, 52], while alkylating agent CT is linked with greatly elevated risk. In cohort analysis of CT-treated patients, the SIRs of leukemia overall tend to be over 20-fold increased compared to the general population, while for AML over 50-fold risk increases are reported [10, 31, 51, 81–84].

Several studies have compared the leukemogenicity of different CT regimens. Where exposure has been quantified, risk appears to be most related to total dose of alkylating agents or nitrosoureas [10, 29, 44, 51, 81, 84]. Risk of AML rises sharply with an increasing number of MOPP (or MOPP-like) cycles [29, 51]. The risk associated with 10–12 MOPP cycles appears to be approximately 3–5 times higher than the risk following six MOPP cycles [29, 51]. Total dose of alkylators and nitrosoureas is likely the explanation of the reports of higher risk associated with salvage CT or maintenance CT [51, 52, 122], but there is evidence that retreatment may be a factor in risk [50, 51, 81, 123]. Among those treated with variations of MOPP that substitute chlorambucil for mechlorethamine, the risks appear similar, but with cyclophosphamide in place of mechlorethamine, the risks are lower [10, 51, 84, 124, 125].

Mechlorethamine and procarbazine are usually given in combination, so it is difficult to disentangle the effects of each. One study showed that mechlorethamine rather than procarbazine had the strongest effect on leukemia risk [51]. Since the 1980s, MOPP-only CT has been gradually replaced by ABV(D) (doxorubicin, bleomycin, vinblastine, and dacarbazine)-containing regimens in many centers. There are only a few reports on AML occurrence following ABV(D) alone. Patients treated with ABVD in the Milan Cancer Institute, where this regimen was designed, were shown to have a significantly lower risk of AML than MOPP-treated patients (15-year cumulative risks of 0.7 and 9.5%, respectively) [91]. Another study showed that HL patients treated with MOPP/ABV(D)-containing regimens in the 1980s had substantially lower risk of AML/MDS than patients treated in the 1970s with MOPP alone (10-year cumulative risks of 2.1 and 6.4%, respectively, $P = 0.07$) [31]. A recent international collaborative study showed that the AER of AML declined significantly after 1984, from 7.0 to 4.2 per 10,000 patients per year in those diagnosed before age 35 years, and from 16.4 to 9.9 per 10,000 patient-years in the $\geq 35$ age group [121].

There is, however, concern about the role of anthracyclines and epipodophyllotoxins (both of which are topoisomerase II inhibitors) in the risk of leukemia. Limited evidence suggests that doxorubicin in combination with higher doses of alkylating agents and/or epidophyllotoxins may have a synergistic effect on the risk of AML. Recent analyses of the German Hodgkin's Lymphoma Study Group also show low risks of AML after COPP/ABVD (mechlorethamine replaced by cyclophosphamide) and standard BEACOPP (bleomycin, etoposide, and doxorubicin combined with COPP), while substantially increased risk of AML was observed for the escalated BEACOPP regimen (actuarial risk at 5 years of 2.5%) [126, 127].

Some studies suggest that RT adds to the leukemia risk associated with CT [85, 128], whereas other large series indicate that the risk of AML after combined treatment is comparable to that after CT alone [29, 48, 51]. The interaction between RT and CT could be evaluated most rigorously in the large case–control study by Kaldor et al. [29] that included 163 cases of leukemia following HL. For each category of radiation dose (<10, 10–20, >20 Gy to the active bone marrow), leukemia risk clearly increased with the number of CT cycles. In contrast, among patients with a given number of CT cycles, risk of leukemia did not consistently increase with higher radiation dose. Taken together, the preponderance of available data does not support the hypothesis that the combination of CT and RT confers a higher risk of leukemia than CT alone.

Therapeutic intensification with autologous stem cell transplantation (ASCT) is increasingly used for lymphoma patients who relapse. In some series, relatively high actuarial risks (4–15% at 5 years) of AML

and MDS have been observed after ASCT for HL [85]. Evidence suggests that much of the risk is related to intensive pretransplant CT. Forrest et al. recently compared the risk of AML/MDS between 202 patients who had undergone ASCT and 1,530 patients who underwent conventional therapy for HL [129]. The 15-year cumulative incidence of developing AML/MDS was 1.1% (95% (CI), 0.6–1.8) for those treated with conventional therapy alone, and 3.6% (95% CI, 0.9–9.6) for those undergoing ASCT ($P = 0.22$). In multivariate analysis, leukemia risk was also not influenced by ASCT [129].

The risk of AML in relation to treatment-associated acute and chronic bone marrow toxicity has been examined in only two studies to date [51]. Significantly increased risks of leukemia were found among patients who developed thrombocytopenia, either in response to initial therapy or during follow-up. After adjustment for type and amount of CT, patients who showed a $\geq 70\%$ decrease in platelet counts after initial treatment had an approximately fivefold higher risk of developing leukemia than patients who showed a decrease of 50% or less [51]. Severe acute thrombocytopenia may indicate greater bioavailability of cytotoxic drugs, which would likely contribute to the development of leukemia. In support of these findings, a study of leukemia risk after autologous bone marrow transplantation found that low platelet counts at the time of transplant were predictive for MDS/AML development in NHL patients who had received intensive pretransplant CT [130].

The prognosis of AML/MDS after HL treatment is extremely poor, with only 15% of patients surviving more than 1 year and no apparent survival benefit from allogenic stem cell transplantation [85, 127].

## 22.5.2 Risk Factors of Non-Hodgkin Lymphoma

Krikorian et al. were the first to demonstrate a clearly elevated cumulative risk of NHL after HL, which amounted to 4.4% at 10 years in patients given both irradiation and CT [131]. Other investigators have confirmed the increased risk of NHL in HL survivors [4, 10, 31, 36, 46, 48–50, 52, 132]. In most studies, the SIR for NHL ranges between 6 and 36 compared to the risk in the general population (Table 22.1).

Because the background risk of NHL in the general population is low, this rather high SIR translates into a relatively low cumulative risk, ranging between 2 and 4% at 20 years [36, 48, 133] in the larger studies. AER in these studies has varied between five and ten excess NHL cases per 10,000 patients per year [46, 48]. The majority of cases of second NHL diagnosed after HL are intermediate or aggressive histology B-cell lymphomas [133–135], and more often arise in extranodal sites than primary NHL [133, 136] and 79% of cases [135].

The causes of the excess risk are not well understood. The results of older studies may in part reflect misclassification of the primary lymphoma in the absence of modern lymphoma immunophenotyping protocols (i.e., NHL misdiagnosed as HL) [133]. Rueffer et al. [133] reported that an expert panel of pathologists reviewing the histology of 4,104 HL patients (German Hodgkin's Lymphoma Study Group) rejected 114 cases (2.1%) initially diagnosed as HL and rediagnosed them as primary NHL. Only very few studies included a review of diagnostic pathology slides of the second NHL and original HL in order to avoid such misclassification [31, 50, 133].

Other investigators argued that the clinical, histologic, and immunophenotypic findings of NHL among HL survivors were analogous to those of NHL arising in immunosuppressed patients, suggesting that immunodeficiency plays a role in the pathogenesis of second NHL in these patients [135]. This view is supported by several studies in which risk did not vary appreciably between treatments [10, 48, 82]. However, in other studies, the risk of NHL was found to be lowest among patients treated with RT alone, and highest among patients who received intensive combined modality treatment, both initially and for relapse [31, 52, 131, 133, 137].

There exists some evidence indicating that transformation to NHL may be part of the natural history of the lymphocyte predominant subtype of HL [136, 138], which might explain the association between lymphocyte predominant HL and NHL risk observed in the International Database on HL [52] and the British National Lymphoma Investigation [139]. It may be that more than one of the above mechanisms operates in the development of NHL following treatment for HL. Although transformation to NHL may be part of the natural history of some types of HL, the role of intensive combined modality treatment and its

associated immunosuppression should be explored further. Future studies should incorporate a review of all slides of the second NHL and the original HL diagnosis by an expert pathologist.

## 22.5.3 Risk Factors for Breast Cancer

For female HL survivors, the strongly elevated risk of breast cancer following RT has become a major concern [36, 46, 79, 140–144]. In several recent studies breast cancer contributes most to the AER of second malignancy in female survivors [4, 36, 49, 61, 145]. The magnitude of the risk of breast cancer after HL and risk factors for its development have been discussed in several review papers [58, 146, 147]. The risk of breast cancer after HL greatly depends on age at treatment, time since treatment, therapies given for HL, and hormonal factors.

The overall SIR of breast cancer in female HL survivors has been only modestly elevated in studies which included all age groups (about 1.5- to 2.2-fold risk increases compared to the general population) (Table 22.1) [28, 31, 46, 48, 52, 125, 148]. Larger SIRs (four- to seven fold) were observed in studies with predominantly young adults, or a large proportion of long-term survivors [4, 35, 36, 79, 132]. AERs for all ages have been around 2–10 per 10,000 HL patients per year [31, 46, 48] (Table 22.2), again with a greater risk (20–60 per 10,000 per year) in recent studies with predominantly young adults and/or a large proportion of long-term survivors [4, 36, 79, 132]. Several studies covering the whole age range have shown that the SIR of developing breast cancer increases dramatically with younger age at first irradiation (or start of treatment) [4, 36, 46, 48, 61, 79, 132, 149] (Fig. 22.2). A strong trend of increasing SIR of breast cancer with decreasing age at exposure has also been observed in other radiation-exposed cohorts [150–153]. In a recent Dutch study, survivors who had radiation treatment before 21 years of age had an 18-fold increased risk of breast cancer compared with the general female population of the same age; women irradiated at ages 21–30 had a seven fold increased risk; women irradiated at ages 31–40 had a 3.2-fold increased risk; and a small, nonsignificant increase was observed for women irradiated at ages 41 or older (SIR, 1.4) [79]. Similar trends have been reported by others [4, 35, 46]. Most studies confirm that breast cancer risk is not elevated compared with the general population in women treated after age 35–40 [4, 46, 48, 79]. In most studies, the AER of breast cancer is also highest after treatment before age 20 [4, 36, 46, 47, 79] (Fig. 22.2), but shows little variation between exposure at ages 20–35.

Three recent studies with long-term follow-up reported that, among women treated before age 20, the SIR compared with age-matched peers from the general population did not consistently vary by age at treatment [49, 69, 154]. It is important to note here that consequently, prepubertal radiation exposure increases the risk to the same extent as exposure during puberty. In the atomic bomb survivors and other radiation-exposed cohorts, the RR also did not vary by exposure age for ages under 20 [155]. The SIR of breast cancer after HL treatment at ages under 16 has ranged from 17 to 458 [82, 83, 156], with most studies showing SIRs around 50–100 [4, 35, 36, 49, 148, 149, 154, 157].

The large variation in breast cancer risks across studies, especially in young patients, is not surprising in view of the large differences between series in important variables such as the proportion of patients irradiated, duration of follow-up, and completeness of follow-up. Studies with more complete follow-up have generally found lower risks of breast cancer [36, 46, 48, 83, 157] than those in which follow-up was less complete, or not addressed [81, 82, 149]

Incomplete follow-up may lead to overestimation of second malignancy risk if patients who remain well lose contact with clinical follow-up, while those with second cancer come to attention because of this. In a recent Dutch study, with (nearly) complete follow-up, the 30-year cumulative incidence of breast cancer (accounting for death as a competing risk) amounted to 26% for women first treated before age 21 and 19% for those treated at ages 20–30 [79]. In pediatric HL survivors, Bhatia et al [49]. estimated a cumulative incidence of breast cancer of 13.9% at age 40 years, reaching 20.1% at age 45 years. Kenney et al. [154] recently reported quite similar risk estimates, i.e., a cumulative incidence of 12.9% (95% CI, 9.3–16.5) at age 40 in the U.S. Childhood Cancer Survivor Study. Travis and collaborators [158] estimated treatment-specific cumulative risks of breast cancer: for a HL survivor who was treated at age 25 with a chest radiation dose of at least 40 Gy without alkylating agents, the cumulative absolute risks of breast cancer by age 35, 45, and 55 years were 1.4% (95% CI, 0.9–2.1),

11.1% (95% CI, 7.4–16.3), and 29.0% (95% CI, 20.2–40.1), respectively [158].

The high risk of breast cancer after HL is largely attributable to chest RT. Since in many cohort studies 80 to over 90% of patients received supradiaphragmatic RT, few studies could estimate RRs associated with such RT compared with no RT [4, 36, 49, 79, 132]. In the British cohort reported by Swerdlow et al. [48], a large proportion of patients had been treated with CT alone, and the risk of breast cancer was increased only after RT without CT. In women treated at ages younger than 25 years, the risk of breast cancer was increased 14.4-fold (95% CI, 5.7–29.3) after RT alone, which was significantly greater than the SIR of 4.6 among those treated with mixed modalities; no breast cancers occurred in women treated solely with CT.

Elevated risk of breast cancer develops late and is typically observed from 15 or more years after first treatment [4, 36, 46, 48, 79, 132] (Fig. 22.6). This strong trend in breast cancer risk by time since treatment strongly indicates of a radiogenic effect. Furthermore, in several cohort studies almost all cases of breast cancer after HL have been in or at the margin of the radiation field: for instance, 16 of 16 cases [83], 22 of 26 cases [35], and all of 42 cases [49] in three publications. In the large, population-based study by Travis et al. [42], 49% of 105 breast cancers occurred in the unblocked chest treatment field, 24% under the lung blocks, 15% at the blocked edge, 8% in the field edge, and 3% out-of-beam, with relative location not known for one patient.

Three case–control studies investigated the effects of RT dose and other treatment factors on breast cancer risk [42, 45, 69]. In all studies, the risk of breast cancer increased significantly with higher RT dose up to the highest dose levels (Table 22.3; see for details Sect. 4.1). A recent, large Dutch study examined the effect of radiation fields (volume) on the risk of breast cancer up to more than 30 years after treatment of HL [79]. Among 1,122 female 5-year survivors treated for HL before age 51 (median follow-up time of 18 years), 120 cases of breast cancer were identified (overall SIR 5.6; AER 57 per 10,000 patients per year). Importantly, mantle field RT (involving the axillary, mediastinal, and neck nodes) was associated with a 2.7-fold (95% CI, 1.1–6.9) increased risk of breast cancer compared to similarly dosed (36–44 Gy) radiation to the mediastinum alone [79] (Fig. 22.5).

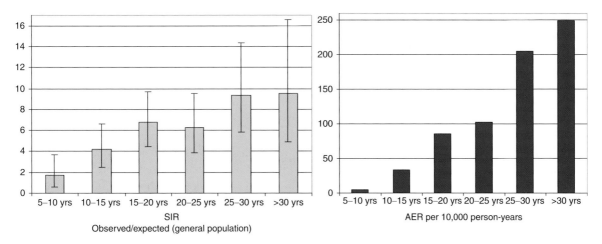

**Fig. 22.6** Risk of breast cancer after HL by follow-up time (1,122 Dutch HL patients). (Adapted from [79])

In three studies, patients who received both CT and RT had significantly decreased risk (about halved) compared to those treated with RT alone, and the RT-related risks were attenuated by treatment with alkylating agents [42, 45, 79]. Risk of breast cancer decreased with increasing number of alkylating agent cycles ($P=0.003$ for trend); the RR associated with nine or more cycles of alkylating CT compared with no alkylating CT was 0.2 (95% CI, 0.1–0.7) [42] (Table 22.3). In the recent large Dutch cohort study [79], CT regimens with higher cumulative procarbazine doses seemed to be associated with a greater reduction of breast cancer risk, with 40 and 60% risk reductions for regimens with less than 8.4 g/m² procarbazine and more than 8.4 g/m² procarbazine, respectively. The substantial risk reduction associated with CT appears to be due to the high frequency of premature menopause in CT-treated patients [45, 79] and the resulting reduction in the exposure to ovarian hormones. In a recent study [79], 30% of all women reached menopause before age 41; such an early menopause was associated with a 60% (95% CI, 20–80%) reduced risk of breast cancer (Table 22.4). A strong decrease in breast cancer risk (about 60%) has also been observed among women who received a castrating dose of 5 Gy or more to the ovaries, compared with those who received lower doses [42, 45, 69, 79] (Fig. 22.4). These results indicate that ovarian hormones are a crucial factor to promote tumorigenesis once RT has produced an initiating event.

In the Dutch study, a long vs. short duration of intact ovarian function after radiation was a strong predictor of subsequent breast cancer risk. Women with less than 10 years of intact ovarian function after RT had a 70% (95% CI, 40–80%) decreased risk of breast cancer compared with women with 10–20 years of ovarian function after irradiation, while those with more than 20 years of intact ovarian function after RT had 5.3-fold (95% CI, 2.9–9.9) increased risk of breast cancer (Table 22.4). These risk reductions were observed both among women treated before age 21, and among those treated between ages 21 and 30. Among women treated between ages 31 and 40, cumulative exposure to endogenous estrogens was not associated with risk for breast cancer, possibly because these women were closer to natural menopause at time of treatment [79].

It is not yet known whether current less gonadotoxic CT, such as ABVD, is also associated with reduced risk of RT-associated breast cancer risk. Furthermore, we do not yet know whether hormone replacement therapy (HRT) for CT-induced premature menopause affects RT-associated breast cancer risk. HRT is an established risk factor for breast cancer [159, 160], and might counteract the protective effect of CT. Remarkably, in the international case–control study by Travis et al. [42], the relation between alkylating agent treatment and breast cancer risk differed between North America and European centers. Within Europe, significant reductions in risk were observed (for six cycles: RR=0.33; 95% CI, 0.15–0.65), while in North America the RR associated with six cycles of alkylating agent therapy was close to unity. These discrepant results may be due to the much higher prevalence of HRT in North America compared with Europe.

**Table 22.4** Effects of fertile lifespan after irradiation to the breast on BC risk (IBC+DCIS) according to age at first treatment[a]

|  | All ages <41 | Age <21 | Age 21–30 | Age 31–40 |
| --- | --- | --- | --- | --- |
| Number of patients | 715 | 201 | 323 | 191 |
| Number of events | 98 | 36 | 40 | 22 |
|  | HR (95% CI) | HR (95% CI) | HR (95% CI) | HR (95% CI) |
| Model 3[b] | | | | |
| *Premature menopause*[c] | | | | |
| Menopause at age 41 or later | 1 (Ref) | 1 (Ref) | 1 (Ref) | 1 (Ref) |
| Menopause before age 41 | 0.4 (0.2–0.8) | 0.2 (0.0–0.8) | 0.1 (0.0–0.5) | 1.3 (0.4–3.6) |
| Model 4[b] | | | | |
| *Years of intact ovarian function*[c] | | | | |
| <10 years | 0.3 (0.2–0.6) | 0.1 (0.0–0.6) | 0.1 (0.0–0.3) | 1.2 (0.4–3.5) |
| 10–20 years | 1 (Ref) | 1 (Ref) | 1 (Ref) | 1 (Ref) |
| >20 years | 5.3 (2.9–9.9 ) | 11.9 (3.7–37.9) | 6.0 (2.3–15.4) | 3.2 (0.3–30.7) |

*BC* breast cancer; *IBC* invasive breast cancer; *DCIS* ductal carcinoma in situ; *HR* hazard ratio; *Ref* referent; *RT* radiation therapy
[a]Adapted from [79]
[b]Adjusted for each other, radiation field size, age at first RT to the breast and time since first RT to the breast, smoking, obesity, nulliparity, oral contraceptive use; calendar-time was used as the time scale
[c]Unknown age at menopause was modeled as a separate category

In summary, chest RT at young ages is associated with a very high risk of breast cancer after 15 years and later, and this hazard needs to be borne in mind both when selecting treatment for girls and young women with HL and when following up patients treated in this way. Reductions of radiation dose and field size (replacement of mantle RT by involved field/ involved node RT) in current treatment protocols are expected to result in lower breast cancer risk. Gonadotoxic CT such as the MOPP regimen appears to reduce the increased risk of breast cancer from RT through the induction of premature menopause. The use of HRT may negate this favorable effect of CT, but direct information about this is lacking.

### 22.5.4 Risk Factors for Lung Cancer

Next to breast cancer, lung cancer accounts in many studies for the largest absolute excess of solid malignancy after HL [46, 48]. An excellent review of risk factors for lung cancer after HL has been published [161]. The risk of lung cancer after HL depends on time since treatment, age at treatment, treatments administered for HL, and smoking.

The SIR of lung cancer is hardly increased in the first 5 years after treatment, with larger SIRs (5 or greater) thereafter, until at least 25 years [4, 13, 36, 46, 48, 132]. SIRs of lung cancer decrease with older age at first treatment [4, 13, 36, 48, 132]. Dores et al. [46] reported that the SIR of lung cancer decreased from a 5.5-fold increase (compared with the general population) for patients diagnosed before age 21 to a 1.5-fold excess for patients diagnosed at age 61 or above. In a British study [48], the SIRs for lung cancer decreased from 20-fold among those diagnosed before age 25 to a 2.2-fold excess for patients diagnosed at age 55 or above.

A large international collaborative case–control study examined lung cancer risk in relation to the radiation dose to the specific location in the lung in which cancer later developed [13]. This study included 222 lung cancer patients and 444 matched controls (patients with HL in whom lung cancer had not been diagnosed) [13, 71]. Case patients developed lung cancer after an average of 10.8 years. The risk increased with increasing radiation dose to the area of the lung in which cancer later developed (*P* for trend <0.001; see also Table 22.3). The risk estimates for the highest dose categories of 30.0–39.9 Gy and ≥40 Gy compared with no RT were 8.5 (95% CI, 3.3–24) and 6.3 (95% CI, 2.2–19), respectively, suggesting that the risk might level off at very high doses [71]. This study also addressed the modifying effects of the patient's smoking habits on RT-associated risks. The increased RRs from smoking appeared to multiply the elevated risks

**Table 22.5** Risk of lung cancer in patients with HL according to type of treatment and smoking category[a]

| Treatment for Hodgkin Lymphoma | | RR (95% CI) by smoking category (number of case patients; control patients)[b] | |
| --- | --- | --- | --- |
| Radiation ≥5 Gy | Alkylating agents | Nonsmoker, light, other[c] | Moderate–heavy[d] |
| No | No | 1.0[e] | 6.0 (1.9–20.4) |
| Yes | No | 7.2 (2.9–21.2) | 20.2 (6.8–68) |
| No | Yes | 4.3 (1.8–11.7) | 16.8 (6.2–53) |
| Yes | Yes | 7.2 (2.8–21.6) | 49.1 (15.1–187) |

*RR* relative risk; *95% CI* 95% confidence interval
[a]Adapted from [13]
[b]Represents estimated tobacco smoking habit 5 years before diagnosis date of lung cancer and corresponding date in control patients, with the use of information recorded up to 1 year before these dates
[c]This group includes nonsmokers, light current cigarette smokers (less than one pack per day), former cigarette smokers, smokers of cigar and pipes only, and patients for whom tobacco smoking habit was not stated
[d]Moderate (one to two packs per day) and heavy (two or more packs per day) current cigarette smokers
[e]Reference group

from radiation (Table 22.5). This implies that there are very large AERs for lung cancer among irradiated patients who smoke.

CT for HL can also increase the risk of lung cancer [13, 48, 50, 161, 162]. The British National Lymphoma Investigation cohort study of 5,519 patients [48] showed a significantly elevated risk of lung cancer following CT alone, with the SIR (3.3; 95% CI, 2.2–4.7) compared with the general population being of similar magnitude to that observed in patients treated with either RT (SIR = 2.9; 95% CI, 1.9–4.1) or mixed modality treatment (SIR = 4.3; 95% CI, 2.9–6.2).

Two large case–control studies have investigated the separate and joint roles of CT, radiation, and smoking in detail [13, 72]. In both reports, there was a clear trend of increasing lung cancer risk with greater number of cycles of alkylating CT (*P* trend <0.001; Table 22.3) [13] or MOPP-CT (*P* trend = 0.07) [72]. In the study by Travis et al. [13], data were also collected on cumulative dose of individual cytotoxic drugs. Among patients treated with MOPP, increasing total dose of mechlorethamine or procarbazine was strongly associated with increasing lung cancer risk when evaluated separately (*P* trend for dose for each <0.001) [13]. Risk of lung cancer after treatment with alkylating agents and radiation together was as expected if individual excess RRs were summed: RRs of 4.2 (95% CI, 2.1–8.8) were observed for patients given alkylating agents alone, 5.9 (95% CI, 2.7–13.5) for patients treated with RT alone (>5 Gy), and 8.0 (95% CI, 3.6–18.5) for those who received combined modality

treatment, compared with the reference group of patients who received no alkylating agents and had less than 5 Gy of radiation [13]. As was observed for the joint effects of smoking and RT, the risks from smoking appeared to at least multiply risks from alkylating CT [13] (Table 22.5).

Smoking remains a major cause of lung cancer in patients treated for HL, as is evident from the observation that only 7 out of 222 cases included in the study by Travis et al. [13] occurred in patients who had never smoked. Further, it was estimated that 9.6% of all lung cancers were due to treatment, 24% were due to smoking, but 63% were due to treatment and smoking in combination; the remainder (3%) represented tumors in which neither smoking nor treatment played a role.

In summary, both supradiaphragmatic RT and CT contribute to the elevated risk of lung cancer after HL. In addition, the above data suggest that patients with HL who smoke will have a considerably greater risk of lung cancer after chest RT and/or CT than those who do not smoke, and this is in accord with experience in other radiation-exposed groups [163]. As a consequence, smokers who have received chest RT should be particularly strongly advised to refrain from smoking. The evidence implicating specific chemotherapeutic agents as carcinogenic to the lung is less clear. It is not yet known whether modern CT regimens other than MOPP also increase the risk of lung cancer. The role of lung cancer screening in HL patients has not yet been assessed; international collaboration is needed to study the efficacy of screening with low dose spiral computer tomography [161].

## 22.6 Clincal Implications

HL survivors who are at high risk of developing second cancers can be identified largely based on their prior treatment exposures, current age, and latency since treatment. Expert opinion-based recommendations have been published advocating the early onset of breast cancer screening starting 8–10 years following mediastinal RT, for women who are aged 25–30 [164, 165]. However, a large proportion of irradiated females do not perceive their risk of breast cancer to be much higher than that of the general population [166–169]. As a consequence, a large proportion of HL survivors do currently not undergo appropriate breast surveillance at young ages, when their risk is already high and comparable to that of carriers of BRCA1/2 mutations. A recent study among irradiated female childhood cancer survivors in the United States showed that 64% of those aged 25–39 years and 24% of those 40–50 years old had not had a mammography in the past 2 years, despite a guideline recommending annual screening [169]. In the UK, in 2003 the Department of Health recalled 5,000 survivors treated with mantle RT before age 35 to educate them about their risk and to recommend breast cancer screening [166]. Although early breast surveillance starting is recommended following mediastinal RT, the efficacy of various screening procedures has not been demonstrated. Two series found that 90% or more of breast cancers after HL were visible on mammography [168, 170] and a recent British study of screening program for women previously treated with supradiaphragmatic RT found that none of the five invasive BCs diagnosed involved axillary lymph nodes, compared with 7 of 13 (54%) diagnosed outside the program [171]. However, in one of these studies, after excluding two cases of incident breast cancer on baseline mammogram, five of the secondary 10 breast cancers in were detected clinically [168], and in another series of female HL survivors undergoing mammographic screening 7 of 12 breast cancers were palpable at the time of detection [172]. Because mammography is less sensitive in young women with dense breast tissue, (MRI) should be considered at younger ages.

Some have recommended that patients who have received para-aortic RT should undergo colorectal cancer screening starting 10–15 years following treatment (www.survivorshipguidelines.org). Screening for secondary lung cancer is more controversial. As noted above, older HL survivors treated with alkylating agents or mantle RT are at significantly increased risk of developing lung cancer, particularly if they are smokers. One important consideration is that the absolute risk of lung cancer is low among non-smoking patients treated before age 30 with contemporary CT (e.g., ABVD, doxorubicin, bleomycin, vinblastine, dacarbazine), and it is unlikely that they would benefit from screening. Risk is highest among those treated with chest RT and alklyator-based CT at ages >40 years, particularly if they are smokers. The results of studies evaluating the efficacy of screening with spiral computer tomography in other high-risk patients may illuminate the potential benefit to HL survivors, but it currently remains investigational.

Physicians should make a special effort to dissuade HL patients from smoking. While most survivors will be aware that smoking increases their risk of lung cancer, they may not understand that their smoking-related risk may be significantly greater than that of others with whom they share the activity, and they are often not aware of the poor prognosis associated with lung cancer. Advice on smoking cessation during an office visit can improve quit rates, and pharmacotherapy improves the probability of success [173].

While retrospective studies describing the RT-related risk of SMNs have been useful in identifying groups of survivors for whom the early utilization of cancer screening may be worthwhile, and have been instrumental in motivating the development of clinical trials, which are now much less reliant on the use of RT, it is important to recognize that they often have limited value in counseling contemporary patients about the risks of modern therapy. For example, most of the widely cited cohort studies of SMN risk among HL survivors include patients treated in the 1960s [31, 46, 48, 49, 62]. At that time, RT was often the sole primary treatment for early stage HL, and the RT fields typically encompassed the whole neck, bilateral axillae, the entire length of the mediastinum, the spleen, and para-aortic nodes. Patients were often prescribed 40–45 Gy and treated without customized lung shielding [174, 175]. Since that time, several important improvements have occurred in the delivery of RT that reduce the normal tissue exposure: prescribed doses are typically 20–30 Gy for adults and 21 Gy for children; in the majority of cases, the axillae can be excluded from mediastinal IFRT, thereby reducing breast and lung dose; it is rarely necessary to irradiate the spleen, which can also be a source of exposure to the left breast, lung, and heart; improved imaging of the target volume, patient immobilization, customized shielding, and compensation for tissue inhomogeneity can reduce the amount of normal tissue exposed and the occurrence of "hot spots" in normal tissues. As noted previously, these changes have been shown to significantly reduce the normal tissue exposure associated with IFRT [78], and early clinical studies of more limited field RT suggest that the RT volume reduction translates into a clinically significant reduction in SMN risk [79, 80].

Similarly, many patients in second cancer studies received MOPP CT, and the increased SMN risks associated with alkylator-based CT do not apply to patients receiving, for example, ABVD CT. The existing SMN studies support the use of abbreviated CT regimens and lower doses of RT for selected patients, for whom excellent rates of lymphoma control have been reported.

As an increasing proportion of patients are treated with CT alone, an emerging issue will be the extent to which contemporary CT regimens contribute to the risk of solid tumors. Patients treated initially with CT alone, even in more recent years, have increased risks of solid cancers [61], though it is unknown what regimens or specific agents might account for this risk. Large studies will be needed to examine whether modern CT regimens affect the risk of specific solid tumors. Similarly, as our understanding of the relationship between radiation dose and SMN risk develops, it should be possible to create predictive models of the SMN risk associated with modern HL treatments. Epidemiologic studies can contribute to the development of accurate predictive models.

As noted above, genetic susceptibility likely plays a role in the development of treatment-related SMNs. It is unlikely that an abnormal allele in a single candidate gene will account for a significant proportion of SMNs. New cohorts should be assembled to create a resource of biologic samples that would facilitate study of the molecular biology of second cancers.

Finally, when interpreting results of second cancer studies, it must be kept in mind that the problem of treatment-induced malignancies has arisen by virtue of the successes of HL treatment. The SMN risk of treatment must be balanced against the potential benefit in terms of curing patients' HL. For example, 10-year follow-up of patients treated with "dose escalated" BEACOPP demonstrated that this regimen increased the risk of secondary AML compared to COPP/ABVD (0.4 vs. 3.0%), but produced a significant improvement in overall survival (75 vs. 86%) [176]. These outcomes highlight both the challenges of improving the cure rate for high-risk patients without adding clinically significant toxicity, and the importance of considering SMN risk in the context of the beneficial effects that the exposures under study may have on curing the primary HL.

# References

1. Aleman BM, van den Belt-Dusebout AW, Klokman WJ, van't Veer MB, Bartelink H, van Leeuwen FE. Long-term cause-specific mortality of patients treated for Hodgkin's disease. J Clin Oncol. 2003;21:3431–9.
2. Arseneau JC, Sponzo RW, Levin DL, Schnipper LE, Bonner H, Young RC, et al. Nonlymphomatous malignant tumors complicating Hodgkin's disease. Possible association with intensive therapy. N Engl J Med. 1972;287:1119–22.
3. Aviles A, Neri N, Cuadra I, Alvarado I, Cleto S. Second lethal events associated with treatment for Hodgkin's disease: a review of 2980 patients treated in a single Mexican institute. Leuk Lymphoma. 2000;39:311–9.
4. Ng AK, Bernardo MV, Weller E, Backstrand K, Silver B, Marcus KC, et al. Second malignancy after Hodgkin disease treated with radiation therapy with or without chemotherapy: long-term risks and risk factors. Blood. 2002;100:1989–96.
5. Bonadonna G, De Lena M, Banfi A, Lattuada A. Secondary neoplasms in malignant lymphomas after intensive therapy. N Engl J Med. 1973;288:1242–3.
6. Canellos GP, Arseneau JC, DeVita VT, Whang-Peng J, Johnson RE. Second malignancies complicating Hodgkin's disease in remission. Lancet. 1975;1:947–9.
7. Coleman CN, McDougall IR, Dailey MO, Ager P, Bush S, Kaplan HS. Functional hyposplenia after splenic irradiation for Hodgkin's disease. Ann Intern Med. 1982;96:44–7.
8. Boivin JF, Hutchison GB, Lyden M, Godbold J, Chorosh J, Schottenfeld D. Second primary cancers following treatment of Hodgkin's disease. J Natl Cancer Inst. 1984;72:233–41.
9. Henry-Amar M. Second cancers after radiotherapy and chemotherapy for early stages of Hodgkin's disease. J Natl Cancer Inst. 1983;71:911–6.
10. Tucker MA, Coleman CN, Cox RS, Varghese A, Rosenberg SA. Risk of second cancers after treatment for Hodgkin's disease. N Engl J Med. 1988;318:76–81.
11. van Leeuwen FE, Somers R, Taal BG, van Heerde P, Coster B, Dozeman T, et al. Increased risk of lung cancer, non-Hodgkin's lymphoma, and leukemia following Hodgkin's disease. J Clin Oncol. 1989;7:1046–58.
12. Boice Jr JD, Storm HH, Curtis RE, Jensen OM, Kleinerman RA, Jensen HS, et al. Introduction to the study of multiple primary cancers. Natl Cancer Inst Monogr. 1985;68:3–9.
13. Travis LB, Gospodarowicz M, Curtis RE, Clarke EA, Andersson M, Glimelius B, et al. Lung cancer following chemotherapy and radiotherapy for Hodgkin's disease. J Natl Cancer Inst. 2002;94:182–92.

14. Kaldor JM, Day NE, Shiboski S. Epidemiological studies of anticancer drug carcinogenicity. IARC Sci Publ. 1986;78: 189–201.
15. Kyle RA, Pierre RV, Bayrd ED. Multiple myeloma and acute myelomonocytic leukemia. N Engl J Med. 1970;283: 1121–5.
16. Rosner F, Grunwald H. Multiple myeloma terminating in acute leukemia. Report of 12 cases and review of the literature [Review]. Am J Med. 1974;57:927–39.
17. Makuch R, Simon R. Recommendations for the analysis of the effect of treatment on the development of second malignancies. Cancer. 1979;44:250–3.
18. Schoenberg BS, Myers MH. Statistical methods for studying multiple primary malignant neoplasms. Cancer. 1977;40: 1892–8.
19. Kaplan EL, Meier P. Non-parametric estimation from incomplete observations. J Am Stat Assoc. 1958;53:457–81.
20. Darrington DL, Vose JM, Anderson JR, Bierman PJ, Bishop MR, Chan WC, et al. Incidence and characterization of secondary myelodysplastic syndrome and acute myelogenous leukemia following high-dose chemoradiotherapy and autologous stem-cell transplantation for lymphoid malignancies. J Clin Oncol. 1994;12:2527–34.
21. Gooley TA, Leisenring W, Crowley J, Storer BE. Estimation of failure probabilities in the presence of competing risks: new representations of old estimators. Stat Med. 1999;18: 695–706.
22. Mauch PM, Kalish LA, Marcus KC, Shulman LN, Krill E, Tarbell NJ, et al. Long-term survival in Hodgkin's disease: relative impact of mortality, second tumors, infection, and cardiovascular disease. Cancer J Sci Am. 1995;1: 33–42.
23. Pepe MS, Mori M. Kaplan-Meier, marginal or conditional probability curves in summarizing competing risks failure time data? Stat Med. 1993;12:737–51.
24. Travis LB, Curtis RE, Glimelius B, Holowaty E, van Leeuwen FE, Lynch CF, et al. Second cancers among long-term survivors of non-Hodgkin's lymphoma. J Natl Cancer Inst. 1993;85:1932–7.
25. Breslow NE, Day NE. Statistical methods in cancer research. Volume II – the design and analysis of cohort studies. IARC Sci Publ. 1987;82:1–406.
26. Cox DR. Regression models and life-tables. J R Stat Soc B. 1972;334:187–202.
27. Boice Jr JD, Day NE, Andersen A, Brinton LA, Brown R, Choi NW, et al. Second cancers following radiation treatment for cervical cancer. An international collaboration among cancer registries. J Natl Cancer Inst. 1985;74:955–75.
28. Kaldor JM, Day NE, Band P, Choi NW, Clarke EA, Coleman MP, et al. Second malignancies following testicular cancer, ovarian cancer and Hodgkin's disease: an international collaborative study among cancer registries. Int J Cancer. 1987;39:571–85.
29. Kaldor JM, Day NE, Clarke EA, van Leeuwen FE, Henry-Amar M, Fiorentino MV, et al. Leukemia following Hodgkin's disease [see Comments]. N Engl J Med. 1990;322:7–13.
30. Storm HH, Prener A. Second cancer following lymphatic and hematopoietic cancers in Denmark, 1943–80. Natl Cancer Inst Monogr. 1985;68:389–409.
31. van Leeuwen FE, Klokman WJ, Hagenbeek A, Noyon R, van den Belt-Dusebout AW, van Kerkhoff EH, et al. Second cancer risk following Hodgkin's disease: a 20-year follow-up study. J Clin Oncol. 1994;12:312–25.
32. Greene MH. Is cisplatin a human carcinogen? [Review]. J Natl Cancer Inst. 1992;84:306–12.
33. Travis LB, Rabkin CS, Brown LM, Allan JM, Alter BP, Ambrosone CB, et al. Cancer survivorship – genetic susceptibility and second primary cancers: research strategies and recommendations. J Natl Cancer Inst. 2006;98:15–25.
34. Coleman CN, Williams CJ, Flint A, Glatstein EJ, Rosenberg SA, Kaplan HS. Hematologic neoplasia in patients treated for Hodgkin's disease. N Engl J Med. 1977;297:1249–52.
35. Hancock SL, Tucker MA, Hoppe RT. Breast cancer after treatment of Hodgkin's disease. J Natl Cancer Inst. 1993; 85:25–31.
36. van Leeuwen FE, Klokman WJ, van't Veer MB, Hagenbeek A, Krol AD, Vetter UA, et al. Long-term risk of second malignancy in survivors of Hodgkin's disease treated during adolescence or young adulthood. J Clin Oncol. 2000;18: 487–97.
37. Boice Jr JD, Blettner M, Kleinerman RA, Stovall M, Moloney WC, Engholm G, et al. Radiation dose and leukemia risk in patients treated for cancer of the cervix. J Natl Cancer Inst. 1987;79:1295–311.
38. Boice Jr JD, Harvey EB, Blettner M, Stovall M, Flannery JT. Cancer in the contralateral breast after radiotherapy for breast cancer [see Comments]. N Engl J Med. 1992;326: 781–5.
39. Curtis RE, Boice Jr JD, Stovall M, Bernstein L, Greenberg RS, Flannery JT, et al. Risk of leukemia after chemotherapy and radiation treatment for breast cancer [see Comments]. N Engl J Med. 1992;326:1745–51.
40. Kaldor JM, Day NE, Pettersson F, Clarke EA, Pedersen D, Mehnert W, et al. Leukemia following chemotherapy for ovarian cancer [see Comments]. N Engl J Med. 1990;322:1–6.
41. Travis LB, Curtis RE, Glimelius B, Holowaty EJ, van Leeuwen FE, Lynch CF, et al. Bladder and kidney cancer following cyclophosphamide therapy for non-Hodgkin's lymphoma. J Natl Cancer Inst. 1995;87:524–30.
42. Travis LB, Hill DA, Dores GM, Gospodarowicz M, van Leeuwen FE, Holowaty E, et al. Breast cancer following radiotherapy and chemotherapy among young women with Hodgkin's disease. JAMA. 2003;290:465–75.
43. Tucker MA, D'Angio GJ, Boice Jr JD, Strong LC, Li FP, Stovall M, et al. Bone sarcomas linked to radiotherapy and chemotherapy in children. N Engl J Med. 1987;317: 588–93.
44. Tucker MA, Meadows AT, Boice Jr JD, Stovall M, Oberlin O, Stone BJ, et al. Leukemia after therapy with alkylating agents for childhood cancer. J Natl Cancer Inst. 1987;78: 459–64.
45. van Leeuwen FE, Klokman WJ, Stovall M, Dahler EC, van't Veer MB, Noordijk EM, et al. Roles of radiation dose, chemotherapy, and hormonal factors in breast cancer following Hodgkin's disease. J Natl Cancer Inst. 2003;95:971–80.
46. Dores GM, Metayer C, Curtis RE, Lynch CF, Clarke EA, Glimelius B, et al. Second malignant neoplasms among long-term survivors of Hodgkin's disease: a population-based evaluation over 25 years. J Clin Oncol. 2002;20: 3484–94.
47. Hodgson DC, Pintilie M, Gitterman L, Dewitt B, Buckley CA, Ahmed S, et al. Fertility among female Hodgkin

lymphoma survivors attempting pregnancy following ABVD chemotherapy. Hematol Oncol. 2007;25:11–5.

48. Swerdlow AJ, Barber JA, Hudson GV, Cunningham D, Gupta RK, Hancock BW, et al. Risk of second malignancy after Hodgkin's disease in a collaborative British cohort: the relation to age at treatment. J Clin Oncol. 2000;18:498–509.

49. Bhatia S, Yasui Y, Robison LL, Birch JM, Bogue MK, Diller L, et al. High risk of subsequent neoplasms continues with extended follow-up of childhood Hodgkin's disease: report from the Late Effects Study Group. J Clin Oncol. 2003; 21:4386–94.

50. Swerdlow AJ, Douglas AJ, Hudson GV, Hudson BV, Bennett MH, MacLennan KA. Risk of second primary cancers after Hodgkin's disease by type of treatment: analysis of 2846 patients in the British National Lymphoma Investigation. BMJ. 1992;304:1137–43.

51. van Leeuwen FE, Chorus AM, van den Belt-Dusebout AW, Hagenbeek A, Noyon R, van Kerkhoff EH, et al. Leukemia risk following Hodgkin's disease: relation to cumulative dose of alkylating agents, treatment with teniposide combinations, number of episodes of chemotherapy, and bone marrow damage. J Clin Oncol. 1994;12:1063–73.

52. Henry-Amar M. Second cancer after the treatment for Hodgkin's disease: a report from the International Database on Hodgkin's disease. Ann Oncol. 1992;3 suppl 4:117–28.

53. Birdwell SH, Hancock SL, Varghese A, Cox RS, Hoppe RT. Gastrointestinal cancer after treatment of Hodgkin's disease. Int J Radiat Oncol Biol Phys. 1997;37:67–73.

54. Constine L, Tarbell N, Hudson M, Schwartz C, Fisher S, Muhs A, et al. Subsequent malignancies in children treated for Hodgkin's disease: associations with gender and radiation dose. Int J Radiat Oncol Biol Phys. 2008;72:24–33.

55. Hancock SL, Tucker MA, Hoppe RT. Factors affecting late mortality from heart disease after treatment of Hodgkin's disease. JAMA. 1993;270:1949–55.

56. Ahsan H, Neugut AI. Radiation therapy for breast cancer and increased risk for esophageal carcinoma. Ann Intern Med. 1998;128:114–7.

57. Antman KH, Corson JM, Li FP, Greenberger J, Sytkowski A, Henson DE, et al. Malignant mesothelioma following radiation exposure. J Clin Oncol. 1983;1:695–700.

58. Clemons M, Loijens L, Goss P. Breast cancer risk following irradiation for Hodgkin's disease. Cancer Treat Rev. 2000;26:291–302.

59. Preston DL, Ron E, Tokuoka S, Funamoto S, Nishi N, Soda M, et al. Solid cancer incidence in atomic bomb survivors: 1958–1998. Radiat Res. 2007;168:1–64.

60. Ron E, Lubin JH, Shore RE, Mabuchi K, Modan B, Pottern LM, et al. Thyroid cancer after exposure to external radiation: a pooled analysis of seven studies. Radiat Res. 1995; 141:259–77.

61. Hodgson DC, Gilbert ES, Dores GM, Schonfeld SJ, Lynch CF, Storm H, et al. Long-term solid cancer risk among 5-year survivors of Hodgkin's lymphoma. J Clin Oncol. 2007; 25:1489–97.

62. Metayer C, Lynch CF, Clarke EA, Glimelius B, Storm H, Pukkala E, et al. Second cancers among long-term survivors of Hodgkin's disease diagnosed in childhood and adolescence. J Clin Oncol. 2000;18:2435–43.

63. Preston DL, Mattsson A, Holmberg E, Shore R, Hildreth NG, Boice Jr JD. Radiation effects on breast cancer risk: a pooled analysis of eight cohorts. Radiat Res. 2002;158: 220–35.

64. Preston DL, Shimizu Y, Pierce DA, Suyama A, Mabuchi K. Studies of mortality of atomic bomb survivors. Report 13: solid cancer and noncancer disease mortality: 1950–1997. Radiat Res. 2003;160:381–407.

65. Ronckers C, Erdmann C, Land C. Radiation and breast cancer: a review of current evidence. Breast Cancer Res. 2005; 7:21–32.

66. Curtis RE, Boice Jr JD, Stovall M, Bernstein L, Holowaty E, Karjalainen S, et al. Relationship of leukemia risk to radiation dose following cancer of the uterine corpus. J Natl Cancer Inst. 1994;86:1315–24.

67. Preston DL, Kusumi S, Tomonaga M, Izumi S, Ron E, Kuramoto A, Kamada N, Dohy H, Matsuo T, Matsui T, et al. Cancer incidence in atomic bomb survivors. Part III. Leukemia, lymphoma and multiple myeloma, 1950–1987. Radiat Res.1994;137:S68–97. [Published erratum appears in Radiat Res. 1994;139(1):129].

68. Boice Jr JD, Engholm G, Kleinerman RA, Blettner M, Stovall M, Lisco H, et al. Radiation dose and second cancer risk in patients treated for cancer of the cervix. Radiat Res. 1988;116:3–55.

69. Inskip PD, Robison LL, Stovall M, Smith SA, Hammond S, Mertens AC, et al. Radiation dose and breast cancer risk in the childhood cancer survivor study. J Clin Oncol. 2009;27: 3901–7.

70. Neglia JP, Robison LL, Stovall M, Liu Y, Packer RJ, Hammond S, et al. New primary neoplasms of the central nervous system in survivors of childhood cancer: a report from the Childhood Cancer Survivor Study. J Natl Cancer Inst. 2006;98:1528–37.

71. Gilbert ES, Stovall M, Gospodarowicz M, van Leeuwen FE, Andersson M, Glimelius B, et al. Lung cancer after treatment for Hodgkin's disease: focus on radiation effects. Radiat Res. 2003;159:161–73.

72. Swerdlow AJ, Schoemaker MJ, Allerton R, Horwich A, Barber JA, Cunningham D, et al. Lung cancer after Hodgkin's disease: a nested case–control study of the relation to treatment. J Clin Oncol. 2001;19:1610–8.

73. Hawkins MM, Wilson LM, Burton HS, Potok MH, Winter DL, Marsden HB, et al. Radiotherapy, alkylating agents, and risk of bone cancer after childhood cancer. J Natl Cancer Inst. 1996;88:270–8.

74. Jenkinson HC, Winter DL, Marsden HB, Stovall MA, Stevens MCG, Stiller CA, et al. A study of soft tissue sarcomas after childhood cancer in Britain. Br J Cancer. 2007;97:695–9.

75. van den Belt-Dusebout AW, Aleman BM, Besseling G, De Bruin ML, Hauptmann M, van't Veer LJ, de Wit R, Ribot JG, Noordijk E, Kerst JM, Gietema JA, van Leeuwen FE. Roles of radiation dose and chemotherapy in the etiology of stomach cancer as a second malignancy. Int J Rad Oncol Biol Phys. 2009;75(5):1420–9.

76. Sigurdson A, Ronckers C, Mertens A, Stovall M, Smith S, Liu Y, et al. Primary thyroid cancer after a first tumour in childhood (the Childhood Cancer Survivor Study): a nested case-control study. Lancet. 2005;365:2014–23.

77. Tucker MA, Jones PH, Boice Jr JD, Robison LL, Stone BJ, Stovall M, et al. Therapeutic radiation at a young age is linked to secondary thyroid cancer. The Late Effects Study Group. Cancer Res. 1991;51:2885–8.

78. Koh E, Tran T, Heydarian M, Sachs R, Tsang R, Brenner D, et al. A comparison of mantle versus involved-field radiotherapy for Hodgkin's lymphoma: reduction in normal tissue dose and second cancer risk. Radiat Oncol. 2007;2:13.

79. De Bruin ML, Sparidans J, van't Veer MB, Noordijk E, Louwman MW, Zijlstra JM, van den Berg H, Russell N, Broeks A, Baaijens MH, Aleman BM, van Leeuwen FE. Breast cancer risk in female survivors of Hodgkin's lymphoma; lower risk after smaller radiation volumes. J Clin Oncol. 2009;27(26):4239–46.

80. Franklin J, Pluetschow A, Paus M, Specht L, Anselmo AP, Aviles A, et al. Second malignancy risk associated with treatment of Hodgkin's lymphoma: meta-analysis of the randomised trials. Ann Oncol. 2006;17:1749–60.

81. Bhatia S, Robison LL, Oberlin O, Greenberg M, Bunin G, Fossati-Bellani F, et al. Breast cancer and other second neoplasms after childhood Hodgkin's disease. N Engl J Med. 1996;334:745–51.

82. Mauch PM, Kalish LA, Marcus KC, Coleman CN, Shulman LN, Krill E, et al. Second malignancies after treatment for laparotomy staged IA-IIIB Hodgkin's disease: long-term analysis of risk factors and outcome. Blood. 1996;87:3625–32.

83. Sankila R, Garwicz S, Olsen JH, Dollner H, Hertz H, Kreuger A, et al. Risk of subsequent malignant neoplasms among 1,641 Hodgkin's disease patients diagnosed in childhood and adolescence: a population-based cohort study in the five Nordic countries. Association of the Nordic Cancer Registries and the Nordic Society of Pediatric Hematology and Oncology. J Clin Oncol. 1996;14:1442–6.

84. Swerdlow AJ, Barber JA, Horwich A, Cunningham D, Milan S, Omar RZ. Second malignancy in patients with Hodgkin's disease treated at the Royal Marsden Hospital. Br J Cancer. 1997;75:116–23.

85. van Leeuwen FE, Swerdlow AJ, Travis LB. Second cancers after treatment of Hodgkin lymphoma. In: Hoppe RT et al., editors. Hodgkin lymphoma. Philadelphia: Lippincott Williams & Wilkins; 2007. p. 347–70.

86. Levine EG, Bloomfield CD. Leukemias and myelodysplastic syndromes secondary to drug, radiation, and environmental exposure [Review]. Semin Oncol. 1992;19:47–84.

87. Michels SD, McKenna RW, Arthur DC, Brunning RD. Therapy-related acute myeloid leukemia and myelodysplastic syndrome: a clinical and morphologic study of 65 cases. Blood. 1985;65:1364–72.

88. Pedersen-Bjergaard J, Philip P, Larsen SO, Jensen G, Byrsting K. Chromosome aberrations and prognostic factors in therapy-related myelodysplasia and acute nonlymphocytic leukemia. Blood. 1990;76:1083–91.

89. Pedersen-Bjergaard J, Sigsgaard TC, Nielsen D, Gjedde SB, Philip P, Hansen M, et al. Acute monocytic or myelomonocytic leukemia with balanced chromosome translocations to band 11q23 after therapy with 4-epi-doxorubicin and cisplatin or cyclophosphamide for breast cancer [see Comments]. J Clin Oncol. 1992;10:1444–51.

90. Sandoval C, Pui CH, Bowman LC, Heaton D, Hurwitz CA, Raimondi SC, et al. Secondary acute myeloid leukemia in children previously treated with alkylating agents, intercalating topoisomerase II inhibitors, and irradiation. J Clin Oncol. 1993;11:1039–45.

91. Valagussa PA, Bonadonna G. Carcinogenic effects of cancer treatment. In: Peckham M, Pinedo H, Veronesi U, editors. Oxford textbook of oncology. Oxford: Oxford University Press; 1995. p. 2348.

92. IARC. Some antiviral and antineoplastic drugs, and other pharmaceutical agents. IARC Monogr Eval Carcinog Risk Chem Hum. 2000;76:177.

93. Pedersen-Bjergaard J, Philip P. Balanced translocations involving chromosome bands 11q23 and 21q22 are highly characteristic of myelodysplasia and leukemia following therapy with cytostatic agents targeting at DNA-topoisomerase II [Letter]. Blood. 1991;78:1147–8.

94. Pedersen-Bjergaard J, Rowley JD. The balanced and the unbalanced chromosome aberrations of acute myeloid leukemia may develop in different ways and may contribute differently to malignant transformation [Review]. Blood. 1994;83:2780–6.

95. Rubin CM, Arthur DC, Woods WG, Lange BJ, Nowell PC, Rowley JD, et al. Therapy-related myelodysplastic syndrome and acute myeloid leukemia in children: correlation between chromosomal abnormalities and prior therapy. Blood. 1991;78:2982–8.

96. Kaldor JM, Day NE, Kittelmann B, Pettersson F, Langmark F, Pedersen D, et al. Bladder tumours following chemotherapy and radiotherapy for ovarian cancer: a case-control study. Int J Cancer. 1995;63:1–6.

97. Kleinerman R, Tucker M, Tarone R, Abramson D, Seddon J, Stovall M, et al. Risk of new cancers after radiotherapy in long-term survivors of retinoblastoma: an extended follow-up. J Clin Oncol. 2005;23:2272–9.

98. Marees T, Moll A, Imhof S, de Boer M, Ringens P, van Leeuwen F. Risk of second malignancies in survivors of retinoblastoma: more than 40 years of follow-up. J Natl Cancer Inst. 2008;100:1771–9.

99. Wong FL, Boice Jr JD, Abramson DH, Tarone RE, Kleinerman RA, Stovall M, et al. Cancer incidence after retinoblastoma. Radiation dose and sarcoma risk [see Comments]. JAMA. 1997;278:1262–7.

100. Andersson A, Enblad G, Tavelin B, Bjorkholm M, Linderoth J, Lagerlof I, et al. Family history of cancer as a risk factor for second malignancies after Hodgkin's lymphoma. Br J Cancer. 2008;98:1001–5.

101. Bhatia S, Meadows AT, Robison LL. Family history of patients with breast cancer after treatment of Hodgkin's disease in childhood. Late Effects Study Group. Lancet. 1997;350:888–9.

102. Kony SJ, de Vathaire F, Chompret A, Shamsaldim A, Grimaud E, Raquin MA, et al. Radiation and genetic factors in the risk of second malignant neoplasms after a first cancer in childhood [see Comments]. Lancet. 1997;350:91–5.

103. Landgren O, Bjorkholm M, Montgomery SM, Hjalgrim H, Sjoberg J, Goldin LR, et al. Personal and family history of autoimmune diabetes mellitus and susceptibility to young-adult-onset Hodgkin lymphoma. Int J Cancer. 2006;118:449–52.

104. Nichols KE, Levitz S, Shannon KE, Wahrer DC, Bell DW, Chang G, et al. Heterozygous germline ATM mutations do not contribute to radiation-associated malignancies after Hodgkin's disease. J Clin Oncol. 1999;17:1259.

105. Prochazka M, Hall P, Granath F, Czene K. Family history of breast cancer and young age at diagnosis of breast cancer

increase risk of second primary malignancies in women: a population-based cohort study. Br J Cancer. 2006;95:1291–5.

106. Goldfrank D, Chuai S, Bernstein J, Cajal T, Lee J, Alonso MC, et al. Effect of mammography on breast cancer risk in women with mutations in BRCA1 or BRCA2. Cancer Epidemiol Biomark Prev. 2006;15:2311–3.

107. Narod S, Lubinski J, Ghadirian P, Lynch H, Moller P, Foulkes W, et al. Screening mammography and risk of breast cancer in BRCA1 and BRCA2 mutation carriers: a case-control study. Lancet Oncol. 2006;7:402–6.

108. Andrieu N, Easton D, Chang-Claude J, Rookus M, Brohet R, Cardis E, et al. Effect of chest X-rays on the risk of breast cancer among BRCA1/2 Mutation Carriers in the International BRCA1/2 Carrier Cohort Study: a report from the EMBRACE, GENEPSO, GEO-HEBON, and IBCCS Collaborators' Group. J Clin Oncol. 2006;24:3361–6.

109. Gronwald J, Cybulski C, Piesiak W, Suchy J, Huzarski T, Byrski T, et al. Cancer risks in first-degree relatives of CHEK2 mutation carriers: effects of mutation type and cancer site in proband. Br J Cancer. 2009;100:1508–12.

110. Broeks A, Russell NS, Floore AN, Urbanus JH, Dahler EC, van't Veer MB, Hagenbeek A, Noordijk EM, Crommelin MA, van Leeuwen FE, van't Veer LJ. Increased risk of breast cancer following irradiation for Hodgkin's disease is not a result of ATM germline mutations. Int J Radiat Biol. 2000;76:693–8.

111. Tabori U, Malkin D. Risk stratification in cancer predisposition syndromes: lessons learned from novel molecular developments in Li-Fraumeni syndrome. Cancer Res. 2008;68:2053–7.

112. Boyle JM, Spreadborough AR, Greaves MJ, Birch JM, Varley JM, Scott D. Delayed chromosome changes in gamma-irradiated normal and Li-Fraumeni fibroblasts. Radiat Res. 2002;157:158–65.

113. Parshad R, Price FM, Pirollo KF, Chang EH, Sanford KK. Cytogenetic response to G2-phase X irradiation in relation to DNA repair and radiosensitivity in a cancer-prone family with Li-Fraumeni syndrome. Radiat Res. 1993;136:236–40.

114. Broeks A, Braaf LM, Wessels LFA, van de Vijver M, De Bruin ML, Stovall M, Russell N, van Leeuwen FE, van't Veer LJ. Radiation-associated breast tumors display a distinct gene expression profile frequently correlated with the basal molecular subtype. Int J Radiat Oncol Biol Phys. 2009 (in press).

115. Worrillow LJ, Smith AG, Scott K, Andersson M, Ashcroft AJ, Dores GM, et al. Polymorphic MLH1 and risk of cancer after methylating chemotherapy for Hodgkin lymphoma. J Med Genet. 2008;45:142–6.

116. Ben-Yehuda D, Krichevsky S, Caspi O, Rund D, Polliack A, Abeliovich D, et al. Microsatellite instability and p53 mutations in therapy-related leukemia suggest mutator phenotype. Blood. 1996;88:4296–303.

117. Zhu YM, Das-Gupta EP, Russell NH. Microsatellite instability and p53 mutations are associated with abnormal expression of the MSH2 gene in adult acute leukemia. Blood. 1999;94:733–40.

118. Felix CA. Chemotherapy-related second cancers. In: Neugut AI, Meadows AT, Robinson E, editors. Multiple primary cancers. Philadelphia: Lippincott Williams & Wilkins; 1999. p. 137–64.

119. Smith MA, McCaffrey RP, Karp JE. The secondary leukemias: challenges and research directions. [Review]. J Natl Cancer Inst. 1996;88:407–18.

120. Andreassen C, Alsner J. Genetic variants and normal tissue toxicity after radiotherapy: a systematic review. Radiother Oncol. 2009;92:299–309.

121. Schonfeld SJ, Gilbert ES, Dores GM, Lynch CF, Hodgson DC, Hall P, et al. Acute myeloid leukemia following Hodgkin lymphoma: a population-based study of 35,511 patients. J Natl Cancer Inst. 2006;98:215–8.

122. Cimino G, Papa G, Tura S, Mazza P, Rossi Ferrini PL, Bosi A, et al. Second primary cancer following Hodgkin's disease: updated results of an Italian multicentric study. J Clin Oncol. 1991;9:432–7.

123. Devereux S, Selassie TG, Vaughan Hudson G, Vaughan Hudson B, Linch DC. Leukaemia complicating treatment for Hodgkin's disease: the experience of the British National Lymphoma Investigation. BMJ. 1990;301:1077–80.

124. Abrahamsen JF, Andersen A, Hannisdal E, Nome O, Abrahamsen AF, Kvaloy S, et al. Second malignancies after treatment of Hodgkin's disease: the influence of treatment, follow-up time, and age [see Comments]. J Clin Oncol. 1993;11:255–61.

125. Boivin JF, Hutchison GB, Zauber AG, Bernstein L, Davis FG, Michel RP, et al. Incidence of second cancers in patients treated for Hodgkin's disease [see Comments]. J Natl Cancer Inst. 1995;87:732–41.

126. Diehl V, Franklin J, Pfreundschuh M, Lathan B, Paulus U, Hasenclever D, et al. Standard and increased-dose BEACOPP chemotherapy compared with COPP-ABVD for advanced Hodgkin's disease. N Engl J Med. 2003;348:2386–95.

127. Josting A, Wiedenmann S, Franklin J, May M, Sieber M, Wolf J, et al. Secondary myeloid leukemia and myelodysplastic syndromes in patients treated for Hodgkin's disease: a report from the German Hodgkin's Lymphoma Study Group. J Clin Oncol. 2003;21:3440–6.

128. Andrieu JM, Ifrah N, Payen C, Fermanian J, Coscas Y, Flandrin G. Increased risk of secondary acute nonlymphocytic leukemia after extended-field radiation therapy combined with MOPP chemotherapy for Hodgkin's disease [see Comments; Review]. J Clin Oncol. 1990;8:1148–54.

129. Forrest DL, Hogge DE, Nevill TJ, Nantel SH, Barnett MJ, Shepherd JD, et al. High-dose therapy and autologous hematopoietic stem-cell transplantation does not increase the risk of second neoplasms for patients with Hodgkin's lymphoma: a comparison of conventional therapy alone versus conventional therapy followed by autologous hematopoietic stem-cell transplantation. J Clin Oncol. 2005;23:7994–8002.

130. Stone RM, Neuberg D, Soiffer R, Takvorian T, Whelan M, Rabinowe SN, et al. Myelodysplastic syndrome as a late complication following autologous bone marrow transplantation for non-Hodgkin's lymphoma. J Clin Oncol. 1994;12:2535–42.

131. Krikorian JG, Burke JS, Rosenberg SA, Kaplan HS. Occurrence of non-Hodgkin's lymphoma after therapy for Hodgkin's disease. N Engl J Med. 1979;300:452–8.

132. Foss Abrahamsen A, Andersen A, Nome O, Jacobsen AB, Holte H, Foss Abrahamsen J, et al. Long-term risk of sec-

ond malignancy after treatment of Hodgkin's disease: the influence of treatment, age and follow-up time. Ann Oncol. 2002;13:1786–91.

133. Rueffer U, Josting A, Franklin J, May M, Sieber M, Breuer K, et al. Non-Hodgkin's lymphoma after primary Hodgkin's disease in the German Hodgkin's Lymphoma Study Group: incidence, treatment, and prognosis. J Clin Oncol. 2001;19:2026–32.

134. Amini RM, Enblad G, Sundstrom C, Glimelius B. Patients suffering from both Hodgkin's disease and non-Hodgkin's lymphoma: a clinico-pathological and immuno-histochemical population-based study of 32 patients. Int J Cancer. 1997;71:510–6.

135. Zarate-Osorno A, Medeiros LJ, Longo DL, Jaffe ES. Non-Hodgkin's lymphomas arising in patients successfully treated for Hodgkin's disease. A clinical, histologic, and immunophenotypic study of 14 cases. Am J Surg Pathol. 1992;16:885–95.

136. Bennett MH, MacLennan KA, Vaughan Hudson G, Vaughan Hudson B. Non-Hodgkin's lymphoma arising in patients treated for Hodgkin's disease in the BNLI: a 20-year experience. British National Lymphoma Investigation. Ann Oncol. 1991;2 suppl 2:83–92.

137. Prosper F, Robledo C, Cuesta B, Rifon J, Borbolla JR, Pardo J, et al. Incidence of non-Hodgkin's lymphoma in patients treated for Hodgkin's disease. Leuk Lymphoma. 1994;12:457–62.

138. Kim H, Zelman RJ, Fox MA, Bennett JM, Berard CW, Butler JJ, et al. Pathology panel for lymphoma clinical studies: a comprehensive analysis of cases accumulated since its inception. J Natl Cancer Inst. 1982;68:43–67.

139. Swerdlow AJ, Douglas AJ, Vaughan Hudson G, Vaughan Hudson B, MacLennan KA. Risk of second primary cancer after Hodgkin's disease in patients in the British National Lymphoma Investigation: relationships to host factors, histology and stage of Hodgkin's disease, and splenectomy. Br J Cancer. 1993;68:1006–11.

140. Donaldson SS, Hancock SL. Second cancers after Hodgkin's disease in childhood [Editorial; Comment] [see Comments]. N Engl J Med. 1996;334:792–4.

141. Goss PE, Sierra S. Current perspectives on radiation-induced breast cancer [see Comments; Review]. J Clin Oncol. 1998;16:338–47.

142. Neglia JP, Friedman DL, Yasui Y, Mertens AC, Hammond S, Stovall M, et al. Second malignant neoplasms in five-year survivors of childhood cancer: childhood cancer survivor study. J Natl Cancer Inst. 2001;93:618–29.

143. Wolden SL, Hancock SL, Carlson RW, Goffinet DR, Jeffrey SS, Hoppe RT. Management of breast cancer after Hodgkin's disease. J Clin Oncol. 2000;18:765–72.

144. Wolf J, Schellong G, Diehl V. Breast cancer following treatment of Hodgkin's disease – more reasons for less radiotherapy? [Editorial; Comment]. Eur J Cancer. 1997;33:2293–4.

145. Yahalom J. Breast cancer after Hodgkin disease: hope for a safer cure. JAMA. 2003;290:529–31.

146. Deniz K, O'Mahony S, Ross G, Purushotham A. Breast cancer in women after treatment for Hodgkin's disease. Lancet Oncol. 2003;4:207–14.

147. Horwich A, Swerdlow AJ. Second primary breast cancer after Hodgkin's disease. Br J Cancer. 2004;90:294–8.

148. Travis LB, Curtis RE, Boice Jr JD. Late effects of treatment for childhood Hodgkin's disease [Letter; Comment]. N Engl J Med. 1996;335:352–3.

149. Aisenberg AC, Finkelstein DM, Doppke KP, Koerner FC, Boivin JF, Willett CG. High risk of breast carcinoma after irradiation of young women with Hodgkin's disease. Cancer. 1997;79:1203–10.

150. Boice Jr JD, Preston D, Davis FG, Monson RR. Frequent chest X-ray fluoroscopy and breast cancer incidence among tuberculosis patients in Massachusetts. Radiat Res. 1991;125:214–22.

151. Hildreth NG, Shore RE, Dvoretsky PM. The risk of breast cancer after irradiation of the thymus in infancy. N Engl J Med. 1989;321:1281–4.

152. Ronckers CM, Land CE, Neglia JP, Meadows AT. Breast cancer. Lancet. 2005;366:1605–6.

153. Tokunaga M, Land CE, Tokuoka S, Nishimori I, Soda M, Akiba S. Incidence of female breast cancer among atomic bomb survivors, 1950–1985. Radiat Res. 1994;138:209–23.

154. Kenney LB, Yasui Y, Inskip PD, Hammond S, Neglia JP, Mertens AC, et al. Breast cancer after childhood cancer: a report from the Childhood Cancer Survivor Study. Ann Intern Med. 2004;141:590–7.

155. Land CE, Tokunaga M, Koyama K, Soda M, Preston DL, Nishimori I, et al. Incidence of female breast cancer among atomic bomb survivors, Hiroshima and Nagasaki, 1950–1990. Radiat Res. 2003;160:707–17.

156. Basu S, Schwartz C, Fisher S, Hudson M, Tarbell N, Muhs A, et al. Unilateral and bilateral breast cancer in women surviving pediatric Hodgkin's disease. Int J Radiat Oncol Biol Phys. 2008;72:34–40.

157. Wolden SL, Lamborn KR, Cleary SF, Tate DJ, Donaldson SS. Second cancers following pediatric Hodgkin's disease [see Comments]. J Clin Oncol. 1998;16:536–44.

158. Travis LB, Hill D, Dores GM, Gospodarowicz M, van Leeuwen FE, Holowaty E, et al. Cumulative absolute breast cancer risk for young women treated for Hodgkin lymphoma. J Natl Cancer Inst. 2005;97:1428–37.

159. Beral V. Breast cancer and hormone-replacement therapy in the Million Women Study. Lancet. 2003;362:419–27.

160. Collaborative Group on Hormonal Factors in Breast Cancer. Breast cancer and hormone replacement therapy: collaborative reanalysis of data from 51 epidemiological studies of 52,705 women with breast cancer and 108,411 women without breast cancer. Lancet. 1997;350:1047–59.

161. Lorigan P, Radford J, Howell A, Thatcher N. Lung cancer after treatment for Hodgkin's lymphoma: a systematic review. Lancet Oncol. 2005;6:773–9.

162. Kaldor JM, Day NE, Bell J, Clarke EA, Langmark F, Karjalainen S, et al. Lung cancer following Hodgkin's disease: a case-control study. Int J Cancer. 1992;52:677–81.

163. National Research Council of the National Academies. Health risks from exposure to low levels of ionizing radiation. Washington: The National Academies Press; 2006.

164. Ralleigh G, Given-Wilson R; on behalf of the Royal College of Radiologists Breast Group working party on Hodgkin's disease and secondary breast cancer. Breast cancer risk and possible screening strategies for young women following supradiaphragmatic irradiation for Hodgkin's disease. Clin Radiol. 2004;59:647–50.

165. Saslow D, Boetes C, Burke W, Harms S, Leach MO, Lehman CD, et al. American Cancer Society guidelines for breast screening with MRI as an adjunct to mammography. CA Cancer J Clin. 2007;57:75–89.

166. Absolom K, Greenfield D, Ross R, Davies H, Hancock B, Eiser C. Reassurance following breast screening recall for female survivors of Hodgkin's lymphoma. Breast. 2007;16: 590–6.

167. Bober SL, Park ER, Schmookler T, Medeiros Nancarrow C, Diller L. Perceptions of breast cancer risk and cancer screening: a qualitative study of young, female Hodgkin's disease survivors. J Cancer Educ. 2007;22:42–6.

168. Diller L, Medeiros Nancarrow C, Shaffer K, Matulonis U, Mauch P, Neuberg D, et al. Breast cancer screening in women previously treated for Hodgkin's disease: a prospective cohort study. J Clin Oncol. 2002;20:2085–91.

169. Oeffinger KC, Ford JS, Moskowitz CS, Diller LR, Hudson MM, Chou JF, et al. Breast cancer surveillance practices among women previously treated with chest radiation for a childhood cancer. JAMA. 2009;301:404–14.

170. Dershaw DD, Yahalom J, Petrek JA. Breast carcinoma in women previously treated for Hodgkin disease: mammographic evaluation. Radiology. 1992;184:421–3.

171. Howell SJ, Searle C, Goode V, Gardener T, Linton K, Cowan RA, et al. The UK national breast cancer screening programme for survivors of Hodgkin lymphoma detects breast cancer at an early stage. Br J Cancer. 2009;101:582–8.

172. Lee L, Pintilie M, Hodgson DC, Goss PE, Crump M. Screening mammography for young women treated with supradiaphragmatic radiation for Hodgkin's lymphoma. Ann Oncol. 2008;19:62–7.

173. Abrams SA. Using stable isotopes to assess the bioavailability of minerals in food-fortification programs. Forum Nutr. 2003;56:312–3.

174. Hoppe RT, Hanlon AL, Hanks GE, Owen JB. Progress in the treatment of Hodgkin's disease in the United States, 1973 versus 1983. The patterns of care study. Cancer. 1994;74:3198–203.

175. Smitt M, Stouffer N, Owen J, Hoppe R, Hanks G. Results of the 1988–1989 patterns of care study process survey for Hodgkin's disease. Int J Radiat Oncol Biol Phys. 1999;43:335–9.

176. Engert A, Diehl V, Franklin J, Lohri A, Dorken B, Ludwig W, et al. Escalated-dose BEACOPP in the treatment of patients with advanced-stage Hodgkin's lymphoma: 10 years of follow-up of the GHSG HD9 study. J Clin Oncol. 2009;27:4548–54.

# Cardiovascular and Pulmonary Late Effects

## 23

### Berthe M.P. Aleman

## Contents

## 23.1 Cardiovascular Toxicity

Both radiotherapy and chemotherapy for Hodgkin lymphoma may cause early and late cardiovascular toxicity. This chapter mainly focuses on long-term effects. While cardiotoxicity following radiotherapy is usually observed 5–10 years after therapy and onward, anthracycline-related toxicity is observed at varying intervals after therapy. Tables 23.1 and 23.2 show standardized mortality rates and standardized incidence rates of several cardiovascular diseases including the absolute excess risks.

### 23.1.1 Chemotherapy-Associated Cardiotoxicity

#### 23.1.1.1 General Aspects of Chemotherapy-Associated Cardiotoxicity

The most relevant cardiotoxic chemotherapeutic agents used in treatment for patients with Hodgkin lymphoma are anthracyclines, especially doxorubicin and epirubicin. Anthracycline-associated toxicity may occur at different intervals after therapy. Cardiotoxicity often presents as electrocardiographic changes and arrhythmias, or as cardiomyopathy leading to congestive heart failure. Anthracycline-associated cardiotoxicity is caused by direct damage to the myoepithelium. Several risk factors for anthracycline-associated cardiotoxicity have been identified (see Table 23.3). The occurrence of anthracycline-associated cardiotoxicity is strongly related to the cumulative dose [1, 2]. Doses less than 500 mg/m² are usually well tolerated. The total dose of anthracyclines during first-line therapy for Hodgkin

B.M.P. Aleman
Department of Radiotherapy, The Netherlands Cancer Institute,
Plesmanlaan 121, 1066 CX, Amsterdam, The Netherlands
e-mail: b.aleman@nki.nl

A. Engert and S.J. Horning (eds.), *Hodgkin Lymphoma*,
DOI: 10.1007/978-3-642-12780-9_23, © Springer-Verlag Berlin Heidelberg 2011

**Table 23.1** Risk of death from myocardial infarction in large cohorts of patients treated for Hodgkin lymphoma

| Authors (years of treatment) | No. in cohort | Age range at treatment in years | Follow-up time in years (range) | Type of treatment | SMR[a] | (95% CI) SMR[a] | AER[b] |
|---|---|---|---|---|---|---|---|
| Boivin [20] (1940–1985) | 4,665 | All ages[c] | Average 7 (–) | Mediastinal RT±CT | 4.1 | (1.5–10.9) | – |
| Hancock [57] and Hoppe [58] (1960–1991) | 2,232 | 1–82 (average 29) | Average 9.5 (–) | 89% including mediastinal RT | 3.2 | (2.3–4.0) | 17.8 |
| King [59] (1954–1989) | 326 | 5–72 (mean 25.6) | Mean 13.3 (3–37) | Mantle RT±CT | 2.8 | (0.7–4.9) | 10.4[d] |
| Glanzmann [60] (1964–1992) | 352 | 4.0–81 (mean 33.8) | Mean 11.2 (1.0–31.5) | Mediastinal RT±CT | 4.2 | (1.8–8.3) | – |
| Brierley [61] (1973–1984) | 611 | 17–90 (median 31) | Median 11.0 (0.7–18.0) | 97% RT±CT | 1.5 | (0.7–3.0) | 5.4 |
| Aleman [19] (1965–1987) | 1,261 | Median 26 | Median 17.8 | 97% RT±CT; 84% mediastinal RT | 4 | (2.3–6.5) | 5.6 |
| Swerdlow [6] (1967–2000) | 7,033 | All ages | Median 11.1 | 72% RT±CT; 34% including mediastinal RT | 2.5 | (2.1–2.9) | 12.6 |

*CT* chemotherapy; *RT* radiotherapy; *SMR* standardized mortality ratio; *CI* confidence interval; *AER* absolute excess risk

[a]Standardized mortality ratio (SMR) as the ratio of the observed (O) and expected (E) numbers of cardiovascular events in the cohort. The expected numbers are calculated based on general population rates

[b]Absolute excess risk (AER) per 10,000 person-years as O minus E, divided by the number of person-years at risk, multiplied by 10,000

[c]62% <40 years

[d]Calculated from the data in the paper: (observed (7) – expected (2.5)/person-years at risk (4,335))×10,000

**Table 23.2** Standardized incidence ratio and absolute excess risks of myocardial infarction, congestive heart failure, stroke and transient ischemic attack by sex, age at start of treatment, follow-up interval, attained age, and treatment in patient treated for Hodgkin lymphoma

| | MI | | CHF | | Stroke | | TIA | |
|---|---|---|---|---|---|---|---|---|
| | SIR | AER | SIR | AER | SIR | AER | SIR | AER |
| Total cohort[a] | 3.6 | 35.7 | 4.9 | 25.6 | 2.2 | 12 | 3.1 | 9 |
| *Sex* | | | | | | | | |
| Male | 4.2 | 60.7 | 3.9 | 21.7 | 2.0 | 10 | 2.7 | 8 |
| Female | 2.1 | 9.4 | 6.4 | 29.8 | 2.4 | 14 | 3.8 | 11 |
| *Age at treatment (years)* | | | | | | | | |
| ≤20 | 5.4 | 15.0 | 18.2 | 27.6 | 3.8 | 7 | 7.6 | 5 |
| 21–30 | 4.9 | 40.1 | 6.8 | 40.5 | 3.1 | 14 | 4.2 | 7 |
| 31–40 | 2.7 | 46.3 | 2.6 | 21.2 | 2.0 | 15 | 3.1 | 13 |
| 41–50 | – | – | – | – | 1.4[b] | 11 | 2.1[b] | 18 |
| *Follow-up period (years)* | | | | | | | | |
| 5–9 | 1.7[b] | 4.3 | 7.1 | 11.0 | 2.1[b] | 5 | 2.3 | 3 |
| 10–14 | 4.4 | 33.9 | 3.4 | 8.7 | 2.3 | 10 | 3.3 | 8 |
| 15–19 | 4.0 | 46.4 | 8.5 | 47.3 | 2.6 | 18 | 4.4 | 17 |
| 20–24 | 4.7 | 84.0 | 2.4[b] | 13.7 | 2.1[b] | 17 | 2.5[b] | 11 |
| ≥25 | 2.9 | 69.2 | 4.5 | 62.5 | 1.9[b] | 26 | 2.8 | 23 |
| *Attained age (years)* | | | | | | | | |
| <51 | 4.1 | 24.8 | 6.9 | 13.8 | 2.5 | 7 | 3.2 | 4 |
| ≥51 | 3.1 | 93.0 | 3.9 | 55.9 | 2.0 | 29 | 3.1 | 30 |
| *Treatment* | | | | | | | | |
| Radiotherapy alone | | | | | 2.0 | 11 | 3.4 | 12 |
| Chemotherapy alone | | | | | 0.4[b] | –6 | – | – |
| Radio/chemotherapy | | | | | 2.6 | 15 | 3.4 | 10 |
| *Treatment* | | | | | | | | |
| Initial RT only | 3.9 | 49.9 | 4.8 | 27.1 | | | | |
| RT+CT, no anthracyclines | 3.9 | 66.0 | 5.3 | 31.8 | | | | |
| RT+CT, anthracyclines | 3.5 | 23.6 | 6.2 | 21.2 | | | | |
| Initial CT only | 1.0[b] | 7.4 | 0.0 | –8.2 | | | | |

*MI* myocardial infarction; *CHF* congestive heart failure; *TIA* transient ischemic attack; *SIR* standardized incidence ratio; *AER* absolute excess risk; *RT* radiotherapy; *CT* chemotherapy;

[a]Adapted from Aleman and van den Belt-Dusebout et al. [3] and De Bruin and Dorresteijn et al. [44]. MI and CHF data from cohort of 1,474 survivors of Hodgkin lymphoma treated before the age of 41 between 1965 and 1995 and stroke and TIA data from cohort of 2,201 5-year survivors of Hodgkin lymphoma treated before the age of 51 between 1965 and 1995

[b]Not statistically significant

**Table 23.3** Risk factors for anthracycline-associated cardiotoxicity in decreasing order of importance

| Risk factor | Features |
|---|---|
| Total cumulative dose | Most significant predictor for abnormal cardiac function |
| Age | For comparable cumulative doses, younger age predisposes to greater cardiotoxicity |
| Length of follow-up | Longer follow-up results in higher prevalence of myocardial impairment |
| Gender | Females more vulnerable than males for comparable doses |
| Concomitant mediastinal irradiation | Enhanced toxicity; not clear whether additive or synergistic |

Adapted from Table 10.4 of Chapter 10, Cardiovascular effects of cancer therapy, by Adams, Constine, Duffy, and Lipshultz (and from [3]) in Survivors of childhood and adolescent cancer (second edition) published by Springer

lymphoma is relatively low compared with treatment regimens for breast cancer and pediatric malignancies. The cumulative dose of eight cycles of doxorubicin, bleomycin, vinblastine, and dacarbazine (ABVD) is 400 mg/m$^2$ and of eight cycles of bleomycin, etoposide, adriamycin, cyclophosphamide, vincristine, procarbazine, and prednisone (escalated BEACOPP) is 280 mg/m$^2$. However, most patients are treated with fewer than eight cycles of anthracycline-containing chemotherapy.

Whether toxicity following chemotherapy and radiotherapy is additive or synergistic remains unclear. Several clinical studies showed that anthracycline-containing therapy may further increase the radiation-related risk of congestive heart failure and valvular disorders by twofold to threefold compared to radiotherapy alone [4, 5]. This effect may also be more than additive [6]. A recent British study also showed that the increased risks for death from myocardial infarction may be related not only to supradiaphragmatic radiotherapy but also to anthracycline and vincristine treatment; the risk of death from myocardial infarction was increased for patients who did not receive supradiaphragmatic radiotherapy but had received vincristine was 2.2 (95% CI = 1.6–3.0) and anthracyclines (SMR = 3.2, 95% CI = 1.9–5.2), especially those who were treated with the ABVD regimen (SMR = 7.8, 95% CI = 1.6–22.7) [7].

The potential role of genetic variability in the pathogenesis of chronic cardiotoxicity including congestive heart failure remains to be elucidated. Only a few studies in humans provide evidence that genetic susceptibility may play an important role in the risk of anthracycline-associated cardiotoxicity [8–10].

### 23.1.1.2 Management of Chemotherapy-Associated Cardiotoxicity

Currently there are no indications that anthracycline-associated congestive heart failure needs a special approach. Treatment generally focuses on correcting underlying abnormalities such as increased afterload and decreased contractility, and frequently includes treatment with angiotensin-converting enzyme (ACE) inhibitors and/or beta-blockers [11]. Several guidelines developed for treating patients with asymptomatic left ventricular dysfunction or heart failure (not specifically after cancer treatment) include beta-blockers, ACE-inhibitors, diuretics, and others [12].

### 23.1.1.3 Prevention of Chemotherapy-Associated Cardiotoxicity

A rather obvious measure to prevent cardiotoxicity is to limit both cardiotoxic chemotherapy (especially anthracyclines) and radiation volume and dose as much as possible. The evidence on the effectiveness of approaches to reduce or prevent anthracycline-associated cardiotoxicity is limited in quantity and quality [13, 14]. The available evidence mainly comes from treatment of children. Attempts have been made to optimize the anthracycline scheduling such as avoiding peak doses. However, results so far have been disappointing [14].

Anthracyclines release free radicals that damage cardiac myocytes, which are especially susceptible to free-radical damage because of their highly oxidative metabolism and poor antioxidant defenses. The free-radical scavenging cardioprotectant, dexrazoxane, has been shown to reduce anthracycline-associated myocardial injury in rats [15] and in selected studies in humans [16]. More information is, however, needed before this agent can be introduced in clinical practice. Furthermore, there are some indications of a possible beneficial effect of ACE-inhibitors and beta-blockers [17] after cardiotoxic chemotherapy [18].

## 23.1.2 Radiation-Associated Cardiotoxicity

### 23.1.2.1 General Aspects of Radiation-Associated Cardiotoxicity

Radiation-associated heart disease in cancer survivors includes a wide spectrum of cardiac pathologies, such as coronary artery disease, myocardial dysfunction, valvular heart disease, pericardial disease, and electrical conduction abnormalities [4, 19]. Radiation-associated heart diseases, except for pericarditis, usually present 10–15 years after exposure, although non-symptomatic abnormalities may develop much earlier. The long delay before expression of serious damage probably explains why radiation sensitivity of the heart has previously been underestimated.

Radiation causes both increased mortality (mainly fatal myocardial infarction) and increased morbidity (see Tables 23.1 and 23.2). Epidemiological studies on Hodgkin lymphoma survivors show relative risk estimates for cardiac deaths in the range of 2–7, depending on patients age (increased risks for irradiation at young age), the radiation therapy methods used, and the follow-up time [7, 19–22]. In a Dutch study of Hodgkin lymphoma patients treated before the age of 41 years, threefold to fivefold increased standardized incidence ratios (SIR) of various heart diseases were observed relative to the general population, even after a follow-up of more than 20 years [4]. The persistence of increased risk over prolonged follow-up time is of concern because this implies increasing absolute excess risks over time, due to the rising incidence of cardiovascular diseases with age.

Prospective screening studies demonstrate that clinically significant cardiovascular abnormalities, like reduced left ventricular dimensions, and valvular and conduction defects, are very common, even in asymptomatic Hodgkin survivors [23]. Hodgkin lymphoma patients also have a significantly higher risk (SIR 8.4) of requiring valve surgery or revascularization procedures 15–20 years after radiotherapy [24]. Furthermore, an increased risk of restenosis after coronary artery stenting has been reported in patients treated with thoracic radiation for lymphoma [25].

There are several risk factors for radiation-associated cardiotoxicity (see Table 23.4). Cardiotoxicity is evidently related to total radiation dose and dose per fraction to the heart [22, 26]. Large doses per fraction are expected to be more damaging to the heart than low doses per fraction. Indeed, increased complication rates were reported for Hodgkin lymphoma patients treated with $3 \times 3.3$ Gy per week, compared with patients treated with $4 \times 2.5$ Gy per week to the same total dose [27].

The heart volume included in the radiation field influences the risk of cardiotoxicity [5, 28], although

**Table 23.4** Risk factors for the different manifestations of radiation-associated cardiotoxicity

| Risk factor | Pericarditis | CM | CAD | Arrhythmia | Valvular disease | All causes of CD | Reference |
|---|---|---|---|---|---|---|---|
| Total dose (>30–35 Gy) | X | X | X | X | X | X | [5, 28, 63] |
| Dose per fraction ( ≥2.0 Gy/day) | X | X | X | Likely | Likely | X | [27] |
| Volume of heart exposed | X | X | X | Likely | Likely | X | [28, 58] |
| Younger age at exposure | – | X | X | Likely | Likely | X | [4, 58] |
| Increased time since exposure | – | X | X | X | X | X | [4] |
| Use of adjuvant cardiotoxic chemotherapy | – | X | – | X | X | X | [4–6] |
| The presence of other known risk factors in each individual such as current age, weight, lipid profile, and habits such as smoking | – | – | X | – | – | X | [4, 61] |

*CM* cardiomyopathy; *CAD* coronary artery disease; *CD* cardiac death

Adapted with permission from Table 10.5 of Chapter 10, Cardiovascular effects of cancer therapy, by Adams, Constine, Duffy, and Lipshultz (and from [3]) in Survivors of childhood and adolescent cancer (second edition) published by Springer there are still many uncertainties regarding dose–effect and volume–effect relationship. A reduction in the increased risk of death from cardiovascular diseases other than myocardial infarction has been reported in Hodgkin lymphoma patients treated after partial shielding of the heart and restriction of the total, fractionated, mediastinal dose to less than 30 Gy [22]. Radiotherapy techniques have greatly improved over the past 20 years, leading to more homogeneous dose distributions and reduced risks of toxicity [29]. For pericarditis, TD 5/5 values (total dose for 5% incidence at 5 years) of 60, 45, and 40 Gy have been calculated when 1/3, 2/3, and the whole heart is irradiated using 2 Gy per fraction [30]. There is also some evidence of a volume effect from studies demonstrating that the extent of left ventricular radiation dose is an adverse prognostic factor of radiation-induced heart disease [31, 32]. Several studies using functional imaging have shown myocardial perfusion changes less than 2 years after radiotherapy. Although a relationship between these abnormalities and subsequent clinical heart disease may be expected, this has not yet been demonstrated [31–33].

### 23.1.2.2 Other Risk Factors for Cardiotoxicity

The risk for cardiovascular disease may also increase through indirect effects of radiotherapy; irradiation of the left kidney during para-aortic and spleen radiotherapy, for example, may lead to hypertension [34].

General risk factors for cardiovascular diseases, such as hypertension, diabetes, hypercholesterolemia, overweight, and smoking [35–39] probably also contribute to the risk for cardiovascular diseases in patients treated for Hodgkin lymphoma [40, 41]. Whether the cardiovascular risk factor profile in patients treated for Hodgkin lymphoma differs from that of the general population is unknown.

### 23.1.2.3 Management of Radiation-Associated Cardiotoxicity

There are currently no indications that treatment-associated ischemic heart disease needs a special approach. Screening for cardiovascular diseases is still a matter of debate. There are uncertainties about the screening modalities. Stress testing may identify asymptomatic individuals at high risk for acute myocardial infarction or sudden cardiac death [26], but this is not common practice yet. Furthermore, there is no evidence for treatment other than management of general risk factors for cardiovascular disease. It is quite likely that among patients treated for Hodgkin lymphoma, subgroups can be identified that have risks similar to patients with recognized risk factors like, for instance, diabetes. In many countries, guidelines have been developed for primary and secondary prevention of cardiovascular diseases [42, 43]. Lifestyle advice should be given, i.e., patients should be advised to refrain from smoking from the start of treatment of Hodgkin lymphoma, maintain a healthy body weight, and exercise regularly. In case cardiovascular surgery is needed, treating physicians should be aware of increased risks due to radiation-induced fibrosis [44].

### 23.1.2.4 Prevention of Radiation-Associated Cardiotoxicity

With respect to radiation it is important to use conventionally fractionated radiation, and to limit both radiation dose and volume. Modern radiation techniques like intensity-modified radiotherapy allow radiation with lower exposure of the heart without compromising the radiation dose in the target volume. Ongoing research is expected to provide more information regarding which structures are most critical and whether it is less harmful to expose a slightly larger volume to a low dose or a smaller volume to a slightly higher dose.

Optimization of treatment choice is still an important subject of study. In the future, we hope to be able to identify survivor groups at high risk of late adverse effects (based on treatment and/or genotype) for which screening should be recommended and/or intervention trials could be designed.

### 23.1.3 Radiation Damage to Major Arteries

### 23.1.3.1 General Aspects of Radiation Damage to Major Arteries

Not only cardiac toxicity has been reported following treatment for Hodgkin lymphoma, also other blood vessels may be damaged by radiation. Damage to the carotid arteries is of special importance. Significantly, increased risks of transient ischemic attack (TIA) and stroke have been described in patients treated with radiotherapy for HL [40, 45].

Recently, the Childhood Cancer Survivor Study (CCSS) published on self-reported incidence and risk factors for stroke among childhood Hodgkin lymphoma survivors [40]. Twenty-four late-occurring strokes were observed in a cohort of 1,926 survivors of childhood Hodgkin lymphoma (RR = 4.32; 95% CI = 2.01–9.29). Patients irradiated with mantle fields even experienced higher relative risks for stroke (RR = 5.62; 95% CI = 2.59–12.25). A Dutch retrospective cohort study among 2,201 5-year Hodgkin lymphoma survivors treated before the age of 51 between 1965 and 1995 showed a substantially increased risk for stroke and TIA that was associated with radiation to the neck and mediastinum [45]. The standardized incidence ratio for stroke was 2.2 (95% CI = 1.7–2.8) and 3.1 for TIA (95% CI = 2.2–4.2). Compared with the general population, these risks remained elevated after prolonged follow-up. The cumulative incidence of ischemic stroke or TIA 30 years after Hodgkin lymphoma treatment was 7% (95% CI = 5–8%).

### 23.1.3.2 Management of Radiation Damage to Major Arteries

There is no proof for the value of screening. Furthermore, there is no evidence for treatment other than management of general risk factors for cardiovascular diseases (as abovementioned). Lifestyle advice should be given, i.e., patients should be advised to refrain from smoking (from the start of treatment of Hodgkin lymphoma), maintain a healthy body weight, and exercise regularly.

### 23.1.3.3 Prevention of Radiation Damage to Major Arteries

Limitation of radiation-dose and volume and the use of adequate radiation techniques leading to homogeneous dose distributions are important. With the current concept used in radiation of patients with Hodgkin lymphoma (like involved-node radiation instead of involved-field radiation) [45], it is likely that the risk of radiation-related

damage to the carotids in patients treated for Hodgkin lymphoma will diminish.

Screening for radiation effects on the carotid arteries is not generally recommended since there are no therapeutic consequences. Intervention studies are difficult to perform because of the relatively low number of patients treated for Hodgkin lymphoma and the long interval between treatment and clinical event. Surrogate endpoints like measurement of intima-media thickness of the carotid arteries could be used. An intervention study is ongoing in the Netherlands, using such an endpoint, but the results of this study will have to be awaited.

## 23.2 Late Pulmonary Toxicity

Several chemotherapeutic agents and radiation may lead to pulmonary morbidity and mortality. Significant mortality may be seen in the first months up to 1 year after chemotherapy [47]. During long-term follow-up, the mortality from second pulmonary neoplasms is significantly increased (see Chapter 23), but not from other pulmonary diseases [20, 48]. Furthermore, higher morbidity may also be seen with longer follow-up.

### 23.2.1 Chemotherapy-Associated Pulmonary Toxicity

#### 23.2.1.1 General Aspects of Chemotherapy-Associated Pulmonary Toxicity

Several frequently used chemotherapeutic agents may cause pulmonary toxicity. Bleomycin is the most frequently used agent in treatment of patients with Hodgkin lymphoma causing pulmonary toxicity.

#### 23.2.1.2 Bleomycin

The pulmonary toxicity of bleomycin has been recognized since it was used in clinical trials in the 1960s for testicular cancer. Acute pulmonary toxicity following bleomycin-containing chemotherapy usually presents with dyspnea, dry cough, and fever. Long-term pulmonary toxicity is predominantly fibrotic and may be

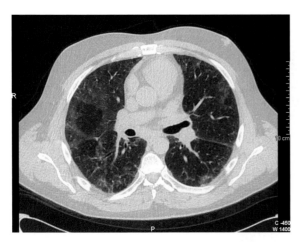

**Fig. 23.1** CT scan of the chest showing interstitial pulmonary changes attributed to bleomycin

associated with pulmonary impairment and a dry cough. The classic radiographic pattern of bleomycin-induced interstitial fibrosis is marked by bibasilar reticular or fine nodular infiltrates. On CT scans, infiltrative changes, nodules, and patchy ground-glass opacities may be seen (see Fig. 23.1). Nowadays, FDG-PET can identify early bleomycin-related pulmonary toxicity and it may also be used for follow-up of this toxicity. Conventional CT scanning is not able to distinguish between residual changes and active inflammation. Thus, PET represents a useful diagnostic tool and, independently of CT, indicates the resolution of disease activity, even in the presence of residual pulmonary scarring [49].

The severity of bleomycin toxicity may vary. Martin et al. [47] recently reported a bleomycin pulmonary toxicity incidence rate of 18% in patients treated with ABVD (25 of 141 patients) and one quarter of the patients with bleomycin pulmonary toxicity died from pulmonary toxicity within 9 months of their Hodgkin lymphoma diagnosis. In this study, a detrimental impact on 5-year overall survival rates in Hodgkin lymphoma patients who developed bleomycin pulmonary toxicity was observed, with a decrease in the median survival from 90 to 63%. In patients who survived the pulmonary toxicity, bleomycin pulmonary toxicity had no effect on outcome.

### 23.2.1.3 Other Agents Leading to Pulmonary Toxicity

Carmustine is used in high-dose regimen such as carmustine, etoposide, cytarabine, and melphalan (BEAM)

and may also induce pulmonary toxicity. The toxic reaction in the lung caused by carmustine usually manifests as chronic interstitial fibrosis that occurs after prolonged treatment and high cumulative doses.

Recently, the substitution of etoposide by gemcitabine in the escalated BEACOPP regimen was reported non-feasible and lead to severe acute pulmonary toxicity. This toxicity was probably related to the concomitant application of gemcitabine and bleomycin [50]. No long-term follow-up is available for this treatment yet. In the same patient population, pulmonary toxicity following radiation was studied as well [51]. No increased toxicity was observed, so the authors concluded that integration of radiotherapy in gemcitabine-containing regimens in Hodgkin lymphoma is feasible provided there is an interval of at least 4 weeks between the two modalities and radiotherapy follows chemotherapy.

### 23.2.1.4 Management of Chemotherapy-Associated Pulmonary Toxicity

There is no accepted standard treatment for acute bleomycin toxicity. Corticosteroids, withholding bleomycin from subsequent chemotherapy, and proceeding with a regimen not containing bleomycin, if possible, is the most common approach [47]. Long-term corticosteroid treatment may be necessary to avoid recall pneumonitis.

### 23.2.1.5 Prevention of Chemotherapy-Associated Pulmonary Toxicity

Information on how to prevent long-term toxicity is scarce. High inspired concentrations of oxygen after prior treatment with bleomycin have been reported to be toxic [52].

## 23.2.2 Radiation-Associated Pulmonary Toxicity

### 23.2.2.1 General Aspects of Radiation-Associated Pulmonary Toxicity

Radiation may not only damage the lung but also the pleura leading to different clinical symptoms. Radiation

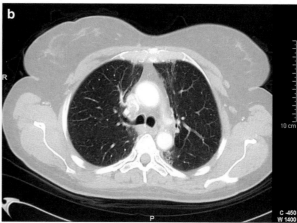

**Fig. 23.2** (**a**) Chest X-ray 11 years after mediastinal radiation showing paramediastinal radiation fibrosis. (**b**) CT scan of the chest of the same patient also 11 years after mediastinal radia-tion showing interstitial pulmonary changes limited to the mediastinal radiation field

can cause a dry cough and shortness of breath in the first months following radiation. The radiological changes after conventional treatment are well known. Changes on chest X-rays and CT scans of the thorax are usually observed 2–3 months following radiotherapy (see Fig. 23.2). In the long term, progressive fibrotic retraction may be observed. Splenic radiation may lead to limited radiation pneumonitis of the left lung base, followed by pleural thickening, often without any clinical symptoms [53]. A Dutch study on breast cancer and Hodgkin lymphoma patients reported a partial recovery from early local perfusion, ventilation, and density changes that were seen between 3 and 18 months after radiotherapy. In lymphoma patients, local lung function did not further improve after 18 months [54].

The risk for radiation-induced pneumonitis is related to the radiation dose and irradiated volume. Generally accepted clinical parameters related to radiation pneumonitis within 1 year after treatment include mean lung dose (MLD) and the volume of lung tissue receiving at least 20 Gy (=V20). Koh et al. reported in their study performed to quantify the incidence of radiation pneumonitis in a modern Hodgkin lymphoma cohort, that a V20 range greater than 36–40% and a mean lung dose range of more than 14–16 Gy, over and above which the risk of RTOG Grade 2 or greater pneumonitis would be considered clinically significant [55].

Although minor pleural changes such as small pleural effusions and pleural thickening may be seen regularly following radiation for Hodgkin lymphoma, clinically significant symptoms are rare [56].

### 23.2.2.2 Management of Radiation-Associated Pulmonary Toxicity

Treatment of radiation pneumonitis, usually occurring within the first year following treatment, generally consists of high-dose corticosteroids. In the long-term, no specific treatment is available since pulmonary fibrosis following radiation is generally irreversible.

### 23.2.2.3 Prevention of Radiation-Associated Pulmonary Toxicity

During treatment the mean lung dose should be kept as low as possible. Patients are advised to refrain from smoking.

### 23.2.2.4 Combined Toxicity

Combined modality treatment is frequently used in patients with Hodgkin lymphoma. Bleomycin dose modification may be required in a substantial number of patients [57]. Since the addition of radiotherapy may further decrease pulmonary function, radiotherapy may have to be adapted as well.

## 23.3 Conclusion

The cure rate of Hodgkin lymphoma patients today amounts to 80% or more with risk-adapted treatment using modern chemotherapy and radiotherapy regimen. Effective chemotherapy combinations have been developed and possibilities to treat acute toxicity have improved significantly. Long-term cardiovascular and pulmonary toxicity currently observed was caused by treatment regimens that are no longer applied. Because of improved knowledge on toxicity and patient-tailored treatment we expect to observe lower risks of cardiovascular and pulmonary toxicity in the majority of patients. However, it is important for treating physicians and patients to remain aware of possible late effects following treatment.

## References

1. Kremer LC, van Dalen EC, Offringa M, et al. Anthracycline-induced clinical heart failure in a cohort of 607 children: long-term follow-up study. J Clin Oncol. 2001;19:191–6.
2. Steinherz LJ. Anthracycline-induced cardiotoxicity. Ann Intern Med. 1997;126:827–8.
3. Simbre VC, Adams MJDSS, Duffy SA, Miller TL, Lipshultz SE. Cardiomyopathy caused by antineoplastic therapies. Curr Treat Options Cardiovasc Med 2001;3:493–505.
4. Aleman BM, van den Belt-Dusebout AW, De Bruin ML, 't Veer MB, Baaijens MH, de Boer JP, et al. Late cardiotoxicity after treatment for Hodgkin lymphoma. Blood. 2007;109:1878–86.
5. Moser EC, Noordijk EM, van Leeuwen FE, et al. Long-term risk of cardiovascular disease after treatment for aggressive non-Hodgkin's lymphoma. Blood. 2005;107:2912–9.
6. Myrehaug S, Pintilie M, Tsang R, et al. Cardiac morbidity following modern treatment for Hodgkin lymphoma: supra-additive cardiotoxicity of doxorubicin and radiation therapy. Leuk Lymphoma. 2008;49:1486–93.
7. Swerdlow AJ, Higgins CD, Smith P, et al. Myocardial infarction mortality risk after treatment for Hodgkin disease: a collaborative British cohort study. J Natl Cancer Inst. 2007; 99:206–14.
8. Blanco JG, Leisenring WM, Gonzalez-Covarrubias VM, et al. Genetic polymorphisms in the carbonyl reductase 3 gene CBR3 and the NAD(P)H:quinone oxidoreductase 1 gene NQO1 in patients who developed anthracycline-related congestive heart failure after childhood cancer. Cancer. 2008;112:2789–95.
9. Deng S, Wojnowski L. Genotyping the risk of anthracycline-induced cardiotoxicity. Cardiovasc Toxicol. 2007;7:129–34.
10. Wojnowski L, Kulle B, Schirmer M, et al. NAD(P)H oxidase and multidrug resistance protein genetic polymorphisms are associated with doxorubicin-induced cardiotoxicity. Circulation. 2005;112:3754–62.
11. Barry E, Alvarez JA, Scully RE, et al. Anthracycline-induced cardiotoxicity: course, pathophysiology, prevention and management. Expert Opin Pharmacother. 2007;8:1039–58.
12. Hunt SA, Abraham WT, Chin MH, et al. ACC/AHA 2005 Guideline Update for the Diagnosis and Management of Chronic Heart Failure in the Adult: a report of the American College of Cardiology/American Heart Association Task Force on Practice Guidelines (Writing Committee to Update the 2001 Guidelines for the Evaluation and Management of Heart Failure): developed in collaboration with the American College of Chest Physicians and the International Society for Heart and Lung Transplantation: endorsed by the Heart Rhythm Society. Circulation. 2005;112:e154–235.
13. van Dalen EC, Caron HN, Dickinson HO, et al. Cardioprotective interventions for cancer patients receiving anthracyclines. Cochrane Database Syst Rev. 2008; CD003917.
14. van Dalen EC, van der Pal HJ, Caron HN, et al. Different dosage schedules for reducing cardiotoxicity in cancer patients receiving anthracycline chemotherapy. Cochrane Database Syst Rev. 2009; CD005008.
15. Herman EH, Zhang J, Rifai N, et al. The use of serum levels of cardiac troponin T to compare the protective activity of dexrazoxane against doxorubicin- and mitoxantrone-induced cardiotoxicity. Cancer Chemother Pharmacol. 2001;48:297–304.
16. Swain SM, Whaley FS, Gerber MC, et al. Cardioprotection with dexrazoxane for doxorubicin-containing therapy in advanced breast cancer. J Clin Oncol. 1997;15:1318–32.
17. Noori A, Lindenfeld J, Wolfel E, et al. Beta-blockade in adriamycin-induced cardiomyopathy. J Card Fail. 2000; 6:115–9.
18. Cardinale D, Colombo A, Sandri MT, et al. Prevention of high-dose chemotherapy-induced cardiotoxicity in high-risk patients by angiotensin-converting enzyme inhibition. Circulation. 2006;114:2474–81.
19. Adams MJ, Lipshultz SE, Schwartz C, et al. Radiation-associated cardiovascular disease: manifestations and management. Semin Radiat Oncol. 2003;13:346–56.
20. Aleman BM, van den Belt-Dusebout AW, Klokman WJ, et al. Long-Term Cause-Specific Mortality of Patients Treated for Hodgkin's Disease. J Clin Oncol. 2003;21:3431–9.
21. Boivin JF, Hutchison GB, Lubin JH, et al. Coronary artery disease mortality in patients treated for Hodgkin's disease. Cancer. 1992;69:1241–7.
22. Hancock SL, Donaldson SS, Hoppe RT. Cardiac disease following treatment of Hodgkin's disease in children and adolescents. J Clin Oncol. 1993;11:1208–15.
23. Adams MJ, Lipsitz SR, Colan SD, et al. Cardiovascular status in long-term survivors of Hodgkin's disease treated with chest radiotherapy. J Clin Oncol. 2004;22:3139–48.
24. Hull MC, Morris CG, Pepine CJ, et al. Valvular dysfunction and carotid, subclavian, and coronary artery disease in survivors of hodgkin lymphoma treated with radiation therapy. JAMA. 2003;290:2831–7.

25. Schomig K, Ndrepepa G, Mehilli J, et al. Thoracic radiotherapy in patients with lymphoma and restenosis after coronary stent placement. Catheter Cardiovasc Interv. 2007; 70:359–65.

26. Heidenreich PA, Schnittger I, Strauss HW, et al. Screening for coronary artery disease after mediastinal irradiation for Hodgkin's disease. J Clin Oncol. 2007;25:43–9.

27. Cosset JM, Henry-Amar M, Girinski T, et al. Late toxicity of radiotherapy in Hodgkin's disease. The role of fraction size. Acta Oncol. 1988;27:123–9.

28. Schultz-Hector S, Trott KR. Radiation-induced cardiovascular diseases: is the epidemiologic evidence compatible with the radiobiologic data? Int J Radiat Oncol Biol Phys. 2007; 67:10–8.

29. Lee SP, Leu MY, Smathers JB, et al. Biologically effective dose distribution based on the linear quadratic model and its clinical relevance. Int J Radiat Oncol Biol Phys. 1995;33: 375–89.

30. Emami B, Lyman J, Brown A, et al. Tolerance of normal tissue to therapeutic irradiation. Int J Radiat Oncol Biol Phys. 1991;21:109–22.

31. Girinsky T, Cordova A, Rey A, et al. Thallium-201 scintigraphy is not predictive of late cardiac complications in patients with Hodgkin's disease treated with mediastinal radiation. Int J Radiat Oncol Biol Phys. 2000;48: 1503–6.

32. Marks LB, Yu X, Prosnitz RG, et al. The incidence and functional consequences of RT-associated cardiac perfusion defects. Int J Radiat Oncol Biol Phys. 2005;63: 214–23.

33. Prosnitz RG, Hubbs JL, Evans ES, et al. Prospective assessment of radiotherapy-associated cardiac toxicity in breast cancer patients: analysis of data 3 to 6 years after treatment. Cancer. 2007;110:1840–50.

34. Verheij M, Dewit LG, Valdes Olmos RA, et al. Evidence for a renovascular component in hypertensive patients with late radiation nephropathy. Int J Radiat Oncol Biol Phys. 1994; 30:677–83.

35. Bakx JC, Veldstra MI, van den Hoogen HM, et al. Blood pressure and cardiovascular morbidity and mortality in a Dutch population: the Nijmegen cohort study. Prev Med. 2001;32:142–7.

36. Chobanian AV, Bakris GL, Black HR, et al. Seventh report of the Joint National Committee on Prevention, Detection, Evaluation, and Treatment of High Blood Pressure. Hypertension. 2003;42:1206–52.

37. Haider AW, Larson MG, Franklin SS, et al. Systolic blood pressure, diastolic blood pressure, and pulse pressure as predictors of risk for congestive heart failure in the Framingham Heart Study. Ann Intern Med. 2003;138:10–6.

38. Kannel WB. Blood pressure as a cardiovascular risk factor: prevention and treatment. JAMA. 1996;275:1571–6.

39. Miura K, Daviglus ML, Dyer AR, et al. Relationship of blood pressure to 25-year mortality due to coronary heart disease, cardiovascular diseases, and all causes in young adult men: the Chicago Heart Association Detection Project in Industry. Arch Intern Med. 2001;161:1501–8.

40. Bowers DC, McNeil DE, Liu Y, et al. Stroke as a late treatment effect of Hodgkin's Disease: a report from the Childhood Cancer Survivor Study. J Clin Oncol. 2005;23: 6508–15.

41. Glanzmann C, Huguenin P, Lutolf UM, et al. Cardiac lesions after mediastinal irradiation for Hodgkin's disease. Radiother Oncol. 1994;30:43–54.

42. Pearson TA, Blair SN, Daniels SR, et al. AHA Guidelines for Primary Prevention of Cardiovascular Disease and Stroke: 2002 Update: Consensus Panel Guide to Comprehensive Risk Reduction for Adult Patients Without Coronary or Other Atherosclerotic Vascular Diseases. American Heart Association Science Advisory and Coordinating Committee. Circulation. 2002;106:388–91.

43. Smith Jr SC, Allen J, Blair SN, et al. AHA/ACC guidelines for secondary prevention for patients with coronary and other atherosclerotic vascular disease: 2006 update: endorsed by the National Heart, Lung, and Blood Institute. Circulation. 2006;113:2363–72.

44. Heidenreich PA, Kapoor JR. Radiation induced heart disease: systemic disorders in heart disease. Heart. 2009;95:252–8.

45. De Bruin ML, Dorresteijn LD, van't Veer MB, et al. Increased risk of stroke and transient ischemic attack in 5-year survivors of Hodgkin lymphoma. J Natl Cancer Inst. 2009;101:928–37.

46. Girinsky T, van der MR, Specht L, et al. Involved-node radiotherapy (INRT) in patients with early Hodgkin lymphoma: concepts and guidelines. Radiother Oncol. 2006;79: 270–7.

47. Martin WG, Ristow KM, Habermann TM, et al. Bleomycin pulmonary toxicity has a negative impact on the outcome of patients with Hodgkin's lymphoma. J Clin Oncol. 2005;23:7614–20.

48. Ng AK, Bernardo MP, Weller E, et al. Long-term survival and competing causes of death in patients with early-stage Hodgkin's disease treated at age 50 or younger. J Clin Oncol. 2002;20:2101–8.

49. Buchler T, Bomanji J, Lee SM. FDG-PET in bleomycin-induced pneumonitis following ABVD chemotherapy for Hodgkin's disease–a useful tool for monitoring pulmonary toxicity and disease activity. Haematologica. 2007;92: e120–1.

50. Bredenfeld H, Franklin J, Nogova L, et al. Severe pulmonary toxicity in patients with advanced-stage Hodgkin's disease treated with a modified bleomycin, doxorubicin, cyclophosphamide, vincristine, procarbazine, prednisone, and gemcitabine (BEACOPP) regimen is probably related to the combination of gemcitabine and bleomycin: a report of the German Hodgkin's Lymphoma Study Group. J Clin Oncol. 2004;22:2424–9.

51. Macann A, Bredenfeld H, Muller RP, et al. Radiotherapy does not influence the severe pulmonary toxicity observed with the administration of gemcitabine and bleomycin in patients with advanced-stage Hodgkin's lymphoma treated with the BAGCOPP regimen: a report by the German Hodgkin's Lymphoma Study Group. Int J Radiat Oncol Biol Phys. 2008;70:161–5.

52. Zaniboni A, Prabhu S, Audisio RA. Chemotherapy and anaesthetic drugs: too little is known. Lancet Oncol. 2005; 6:176–81.

53. Cosset JM, Hoppe RT. Pulmonary late effects after treatment of Hodgkin's disease. In: Mauch PM, Armitage JO, Diehl V, Hoppe RT, Weiss LM, editors. Hodgkin's Disease. Philadelphia: Lippincott Williams and Wilkins; 1999. p. 633.

54. Theuws JC, Kwa SL, Wagenaar AC, et al. Prediction of overall pulmonary function loss in relation to the 3-D dose distribution for patients with breast cancer and malignant lymphoma. Radiother Oncol. 1998;49:233–43.

55. Koh ES, Sun A, Tran TH, et al. Clinical dose-volume histogram analysis in predicting radiation pneumonitis in Hodgkin's lymphoma. Int J Radiat Oncol Biol Phys. 2006; 66:223–8.

56. Brice P, Tredaniel J, Monsuez JJ, et al. Cardiopulmonary toxicity after three courses of ABVD and mediastinal irradiation in favorable Hodgkin's disease. Ann Oncol. 1991;2 Suppl 2:73–6.

57. Hirsch A, Vander EN, Straus DJ, et al. Effect of ABVD chemotherapy with and without mantle or mediastinal irradiation on pulmonary function and symptoms in early-stage Hodgkin's disease. J Clin Oncol. 1996;14: 1297–305.

58. Hancock SL, Tucker MA, Hoppe RT. Factors affecting late mortality from heart disease after treatment of Hodgkin's disease. JAMA. 1993;270:1949–55.

59. Hoppe RT. Hodgkin's disease: complications of therapy and excess mortality. Ann Oncol. 1997;8 Suppl 1:115–8.

60. King V, Constine LS, Clark D, et al. Symptomatic coronary artery disease after mantle irradiation for Hodgkin's disease. Int J Radiat Oncol Biol Phys. 1996;36:881–9.

61. Glanzmann C, Kaufmann P, Jenni R, et al. Cardiac risk after mediastinal irradiation for Hodgkin's disease. Radiother Oncol. 1998;46:51–62.

62. Brierley JD, Rathmell AJ, Gospodarowicz MK, et al. Late effects of treatment for early-stage Hodgkin's disease. Br J Cancer. 1998;77:1300–10.

63. Heidenreich PA, Hancock SL, Lee BK, et al. Asymptomatic cardiac disease following mediastinal irradiation. J Am Coll Cardiol. 2003;42:743–9.

# Gonadal Dysfunction and Fertility Preservation in Hodgkin Lymphoma Patients

# 24

Karolin Behringer, Michael von Wolff, and Graham M. Mead

## Contents

K. Behringer (✉)
First Department of Internal Medicine, German Hodgkin Study Group (GHSG), University Hospital Cologne, Cologne, Germany
e-mail: karolin.behringer@uk-koeln.de

M. von Wolff
Department of Gynecological Endocrinology and Reproductive Medicine, University Hospital – Inselspital Berne, Berne, Switzerland

G.M. Mead
Cancer Research UK Clinical Centre, Southampton General Hospital, Southampton University Hospitals NHS Trust, Southampton, Hampshire, UK

## 24.1 Gonadal Dysfunction in Men

### 24.1.1 Male Reproductive Physiology

Sperm production in males is stimulated via secretion of follicle-stimulating hormone (FSH) by the pituitary gland, regulated by a negative feedback mechanism via inhibin produced from the Sertoli cells and/or seminiferous tubules. Impaired or absent sperm production can be anticipated based on progressive elevation of FSH levels. Testicular androgen production is regulated by pituitary secretion of luteinizing hormone (LH) and controlled by a comparable feedback mechanism via testosterone production of the testicular Leydig cells.

Gonadal function can be evaluated by measuring FSH and LH together with the morning testosterone level. A semen analysis is a more definitive test of fertility, with normal values of $>20 \times 10^6$/mL, a sperm motility of $>50\%$, and with $>14\%$ of normal forms.

### 24.1.2 Hodgkin Lymphoma and Male Gonadal Dysfunction

Seventy-eighty percent of male HL patients have inadequate pre-treatment semen quality due to the lymphoma itself [1–4]. The mechanisms involved are

A. Engert and S.J. Horning (eds.), *Hodgkin Lymphoma*,
DOI: 10.1007/978-3-642-12780-9_24, © Springer-Verlag Berlin Heidelberg 2011

still unknown, however, possible factors include damage to the germinal epithelium, disturbances in the hypothalamic–hypophysial axis, immunological processes associated with cancer that impair spermatogenesis, and the impact of cytokines [2, 5–9]. In a recent study by the German Hodgkin Study Group (GHSG), male fertility was assessed in a total of 243 patients. In pre-treatment semen analysis, only 20% of patients had normal sperms. Azoospermia was observed in 11% of patients and dysspermia in 69% [3].

### 24.1.3 Treatment-Related Gonadal Dysfunction

Post-treatment gonadal damage is most often associated with chemotherapy regimens that include alkylating agents such as cyclophosphamide and procarbazine. The degree of damage and recovery of spermatogenesis depends on the choice of drugs and the dose given. In multiple analyses, the rate of azoospermia after cyclophosphamide, vincristine, procarbazine, and prednisone (COPP); mustargen, vincristine, procarbazine, and prednisone (MOPP); or cyclophosphamide, vincristine, procarbazine, prednisone, adriamycin, bleomycin, vinblastine, and dacarbazine (COPP/ABVD) is high, ranging from 80 to 100% [4, 10–14]. Recovery of spermatogenesis can occur, and has been recorded in 11–14% of males after these regimens [4, 13–15]. This rate was 40% when dysspermia was included [4]. Da Cunha and colleagues assessed MOPP-induced gonadotoxicity, demonstrating a significantly higher rate of azoospermia in patients treated with more than five cycles of MOPP compared to those receiving three or fewer cycles [16]. Newer and more intensive alkylating agent based combinations such as bleomycin, etoposide, adriamycin, cyclophosphamide, vincristine, procarbazine, and prednisone (BEACOPP) are highly gonadotoxic in males. In a recent study, post-treatment sperm analyses performed at a median of 17.4 months after the end of therapy revealed azoospermia in 64% of patients, other forms of dysspermia in 30%, and normal sperm analysis results in only 6% of cases [3]. Thirty-eight patients with advanced stage disease were examined and 89% were azoospermic after treatment. None of these patients had a normal sperm status. There was no statistically significant difference in the post-treatment fertility status between a group of patients treated with eight cycles of BEACOPP baseline (with a cumulative cyclophosphamide dose of 5,200 mg/m²) and a group treated with eight cycles of BEACOPP escalated regimens (with a cumulative cyclophosphamide dose of 10,000 mg/m²) [3].

In contrast, the probably most widely used standard treatment for HL, ABVD, is less gonadotoxic, with gonadal damage that might be only transient [13, 17, 18].

Pelvic radiotherapy is now infrequently used in the management of HL. The testes are highly sensitive to irradiation in a dose-dependent manner. Doses above 4–6 Gy can result in permanent azoospermia and doses of more than 6 Gy have a significant risk of this complication. Direct testicular irradiation is usually not necessary in HL patients, and scattered irradiation can be reduced by shielding the testes.

### 24.1.4 Predictive Factors for Gonadal Dysfunction and Damage

In a multivariate analysis of HL patients at initial diagnosis, Rueffer and colleagues described an elevated erythrocyte sedimentation rate (ESR) and poor prognostic risk groups as predictive for severe dysspermia [2]. A comparable study by Gandini and colleagues evaluated the semen quality in 106 untreated HL patients and showed a significant decrease in sperm concentration, total sperm count, and forward motility in the later stages of HL (stage III–IV) compared to early stages (stage I–II). Interestingly, of 53 patients with elevated ESR, 79.2% had a normal sperm count, suggesting this parameter was not predictive for semen quality or potential infertility [19]. In a recent analysis of the GHSG risk groups, extranodal involvement, treatment with chemotherapy and BEACOPP were predictive factors for post-treatment azoospermia only in a univariate model. The fertility status prior to therapy was not predictive for post-treatment fertility [4, 20].

### 24.1.5 Hormonal Analyses to Assess Testicular Function After Therapy

Achievement of paternity and sperm counts provide the strongest evidence of male fertility; however, gonadotropin measurement can also provide useful surrogate information. Most studies in male patients show that the FSH levels correlate with testicular function after treatment [3, 4, 11, 18, 21]. In a recent study by van der Kaaij and colleagues, FSH was measured in a total of 355 patients with early-stage disease at least 12 months after the end of treatment. FSH was elevated in 35% of all patients and in 3% of those receiving radiotherapy only. In contrast, 60% of patients treated with alkylating agents had elevated FSH levels whereas this was observed in only 8% of patients receiving chemotherapy without alkylators. Recovery of fertility was also poorer in patients treated with alkylating-agent-containing chemotherapy [21]. Kreuser and colleagues reported increased FSH levels in 80% of patients after treatment with COPP/ABVD [11]. In a retrospective GHSG analysis, abnormal FSH levels after chemotherapy were found in 79%. In this group, the majority of patients were azoospermic (78%; $p = 0.001$), suggesting an indirect correlation between FSH level and testicular dysfunction after therapy [3]. In contrast, normal levels of LH and testosterone were found in 86 and 63% of patients after treatment. This underlines the hypothesis that spermatogonia cells are sensitive, whereas Leydig cells are more resistant to the toxic effects of cytostatic drugs [3, 11, 14]. A further important hormone in the assessment of infertility in men is inhibin B, which is produced by the Sertoli cells. Some studies support the use of inhibin B and inhibin B/FSH ratios as markers of male infertility [22, 23]. According to the results of a recent study, 65% of male cancer survivors had low inhibin B values as compared to 26% in the control group [24]. Inhibin B levels correlated significantly with sperm concentration [24–26].

### 24.1.6 Endocrine Hypogonadism After Chemotherapy in Men

Little is known on the endocrine status of men after chemotherapy for HL. A recent study by Kiserud and colleagues investigated post-treatment exocrine and endocrine gonadal function in 165 HL and 129 non-Hodgkin lymphoma (NHL) patients. In almost one-third of the patients, the hormone levels were compatible with endocrine hypogonadism, defined as low testosterone with or without elevated LH, or

elevated LH and normal testosterone. Interestingly, only three patients were receiving testosterone replacement at the time of analysis [27]. Comparable findings after chemotherapy for testicular cancer in young males were linked with a subsequent risk of developing metabolic syndrome [28].

### 24.1.7 Fertility Preservation in Men: Preventative Pretreatment Strategies and Management After Chemotherapy

Sperm banking is a widely available and successful pre-treatment preventative strategy. All postpubertal males should be offered sperm banking prior to potentially gonadotoxic chemotherapy. This also needs to include patients planned for ABVD, although this regimen has a rather low risk of treatment-related infertility. The reason for this is that in the event of early relapse, sperm quality and quantity might not have recovered, rendering banking impossible prior to gonadotoxic salvage treatment. Sperm should be banked regardless of count as intracytoplasmic sperm injection can be successfully used as part of in vitro fertilization (IVF) where counts are low. If azoospermia is present and time permits, testicular sperm retrieval can be successful, particularly in the presence of a normal or only modestly elevated FSH level.

## 24.2 Gonadal Dysfunction in Women

### 24.2.1 Female Reproductive Physiology

In premenopausal menstruating women, ovarian function is controlled by pituitary secretion of FSH and LH. FSH activates the granulosa cells of growing ovarian follicles which in turn begin to proliferate and to produce estradiol. This reduces the FSH levels by feedback inhibition, maintaining them at low levels. A mid-cycle LH surge induces ovulation following the formation of the luteal body that produces progesterone. Follicle development takes place over several months prior to ovulation. The growing follicles produce not only estradiol, but also inhibin, which prevents the growth of too many follicles by downregulating FSH.

At puberty, approximately 300,000 follicles are present in the ovary. This number declines with age to around 1,000 at menopause (around 50–52 years of age), when FSH levels are insufficiently suppressed due to declining estrogen levels and therefore rise. The decline accelerates after the age of 35.

The number of follicles present in the ovary is known as the ovarian reserve and reflects reproductive capacity. Anti-Müllerian hormone (AMH) is produced by early, developing follicles, and its levels vary slightly during the menstrual cycle. It acts directly on other follicles in the ovary and inhibits the growth of too many follicles. The levels of this hormone are increasingly used in clinical studies to assess long-term gonadal damage and ovarian reserve.

## 24.2.2 Treatment-Related Infertility

While the mechanisms underlying the ovariotoxic effects of cytostatic drugs are still largely unknown, it is clear that the development of primary ovarian failure after chemotherapy is caused by accelerated attrition of the ovarian primordial follicles. As described above, this is age-dependent in relation to the ovarian reserve. For alkylating agents, a direct dose-dependent cytotoxic effect has been described. Acute toxicity reduces the number of follicles, whereas chronic toxicity affects the quality of follicles resulting in early atresia [29].

Very similar to male patients, alkylating agents are most commonly involved in female gonadal damage. This is well documented after treatment with older chemotherapy regimens such as MOPP or MVPP (mustargen, vinblastine, procarbazine, and prednisone). In an early study, only 17 of 44 women maintained regular menses when either of these regimens was used [30]. In a similar study, Schilsky and colleagues investigated ovarian function after treatment with MOPP and documented persistent amenorrhea in 11 of 24 women [31]. Similarly, after treatment with alternating COPP/ABVD for advanced-stage HL, therapy-induced ovarian failure was described in 17 of 22 women (77%) [11]. A more recent analysis included a total of 84 female patients with HL and NHL treated with at least three cycles of chemotherapy including alkylating agents. Premature ovarian failure (POF) was

defined as persistent amenorrhea for at least 2 years after the end of chemotherapy and elevated FSH levels. After a median follow-up of 100 months, 31 (37%) women with preserved fertility achieved natural pregnancy; in 34 women (40.5%), premature ovarian failure was reported [32]. A study by Haukvik and colleagues reported POF (in this study defined as persistent amenorrhea before the age of 41) in 37% of women after HL treatment. This occurred more commonly in alkylating-agent-treated patients [33]. In a retrospective GHSG analysis, the menstrual status after HL treatment of 405 female patients younger than 40 years was analyzed. With a median follow-up of 3.2 years, 51.4% of women who received eight cycles of escalated BEACOPP had continuous amenorrhea. Amenorrhea was significantly less common in women treated with two cycles of ABVD (3.9%), two cycles of alternating COPP/ABVD (6.9%), four cycles of alternating COPP/ABVD (37.5%), or eight cycles of BEACOPP baseline (22.6%). In a multivariate analysis, amenorrhea was most pronounced in women with advanced-stage HL, women older than 30 years of age at treatment, and women who did not take oral contraceptives during chemotherapy [34].

After ABVD alone, chemotherapy-induced ovarian failure is less likely, especially when women are younger than 30 years at the time of treatment [17, 35–38].

Older women have a significantly lower likelihood of ovarian recovery than those of younger age [11, 30–32, 34, 39, 40]. In the GHSG analysis, 40% of women younger than 30 years of age experienced amenorrhea after treatment with eight cycles of escalated BEACOPP, compared to 70% of women aged 30 years or older [34] (Table 24.1). Interestingly, the study by Haukvik and colleagues demonstrated a high cumulative percentage of POF in the youngest group of women. Compared to women diagnosed at the age of 30 years or older, those younger than 30 years developed POF approximately 5 years later. These findings suggest that younger age at HL treatment delays the

Table 24.1 Chemotherapy-induced amenorrhea depending on chemotherapy regimen in advanced stages and age at treatment (Behringer et al., 2005)

| Age | Chemotherapy regimen | Amenorrhea (%) |
| --- | --- | --- |
| <30 years | 8×BEACOPP baseline | 11.8 |
| ≥30 years | | 42.1 |
| <30 years | 8×BEACOPP escalated | 40.4 |
| ≥30 years | | 70.4 |

development of POF, but that the life-time risk of POF is not decreased [33].

### 24.2.3 Post-treatment Assessment of Ovarian Reserve with Anti-Müllerian Hormone Levels

In the literature, the definition of gonadal toxicity varies. As described in the prior section, gonadal toxicity is in some reports defined by amenorrhea only, whereas in others also hormonal parameters such as FSH or LH were used. However, all of these parameters only measure the ovarian reserve indirectly and have little sensitivity. Recent studies suggested that AMH is the most sensitive marker of gonadal function. This hormone is produced by the granulosa cells of early developing pre-antral and antral follicles in the ovary. The serum AMH levels can be used as a marker for the number of growing follicles – the levels decrease when the number of follicles decline. The AMH levels are not influenced by the day of the menstrual cycle. They are therefore a potentially convenient and useful marker [41–43]. Recently, AMH has been tested to identify subgroups of childhood cancer survivors at risk for premature ovarian failure [44].

### 24.2.4 Radiation Therapy

Due to the increasing use of combined modality or chemotherapy-only approaches, infradiaphragmatic radiation is rarely used in the treatment of HL. According to a mathematic model described by Wallace and colleagues, the dose of radiation required to destroy approximately 50% of oocytes has been estimated to be less than 2 Gy [45]. The estimated effective sterilizing radiation dose to the ovary for 20-year-old patients is 16.5 Gy [46]. The uterus is more radioresistant than are the ovaries. Nonetheless, partial or complete uterine irradiation, though rarely required, can result in uterine fibrosis with an increased rate of miscarriage. Gonadal and organ damage can be reduced by shielding and other techniques, and pre-treatment oophoropexy may also have a role in this process.

### 24.2.5 Preventative Treatment Strategies in Women

After HL diagnosis, strategies for ovarian protection should be offered to all women who have not completed their family planning. Women should be referred to an experienced center for counseling on protective procedures, after which management approaches should also be discussed with the attending oncologist. Figure 24.1 summarizes the options to preserve fertility in women with HL [47].

### 24.2.6 Pharmacological Prevention of Gonadal Damage

Gonadotoxic chemotherapy destroys ovarian follicles and leads to decreased estrogen and inhibin secretion. Due to the negative feedback mechanism, the FSH levels increase and induce an increased recruitment of follicles, which are also potentially destroyed by chemotherapy. Pharmacological methods to protect fertility aim at suppressing pituitary gonadotropin secretion and cyclic ovarian function with the use of GnRH agonists, antagonists, and oral contraceptives.

The following putative protective mechanisms using GnRH analogues have been suggested [48].

1. Creating a prepubertal, hypogonadotropic milieu: Injected GnRH analogues cause an initial stimulation ("flare up") of the pituitary LH and FSH secretion. As a consequence of the downregulation of the pituitary GnRH receptors, the FSH and LH secretion then declines to low, prepubertal serum levels. This mechanism prevents the FSH levels from increasing and can stop the enhanced recruitment of follicles, thereby rescuing them from accelerated atresia.

2. Decreased utero-ovarian perfusion: Due to the hypo-estrogenic milieu, utero-ovarian perfusion is decreased. This may lead to a lower total cumulative exposure of the ovaries to gonadotoxic chemotherapy.

3. A direct effect on GnRH receptors: GnRH-a may directly decrease gonadotoxicity of chemotherapy.

4. Possible role of sphingosine-1-phosphate: Spingosine-1-phosphate (S-1-P) is a lipid mediator of cell growth, survival, invasion, vascular maturation, and angiogenesis, which are all processes that are involved in

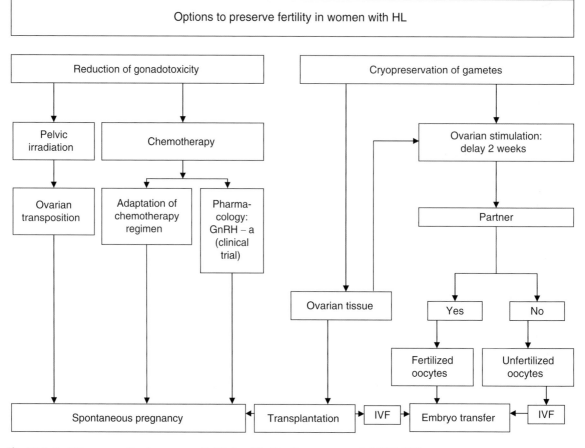

**Fig. 24.1** Fertility preservation in women with HL (modified by Demeestere et al. (2007) [47])

cell viability and cancer progression. It is speculated that GnRH-a may increase intragonadal S-1-P, thus preventing the ovarian follicles from destruction.

5. Possible protection of ovarian stem cells: It is speculated that GnRH-a may protect undifferentiated germ line stem cells that are capable of generating de novo primordial follicles.

Others have challenged the putative protective effect of GnRH-a, as the primordial follicle growth is an FSH-independent process and alkylating agents are not cell-cycle specific. Thus, they might damage resting primordial follicles. It is speculated that GnRH-a might halt the growth of developing follicles, resulting in a resumption of the menstrual cycle in the short term, which might give the false impression that ovarian function is preserved [49].

Two retrospective reviews have recently examined the possible gonadal protective effect of GnRH-a in chemotherapy-treated patients. Beck-Fruchter and colleagues reviewed a total of 12 journal articles (two of which

referred to small prospectively randomized trials), which included 345 women receiving GnRH-a co-treatment with chemotherapy and 234 women who did not receive GnRH-a during cancer treatment. Premature ovarian failure (POF) or persistent amenorrhea was reported in 9% of the GnRH-a co-treatment group and in 59% in the control group [50]. Similar results were reported by Blumenfeld and von Wolff after reviewing a total of nine clinical trials in which the POF rate was 11.1% in the GnRH-a group ($n=225$) compared to 55.5% in the control group ($n=189$) [48]. Despite these data, both authors concluded that the results should be regarded inconclusive and recommended conducting large, well-designed, prospective randomized trials.

Recently, preliminary data from a randomized study in 80 women with breast cancer undergoing 5-fluorouracil, adriamycin, cyclophosphamide (FAC) chemotherapy was reported. After 8 months, menstruation was documented in 89.6% of the GnRH-a co-treatment group compared to 33.3% in the control group [51]. A study by Huser and colleagues investigating the protective effect of GnRH-a in a total of 117 female HL patients suggested that GnRH-a might only be effective in women receiving less aggressive chemotherapy. No significant protection with GnRH-a was achieved in women receiving eight cycles of escalated BEACOPP [52].

Between 2004 and 2007, the GHSG conducted a prospective randomized trial (PROFE) to analyze the protective effect of GnRH-a. This trial was designed for young female patients (18–40 years) with advanced-stage HL, receiving eight cycles of escalated BEACOPP. Patients were randomly assigned either to daily oral contraceptives (OC) or the GnRH-analogue (GnRH-a) goserelin, given monthly during eight cycles of poly-chemotherapy with escalated BEACOPP. The study was closed early after an interim analysis of 23 patients. Twelve patients were enrolled into arm A (OC) and 11 into arm B (GnRH-a). The women's median age was 26 years in arm A and 25 years in arm B. The AMH level after at least 12 months was reduced in all women. Combining both treatment arms, the respective ovarian follicle preservation rate was 0% (95% CI: 0–12%); thus, continuation of the study was not justified.

Clinically relevant side effects of GnRH-a include menopausal symptoms such as hot flushes, headaches, mood changes, and decreased bone density [50, 53].

## 24.2.7 Cryopreservation of Oocytes/Ovarian Tissue

In the field of cryopreservation of oocytes and ovarian tissue, there have been remarkable advances in recent years. But which technique (if any) should be recommended to a young woman before chemotherapy? This depends on the treatment to be used, age, availability of a partner, and the clinical condition of the patient and time available. It should be emphasized that results are likely to significantly improve during the reproductive span of patients currently undergoing harvest and storage.

### 24.2.7.1 Ovarian Stimulation and Cryopreservation of Fertilized and Unfertilized Oocytes

A minimum period of 2 weeks is required for both procedures. This is largely due to the time needed for ovarian stimulation. Modified stimulation regimens requiring 2 weeks have been successfully evaluated [54]. The

cryopreservation of fertilized oocytes is a well-established method. If sufficient numbers of oocytes can be retrieved and all cryopreserved fertilized oocytes are transferred, the average cumulative pregnancy rate can be up to 40%. The success rate of the cryopreservation of unfertilized oocytes seems to depend on the freezing methodology and thus strongly depends on the expertise of the fertility center.

### 24.2.7.2 Embryo Cryopreservation

Embryo cryopreservation and retrieval are validated and successful techniques. Like in oocyte preservation, time is needed to achieve ovarian stimulation. A partner is also required. This is the preferred technique in ideal circumstances.

### 24.2.7.3 Cryopreservation of Ovarian Tissue

Cryopreservation of ovarian tissue is an alternative, especially for young patients without a partner. This method requires little or no preparative time but does require a laparoscopy. A combination of this technique with other invasive methods is possible.

The ovarian tissue is retrieved from one ovary and subsequently prepared and preserved using cryoprotective agents. If ovarian function insufficiency develops while relapse-free on follow-up, the cryopreserved tissue can be transplanted orthotopically to the remaining ovary or heterotopically. Currently, 12 live births and several ongoing pregnancies have been reported using this approach [55]. Work in mice models led to concern about possible tumor re-implantation from ovaries infiltrated with lymphoma [56]. In practice, however, HL rarely involves the ovaries; the tumor cells are extremely fragile and so far there are no recorded events of tumor cell reimplantation [55, 57].

## 24.2.8 Premature Menopause

Early onset of menopause in female patients after treatment for childhood cancer is well described [58, 59], and recent data shows a higher cumulative incidence of premature menopause by the age of 40 for survivors compared to control siblings (8 vs. 0.8%) [60]. Alkylating-agent-based combination chemotherapy will very likely lead to premature menopause in female patients. It is important to note that occasionally transient cessation of menses, with or without hot flushes, can occur. Hormone replacement may be indicated to reduce symptoms and prevent osteoporosis. If fertility is desired in younger women and conventional low-dose HRT is used, it is possible to monitor ovarian recovery with FSH levels. If oral contraceptives are used, treatment breaks with re-evaluation of ovarian function may be reasonable.

## 24.3 Conclusions

Remarkable advances have occurred in the management of HL, and today cure can be anticipated for the vast majority of young adults. When alkylating-agent-based combination chemotherapy was first devised in the 1960s, almost any late effect on fertility was acceptable in the context of the hitherto grim prognosis of HL, particularly in advanced stages. Then, regimens such as ABVD proved to be equivalent or superior, inducing much less gonadotoxic effects. After the more recent introduction of highly effective alkylating-agent-based therapy such as BEACOPP, impressive failure-free survival rates were achieved, but were associated with substantial gonadal toxicity, necessitating the development of adjunctive fertility supporting technology. Current trials evaluate risk-adapted treatment, reserving more effective but more toxic treatment for subgroups of patients with poorer prognosis as judged by positron emission tomography (PET) scanning.

The remarkable advances in the management of HL are paralleled by advances in fertility preservation techniques. It is of particular importance that these are considered and discussed as early as possible after diagnosis in the context of the patient's wishes with regard to treatment and future fertility.

## References

1. Lee SJ et al. American Society of Clinical Oncology recommendations on fertility preservation in cancer patients. J Clin Oncol. 2006;24(18):2917–31.
2. Rueffer U et al. Male gonadal dysfunction in patients with Hodgkin's disease prior to treatment. Ann Oncol. 2001;12(9): 1307–11.
3. Sieniawski M et al. Assessment of male fertility in patients with Hodgkin's lymphoma treated in the German Hodgkin Study Group (GHSG) clinical trials. Ann Oncol. 2008;19(10): 1795–801.
4. Viviani S et al. Testicular dysfunction in Hodgkin's disease before and after treatment. Eur J Cancer. 1991;27(11): p1389–92.
5. Agarwal A, Allamaneni SS. Disruption of spermatogenesis by the cancer disease process. J Natl Cancer Inst Monogr. 2005;(34):9–12.
6. Barr RD, Clark DA, Booth JD. Dysspermia in men with localized Hodgkin's disease. A potentially reversible, immune-mediated disorder. Med Hypotheses. 1993;40(3): 165–8.
7. Dousset B et al. Seminal cytokine concentrations (IL-1beta, IL-2, IL-6, sR IL-2, sR IL-6), semen parameters and blood hormonal status in male infertility. Hum Reprod. 1997;12(7): 1476–9.
8. Huleihel M et al. Distinct expression levels of cytokines and soluble cytokine receptors in seminal plasma of fertile and infertile men. Fertil Steril. 1996;66(1):135–9.
9. Redman JR et al. Semen cryopreservation and artificial insemination for Hodgkin's disease. J Clin Oncol. 1987;5(2): 233–8.
10. Chapman R, Sutcliffe S, Malpas J. Male gonadal dysfunction in Hodgkin's disease. A prospective study. JAMA. 1981;245(13):p1323–8.
11. Kreuser E et al. Long-term gonadal dysfunction and its impact on bone mineralization in patients following COPP/ABVD chemotherapy for Hodgkin's disease. Ann Oncol. 1992;3 Suppl 4:105–10.
12. Kreuser ED et al. Reproductive and endocrine gonadal capacity in patients treated with COPP chemotherapy for Hodgkin's disease. J Cancer Res Clin Oncol. 1987;113(3): 260–6.
13. Viviani S et al. Gonadal toxicity after combination chemotherapy for Hodgkin's disease. Comparative results of MOPP vs ABVD. Eur J Cancer Clin Oncol. 1985;21(5):p601–5.
14. Waxman J et al. Gonadal function in Hodgkin's disease: long-term follow-up of chemotherapy. Br Med J (Clin Res Ed). 1982;285(6355):1612–3.
15. Andrieu J et al. Male fertility in Hodgkin's disease before and after chemotherapy (author's transl). Nouv Presse Méd. 1981;10(25):p2085–8.
16. da Cunha MF et al. Recovery of spermatogenesis after treatment for Hodgkin's disease: limiting dose of MOPP chemotherapy. J Clin Oncol. 1984;2(6):571–7.
17. Bonadonna G et al. Gonadal damage in Hodgkin's disease from cancer chemotherapeutic regimens. Arch Toxicol Suppl. 1984;7:140–5.
18. Kulkarni S et al. Gonadal function following ABVD therapy for Hodgkin's disease. Am J Clin Oncol. 1997;20(4): p354–7.
19. Gandini L et al. Testicular cancer and Hodgkin's disease: evaluation of semen quality. Hum Reprod. 2003;18(4):796–801.
20. Sieniawski M et al. Fertility in male patients with advanced Hodgkin lymphoma treated with BEACOPP: a report of the German Hodgkin Study Group (GHSG). Blood. 2008;111(1): 71–6.
21. van der Kaaij MA et al. Gonadal function in males after chemotherapy for early-stage Hodgkin's lymphoma treated in

four subsequent trials by the European Organisation for Research and Treatment of Cancer: EORTC Lymphoma Group and the Groupe d'Etude des Lymphomes de l'Adulte. J Clin Oncol. 2007;25(19):2825–32.

22. Andersson AM et al. Serum inhibin B and follicle-stimulating hormone levels as tools in the evaluation of infertile men: significance of adequate reference values from proven fertile men. J Clin Endocrinol Metab. 2004;89(6): 2873–9.

23. Bordallo MA et al. Decreased serum inhibin B/FSH ratio as a marker of Sertoli cell function in male survivors after chemotherapy in childhood and adolescence. J Pediatr Endocrinol Metab. 2004;17(6):879–87.

24. van Casteren NJ et al. Effect of childhood cancer treatment on fertility markers in adult male long-term survivors. Pediatr Blood Cancer. 2009;52(1):108–12.

25. Kumanov P et al. Inhibin B is a better marker of spermatogenesis than other hormones in the evaluation of male factor infertility. Fertil Steril. 2006;86(2):332–8.

26. van Beek RD et al. Inhibin B is superior to FSH as a serum marker for spermatogenesis in men treated for Hodgkin's lymphoma with chemotherapy during childhood. Hum Reprod. 2007;22(12):3215–22.

27. Kiserud CE et al. Gonadal function in male patients after treatment for malignant lymphomas, with emphasis on chemotherapy. Br J Cancer. 2009;100(3):455–63.

28. Nuver J et al. The metabolic syndrome and disturbances in hormone levels in long-term survivors of disseminated testicular cancer. J Clin Oncol. 2005;23(16):3718–25.

29. Familiari G et al. Ultrastructure of human ovarian primordial follicles after combination chemotherapy for Hodgkin's disease. Hum Reprod. 1993;8(12):p2080–7.

30. Whitehead E et al. The effect of combination chemotherapy on ovarian function in women treated for Hodgkin's disease. Cancer. 1983;52(6):988–93.

31. Schilsky RL et al. Long-term follow up of ovarian function in women treated with MOPP chemotherapy for Hodgkin's disease. Am J Med. 1981;71(4):552–6.

32. Franchi-Rezgui P et al. Fertility in young women after chemotherapy with alkylating agents for Hodgkin and non-Hodgkin lymphomas. Hematol J. 2003;4(2):116–20.

33. Haukvik UK et al. Treatment-related premature ovarian failure as a long-term complication after Hodgkin's lymphoma. Ann Oncol. 2006;17(9):1428–33.

34. Behringer K et al. Secondary amenorrhea after Hodgkin's lymphoma is influenced by age at treatment, stage of disease, chemotherapy regimen, and the use of oral contraceptives during therapy: a report from the German Hodgkin's Lymphoma Study Group. J Clin Oncol. 2005;23(30): 7555–64.

35. Andre M et al. Results of three courses of adriamycin, bleomycin, vindesine, and dacarbazine with subtotal nodal irradiation in 189 patients with nodal Hodgkin's disease (stage I, II and IIIA). Hematol Cell Ther. 1997;39(2):p59–65.

36. Bonadonna G. Modern treatment of malignant lymphomas: a multidisciplinary approach? The Kaplan Memorial Lecture. Ann Oncol. 1994;5 Suppl 2:5–16.

37. Brusamolino E et al. Treatment of early-stage Hodgkin's disease with four cycles of ABVD followed by adjuvant radio-therapy: analysis of efficacy and long-term toxicity. Haematologica. 2000;85(10):1032–9.

38. Hodgson DC et al. Fertility among female Hodgkin lymphoma survivors attempting pregnancy following ABVD chemotherapy. Hematol Oncol. 2007;25(1):11–5.

39. Horning SJ et al. Female reproductive potential after treatment for Hodgkin's disease. N Engl J Med. 1981;304(23): 1377–82.

40. Howell SJ, Shalet SM. Fertility preservation and management of gonadal failure associated with lymphoma therapy. Curr Oncol Rep. 2002;4(5):443–52.

41. Tsepelidis S et al. Stable serum levels of anti-Mullerian hormone during the menstrual cycle: a prospective study in normo-ovulatory women. Hum Reprod. 2007;22(7):1837–40.

42. van Beek RD et al. Anti-Mullerian hormone is a sensitive serum marker for gonadal function in women treated for Hodgkin's lymphoma during childhood. J Clin Endocrinol Metab. 2007;92(10):3869–74.

43. Visser JA et al. Anti-Mullerian hormone: a new marker for ovarian function. Reproduction. 2006;131(1):1–9.

44. Lie Fong S et al. Assessment of ovarian reserve in adult childhood cancer survivors using anti-Mullerian hormone. Hum Reprod. 2009;24(4):982–90.

45. Wallace WH, Thomson AB, Kelsey TW. The radiosensitivity of the human oocyte. Hum Reprod. 2003;18(1):117–21.

46. Wo JY, Viswanathan AN. Impact of radiotherapy on fertility, pregnancy, and neonatal outcomes in female cancer patients. Int J Radiat Oncol Biol Phys. 2009;73(5):1304–12.

47. Demeestere I et al. Fertility preservation: successful transplantation of cryopreserved ovarian tissue in a young patient previously treated for Hodgkin's disease. Oncologist. 2007;12(12):1437–42.

48. Blumenfeld Z, von Wolff M. GnRH-analogues and oral contraceptives for fertility preservation in women during chemotherapy. Hum Reprod Update. 2008;14(6):543–52.

49. Oktay K et al. Absence of conclusive evidence for the safety and efficacy of gonadotropin-releasing hormone analogue treatment in protecting against chemotherapy-induced gonadal injury. Oncologist. 2007;12(9):1055–66.

50. Beck-Fruchter R, Weiss A, Shalev E. GnRH agonist therapy as ovarian protectants in female patients undergoing chemotherapy: a review of the clinical data. Hum Reprod Update. 2008;14(6):553–61.

51. Badawy A et al. Gonadotropin-releasing hormone agonists for prevention of chemotherapy-induced ovarian damage: prospective randomized study. Fertil Steril. 2009;91(3):694–7.

52. Huser M et al. Prevention of ovarian function damage by a GnRH analogue during chemotherapy in Hodgkin lymphoma patients. Hum Reprod. 2008;23(4):863–8.

53. Del Mastro L et al. Prevention of chemotherapy-induced menopause by temporary ovarian suppression with goserelin in young, early breast cancer patients. Ann Oncol. 2006; 17(1):74–8.

54. von Wolff M et al. Ovarian stimulation to cryopreserve fertilized oocytes in cancer patients can be started in the luteal phase. Fertil Steril. 2009;92(4):1360–5.

55. von Wolff M et al. Cryopreservation and autotransplantation of human ovarian tissue prior to cytotoxic therapy–a technique in its infancy but already successful in fertility preservation. Eur J Cancer. 2009;45(9):1547–53.

56. Shaw JM et al. Fresh and cryopreserved ovarian tissue samples from donors with lymphoma transmit the cancer to graft recipients. Hum Reprod. 1996;11(8):1668–73.

57. Seshadri T et al. Lack of evidence of disease contamination in ovarian tissue harvested for cryopreservation from patients with Hodgkin lymphoma and analysis of factors predictive of oocyte yield. Br J Cancer. 2006;94(7):1007–10.

58. Byrne J. Infertility and premature menopause in childhood cancer survivors. Med Pediatr Oncol. 1999;33(1):24–8.

59. Larsen EC et al. Reduced ovarian function in long-term survivors of radiation- and chemotherapy-treated childhood cancer. J Clin Endocrinol Metab. 2003;88(11):5307–14.

60. Sklar CA et al. Premature menopause in survivors of childhood cancer: a report from the childhood cancer survivor study. J Natl Cancer Inst. 2006;98(13):890–6.

61. Behringer K, Wildt L, Mueller H, Mattle V, Ganitis P, van den Hoonaard B, Ott HW, Hofer S, Pluetschow A, Diehl V, Engert A, Borchmann P; on behalf of the German Hodgkin Study Group. Ann Oncol. 2010 Mar 19. [Epub ahead of print]

# What Will We Learn from Genomics and Proteomics in Hodgkin Lymphoma?

## 25

Christian Steidl and Randy D. Gascoyne

## Contents

## 25.1  Introduction

Genome-wide strategies have been developed in recent years to comprehensively detect changes in DNA, RNA, and proteins. These technologies are in constant flux, as improvements in nanotechnology combined with innovation in the fields of genomics and bioinformatics improve our ability to interrogate single cells at a resolution not seen previously. Next-generation sequencing technology and microarray approaches allow an unparalleled ability to explore genomes, transcriptomes, and proteomes at a depth of coverage and resolution at which novel discovery is possible. The phenotypic consequences of these genetic changes can now be more fully understood. By applying these technologies to Hodgkin lymphoma, major advances have been made and more yet to be realized, all of which improve our understanding of the complex biology of this unique cancer. Despite major advances, numerous obstacles remain that prevent direct clinical translation and meaningful improvements in diagnosis, predicting prognosis and patient care. For both scientists and clinicians interested in the pathogenesis of Hodgkin lymphoma and the identification of new targets for therapy, these obstacles include: (a) the scarcity of the malignant Hodgkin Reed-Sternberg (HRS) cells in diagnostic biopsies; (b) the complex interaction of these cells with non-neoplastic immune cells in the tumor microenvironment; (c) the lack of good in vitro and animal models; (d) sophisticated bioinformatics tools required to properly analyze the large amounts of data that result from high-resolution genomic experiments and finally; (e) systematic clinical data and/or randomized clinical trials material needed to translate novel findings into clinically useful biomarkers.

The focus of this chapter is largely a subject of speculation. Before peering into the future and addressing the question of "what will we learn from genomics

C. Steidl and R.D. Gascoyne (✉)
Department of Pathology and Laboratory Medicine, British Columbia Cancer Agency and the BC Cancer Research Centre, Vancouver, BC, Canada
e-mail: rgascoyn@bccancer.bc.ca

A. Engert and S.J. Horning (eds.), *Hodgkin Lymphoma*,
DOI: 10.1007/978-3-642-12780-9_25, © Springer-Verlag Berlin Heidelberg 2011

and proteomics," we will first examine what useful data these approaches have already provided. We will then turn our attention to a discussion of whether these strategies will ultimately lead to significant insight that will result in unraveling the biology of Hodgkin lymphoma, with the goal of developing new therapies that translate into cures and improved quality of life for patients suffering from this disease.

## 25.2 What Have We Learned Thus Far?

### 25.2.1 HRS Cells or the Microenvironment?

The clinical and pathological features of Hodgkin lymphoma reflect an abnormal immune response that is thought to be due to expression of a variety of cytokines by the HRS cells altering the surrounding microenvironment [1]. Cytokines are low-molecular-weight proteins with a wide variety of functions that work either in a paracrine manner to modulate the activity of surrounding cells or in an autocrine fashion to affect the cells that produce them. Furthermore, it is a widely accepted concept that the overexpression of Th2 cytokines and TGFβ leads to a microenvironment that suppresses cell-mediated immunity and in return favors HRS cell survival, highlighting the bidirectional crosstalk of cells involved in the pathogenesis of Hodgkin lymphoma [2, 3]. To dissect and simplify this complex interaction of the malignant HRS cells with their microenvironment, two types of experiments have been performed, including those focusing on (1) cell lines and enriched HRS cells (by microdissection or fluorescence-activated flow sorting) and (2) the reactive microenvironment. In addition, targeted gene polymorphism studies have established a link to the host-specific genetic background modulating Hodgkin lymphoma susceptibility and treatment outcome [4–6].

### 25.2.2 Array Comparative Genomic Hybridization (aCGH)

Studies of gene copy number changes using conventional chromosomal CGH helped to establish the clonal relationship of HRS cells and revealed that many cases shared common chromosomal imbalances during tumor evolution. In brief, a Hodgkin lymphoma characteristic profile of recurrent copy number gains and losses has been described, including gains of chromosomes 2p, 9p, 16p, 17q, and losses of 13q, 6q, and 11q [7, 8]. These studies for the first time used laser capture microdissection followed by whole-genome amplification (WGA). In one of these studies, the authors also found a correlation of 13q losses with poor outcome; however, the major contribution of these data encompassed an improved understanding of the underlying pathobiology as exemplified by the detailed characterization of the two most prominent alterations, gains of 2p and 9p, recognizing the oncogenes c-REL and JAK2 as putative target genes [9–11]. While these studies were primarily limited because of low resolution (approximately 2–5 Mb for high-level amplifications and 10–20 Mb for deletions), the two most recent studies used oligonucleotide and BAC arrays providing a much higher resolution. In these studies, novel copy number changes were identified including amplification of STAT6, NOTCH1, JUNB, IKBKB, CD40, and MAP3K14 [12, 13]. Remarkably, the smallest detected deletion spanned only 156 kb targeting CDKN2B, emphasizing the improved detection sensitivity over conventional chromosomal CGH. Furthermore, for the first time a correlation of chromosome 16p gains with primary treatment failure could be described [13]. Interestingly, in the therapy-resistant Hodgkin lymphoma cell line KMH2 genomic gains and overexpression of the multidrug resistance gene ABCC1 mapping to cytoband 16p13.11 were found contributing to the drug-resistance phenotype of this cell line.

Characterization of commonly used Hodgkin lymphoma cell lines by high-resolution aCGH further contributed to the inventory of imbalances found in relapsed Hodgkin lymphoma [14].

### 25.2.3 Gene Expression Profiling

Overall, gene expression profiling experiments have contributed substantially to an improved understanding of the disease with respect to the inherent phenotypic features of the malignant HRS cells and the specific composition of the microenvironment. Moreover, first steps could be made to establish outcome correlations with the potential to improve prediction of treatment response. However, many questions remain including often contradictory results derived from different patient cohorts. Focusing on HRS cells, the first major contribution of gene expression profiling was made by investigating Hodgkin lymphoma cell lines. These pivotal studies first established a transcriptome-wide view of the malignant cell compartment describing a unifying gene signature for classical Hodgkin lymphoma [15]. Together with other important similar studies, this gene expression work helped to elucidated the loss of the B cell signature phenotype and the deregulated expression of transcription factor networks in comparison to normal germinal center B cell counterparts [16–19]. Only two gene expression studies have been published examining microdissected HRS cells from clinical biopsy material that further characterized transcriptional changes in these cells [20, 21]. One of these studies for the first time also focused on gene expression profiling of microdissected cells from nodular lymphocyte predominant Hodgkin lymphoma, describing a close relationship to classical Hodgkin lymphoma and T cell–rich B cell lymphoma. However, in both studies correlation of the findings with outcome was not possible due to lack of clinical data and relatively small sample size.

Four major genome-wide gene expression studies have been published to date analyzing whole-tissue lymph node biopsy material. Since the HRS cells are largely outnumbered by reactive cells in most biopsies, these studies using whole frozen biopsies are regarded as largely a reflection of the microenvironment [22–25]. However, some of these data provide evidence that at least part of the apparent signatures are derived from HRS cells [23, 25]. In one study, a specific gene expression signature could be linked to EBV-positivity with genes overexpressed, indicative of an increased Th1/antiviral response in comparison to the EBV-negative cases [24]. In addition to a better characterization of certain Hodgkin lymphoma subtypes defined by specific gene signatures, these experiments also allowed for the study of outcome correlations using supervised analyses. All studies have used dichotomized clinical data sets based on slightly different definitions of clinical extremes according to outcome after systemic treatment (i.e., treatment success vs. treatment failure). However, these types of analyses have in part yielded conflicting results regarding the specific signatures that best define these clinical extremes. While one study found overexpression of genes involved in fibroblast activation, angiogenesis, extracellular matrix remodeling, and downregulation of tumor suppressor genes to be linked with an unfavorable prognosis, another study found a correlation of fibroblast activation, fibroblast

chemotaxis, and matrix remodeling with improved outcome [22, 23]. While small sample sizes in both studies might have hampered interpretation, the most recent study investigated gene expression profiles of 130 patients including 38 patients whose primary treatments failed representing the largest gene expression cohort published to date [25]. This study could validate previously reported outcome correlations, and furthermore showed that a gene signature of macrophages was linked to primary treatment failure. In validation experiments the authors could demonstrate that the enumeration of CD68+ macrophages in lymph node biopsies was a strong and independent predictor of disease-specific survival in an independent set of patients. These data provide proof of principle that clinically relevant findings can be derived from genome-wide profiling platforms and raise hope that better outcome prediction can be achieved in Hodgkin lymphoma.

### 25.2.4 Proteomics

Proteomic studies in lymphoid malignances and in Hodgkin lymphoma in particular are still in their infancy. The application of proteomic techniques has been shown to be a useful tool for detection of biomarkers in other diseases; however, clinically relevant findings are largely lacking in Hodgkin lymphoma [26]. Two approaches have been chosen thus far: one using total cell lysates and the other analyzing the secretome of HRS cells [27–30]. These studies were aimed at developing novel candidate biomarkers and diagnostic tools by identifying specific protein profiles linked to certain lymphoma entities, but also sought to determine an inventory of secreted proteins that are critically involved in the crosstalk of HRS cells with their microenvironment. While these experiments demonstrated the feasibility of proteomic studies in HL cell lines, the literature is still lacking studies using primary lymph node tissues in this disease. In addition, reproducibility of proteomics experiments, in particular, reproducibility of time-of-flight mass spectrometry (TOF-MS), is of general concern for its potential clinical applicability [31]. However, recently developed proteomic approaches using nanoscale reversed-phase liquid chromatograph tandem mass spectrometry (LC-MS/MS) has shown to be a major advance by identifying a large number of secreted proteins using Hodgkin lymphoma cell lines, including candidate molecules such as CCL5, CCL17, CTCS, CTSS, CX3CL1, and MIF. Moreover, these results were validated using independent techniques including enzyme-linked immunosorbent assays (ELISA) and immunohistochemistry (IHC) [29]. Additional efforts are needed to translate these findings into clinically useful biomarkers in Hodgkin lymphoma.

## 25.3 What Will We Learn?

Meaningful separation of clinical Hodgkin lymphoma cases into limited vs. advanced-stage disease, classical Hodgkin lymphoma vs. nodular lymphocyte predominant Hodgkin lymphoma, and finally distinguishing

patients based on the International Prognostic Scoring (IPS) system for advanced-stage disease are still considered the gold standard for risk assessment and stratification used to guide treatment decisions. Despite advances in genomics and proteomics research, none of the findings derived from the various aforementioned platforms have found their way into clinical practice in the form of accepted biomarkers. Similarly, the goal of developing novel targeted therapies has essentially not been achieved. However, as many necessary steps in this direction have already been made, we can hopefully anticipate important advances in the near future. In the following discussion, we will substantiate our optimism and discuss the "ingredients" required for successful clinical translation of genomic and proteomic discovery (Fig. 25.1).

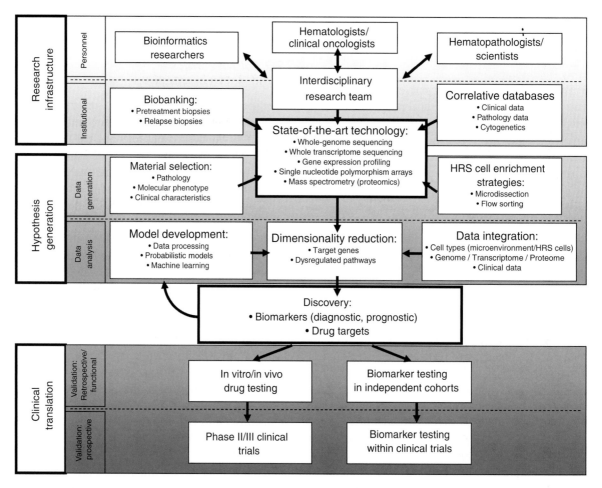

**Fig. 25.1** Flowchart outlining the necessary ingredients for state-of-the-art genomics and proteomics research and clinical translation in Hodgkin lymphoma. The figure details the required

research infrastructure, the technologies needed to test hypotheses, and the clinical requirements for biomarker discovery and clinical application

## 25.3.1 Enrichment Strategies for the Malignant HRS Cells

Research in Hodgkin lymphoma has moved beyond the investigation of whole lymph node biopsies and Hodgkin lymphoma cell lines. Many studies have demonstrated using laser capture microdissection [7, 20, 32] or fluorescence-activated cell sorting (FACS) [33, 34] that the study of isolated HRS cells separated from their microenvironment is both feasible and of value for improved biological understanding. In particular, the technical approach of enriching for HRS by flow sorting has been "revitalized" and can be added to the inventory of methods needed to isolate and study the malignant cell compartment. Although flow sorting in general is an established method used to purify small cell populations, only recently have HRS cells been successfully enriched using a cocktail of unlabeled antibodies to adhesion molecules that block the interaction of HRS cells with rosetting T-cells, unmasking HRS cell antigens such as CD15 or CD30.

Successful application of novel genome-wide applications, however, will be dependent on sophisticated strategies to amplify often small amounts of nucleic acids derived from a small number of enriched HRS cells. Taking advantage of large numbers of clinical samples should allow clinical correlations to be realized. Combining enrichment strategies with state-of-the art genomics platforms including single nucleotide polymorphism (SNP) analyses, gene expression profiling, and whole-genome or whole-transcriptome analysis would seem to be a likely paradigm for new gene discovery tools in the future.

## 25.3.2 Hodgkin Lymphoma Genomics in the Future: What Platforms?

Significant technological advances have been made in the recent past. At the level of the genome, the most striking improvements have been made by introducing massively parallel sequencing approaches (whole-genome and whole-transcriptome sequencing), so-called next generation sequencing, that allow for genome-wide genotyping at base pair resolution with unprecedented depth of genomic coverage. This technology not only maximizes resolution, but also provides the sensitivity for detecting single nucleotide variants, genomic insertions, deletions, and translocations. Similarly, at the transcriptome level (entirety of the transcribed genome) this technology will lead to the detection of novel gene mutations, fusion transcripts, and an improved understanding of RNA editing and the role of noncoding RNAs. However, methods investigating copy number variations (CNVs) of tumor genomes (by SNP arrays) and epigenetics by genome-wide methylation studies (methylated DNA immunoprecipitation [MeDIP], genome-wide bisulfite sequencing) will be needed to complement this comprehensive overview of the molecular genetics of HRS cells. All of these approaches are still largely unexplored in Hodgkin lymphoma and their routine application to small numbers of enriched HRS cells will be technically challenging. Nevertheless, we expect major and novel discoveries once the technical obstacles are solved.

## 25.3.3 Data Integration

Gene expression profiling studies and array CGH have yielded valuable information about the specific biology of HRS cells and their microenvironment, but both cell compartments have only been examined separately thus far on a genome-wide scale. However, such characterization of copy number and transcriptional changes in the malignant cells and in the nonmalignant cellular compartment should ideally be viewed and analyzed together. Experimental designs using matching genome-wide profiles of the same cases will allow for data integration and an in-depth look at the multiple interactions between neoplastic HRS cells and the microenvironment at the molecular level. Bioinformatics tools are already in place to analyze large amounts of data and to detect common patterns of deregulated gene expression that might reflect specific ligand–receptor interactions and cytokine expression patterns. Furthermore, the consequence of genomic copy number changes that might underlie altered gene expression changes can be explored as has been demonstrated in Hodgkin lymphoma cell lines [35]. Linkage of these findings to treatment outcome will be useful for biomarker discovery and will likely shed more light on the specific cellular interactions found in patients who are destined to fail primary or subsequent treatment.

### 25.3.4 Biobanking and Large Correlative Databases

Translation of genomics findings into clinically useful biomarkers is not possible without the availability of well-annotated clinical data sets and linked frozen biopsy samples. These large correlative databases will undoubtedly provide the foundation for translational genomics for years to come. Linkage of fresh frozen lymph node specimens, peripheral blood lymphocyte collections representing constitutional or host genetics, formalin-fixed material, classical cytogenetic and cell culture material, and archived single-cell suspensions all linked with clinical parameters, particularly treatment outcome data, will be crucial for discovery of novel biomarkers, predictive factors, and revised pathological classifications. Ideally, collection of this material must be included in the design of randomized phase III clinical trials where important clinical questions are being addressed. Clearly this represents a major challenge, both in terms of logistics and funding, but must be made an important objective for all clinical trial groups into the future.

A parallel strategy should also be considered using population-based registries, where some of the pitfalls associated with accrual to clinical trials, such as selection and referral bias, are avoided. The experience at the British Columbia Cancer Agency shows that a centralized and representative population-based collection of lymph node material and clinical data provides an ideal platform to assess biomarkers using a retrospective approach. Advantages include large numbers of study cases, lack of substantial selection bias, standardized and homogeneous treatment of the study cohorts, and standardized diagnostic procedures. However, special attention has to be paid to ethical considerations in the era of whole-genome sequencing as systems have to be in place that respect privacy rights and genomic analysis of diagnostic material that has been initially collected for different purposes. With respect to Hodgkin lymphoma, the merging of genomics and proteomics data with established clinical risk factors and clinical outcome correlations of patients that have been homogeneously treated will undoubtedly lead to major improvements in outcome prediction.

Systematic and comprehensive biobanking would include snap-freezing lymph node material obtained at the time of relapse, an inventory that has not been properly collected and thus has been largely unexamined in

the published literature. While in the past, most studies have focused on pretreatment diagnostic biopsies, a detailed investigation of relapse biopsies will likely answer questions related to disease progression and the development of therapy resistance. Moreover, genome-wide approaches using paired pretreatment and relapse biopsies are ideally suited to investigate clonal evolution and tumor progression under the influence of therapy.

### 25.3.5 Interdisciplinary Research

Genomics research in the modern era requires interaction of researchers on many different levels. Fundamental infrastructure for sample acquisition and selection by hematologists, clinical oncologists, and hematopathologists are essential prerequisites; however, data generation in state-of-the-art equipped genome research centers and its proper processing and analysis is becoming increasingly critical. Development and application of specific algorithms and models by specialized bioinformatics research teams are needed to handle and make interpretable large amounts of data generated in genome-wide SNP or whole-genome sequencing experiments. Furthermore, biological and clinical interpretation of genomics research as well as validation of the results by interdisciplinary research groups remains equally critical. In summary, close interaction of clinicians, pathologists, scientists, basic genome researchers, and bioinformaticians provide the important ingredients for novel discoveries in translational research. Thus far, the fruits of interdisciplinary research in lymphoma is best evidenced by the revised WHO classification of tumors of hematopoietic and lymphoid tissues [36] in which much emphasis has been placed on defining entities that can be recognized by (1) pathologists according to morphology, immunophenotype, and genetic features and (2) clinicians who have to ensure its utility and acceptance in daily practice. In the case of Hodgkin lymphoma, biological and clinical studies have lead to subclassification into lymphocyte predominant Hodgkin lymphoma and classical Hodgkin lymphoma, histological distinctions that affect treatment decisions and subsequent clinical management. No genomics data generated thus far have lead to a change or refinement of this distinction. However, overlap of Hodgkin lymphoma with related lymphoma entities exist, including T cell/histiocyte-rich large B cell lymphoma (TCRBCL) and lymphocyte predominant Hodgkin lymphoma, primary mediastinal large B cell lymphoma (PMBCL) and nodular sclerosis Hodgkin lymphoma, or anaplastic large cell lymphoma and classical Hodgkin lymphoma, where gene expression studies of microdissected cells have already yielded further insight into the relatedness of these diseases [20, 37, 38]. We hypothesize that genomics and proteomics approaches will increasingly refine the similarities and differences at the molecular level and ultimately provide the molecular underpinnings of modified classifications in the future. As a consequence, new molecularly defined diseases will likely be recognized with the possibility of candidate gene discovery and new targeted therapies becoming routine in clinical practice.

## 25.4   Will These Advances Lead to a Cure of Hodgkin Lymphoma?

Currently, Hodgkin lymphoma is a very treatable disease and the majority of patients are cured following primary therapy. However, current therapies fail to cure about 20% of patients and reasonable estimates suggest that a similar proportion of patients are overtreated [39], which suggests that the clinical management of Hodgkin lymphoma is far from being satisfactory for typically young patients who suffer from relapse or "off-target" therapy effects. Thus, an answer to this provocative question is not only contingent on further characterization of treatment failure and its underlying mechanisms, but also on strategies to reduce treatment and the far too frequent occurrence of treatment-related long-term sequelae. These two clinical scenarios dictate that we focus on strategies aiming at improved overall survival: (1) the development of prognostic biomarkers for predicting treatment outcome and (2) the definition of unfavorable subtypes according to underlying pathobiology and the development of targeted therapy against these important subgroups. To realize both goals, the analysis of the whole-genome, transcriptome, or proteome seems ideally suited as discovery platforms with the potential to find candidate molecules and molecular pathways that are targetable by modern drugs or alternatively, reliably predict treatment failure with the use of existing therapies.

At the present time, gene expression profiling and aCGH profiles have been linked to treatment outcome, but none of these findings has yet lead to improvements in our existing prognostic systems. Small case numbers and heterogeneity of the underlying mechanisms might only be two of many reasons why clinical translation has not been successful. Furthermore, to substantiate hope for a cure of Hodgkin lymphoma, one would need to anticipate a virtually perfect short list of prognostic biomarkers that in aggregate define with certainty treatment outcome. Despite much work, the existing data is somewhat disappointing in this regard. Nevertheless, the increased resolution of newly developed genomics applications and the feasibility of HRS cell enrichment might at long last improve our predictive ability to an extent that the majority of patients whose treatments are destined to fail can be identified at diagnosis. Establishing favorable biomarkers and improving prediction of treatment success would likewise be of considerable benefit for patients as they might be spared from dose-escalation or be candidates for dose de-escalation to decrease early- and/or late therapy–related toxicities.

The published literature regarding genome-wide experiments, especially from gene expression profiling in Hodgkin lymphoma, provides many phenotypic features that are potential targets for novel therapeutic approaches. However, development of suitable pathway inhibitors, immunotherapeutic approaches, and preclinical/clinical testing of these treatments is a slow and laborious process. Thus, any assessment of the success of novel biomarker discovery and clinical translation will similarly take time. Moreover, with comparably effective standard therapy that is able to cure the majority of patients, changes to standard procedures are harder to justify. Therefore, the focus has to be shifted to the specific biology of treatment failure and the expected unique biology of clinical relapsed disease. Unfortunately, there is only very limited data available for these clinical scenarios. It has to be anticipated that genomics and proteomics will discover further heterogeneity within the generic group of treatment failure. Provided that effective treatment is available, only a subgroup of patients will benefit from these advances, nevertheless leading to improved overall survival and cure rates. Therefore, the hope to cure all patients with Hodgkin lymphoma may be unrealistic.

## 25.5 Summary

In summary, novel genomics and proteomics applications in Hodgkin lymphoma will likely substantially change our understanding of the disease, improve our current prognostic systems used to predict treatment outcome, and identify novel targets for drug intervention. Furthermore, with the help of sophisticated bioinformatics tools we will learn more about the specific crosstalk between the malignant HRS cells and the non-neoplastic cells in the tumor microenvironment. The success of clinical translation of these experiments will depend on continued progress using genomic platforms with increasing resolution and sensitivity, the technical feasibility of these applications using enriched malignant HRS cell, and the availability of clinical and treatment outcome data. The anticipated heterogeneity of the tumor biology linked to treatment failure will remain a major challenge for future research, but we are hopeful that the persistent efforts of interdisciplinary research and clinical teams dedicated to achieving meaningful cures and improving long-term survival in Hodgkin lymphoma will overcome this challenge.

## References

1. Skinnider BF, Mak TW. The role of cytokines in classical Hodgkin lymphoma. Blood. 2002;99(12):4283–97.
2. Kuppers R. The biology of Hodgkin's lymphoma. Nat Rev Cancer. 2009;9(1):15–27.
3. Marshall NA, Christie LE, Munro LR, Culligan DJ, Johnston PW, Barker RN, et al. Immunosuppressive regulatory T cells are abundant in the reactive lymphocytes of Hodgkin lymphoma. Blood. 2004;103(5):1755–62.
4. Hohaus S, Giachelia M, Di Febo A, Martini M, Massini G, Vannata B, et al. Polymorphism in cytokine genes as prognostic markers in Hodgkin's lymphoma. Ann Oncol. 2007; 18(8):1376–81.
5. Ribrag V, Koscielny S, Casasnovas O, Cazeneuve C, Brice P, Morschhauser F, et al. Pharmacogenetic study in Hodgkin lymphomas reveals the impact of UGT1A1 polymorphisms on patient prognosis. Blood. 2009;113(14):3307–13.
6. Casasnovas RO, Mounier N, Brice P, Divine M, Morschhauser F, Gabarre J, et al. Plasma cytokine and soluble receptor signature predicts outcome of patients with classical Hodgkin's lymphoma: a study from the Groupe d'Etude des Lymphomes de l'Adulte. J Clin Oncol. 2007;25(13):1732–40.
7. Joos S, Menz CK, Wrobel G, Siebert R, Gesk S, Ohl S, et al. Classical Hodgkin lymphoma is characterized by recurrent copy number gains of the short arm of chromosome 2. Blood. 2002;99(4):1381–7.
8. Chui DT, Hammond D, Baird M, Shield L, Jackson R, Jarrett RF. Classical Hodgkin lymphoma is associated with frequent gains of 17q. Genes Chromosomes Cancer. 2003;38(2): 126–36.
9. Barth TF, Martin-Subero JI, Joos S, Menz CK, Hasel C, Mechtersheimer G, et al. Gains of 2p involving the REL locus correlate with nuclear c-Rel protein accumulation in neoplastic cells of classical Hodgkin lymphoma. Blood. 2003;101(9):3681–6.
10. Martin-Subero JI, Gesk S, Harder L, Sonoki T, Tucker PW, Schlegelberger B, et al. Recurrent involvement of the REL and BCL11A loci in classical Hodgkin lymphoma. Blood. 2002;99(4):1474–7.
11. Joos S, Granzow M, Holtgreve-Grez H, Siebert R, Harder L, Martin-Subero JI, et al. Hodgkin's lymphoma cell lines are characterized by frequent aberrations on chromosomes 2p and 9p including REL and JAK2. Int J Cancer. 2003;103(4): 489–95.
12. Hartmann E, Fernandez V, Moreno V, Valls J, Hernandez L, Bosch F, et al. Five-gene model to predict survival in mantle-cell lymphoma using frozen or formalin-fixed, paraffin-embedded tissue. J Clin Oncol. 2008;26(30):4966–72.
13. Steidl C, Telenius A, Shah SP, Farinha P, Barclay L, Boyle M, et al. Genome-wide copy number analysis of Hodgkin Reed-Sternberg cells identifies recurrent imbalances with correlations to treatment outcome. Blood. 2010;116(3):418–27.
14. Feys T, Poppe B, De Preter K, Van Roy N, Verhasselt B, De Paepe P, et al. A detailed inventory of DNA copy number alterations in four commonly used Hodgkin's lymphoma cell lines. Haematologica. 2007;92(7):913–20.
15. Kuppers R, Klein U, Schwering I, Distler V, Brauninger A, Cattoretti G, et al. Identification of Hodgkin and Reed-Sternberg cell-specific genes by gene expression profiling. J Clin Invest. 2003;111(4):529–37.
16. Schwering I, Brauninger A, Klein U, Jungnickel B, Tinguely M, Diehl V, et al. Loss of the B-lineage-specific gene expression program in Hodgkin and Reed-Sternberg cells of Hodgkin lymphoma. Blood. 2003;101(4):1505–12.
17. Mathas S, Janz M, Hummel F, Hummel M, Wollert-Wulf B, Lusatis S, et al. Intrinsic inhibition of transcription factor E2A by HLH proteins ABF-1 and Id2 mediates reprogramming of neoplastic B cells in Hodgkin lymphoma. Nat Immunol. 2006;7(2):207–15.
18. Stein H, Marafioti T, Foss HD, Laumen H, Hummel M, Anagnostopoulos I, et al. Down-regulation of BOB.1/OBF.1 and Oct2 in classical Hodgkin disease but not in lymphocyte predominant Hodgkin disease correlates with immunoglobulin transcription. Blood. 2001;97(2):496–501.
19. Jundt F, Kley K, Anagnostopoulos I, Schulze Probsting K, Greiner A, Mathas S, et al. Loss of PU.1 expression is associated with defective immunoglobulin transcription in Hodgkin and Reed-Sternberg cells of classical Hodgkin disease. Blood. 2002;99(8):3060–2.
20. Brune V, Tiacci E, Pfeil I, Doring C, Eckerle S, van Noesel CJ, et al. Origin and pathogenesis of nodular lymphocyte-predominant Hodgkin lymphoma as revealed by global gene expression analysis. J Exp Med. 2008;205(10):2251–68.
21. Karube K, Ohshima K, Suzumiya J, Kawano R, Kikuchi M, Harada M. Gene expression profile of cytokines and chemokines in microdissected primary Hodgkin and Reed-Sternberg (HRS) cells: high expression of interleukin-11 receptor alpha. Ann Oncol. 2006;17(1):110–6.

22. Devilard E, Bertucci F, Trempat P, Bouabdallah R, Loriod B, Giaconia A, et al. Gene expression profiling defines molecular subtypes of classical Hodgkin's disease. Oncogene. 2002; 21(19):3095–102.

23. Sanchez-Aguilera A, Montalban C, de la Cueva P, Sanchez-Verde L, Morente MM, Garcia-Cosio M, et al. Tumor microenvironment and mitotic checkpoint are key factors in the outcome of classic Hodgkin lymphoma. Blood. 2006; 108(2):662–8.

24. Chetaille B, Bertucci F, Finetti P, Esterni B, Stamatoullas A, Picquenot JM, et al. Molecular profiling of classical Hodgkin lymphoma tissues uncovers variations in the tumor microenvironment and correlations with EBV infection and outcome. Blood. 2009;113(12):2765–3775.

25. Steidl C, Lee T, Shah SP, Farinha P, Han G, Nayar T, et al. Tumor-associated macrophages and survival in classic Hodgkin's lymphoma. N Engl J Med. 2010;362(10):875–85.

26. Hanash S. Disease proteomics. Nature. 2003;422(6928): 226–32.

27. Fujii K, Kondo T, Yokoo H, Yamada T, Matsuno Y, Iwatsuki K, et al. Protein expression pattern distinguishes different lymphoid neoplasms. Proteomics. 2005;5(16):4274–86.

28. Fujii K, Kondo T, Yamada M, Iwatsuki K, Hirohashi S. Toward a comprehensive quantitative proteome database: protein expression map of lymphoid neoplasms by 2-D DIGE and MS. Proteomics. 2006;6(17):4856–76.

29. Ma Y, Visser L, Roelofsen H, de Vries M, Diepstra A, van Imhoff G, et al. Proteomics analysis of Hodgkin lymphoma: identification of new players involved in the cross-talk between HRS cells and infiltrating lymphocytes. Blood. 2008;111(4):2339–46.

30. Carvalho PC, Carvalho Mda G, Degrave W, Lilla S, De Nucci G, Fonseca R, et al. Differential protein expression patterns obtained by mass spectrometry can aid in the diagnosis of Hodgkin's disease. J Exp Ther Oncol. 2007;6(2):137–45.

31. Kiehntopf M, Siegmund R, Deufel T. Use of SELDI-TOF mass spectrometry for identification of new biomarkers:

potential and limitations. Clin Chem Lab Med. 2007;45(11): 1435–49.

32. Kuppers R, Rajewsky K, Zhao M, Simons G, Laumann R, Fischer R, et al. Hodgkin disease: Hodgkin and Reed-Sternberg cells picked from histological sections show clonal immunoglobulin gene rearrangements and appear to be derived from B cells at various stages of development. Proc Natl Acad Sci U S A. 1994;91(23):10962–6.

33. Fromm JR, Kussick SJ, Wood BL. Identification and purification of classical Hodgkin cells from lymph nodes by flow cytometry and flow cytometric cell sorting. Am J Clin Pathol. 2006;126(5):764–80.

34. Fromm JR, Thomas A, Wood BL. Flow cytometry can diagnose classical hodgkin lymphoma in lymph nodes with high sensitivity and specificity. Am J Clin Pathol. 2009;131(3):322–32.

35. Giefing M, Arnemann J, Martin-Subero JI, Nielander I, Bug S, Hartmann S, et al. Identification of candidate tumour suppressor gene loci for Hodgkin and Reed-Sternberg cells by characterisation of homozygous deletions in classical Hodgkin lymphoma cell lines. Br J Haematol. 2008;142(6):916–24.

36. Swerdlow SH, Campo E, Harris NL, Jaffe ES, Pileri SA, Stein H, et al., editors. WHO classification of tumours of haematopoietic and lymphoid tissues. Lyon, France: IARC; 2008.

37. Rosenwald A, Wright G, Leroy K, Yu X, Gaulard P, Gascoyne RD, et al. Molecular diagnosis of primary mediastinal B cell lymphoma identifies a clinically favorable subgroup of diffuse large B cell lymphoma related to Hodgkin lymphoma. J Exp Med. 2003;198(6):851–62.

38. Eckerle S, Brune V, Doring C, Tiacci E, Bohle V, Sundstrom C, et al. Gene expression profiling of isolated tumour cells from anaplastic large cell lymphomas: insights into its cellular origin, pathogenesis and relation to Hodgkin lymphoma. Leukemia. 2009;23:2129–38.

39. Bjorkholm M, Axdorph U, Grimfors G, Merk K, Johansson B, Landgren O, et al. Fixed versus response-adapted MOPP/ABVD chemotherapy in Hodgkin's disease. A prospective randomized trial. Ann Oncol. 1995;6(9):895–9.

# Personalized Medicine in Hodgkin Lymphoma?

**26**

Dennis A. Eichenauer and Andreas Engert

## Contents

D.A. Eichenauer (✉) and A. Engert
Department I of Internal Medicine, Uniklinik Köln,
Kerpener Strasse 62, 50937, Köln, Germany
e-mail: dennis.eichenauer@uk-koeln.de;
a.engert@uni-koeln.de

## 26.1 Stage and Risk Factor–Adapted Strategies

At present, treatment of HL is stage-adapted and includes chemo- and radiotherapy. Patients are divided into early favorable, early unfavorable, and advanced stages. Allocation to one of these groups depends on clinical stage and the presence or absence of risk factors. These risk factors include the number of involved nodal areas, erythrocyte sedimentation rate (ESR), and extranodal and bulky disease. This allocation to treatment groups varies only slightly between larger study groups such as the German Hodgkin Study Group (GHSG), the European Organization for Research and Treatment of Cancer (EORTC), and the Eastern Cooperative Oncology Group (ECOG). In addition, an International Prognostic Score (IPS) was established for advanced-stage HL patients in 1998 (1). This score includes seven factors with similar independent prognostic impact: low serum albumin (less than 4 g/dL), low hemoglobin (less than 10.5 g/dL), male sex, age of 45 or above, stage IV disease (according to the Ann Arbor classification), leukocytosis (white-cell count of at least 15,000/mm$^3$), and lymphocytopenia (less than 600/mm$^3$ or a count of less than 8% of the white-cell count or both). This score is based on data from 5,141 patients with advanced HL who received non-BEACOPP (bleomycin, etoposide, adriamycin, cyclophosphamide, vincristine, procarbazine, prednisone) multiagent chemotherapy. The vast majority of these patients were treated between 1983 and 1992. Among the patients included in the analysis, those not presenting any risk factor had a freedom from disease progression rate of 84% while patients with five or more risk factors had a freedom from disease progression rate of only 42% [1]. Novel treatment strategies such

A. Engert and S.J. Horning (eds.), *Hodgkin Lymphoma*,
DOI: 10.1007/978-3-642-12780-9_26, © Springer-Verlag Berlin Heidelberg 2011

as BEACOPP escalated improved results especially in patients with high IPS but in general the score is still valid and can be used for some risk stratification.

## 26.2 Response-Adapted Treatment Strategies

In the past decades, treatment results for all HL patients have improved continuously. The standard of care consists of two cycles of chemotherapy plus involved-field radiotherapy (IF-RT) for early favorable stages and four cycles plus IF-RT for early unfavorable stages [2,3]. The most widely used chemotherapy regimen is ABVD (adriamycin, bleomycin, vinblastine, dacarbazine). By default, patients with advanced HL are treated with six to eight cycles of chemotherapy followed by radiation of larger residual tumor masses. For years, ABVD was accepted standard of care for these patients but it has recently been challenged by novel regimens such as the multiagent Stanford V protocol or intensified BEACOPP [4–6].

With current standard approaches, 60–90% of HL patients can be cured. These cure rates result in a steadily increasing number of long-time survivors who often suffer from treatment-related late side effects such as cardiac failure, infertility, or secondary malignancies [7]. Therefore, the main goal of current trials is to establish treatment strategies associated with reduced toxicity without being therapeutically less effective.

The most promising tool to distinguish between patients who are sufficiently treated with a less toxic therapy and those who require standard or even more aggressive treatment is the positron emission tomography (PET). PET might be an even more precise predictor for treatment failure than the IPS in patients receiving ABVD (see also Chap. 6: PET) [8]. The question whether it is possible to stratify treatment on the basis of an interim PET scan is a matter of ongoing clinical trials. In the EORTC H10 trial, patients with early HL are divided into a favorable and an unfavorable risk group. Standard treatment consists of three and four cycles of ABVD, respectively, followed by involved-node radiotherapy (IN-RT). In the experimental arms of the study, a PET scan is performed after two cycles of ABVD and further treatment depends on the PET result. In case of PET negativity, patients with favorable risk profiles receive two more

cycles of ABVD; patients with unfavorable risk profiles receive four additional cycles. These patients receive no radiotherapy. In case of PET positivity, treatment is continued with two cycles of BEACOPP escalated followed by IN-RT. The GHSG HD16 and HD17 trials for early favorable and early unfavorable disease also evaluate omitting radiotherapy in patients with a negative PET after standard chemotherapy. It would be a substantial improvement if PET could be shown to be a reliable predictor in deciding whether patients with early stages require radiation since radiation is known to be associated with severe late effects such as secondary solid tumors.

The possibility of stratifying therapy on the basis of interim PET is also under investigation in patients with advanced HL. In the ongoing GHSG HD18 trial, all patients receive two cycles of escalated BEACOPP as standard regimen for this group, followed by PET. Patients with a negative PET scan are randomly assigned to either standard treatment consisting of a total of eight cycles of escalated BEACOPP or four cycles of escalated BEACOPP. Patients with positive PET are randomized between a total of eight cycles of escalated BEACOPP or eight cycles of escalated BEACOPP plus the anti-CD20 antibody rituximab. This aims at reducing treatment in patients with good metabolic response after the first two cycles of chemotherapy and intensifying therapy in patients still PET-positive in affected localizations at that time.

In an Italian study, patients with advanced disease receive two cycles of ABVD before a PET scan is performed (ClinicalTrials.gov Identifier: NCT00795613). Patients with a negative PET scan continue to receive ABVD, the standard regimen in this group; patients with positive PET switch to the more intensive BEACOPP regimen for the remaining treatment.

Sequential treatment stratification combining pretreatment IPS and early interim PET to tailor treatment was used by a group from Israel. First, patients were assigned to receive either two cycles of BEACOPP in baseline or escalated dose depending on their IPS. Patients with an IPS ranging from zero to two received the baseline dose while patients with an IPS of three or higher received the escalated dose. Then a gallium or PET scan was performed. Patients with positive interim scan completed treatment with four cycles of escalated BEACOPP and patients with negative scan received four cycles of BEACOPP in baseline dose. This trial suggests that gallium or PET scan-based treatment stratification after IPS-dependent choice of initial chemotherapy results in comparable event-free survival (EFS) and overall survival (OS) rates in both IPS groups [9].

The current questions regarding PET-based treatment stratification including possible differences in the impact of early interim PET with different chemotherapy regimens, the optimal timing, and the definition of adequate therapeutic consequences of a positive or negative PET will probably be answered in a few years. Then, an early interim PET scan might become the standard tool to discriminate between low-, normal-, and high-risk patients. This would be another step toward individually tailoring treatment according to the patient's risk profile.

## 26.3 Strategies to Personalize Treatment

To individualize treatment is one of the current major goals in the field of hemato-oncology. In some malignancies, treatment stratification on the basis of certain mutations or the existence of minimal residual disease (MRD) has already been implemented in clinical trials. Non-small-cell lung cancer (NSCLC) and acute lymphoblastic leukemia (ALL) can serve as examples for risk and treatment stratification according to results of genetic analyses and will be shortly introduced here.

For NSCLC, a large randomized phase III trial showed that patients with a mutated epidermal growth factor receptor (EGFR) gene have an improved outcome when treated with the EGFR kinase inhibitor gefitinib (IRESSA). In contrast, patients without mutation in the EGFR gene did not benefit from gefitinib and had a better outcome when treated with conventional chemotherapy [10].

In ALL, treatment has improved considerably over the last decades, which was in part due to the increased precision of risk stratification. Besides classical risk factors such as age, white blood cell count, and immunophenotype, MRD was added as a novel relevant prognostic factor. In the GMALL 07/2003 trial, treatment after consolidation therapy is stratified based on the MRD risk profile. Treatment options include the end of treatment for low-risk patients and allogeneic stem cell transplantation (aSCT) for high-risk patients. In addition, the advent of the tyrosine kinase inhibitor imatinib led to a substantial improvement of prognosis

in very high-risk ALL patients who are Philadelphia chromosome-positive. By combining imatinib with conventional chemotherapy, the complete remission rate prior to aSCT could be significantly improved. Furthermore, consolidation treatment with imatinib or follow-up products might reduce the risk of relapse after aSCT [11].

### 26.3.1 Approaches to Personalize Treatment in HL

In HL, no genetic markers with the potential for treatment stratification are known to date. However, besides clinical stage and clinical risk factors, there are several factors that might possibly be implemented in future risk and treatment stratification. A universally valid biological score including serum markers might be helpful. To this end, a comprehensive analysis of 519 HL patients was conducted by Casasnovas and colleagues from the Groupe d'Etude des Lymphomes de l'Adulte (GELA). They identified interleukin-1 receptor antagonist (IL-1-RA), interleukin-6 (IL-6), and soluble CD30 (sCD30) as independent negative prognostic factors. Existence of negative prognostic factors was correlated with patients' outcome. Patients without any risk factor had a 5-year OS rate of 92% while patients with one, two, or three risk factors had 5-year OS rates of 85%, 75%, and 15%, respectively [12]. Another French group retrospectively analyzed tissue samples of 59 patients with either refractory or early relapse of disease. They showed that expression of bcl-2 and CD20 on Hodgkin and Reed-Sternberg (H-RS) cells as well as TiA1 expression in lymphocytes and c-kit positivity in mast cells of the microenvironment were independent prognostic markers [13]. Other reports revealed interleukin-10 and other serum cytokines to be predictors for a poor outcome. In a proteomics analysis, proteins secreted by different HL cell lines were evaluated and 16 of them were eventually validated. Seven of these 16 proteins were found to be significantly elevated in the serum of HL patients. They include CD26, CD44, MIF, and TARC [14]. Despite these results, there are currently no prognostic scores incorporating biomarkers used to stratify treatment. However, there is a plethora of cytokines and surface molecules with prognostic significance but none of them has been validated in prospective trials to date.

Several receptor tyrosine kinases (RTK) are over-expressed in H-RS cells (Fig. 26.1) and probably being activated by paracrine and autocrine mechanisms. Since RTK play a role in the regulation of many metabolic cellular processes, their dysregulation or aberrant activation can have extensive consequences for the cell homeostasis and promote tumor growth. Therefore, there is a rationale for the use of tyrosine kinase inhibitors in HL. However, usually several overexpressed RTK are active so that either a combination of different tyrosine kinase inhibitors each selectively targeting one RTK or broad spectrum tyrosine kinase inhibitors would be necessary. Both possibilities are rather unrealistic since it does not seem practicable to apply various tyrosine kinase inhibitors in a given patient on one hand but on the other, the use of broad spectrum inhibitors would probably also affect physiological processes and, therefore, potentially cause severe side effects.

Genotyping of primary H-RS cells is complicated due to their paucity in affected lymph nodes. Single cell picking would be necessary but is technically difficult. Thus, there is only limited knowledge on genetic

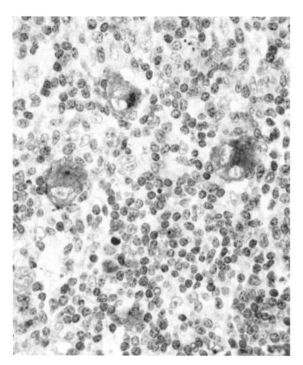

**Fig. 26.1** Immunohistochemical detection of proteins phosphorylated by kinase activity in H-RS cells. (Adapted from [20])

alterations in H-RS cells that are predictive for a certain outcome and appropriate as possible stratification tool for treatment planning.

Besides the identification of mutations in H-RS cells predicting the course of disease and allowing for the allocation of patients to certain risk groups, it would be of interest to identify patients who are at increased risk of developing unacceptable toxicities, for example, to heart or lung. Furthermore, a tool predicting the risk of developing secondary malignancies, secondary acute myeloid leukemia (AML) in particular, is desirable since most patients diagnosed with secondary AML die [15]. A possible way of identifying those patients could be the detection of specific predictive single nucleotide polymorphisms (SNP). However, search for SNP predicting outcome, toxicity, or secondary malignancy risk has only recently begun and there is currently limited knowledge on this topic.

Despite the fact that establishment of novel markers is not as advanced as in other malignancies, there is preclinical and clinical research activity in HL aimed at more specific treatment. In recent years, a multitude of new drugs specifically targeting molecules or signaling pathways that are dysregulated or misdirected in HL have been developed and already brought to early phase clinical trials.

CD30 is a surface molecule selectively overexpressed on H-RS cells and, therefore, well suited for antibody-based targeted treatment. However, results of clinical trials with naked anti-CD30 antibodies so far have been disappointing. Recently, first results from a trial with an antibody-drug conjugate consisting of an anti-CD30 antibody and monomethyl-auristatin (SGN-35, brentuximab vedotin) were reported. In patients who had received a median of three prior treatments, response rate was 46%. Treatment was generally well tolerated and severe side effects were less common than with conventional chemotherapy [16]. Therefore, further investigation of this substance is ongoing.

Small molecules represent another class of drugs that showed promising activity in preclinical studies and are currently under evaluation in HL patients. The pan deacetylase (DAC) inhibitor LBH589 (panobinostat) is one example [17]. Besides its effect as a DAC inhibitor, other modes of action such as inhibition of nuclear factor kappa-b (Nf-kappa-B) might play a role in HL. Vorinostat, another DAC inhibitor, was shown to decrease the phosphorylation of STAT6. In HL, an increased JAK-mediated phosphorylation activates several STAT factors including STAT6 and thus promotes tumor cell survival [18]. Inhibition of STAT activity might therefore have an antitumor effect. Hence, DAC inhibitors target diverse signaling pathways that are misdirected in H-RS cells and represent a drug class that will potentially be of value for future treatment strategies.

Since most of the recently developed drugs show a more favorable side effect profile than conventional chemotherapy, they might be combined with established protocols, used as maintenance therapy for high-risk patients, and thus, in part, replace components of traditional treatment protocols in the future. However, well-conducted clinical trials are required before drawing final conclusions (Table 26.1) (see also Chap. 20).

In addition to more sophisticated risk stratification, there is also room to individualize treatment on the basis of conventional patient characteristics such as age and histology. For instance, it is still unclear how adolescent and elderly patients should ideally be treated. Adolescents represent a relevant portion of patients and are currently inconsistently treated with either pediatric or adult protocols but a direct comparison of both approaches in this ambiguously defined age group has never been undertaken. Even subgroup analyses on adolescents in publications reporting pediatric or adult trials can rarely be found and would be needed to better define this group of patients.

Elderly patients aged 60 and above have a significantly poorer outcome than younger adults. This is in part due to comorbidities that avoid treatment according to standard protocols. Therefore, novel and less toxic regimens possibly containing new substances such as antibodies or small molecules with an improved side effect profile might be helpful in these patients [19].

Treatment of the rare subtype of nodular lymphocyte predominant HL (LPHL), which accounts for about 5% of HL patients, represents another field requiring further analyses and clinical trials. Although immunophenotype and genotype of LPHL substantially differ from classical HL (cHL), it is traditionally treated according to cHL protocols. Consistent and strong expression of CD20 and a more indolent course of disease could be indicators that treatment strategies with reduced chemotherapy supplemented by rituximab might be sufficient in LPHL.

In summary, future research on HL will ideally lead to a more accurate risk and treatment stratification than available today. Patients might be treated on the basis of a scoring system including classical staging and risk factors as well as biological and response-adapted elements. This will allow a therapy more precisely adjusted to the individual patient with reduced treatment for low-risk and intensified treatment, potentially followed by antibody or small molecule maintenance for high-risk patients.

**Table 26.1** Currently ongoing or recently completed phase I and II clinical trials with agents targeting specific pathways or antigens

| Agent | Supplier | Target pathway | Clinical trial |
|---|---|---|---|
| SGN-35 | Seattle Genetics | Anti-CD30 antibody–drug conjugate | NCT00848926 |
| MDX-1401 | Medarex | Anti-CD30 antibody | NCT00634452 |
| XmAb2513 | Xencor | Anti-CD30 antibody | NCT00606645 |
| HCD122 | Novartis | Anti-CD40 antibody | NCT00670592 |
| Lenalidomide | Celgene | Immunomodulatory drug | NCT00478959 |
| Panobinostat | Novartis | HDAC inhibitor | NCT00742027 |
| Entinostat | Syndax | HDAC inhibitor | NCT00866333 |
| Temsirolimus | Wyeth | mTOR inhibitor | NCT00838955 |
| ABVD + Bevacizumab | Roche | Anti-VEGF antibody | NCT00722865 |
| ABVD + Rituximab | Roche | Anti-CD20 antibody | NCT00654732 |

# References

1. Hasenclever D, Diehl V. A prognostic score for advanced Hodgkin's disease. International prognostic factors project on advanced Hodgkin's disease. N Engl J Med. 1998;339: 1506–14.
2. Engert A, Pluetschow A, Eich HT, et al. Combined modality treatment of two or four cycles of ABVD followed by involved field radiotherapy in the treatment of patients with early stage Hodgkin's lymphoma: Update Interim Analysis of the Randomised HD10 Study of the German Hodgkin Study Group (GHSG). Blood (ASH Annual Meeting Abstracts) 2005;106:Abstract 2673.
3. Ferme C, Eghbali H, Meerwaldt JH, et al. Chemotherapy plus involved-field radiation in early-stage Hodgkin's disease. N Engl J Med. 2007;357:1916–27.
4. Canellos GP, Anderson JR, Propert KJ, et al. Chemotherapy of advanced Hodgkin's disease with MOPP, ABVD, or MOPP alternating with ABVD. N Engl J Med. 1992;327: 1478–84.
5. Horning SJ, Hoppe RT, Breslin S, et al. Stanford V and radiotherapy for locally extensive and advanced Hodgkin's disease: mature results of a prospective clinical trial. J Clin Oncol. 2002;20:630–7.
6. Engert A, Diehl V, Franklin J, et al. Escalated-dose BEACOPP in the treatment of patients with advanced-stage Hodgkin's lymphoma: 10 years of follow-up of the GHSG HD9 Study. J Clin Oncol. 2009;27:4548–54.
7. Friedman DL, Constine LS. Late effects of treatment for Hodgkin lymphoma. J Natl Compr Canc Netw. 2006;4:249–57.
8. Gallamini A, Hutchings M, Rigacci L, et al. Early interim 2-[18F]fluoro-2-deoxy-D-glucose positron emission tomography is prognostically superior to international prognostic score in advanced-stage Hodgkin's lymphoma: a report from a joint Italian-Danish study. J Clin Oncol. 2007;25:3746–52.
9. Dann EJ, Bar-Shalom R, Tamir A, et al. Risk-adapted BEACOPP regimen can reduce the cumulative dose of chemotherapy for standard and high-risk Hodgkin lymphoma with no impairment of outcome. Blood. 2007;109:905–9.
10. Friedrich MJ. Using EGFR status to personalize treatment: lung cancer researchers reach a milestone. J Natl Cancer Inst. 2009;101:1039–41.
11. Gokbuget N, Hoelzer D. Treatment of adult acute lymphoblastic leukemia. Semin Hematol. 2009;46:64–75.
12. Casasnovas RO, Mounier N, Brice P, et al. Plasma cytokine and soluble receptor signature predicts outcome of patients with classical Hodgkin's lymphoma: a study from the Groupe d'Etude des Lymphomes de l'Adulte. J Clin Oncol. 2007;25:1732–40.
13. Canioni D, Deau-Fischer B, Taupin P, et al. Prognostic significance of new immunohistochemical markers in refractory classical Hodgkin lymphoma: a study of 59 cases. PLoS One. 2009;4:e6341.
14. Ma Y, Visser L, Roelofsen H, et al. Proteomics analysis of Hodgkin lymphoma: identification of new players involved in the cross-talk between HRS cells and infiltrating lymphocytes. Blood. 2008;111:2339–46.
15. Josting A, Wiedenmann S, Franklin J, et al. Secondary myeloid leukemia and myelodysplastic syndromes in patients treated for Hodgkin's disease: a report from the German Hodgkin's Lymphoma Study Group. J Clin Oncol. 2003; 21:3440–6.
16. Younes A, Forero-Tores A, Bartlett NL, et al. Multiple complete Responses in a phase i dose-escalation study of the antibody-drug conjugate SGN-35 in patients with relapsed or refractory CD30-positive lymphomas. Blood (ASH Annual Meeting Abstracts) 2008;112:Abstract 1006.
17. Dickinson M, Ritchie D, Deangelo DJ, et al. Preliminary evidence of disease response to the pan deacetylase inhibitor panobinostat (LBH589) in refractory Hodgkin Lymphoma. Br J Haematol 2009;147:97–101.
18. Buglio D, Georgakis GV, Hanabuchi S, et al. Vorinostat inhibits STAT6-mediated TH2 cytokine and TARC production and induces cell death in Hodgkin lymphoma cell lines. Blood. 2008;112:1424–33.
19. Proctor SJ, Wilkinson J, Sieniawski M. Hodgkin lymphoma in the elderly: a clinical review of treatment and outcome, past, present and future. Crit Rev Oncol Hematol. 2009; 71:222–32.
20. Renné C, Hansmann ML, Bräuninger A. Receptor tyrosine kinases in Hodgkin lymphoma as possible therapeutic targets. Pathologe. 2009; 30(5):393–400.

# Index